DUAL-PROCESS THEORIES OF THE SOCIAL MIND

Also available

Cognitive Consistency:
A Fundamental Principle in Social Cognition
Bertram Gawronski and Fritz Strack, Editors

Handbook of Implicit Social Cognition:
Measurement, Theory, and Applications
Bertram Gawronski and B. Keith Payne, Editors

Social Cognition: The Official Journal
of the International Social Cognition Network
Jeffrey W. Sherman, Editor

Dual-Process Theories of the Social Mind

EDITED BY

JEFFREY W. SHERMAN

BERTRAM GAWRONSKI

YAACOV TROPE

THE GUILFORD PRESS

New York London

A Division of Guilford Publications, Inc.
72 Spring Street, New York, NY 10012
www.guilford.com

Printed in the United States of America

This book is printed on acid-free paper.

Last digit is print number: 9 8 7 6 5 4 3 2 1

Library of Congress Cataloging-in-Publication Data is available from the publisher.

ISBN 978-1-4625-1439-7

About the Editors

Jeffrey W. Sherman, PhD, is Professor of Psychology at the University of California, Davis. His research investigates the cognitive processes underlying social psychology and behavior, with particular interests in attitude formation and change and how stereotypes and prejudice affect social perception. Dr. Sherman is Editor of the journal *Social Cognition.* A Fellow of the Association for Psychological Science (APS), the Society for Personality and Social Psychology (SPSP), and the Society for Experimental Social Psychology (SESP), he is a recipient of other honors including the Theoretical Innovation Prize from SPSP and the Anneliese Maier Research Award from the Alexander von Humboldt Foundation and the German Federal Ministry of Education.

Bertram Gawronski, PhD, is Professor of Psychology at the University of Texas at Austin. His research investigates the mental underpinnings and behavioral consequences of spontaneous and deliberate evaluations of objects, individuals, groups, and social issues. Dr. Gawronski's work has been recognized with honors including the Theoretical Innovation Prize from SPSP, the Career Trajectory Award from SESP, the Early Career Award from the International Social Cognition Network, the Early Researcher Award from the Ministry of Research and Innovation of Ontario, and the Charlotte and Karl Bühler Award from the German Psychological Society. He is a fellow of APS, SESP, and SPSP.

Yaacov Trope, PhD, is Professor of Psychology at New York University. His research investigates the interrelations among cognition, motivation, and self-regulation in the social context. Particular interests include how psychological distance influences the representations of objects, and, thereby, the predictions, evaluations, and choices individuals make regarding those objects; self-control processes; and the role of affective states and personal desires in social judgment and decision making. Dr. Trope is a Fellow of the American Association for the Advancement of Science, APS, SESP, and SPSP. His research has been funded by the National Institutes of Health and the National Science Foundation.

Contributors

Henk Aarts, PhD, Department of Social and Organizational Psychology, Utrecht University, Utrecht, The Netherlands

Nalini Ambady (deceased), PhD, Department of Psychology, Stanford University, Stanford, California

Elinor Amit, PhD, Department of Psychology, Harvard University, Cambridge, Massachusetts

David M. Amodio, PhD, Department of Psychology, New York University, New York, New York

John A. Bargh, PhD, Department of Psychology, Yale University, New Haven, Connecticut

Roy F. Baumeister, PhD, Department of Psychology, Florida State University, Tallahassee, Florida

Galen V. Bodenhausen, PhD, Department of Psychology, Northwestern University, Evanston, Illinois

Maarten W. Bos, PhD, Negotiation, Organizations and Markets, Harvard Business School, Boston, Massachusetts

Pablo Briñol, PhD, Faculty of Psychology, Autonomous University of Madrid, Madrid, Spain

Jimmy Calanchini, BA, Department of Psychology, University of California, Davis, Davis, California

C. Daryl Cameron, PhD, Department of Psychology, University of Iowa, Iowa City, Iowa

William A. Cunningham, PhD, Department of Psychology, The Ohio State University, Columbus, Ohio

Ruud Custers, PhD, Department of Cognitive, Perceptual, and Brain Sciences, University College London, London, United Kingdom

Jan De Houwer, PhD, Department of Psychology, University of Ghent, Ghent, Belgium

Roland Deutsch, PhD, Institute of Psychology, Technical University of Dresden, Dresden, Germany

Patricia G. Devine, PhD, Department of Psychology, University of Wisconsin–Madison, Madison, Wisconsin

Ap Dijksterhuis, PhD, Behavioral Science Institute, Radboud University, Nijmegen, The Netherlands

Ana Rita Farias, PhD, Lisbon University Institute, Lisbon, Portugal, and Utrecht University, Utrecht, The Netherlands

Russell H. Fazio, PhD, Department of Psychology, The Ohio State University, Columbus, Ohio

Melissa J. Ferguson, PhD, Department of Psychology, Cornell University, Ithaca, New York

Klaus Fiedler, PhD, Department of Psychology, University of Heidelberg, Heidelberg, Germany

Ayelet Fishbach, PhD, Booth School of Business, University of Chicago, Chicago, Illinois

Patrick S. Forscher, BA, Department of Psychology, University of Wisconsin–Madison, Madison, Wisconsin

Jens Förster, PhD, Department of Social Psychology, University of Amsterdam, Amsterdam, The Netherlands

Jonathan B. Freeman, PhD, Department of Psychological and Brain Sciences, Dartmouth College, Hanover, New Hampshire

Kentaro Fujita, PhD, Department of Psychology, The Ohio State University, Columbus, Ohio

Margarida V. Garrido, PhD, Department of Social and Organizational Psychology, University Institute of Lisbon, Lisbon, Portugal

Bertram Gawronski, PhD, Department of Psychology, University of Texas at Austin, Austin, Texas

Sara Gottlieb, BA, Department of Psychology, University of California, Berkeley, Berkeley, California

Joshua D. Greene, PhD, Department of Psychology, Harvard University, Cambridge, Massachusetts

Rainer Greifeneder, PhD, Department of Psychology, University of Basel, Basel, Switzerland

James J. Gross, PhD, Department of Psychology, Stanford University, Stanford, California

Ran R. Hassin, PhD, Psychology Department, The Hebrew University, Jerusalem, Israel

E. Tory Higgins, PhD, Department of Psychology, Columbia University, New York, New York

Mandy Hütter, PhD, Department of Psychology, University of Heidelberg, Heidelberg, Germany

Karl Christoph Klauer, PhD, Institute for Psychology, University of Freiburg, Freiburg, Germany

Kristen M. Klein, PhD, Analytic Services, Inc., Falls Church, Virginia

Stanley B. Klein, PhD, Department of Psychology, University of California, Santa Barbara, Santa Barbara, California

Regina Krieglmeyer, PhD, Department of Psychology, University of Würzburg, Würzburg, Germany

Arie W. Kruglanski, PhD, Department of Psychology, University of Maryland, College Park, College Park, Maryland

Jennifer S. Labrecque, MA, Department of Psychology, University of Southern California, Los Angeles, California

Nira Liberman, PhD, Department of Psychology, Tel Aviv University, Tel Aviv, Israel

Matthew D. Lieberman, PhD, Department of Psychology, University of California, Los Angeles, Los Angeles, California

Pei-Ying Lin, MA, Department of Psychology, University of Southern California, Los Angeles, California

C. Neil Macrae, PhD, School of Psychology, University of Aberdeen, Aberdeen, Scotland

Thomas C. Mann, BS, Department of Psychology, Cornell University, Ithaca, New York

Lucia Mannetti, PhD, Department of Developmental and Social Psychology, Sapienza University, Rome, Italy

Randy J. McCarthy, PhD, Center for the Study of Family Violence and Sexual Assault, Northern Illinois University, DeKalb, Illinois

Allen R. McConnell, PhD, Department of Psychology, Miami University, Oxford, Ohio

Agnes Moors, PhD, Department of Experimental Clinical and Health Psychology, Ghent University, Ghent, Belgium

Gordon B. Moskowitz, PhD, Department of Psychology, Lehigh University, Bethlehem, Pennsylvania

Thomas Mussweiler, PhD, Department of Psychology, University of Cologne, Cologne, Germany

Loran F. Nordgren, PhD, Kellogg School of Management, Northwestern University, Evanston, Indiana

Michael A. Olson, PhD, Department of Psychology, University of Tennessee, Knoxville, Tennessee

B. Keith Payne, PhD, Department of Psychology, University of North Carolina at Chapel Hill, Chapel Hill, North Carolina

Richard E. Petty, PhD, Department of Psychology, The Ohio State University, Columbus, Ohio

Antonio Pierro, PhD, Department of Developmental and Social Psychology, Sapienza University, Rome, Italy

Kimberly A. Quinn, PhD, Department of Psychology, DePaul University, Chicago, Illinois

Dennis Rünger, PhD, Department of Psychology, University of Southern California, Los Angeles, California

Robert J. Rydell, PhD, Department of Psychological and Brain Sciences, Indiana University, Bloomington, Indiana

Norbert Schwarz, PhD, Department of Psychology, University of Southern California, Los Angeles, California

Gün R. Semin, PhD, Faculty of Social and Behavioral Sciences, Utrecht University, Utrecht, The Netherlands

Luxi Shen, BS, Chinese University of Hong Kong, Hong Kong, China

Gal Sheppes, PhD, School of Psychological Sciences, Tel Aviv University, Tel Aviv, Israel

Jeffrey W. Sherman, PhD, Department of Psychology, University of California, Davis, Davis, California

Asael Y. Sklar, MA, Department of Psychology, The Hebrew University, Jerusalem, Israel

John T. Skowronski, PhD, Department of Psychology, Northern Illinois University, DeKalb, Illinois

Steven Sloman, PhD, Department of Cognitive, Linguistic, and Psychological Sciences, Brown University, Providence, Rhode Island

Robert P. Spunt, PhD, Division of Humanities and Social Sciences, California Institute of Technology, Pasadena, California

Keith A. Stanovich, PhD, Department of Human Development and Applied Psychology, University of Toronto, Toronto, Ontario, Canada

Fritz Strack, PhD, Department of Psychology, University of Würzburg, Würzburg, Germany

Madelijn Strick, PhD, Social and Organizational Psychology, Utrecht University, Utrecht, The Netherlands

Maggie E. Toplak, PhD, Department of Psychology, York University, Toronto, Ontario, Canada

Yaacov Trope, PhD, Department of Psychology, New York University, New York, New York

Richard F. West, PhD, Department of Graduate Psychology, James Madison University, Harrisonburg, Virginia

Michael T. Wojnowicz, PhD, Department of Statistics, University of California, Irvine, Irvine, California

Wendy Wood, PhD, Department of Psychology, University of Southern California, Los Angeles, California

Preface

The emergence of dual-process theories has been one of the most significant developments in the history of scientific psychology. The overarching assumption of these theories is that psychological processes can be divided into two distinct categories depending on whether they operate in an automatic or controlled fashion. In recent years, this distinction between "fast" and "slow" modes of thought has even permeated the popular press and the lay public's understanding of psychology.

The publication of Shelly Chaiken and Yaacov Trope's *Dual-Process Theories in Social Psychology* in 1999 played a central role in placing the distinction between automatic and controlled processes at the center of social psychological theory. In so doing, the book captured a critical turning point in how the field of social psychology reconciled competing metatheoretical models of the rational, intuitive scientist versus the satisficing cognitive miser. It also helped to inspire waves of conceptual, methodological, and empirical refinements to dual-process thinking and research that have led to a fundamental reorganization of the theoretical landscape within the field of social psychology.

In this volume, we have tried to capture the most important developments in the 15 years since the publication of Chaiken and Trope's seminal book and to organize and integrate those developments in a novel and coherent manner. Toward this end, we have invited leading authorities to address the pivotal role of automatic and controlled processes across many areas of inquiry. The scope of this volume encompasses the core assumptions and conceptual foundations of dual-process theories, their applications to a wide range of social phenomena, and contemporary critiques of the duality approach. Our goals in this book were to describe the ubiquity of dual-process theories; identify current directions of research on the topic; present key theoretical, methodological, and empirical developments; and raise important questions for future research.

The book is divided into nine major parts. The chapters in Part I explore the conceptual foundations of dual-process theories, analyzing the theoretical basis for distinguishing between two kinds of psychological processes. Part II documents the emerging trend of extending dual-process to dual-system theorizing, reviewing the core assumptions of theories that propose two dissociable mental systems. The chapters in Part III address conceptual issues in the measurement of dual processes and illustrate recent advances in the development of formal process models to investigate automatic and controlled underpinnings of social behavior. The chapters in Parts IV through VIII review the insights that have been gained by applying dual-process theories to a wide range of questions in social psychology, including research on attitudes and evaluation; social perception; thinking and reasoning; the interplay among habits, goals, and motivations; and the range and limits of self-regulation and cognitive control. Finally, the chapters in Part IX address conceptual criticism of and theoretical alternatives to the dual-process approach.

In order to provide some common ground and coherence to the chapters in the book, we requested that the authors of each chapter address three issues that we believe are critical in contemporary thinking about dual-process models. First, we asked the authors to clearly define the central features of their model, including the type of duality addressed by the model, the specific processes proposed in the model, the defining characteristics of those processes, and any assumptions about the extent to which the processes are grounded in distinct mental representations or mental systems. Second, we asked the authors to describe how the processes in their model relate to the distinction between automatic and controlled processes, and to specify the particular features of automaticity (e.g., awareness, intention, efficiency, control) that are central to their model. Finally, we asked the authors to detail the relationship between the proposed processes, including whether the processes are thought to be mutually exclusive, to operate in isolation or in parallel, or to interact with one another. Although the chapters of this volume emphasize different aspects of these issues, the three questions provide a common framework for much of the material, helping to clarify points of consensus, contention, and uncertainty.

Given the ubiquity of the dual-process approach in virtually all areas of social psychology, we hope that the current volume provides an indispensable resource for researchers interested in the contribution of automatic and controlled processes to social judgments and social behavior. The book may serve as a valuable supplement for graduate-level and advanced undergraduate courses on social cognition, judgment and decision making, attitudes and persuasion, social perception, and self-regulation. By providing an up-to-date review of contemporary dual-process theories, the book will be of great interest for any scholar who is interested in the psychological underpinnings of social behavior.

Contents

PART III. MEASUREMENT AND FORMAL MODELING

PART IV. ATTITUDES AND EVALUATION

PART V. SOCIAL PERCEPTION

PART VI. THINKING AND REASONING

PART VII. HABITS, GOALS, AND MOTIVATION

PART VIII. SELF-REGULATION AND CONTROL

PART IX. CRITICISM AND ALTERNATIVES

PART I

THE BASICS

CHAPTER 1

Two of What?

A Conceptual Analysis of Dual-Process Theories

Bertram Gawronski, Jeffrey W. Sherman, and Yaacov Trope

The emergence of dual-process theories is probably one of the most significant theoretical developments in the history of social psychology. The overarching assumption of dual-process theorizing is that the mental processes underlying social phenomena can be divided into two distinct categories depending on whether they operate in an automatic or nonautomatic fashion.[1] Over the past decades, dual-process theories have made important contributions in virtually all areas of social psychology, and this volume showcases the most recent developments since Chaiken and Trope's (1999) seminal volume, *Dual-Process Theories in Social Psychology.*

Despite the ubiquity of dual-process theories in social psychology, their conceptual foundations have also been the subject of ongoing debates. In this chapter, we provide a metatheoretical analysis that aims at clarifying the explanatory function of dual-process theories, the conceptual nature of their underlying dualities, and structural features that characterize different types of dual-process theories. Expanding on this analysis, we discuss the criticism that dual-process theories are unfalsifiable and whether the realm of mental processes can indeed be divided into two distinct categories. Our conclusion is that dual-process theories have provided vital insights into the mental underpinnings of social phenomena. However, their explanatory and predictive value depends on (1) a clear distinction between operating principles and operating conditions, (2) conceptual rigor in the definition of the proposed dualities, (3) precise formulations of empirical hypotheses about covariations between processing dualities, and (4) clearly specified links between the hypothesized mental processes and the causal relations between stimuli and behavior they are supposed to explain. Expanding on this analysis, we conclude with a brief outlook on emerging themes and future directions in dual-process theorizing.

EXPLANATORY FUNCTION

A useful framework to clarify the explanatory function of dual-process theories is Marr's (1982) distinction among three levels of analysis in psychological research: the computational level, the algorithmic level, and the implementational level. According to Marr, research at the *computational level* is concerned with identifying relations between inputs (i.e., stimuli and their broader contexts) and outputs (i.e., judgments and behavior). The overarching goal of research at the computational level is to identify which types of inputs produce which kinds of outputs under which contextual conditions. For example, a large body of research on behavioral priming can be described as computational, in that it focuses on the particular behaviors that are elicited by exposure to various kinds of prime stimuli (for a review, see Bargh, 2006). Research of this kind differs from research at the *algorithmic level*, which is concerned with the mechanisms that translate inputs into outputs. This level of analysis resonates with the goal of social-cognitive research, which aims at identifying the mental processes and representations underlying social behavior. For example, expanding on the identification of input–output relations in studies on behavioral priming, a considerable body of research investigated the mental mechanisms that mediate the effects of prime exposure on overt behavior, including motivational (e.g., Cesario, Plaks, & Higgins, 2006), misattribution (e.g., Loersch & Payne, 2011) and self-related (e.g., Wheeler, DeMarree, & Petty, 2007) processes. Finally, research at the *implementational level* is concerned with the physical systems that implement the mechanisms identified at the algorithmic level. In social psychology, this approach is prominently reflected in the emerging field of social neuroscience, which is concerned with the neural underpinnings of social judgments and social behavior (Cacioppo, Berntson, Sheridan, & McClintock, 2000; Ochsner & Lieberman, 2001). For example, expanding on mental process theories of prime-to-behavior effects (e.g., Cesario et al., 2006; Loersch & Payne, 2011; Wheeler et al., 2007), research at the implementational level may investigate the neural underpinnings of the mechanisms that mediate observed relations between certain kinds of primes and overt behavior.

Dual-process theories are located at Marr's (1982) algorithmic level of analysis, in the sense that they identify mental mechanisms that translate inputs into outputs. A central feature of dual-process theories is that they postulate two qualitatively distinct (sets of) mental processes that mediate between inputs and outputs. Some dual-process theories go beyond the algorithmic level by including assumptions about the neural substrates that implement the hypothesized processes (e.g., Lieberman, Gaunt, Gilbert, & Trope, 2002). Yet even these theories have their theoretical core at the algorithmic level, in that the identified substrates are directly linked to two (sets of) mechanisms that are claimed to translate inputs into outputs.

Although the proposed positioning of dual-process theories at Marr's (1982) algorithmic level may seem rather trivial, it helps to clarify the explanatory function of dual-process theories by specifying the empirical phenomena that dual-process theories aim to explain (*explanandum*) and the theoretical assumptions that are proposed to explain these phenomena (*explanans*). From an epistemological point of view, one could argue that research at the computational level aims to explain observed outputs by relating them to inputs that cause these outputs. Using the previous example of behavioral priming, exposure to a particular stimulus may serve as an explanation for an observed behavioral response to the extent that the stimulus can be said to cause the behavioral response. In other words, the observed behavior represents the phenomenon that needs to be explained, and exposure to the prime stimulus serves as the event that is supposed to explain the behavior (*causal explanation*). However, stating that exposure to the prime explains the behavioral response does not say anything about *how* the prime caused the observed behavior. This question is central in research at the algorithmic level, in which the causal relation between prime exposure and behavior represents a phenomenon that is in need of further explanation (De Houwer, 2011). Research at the algorithmic level provides an answer to this question by identifying the mental mechanisms that mediate the link between prime exposure and overt behavior (*mechanistic explanation*). In this sense, dual-process theories offer explanations of observed input–output relations by specifying the mental mechanisms that translate inputs into outputs. As we outline in the following sections, this conceptualization has important implications for dual-process theorizing in social psychology.

OPERATING PRINCIPLES VERSUS OPERATING CONDITIONS

The first important insight that can be gained from relating dual-process theories to Marr's (1982) algorithmic level of analysis is that it resolves the common conflation of operating principles and operating conditions. Whereas the concept of *operating principles* refers to the mental mechanisms that translate inputs into outputs, the concept of *operating conditions* refers to the conditions under which a given process operates (Gawronski & Bodenhausen, 2009). A central characteristic of dual-process theories is that they are concerned with the question of whether the mental processes underlying social behavior operate in an automatic or nonautomatic fashion. This emphasis has sometimes led to the misunderstanding that labeling a process as automatic or nonautomatic is sufficient to characterize the intrinsic nature of that process. However, stating that a process operates in an automatic or nonautomatic fashion simply specifies *when* the process is assumed to operate; it does not specify *how* the process translates inputs into outputs. That is, characterizing a mental process as automatic versus nonautomatic specifies whether the process does or does not operate (1) when there is no conscious awareness, (2) when there is no goal to start the process, (3) when cognitive resources are reduced, and (4) when there is a goal to alter or stop the process (Bargh, 1994). Thus, although research investigating the unawareness, unintentionality, efficiency, and uncontrollability of a given process is essential to understand the boundary conditions of observed input–output relations (e.g., does a given input lead to a particular output when cognitive resources are reduced?), such research by itself does not address the question of *how* the human mind translates certain inputs into particular outputs.

In terms of Marr's (1982) framework, research on operating conditions is located at the computational level, in that it aims at identifying which types of inputs produce which kinds of outputs under which contextual conditions (e.g., does input *X* produce output *Y* when participants simultaneously perform a secondary task?). Although such research is essential to the concern with automaticity, the explanatory goal of dual-process theories goes beyond the computational level, in that they aim at specifying the mental mechanisms that translate inputs into outputs (e.g., what are the mental operations that translate input *X* into output *Y*?). From the perspective of Marr's algorithmic level, characterizations of a given process as automatic versus nonautomatic are not sufficient as a conceptual foundation of dual-process theories, because they fail to specify the nature of the processes that translate inputs into outputs. An illustrative example is the conscious–unconscious duality, which has been used in a manner suggesting that it refers to two qualitatively distinct mental processes (e.g., Baumeister, Masicampo, & Vohs, 2011; Dijksterhuis & Nordgren, 2006). Of course, it is possible that conscious and unconscious processing of input stimuli produces different behavioral outputs via two qualitatively distinct mechanisms. However, it is also possible that conscious and unconscious processes operate on the basis of the same mental structures involving the same mental operations (Huang & Bargh, in press). Simply stating that a mental process is conscious or unconscious does not specify *how* this process translates inputs into outputs, nor does it specify whether conscious and unconscious processing involve the same or different mental structures and operations. Thus, although dual-process theorizing is often equated with research on awareness, intentionality, efficiency, and controllability (i.e., operating conditions), its explanatory goal at the algorithmic level requires clear specifications of the mental mechanisms that translate inputs into outputs (i.e., operating principles).[2]

Another important caveat in this context is that different features of automatic processing do not necessarily co-occur (Bargh, 1994; Moors & De Houwer, 2006). Counter to early *dual-mode conceptualizations* assuming an all-or-none relation between different features of automaticity, the available evidence indicates that there is virtually no process that is characterized by all four features of automaticity. Instead, most processes studied within social psychology involve combinations of selected features, making them automatic in one sense and nonautomatic in another (Bargh, 1992). For example, a process may be unintentional and controllable, intentional and efficient, unintentional and resource-dependent, conscious and uncontrollable, unconscious and resource-dependent, controllable and resource-independent, and so forth (e.g., Fujita, 2011; Gawronski & Bodenhausen, 2011; Hassin, Bargh, Engell, & McCulloch, 2009). This insight has inspired *disjunctive conceptualizations* of automaticity, according to which a process can be characterized as automatic if it meets at least one of the four criteria of automaticity. According to this view, a process can be described as automatic if it is (1) unconscious, (2) unintentional, (3) efficient, or (4) uncontrollable.

Although disjunctive treatments of automaticity are rather common in social psychology, they involve a number of problems (Gawronski & Creighton, 2013). First, if the presence of a single feature is sufficient to call a process automatic, it is possible that a given process has to be described as automatic and nonautomatic at the same time. Needless to say, such a description can cause considerable confusion if it does not specify in which particular sense the process is automatic and in which sense it is nonautomatic. Second, generic use of the term *automatic* to describe any of the four operating conditions can lead to confusion about conceptually distinct findings that are described with the same term. For example, a given Process A may be described as automatic because it is elicited unintentionally, whereas another Process B may be described as automatic because it does not require a large amount of cognitive resources. Yet despite their common description as automatic, the two processes may be fundamentally different, for example, if Process A is resource dependent and Process B is intentional.

Based on these considerations, several theorists recommended that researchers should be more precise in their use of terminology by describing each feature of automaticity with its proper label (i.e., unconscious, unintentional, efficient, or uncontrollable; Bargh, 1994; Moors & De Houwer, 2006). Importantly, such *decompositional conceptualizations* prohibit simple binary categorizations of mental processes as automatic or nonautomatic. Because the four features of automaticity do not necessarily co-occur, a decompositional classification schema involves 16 rather than two categories of potential operating conditions. On the basis of this conclusion, the assumption that the mental processes underlying social phenomena can be divided into two internally coherent categories depending on whether they operate in an automatic or nonautomatic fashion should be treated with caution. Of course, dual-process theories share the explanatory goal to identify the mental mechanisms that translate inputs into outputs and the assumption that input–output relations are mediated by two qualitatively distinct (sets of) processes that operate under different processing conditions. However, different theories emphasize different features of automaticity, and the nature of the proposed mechanisms is not necessarily equivalent.

TYPES OF DUAL-PROCESS THEORIES

Despite the concerns about generic treatments, the term *dual-process theory* is sometimes used in the singular to refer to an overarching theoretical idea that could be boiled down to a single theory (see Evans & Frankish, 2009). However, as the variety of contributions to this volume illustrates, there is not really a unifying "essence" that captures what might be regarded as the prototype of dual-process theories. Instead, there are important nuances that are easy to miss if different theories are treated as minor variations of the same prototype theory. Nevertheless, it seems possible to classify dual-process theories in terms of a few general characteristics, such as the phenomena they aim to explain (*explanandum*), the theoretical constructs they propose to explain these phenomena (*explanans*), and their mathematical formalization.

Explanandum

When dual-process theories started to emerge in the 1980s, their focus was mainly domain-specific, in that they aimed at explaining phenomena in particular areas of inquiry. Although some of these theories were based on general processing principles from cognitive psychology (e.g., Chaiken, 1987; Trope, 1986), their applications were specific to particular content domains within social psychology. Prominent examples include dual-process theories of persuasion (e.g., Chaiken, 1987; Petty & Cacioppo, 1986), attitude–behavior relations (e.g., Fazio, 1990), dispositional attribution (e.g., Gilbert, 1989; Trope, 1986), prejudice and stereotyping (e.g., Devine, 1989), and impression formation (e.g., Brewer, 1988; Fiske & Neuberg, 1990). A shared feature of these theories is that they explain particular instances of input–output relations (*explanandum*) by postulating two (sets of) mechanisms by which the human mind translates inputs into outputs (*explanans*). For example, dual-process theories of persuasion aim at explaining the effects of different features of persuasive messages on attitudes. Their overarching goal is to understand the mental mechanisms by which different kinds of inputs (e.g., argument strength, source characteristics) are translated into outputs (i.e., attitude change). Similarly, dual-process theories of dispositional attribution aim at explaining the effects of different kinds of information about potential causes of a person's behavior on perceivers' trait impressions. Again, the overarching goal is to understand the mental mechanisms by which different kinds of inputs (e.g., behavioral information, situational information) are translated into outputs (i.e., dispositional attributions). In general, domain-specific dual-process theories differ in terms of the phenomena they aim to explain, in that they focus on input–output relations in different content areas (*explanandum*). Although the proposed explanations are specific to the phenomena of interest, their shared assumption is that different kinds of input–output relations are mediated by two (sets of) qualitatively distinct processes that operate under different conditions (*explanans*).

With the beginning of the new millennium, the focus of dual-process theorizing shifted toward the development of integrative theories that aim at identifying general principles that are independent of particular content domains. A seminal contribution in this regard was Smith and DeCoster's (2000) conceptual integration of various domain-specific theories within a single dual-process framework. The central argument of their integrative account is that the multiple dualisms proposed by domain-specific theories reflect the operation of two basic processes that characterize any kind of human thought irrespective of its content: associative versus rule-based processes (cf. Sloman, 1996). This distinction has become the common denominator of various generalized dual-process theories, including theories that distinguish between reflective and impulsive processing (Strack & Deutsch, 2004), reflective and reflexive processing (Lieberman et al., 2002), and System 1 versus System 2 processing (Kahneman, 2003; Stanovich & West, 2000). Deviating from the initial focus on domain-specific phenomena, generalized dual-process theories are concerned with the basic architecture of information processing (Carruthers, 2009; Samuels, 2009). Thus, generalized dual-process theories differ from domain-specific dual-process theories in terms of the breadth of their *explanandum*, such that the latter aim at explaining input–output relations in particular content areas, whereas the former aim at providing a general account of the workings of the human mind.

Explanans

Beyond differences in terms of the phenomena that dual-process theories aim to explain, there are nontrivial differences in the mental constructs they propose to explain the phenomena of interest. Whereas some theories emphasize functionally distinct mental processes (*dual-process theories*), other theories attribute different behavioral outcomes to functionally distinct mental representations (*dual-representation theories*). Moreover, some theories include assumptions about both process and representation, assuming that different outcomes are the product of two functionally distinct processing systems (*dual-system theories*).

A defining feature of *dual-process theories* is that they explain different kinds of input–output relations on the basis of two (sets of) mental mechanisms. For example, Fiske and Neuberg's (1990) continuum model of impression formation distinguishes between categorization processes and piecemeal integration of individuating attributes. Similarly, Trope's (1986) two-stage model of dispositional attribution distinguishes between perceptual identification of trait-relevant cues and subsequent inference of dispositions. Many of these theories include empirical hypotheses about systematic covariations between operating principles and operating conditions, in that the proposed mechanisms are assumed to operate under different conditions. For example, Fiske and Neuberg's (1990) continuum model assumes that the initial categorization of a target person requires little amounts of cognitive resources, whereas the piecemeal integration of individuating attributes is assumed to be resource-dependent. Similarly, Trope's (1986) two-stage model assumes that the perceptual identification of trait-relevant cues occurs unintentionally, whereas dispositional inference is assumed to be an intentional process (for a review, see Gawronski & Creighton, 2013). Thus, in addition to differences in the particular phenomena they aim to explain, dual-process theories can be characterized by their assumptions about the nature of the two processes they propose to explain these phenomena (i.e., operating principles) and the particular conditions under which each of the two processes is assumed to operate (i.e., operating conditions).

Deviating from the emphasis on processes, *dual-representation theories* attribute different behavioral outcomes to distinct mental representations. A useful example to illustrate the difference between dual-process and dual-representation theories is research comparing evaluative responses on traditional self-report measures to responses on performance-based tasks, such as the Implicit Association Test (Greenwald, McGhee, & Schwartz, 1998) or the evaluative priming task (Fazio, Jackson, Dunton, & Williams, 1995). A common finding in this area is that evaluative responses on the two kinds of measures show various dissociations, including different antecedents, different consequences, and discrepant evaluations of the same object (for reviews, see Friese, Hofmann, & Schmitt, 2008; Gawronski & Bodenhausen, 2006). Such dissociations have led some researchers to conclude that self-report measures reflect conscious, "explicit" attitudes, whereas performance-based tasks reflect unconscious, "implicit" attitudes (e.g., Greenwald & Banaji, 1995; Rydell & McConnell, 2006; see also Wilson, Lindsey, & Schooler, 2000). Yet counter to such dual-representation accounts, dual-process accounts assume that the two kinds of measures capture the same attitudinal representation, the primary difference being the reduced opportunity to control responses on performance-based measures (e.g., Fazio, 2007). Whereas dual-representation accounts are based on presumed parallels to the distinction between explicit and implicit memory, dual-process accounts emphasize the unintentional activation of attitudes and their reduced impact on overt responses when people have the motivation and opportunity to deliberate about specific attributes of the attitude object (for a more detailed discussion, see Payne & Gawronski, 2010).

A third category of theories explains different behavioral outcomes by the operation of two distinct processing systems. The shared assumption of such *dual-system theories* is that multiple psychological dualities are systematically correlated, thereby constituting two functionally distinct mental systems. Although dual-system theories differ in their assumptions about which dualities represent core features of the proposed systems, the hypothesized correlations between dichotomous characteristics are often depicted in lists of features that describe one of the two systems as *associative*, *automatic*, *slow-learning*, *experiential*, *affective*, *parallel*, and *holistic*, and the other one as *rule-based*, *nonautomatic*, *fast-learning*, *rational*, *cognitive*, *sequential*, and *analytic* (e.g., Epstein, 1994; Kahneman, 2003; Sloman, 1996; Smith & DeCoster, 2000). Although some dual-system theories limit their focus to particular content domains (e.g., Rydell & McConnell, 2006), the majority falls into the category of generalized theories that aim at providing a domain-independent account of the workings of the human mind (e.g., Smith & DeCoster, 2000; Strack & Deutsch, 2004).

Formalization

The different types of dual-process theories discussed so far share the feature that they rely only on the informal logic of verbally formulated propositions rather than mathematical formalization (for a notable exception, see Trope, 1986). Over the past decade, some researchers have started to develop formalized theories in which the mechanisms that are assumed to mediate input–output relations are specified in mathematical terms. The most prominent example is Jacoby's (1991) process dissociation (PD) model (for a review, see Payne & Bishara, 2009). Other, more complex theories rely on multinomial modeling (e.g., Conrey, Sherman, Gawronski, Hugenberg, & Groom, 2005; Krieglmeyer & Sherman, 2012; Meissner & Rothermund, 2013; Nadarevic & Erdfelder, 2010; Payne, Hall, Cameron, & Bishara, 2010; Stahl & Degner, 2007) and applications of random-walk and diffusion modeling (e.g., Klauer, Voss, Schmitz, & Teige-Mocigemba, 2007). Regardless of the specifics of their mathematical underpinnings, formalized dual-process theories have at least three advantages over nonformalized theories.

First, formalized theories allow researchers to quantify the contribution of multiple distinct processes to a given behavioral outcome, which is not possible on the basis of verbally formulated theories. The significance of this characteristic is reflected in the principle of *equifinality,* which refers to cases in which combinations of different processes produce the same behavioral outcome. For example, in research on self-regulation, two people may show the same behavioral response when (1) the initial impulse and inhibitory control are weak or (2) the initial impulse and inhibitory control are strong (Sherman et al., 2008). Formalized theories are able to capture such complex interplays by providing quantitative estimates for each of the proposed processes.

Second, formalized theories have the advantage that their logical coherence can be tested by means of their mathematical constraints (Klauer, in press). For many verbally formulated theories it can be very difficult to identify logical inconsistencies between their core assumptions, particularly when they involve a large number of theoretical claims. To illustrate this problem, consider a theory that includes a set of N propositions. Logically, any subset of $N - 1$ of these propositions could be internally consistent even if the entire set N is inconsistent. This possibility implies that an exhaustive consistency assessment of N propositions requires scrutiny of 2^N cases. The resulting capacity problem is illustrated by the fact that, even if each case could be examined in a millionth of a second, an exhaustive consistency check for a theory including 100 propositions would take longer than the universe has existed (see Johnson-Laird, 2012). Formalized theories avoid this problem, because their underlying mathematical constraints help to identify inconsistent assumptions at various stages of the research process, including the initial specification of a theory, the generation of predicted data patterns, the estimation of model parameters from observed data, and the assessment of fit between predicted and observed data (Klauer, in press).

Third, formalized theories have the advantage that they directly link the proposed processes to relations between inputs and outputs. In a strict sense, psychological measures do not assess mental processes or mental representations, but their behavioral outcomes (De Houwer, 2011). Although it is rather common to treat behavioral outcomes as "proxies" for mental constructs, such treatments involve the logical fallacy of *affirming the consequent*, also known as *reverse inference* (Gawronski & Bodenhausen, in press-a). One possibility to avoid this problem is to distinguish clearly between the behavioral outputs captured by psychological measures and the mental constructs that are proposed to explain input–output relations. The validity of dual-process theories (like any other mental process theory) can then be tested by deriving predictions about input–output relations and the particular conditions under which they should emerge (Gawronski & Bodenhausen, in press-b). Yet the derivation of such predictions requires "bridging" assumptions that link the proposed mental constructs to inputs and outputs (McGrath, 1981). Domain-specific dual-process theories typically include such assumptions, but these theories have been criticized for referring to particular contents (e.g., argument strength vs. source characteristics) in linking phenomenon-relevant inputs to the proposed processes (e.g., central/systematic vs. peripheral/heuristic processing). This strategy seems problematic to the extent that the processing of different information involves the same mental operations irrespective of its content (see Kruglanski, Erb, Pierro, Mannetti, & Chun, 2006; Sherman, 2006). Generalized dual-process theories avoid this problem by postulating two (sets of) content-independent processes. However, many of these theories focus primarily on the internal architecture of the human mind, without specifying links between the proposed processes and the relevant inputs. Formalized dual-process theories avoid both problems by (1) proposing general processes that are independent of particular contents and (2) directly linking the proposed processes to observed input–output relations in their mathematical formulations.

An important aspect of formalized dual-process theories is the relation between their processing parameters and the concept of automaticity. For example, the processing parameters of Jacoby's (1991) PD model have sometimes been interpreted as capturing automatic and nonautomatic processes by virtue of its underlying mathematical structure. This interpretation is reflected in the common depiction of the two parameter estimates as *automatic* (using the acronym A) and *controlled* (using the acronym C). However, such depictions conflate the difference between operating principles and operating conditions. Although formalized theories provide clear specifications of *how* inputs are translated into outputs, their mathematical underpinnings do not have any implications for *when* the proposed processes operate (i.e., when there is no conscious awareness; when cognitive resources are reduced; when there is no goal to start the process; when there is a goal to alter or stop the process). Questions about the conditions under which a given process operates cannot be addressed by mathematical formalizations but have to be answered on the basis of empirical data. For example, whether the particular processes captured by the two PD parameters depend on the availability of cognitive resources has to be investigated by testing effects of cognitive load or time pressure on the two parameters, and there is nothing in the underlying PD formulas that would guarantee one or the other outcome. The same is true for all other features of automaticity, including unawareness, unintentionality, and uncontrollability (for a more detailed discussion, see Gawronski & Creighton, 2013).

COVARIATION OF DUALITIES

Many dual-process theories hypothesize systematic covariations between two or more psychological dualities (Samuels, 2009). At the most basic level, these covariations involve empirical relations between functionally distinct processes and the conditions under which these processes operate. For example, a common assumption of domain-specific dual-process theories is that the processes underlying the effects of certain kinds of inputs are intentional and resource-dependent, whereas those underlying the effects of other kinds of inputs are unintentional and resource-independent. Examples include processing constraints on the effects of central versus peripheral cues in dual-process theories of persuasion (e.g., Petty & Cacioppo, 1986), behavioral versus situational information in dual-process theories of dispositional attribution (e.g., Gilbert, 1989), and category versus individuating information in dual-process theories of impression formation (e.g., Fiske & Neuberg, 1990). Similarly, dual-representation theories often attribute a particular feature of automatic processing (e.g., unconscious) to one representation and the opposite feature (e.g., conscious) to the other representation (e.g., Greenwald & Banaji, 1995). Yet the idea of covariation between dualities is most explicit in dual-system theories, which propose systematic relations between multiple distinct dualities (e.g., Epstein, 1994; Kahneman, 2003; Lieberman et al., 2002; Sloman, 1996; Smith & DeCoster, 2000; Stanovich & West, 2000; Strack & Deutsch, 2004).

Although assumptions about covariations between psychological dualities are very common, their epistemic value depends on two conceptual issues (see Moors, Chapter 2, this volume). First, it is important that the two categories underlying a given duality are characterized by a clear demarcation, so that they constitute nonoverlapping categories. For example, the distinction between categorical and individuating information in dual-process theories of impression formation has been criticized for being ambiguous as to whether a given target characteristic should be regarded as categorical information (e.g., man vs. woman; adolescent vs. elderly) or as an individuating attribute (e.g., male vs. female; young vs. old) (see Kunda & Thagard, 1996). Second, it is important to distinguish between conceptual definitions and empirical hypotheses when proposing systematic relations between two or more dualities. For example, to the extent that associative processes are *defined* as unconscious and propositional processes are *defined* as conscious (e.g., Mitchell, De Houwer, & Lovibond, 2009), the relation between the two dualities would be purely semantic rather than empirical (cf. Smedslund, 2000; Wallach & Wallach, 1994). In this case, it would make no sense to test empirically whether propositional processes require conscious awareness, because that is how propositional processes are defined in the first place. Any process that is conscious would be propositional by definition. Yet, if the associative–propositional dualism is defined without reference to the unconscious–conscious dualism (e.g., Gawronski & Bodenhausen, 2011), assumptions about systematic covariations between the two dualities could be subject to empirical tests to the extent that (1) the associative–propositional distinction specifies particular input–output relations that can be expected on the basis of the two processes (operating principles), and (2) the unconscious–conscious distinction specifies the conditions under which these input–output relations should emerge (operating conditions). Thus, a basic requirement for conceptually sound dual-process theorizing is that the categories of conceptually distinct dualities are defined in a manner that avoids semantic overlap between these dualities (Moors, Chapter 2, this volume). Moreover, although conceptual definitions and empirical hypotheses are often conflated in claims about covariations between multiple dualities, it is important that the categories constituting a given duality are defined in a manner that allows unambiguous demarcations between these categories.

ARE DUAL-PROCESS THEORIES UNFALSIFIABLE?

The quest to distinguish clearly between conceptual definitions and empirical hypotheses is particularly important in the context of criticism that dual-process theories are unfalsifiable (e.g., Keren & Schul, 2009). If there is no demarcation between the conceptual definitions of the proposed dualities and empirical hypotheses about covariations between dualities, there is a considerable risk that the value of dual-process theories will be reduced to post hoc categorizations of empirical effects. An illustrative example is the common equation of System 1 processing with resource-independence and System 2 processing with resource-dependence (e.g., Dhar & Gorlin, 2013). The problem is that such an equation does not offer anything beyond post hoc classifications of observed effects (Gawronski, 2013). To the extent that a given effect is resource-independent it will be categorized as being due to System 1, but it will be attributed to System 2 if it is resource dependent. Moreover, if an effect that was initially attributed to System 1 turns out to depend on cognitive resources, this effect would simply be recategorized as the product of System 2, and vice versa. Without a clear specification of the operating principles of System 1 and System 2 processing, the theory does not impose any constraints on the interpretation of a given result. Thus, criticism of dual-process theories as being unfalsifiable can be avoided by (1) conceptually precise definitions of the proposed dualities and (2) clear formulations of empirical hypotheses about their covariations.

To the extent that the two requirements are met, dual-process theories are in fact highly falsifiable, counter to the common criticism that they are unfalsifiable. According to Popper (1934), the falsifiability of a given theory increases with the number of events that are prohibited by the theory (see Gawronski & Bodenhausen, in press-a). Thus, by assuming systematic overlap between two conceptually distinct dualities, dual-process theories can be said to prohibit two out of four possible events. For example, dual-process theories of dispositional attribution claiming that the impact of situational information is mediated by a resource-dependent process, whereas the impact of behavioral information is mediated by a resource-independent process, would be disconfirmed by any finding showing that either (1) the impact of behavioral information is resource-dependent or (2) the impact of situational information is resource-independent (e.g., Krull, 1993; Trope & Gaunt, 2000). Importantly, the number of events prohibited by dual-process theories—and thus their falsifiability—increases with the number of proposed covariations between dualities. For example, a dual-systems theory assuming systematic overlap between four conceptually distinct dualities would prohibit 14 out of 16 possible combinations. Such a theory would be highly falsifiable, because it would be disconfirmed by any one of the 14 cases that are prohibited by the theory. To be sure, certain assumptions about systematic overlap between multiple dualities may be rejected as empirically implausible or inconsistent with the available evidence (Keren & Schul, 2009; Kruglanski & Gigerenzer, 2011). For example, the assumption that the associative–propositional, affective–cognitive, and unconscious–conscious dualities have systematic overlap may be rejected on the grounds that there are cognitive associative processes, unconscious cognitive processes, conscious affective processes, and so forth. However, because such rejections are based on empirical arguments, they invalidate rather than support the common contention that dual-process theories are unfalsifiable.

Despite our rejection of generalized claims of unfalsifiability, we believe that there is another, less obvious feature that can make dual-process theories unfalsifiable. Many domain-specific dual-process theories were formulated in a manner such that the relevant inputs were specified at the level of external stimuli (e.g., source characteristics, situational information, category membership). The same was true for the proposed outputs, which were clearly specified at the level of overt responses (e.g., evaluative judgments, trait judgments). These specifications made it relatively easy to determine whether a theoretically derived prediction about input–output relations is consistent or inconsistent with a given finding. With the emergence of generalized dual-process theories, the focus shifted toward properties of the mind's internal architecture. In these theories, many of the core assumptions are specified at the mental level, without reference to external stimuli and overt responses. For example, in Kahneman's (2003) dual-system theory of judgment and choice, System 1 processing is claimed to involve a process of attribute substitution, in which a target attribute is substituted by a heuristic attribute that comes more readily to mind. Moreover, System 2 processing is assumed to monitor and, if necessary, modify or override the outputs of System 1. However, the theory itself does not specify which stimulus attributes count as target attributes and which ones should be regarded as heuristic attributes.[3] Thus, enhanced effects of any given attribute may be explained by either (1) dominance of System 1 processing involving the replacement of a target attribute by another heuristic attribute or (2) dominance of System 2 processing involving the replacement of the output of System 1 processing. In the absence of "bridging" assumptions that link the hypothesized mental constructs to external inputs and overt outputs, it can be rather difficult to determine whether a given theory is consistent or inconsistent with a particular finding (McGrath, 1981). This difficulty can lead to the impression that dual-process theories are unfalsifiable, although their assumptions about covariations between two or more dualities clearly prohibit a large number of possible events. In other words, although dual-process theories are falsifiable *in principle* if they are evaluated in terms of Popper's (1934) structural criterion, some of them are *practically* unfalsifiable, because they are formulated in a manner that makes it difficult to determine which relations between external stimuli and overt behavioral responses would be inconsistent with these theories. This feature allows researchers to apply some dual-process theories to virtually every empirical outcome in a post hoc fashion (e.g., post hoc categorizations of a given effect as being driven by System 1 vs. System 2). However, it is rather difficult to derive a priori predictions that could pose a strong challenge to these theories.

HOW MANY PROCESSES ARE THERE?

A common question about dual-process theories is whether the realm of mental processes can indeed be meaningfully divided into two distinct categories. Whereas some theorists have argued that dual-process theories clearly demonstrated their explanatory and predictive value (Deutsch & Strack, 2006), others have argued for the superiority of single-process (e.g., Kruglanski et al., 2006) or multiple process alternatives (e.g., Sherman, 2006). Yet when discussing the question of how many processes there "really" are, it is important to note that existence claims—including claims about the existence of one, two, or multiple processes—are ontological in nature. In the philosophy of science, ontological claims fall into the realm of metaphysics, which means that they cannot be tested empirically (e.g., Popper, 1934; Quine, 1960). From this perspective, it is not possible to test whether there are one, two, or multiple processes. However, researchers can make decisions about the usefulness of ontological claims by empirically testing assumptions *about* the proposed processes. To the extent that dual-process theories help us to understand past observations of input–output relations (*explanation*) and correctly forecast future observations of input–output relations (*prediction*), there is reason to believe that their assumptions are correct, including their ontological assumptions about the existence of certain mental processes. However, if the predictions of a given theory are continuously disconfirmed, it seems likely that researchers will at some point reject its underlying ontological claims (cf. Peters & Gawronski, 2011). Note, however, that in such cases it is not the existence-claim itself that is confirmed or disconfirmed, but the assumptions that are made about the proposed entities. In this sense, the number of mental processes is not an objective fact that can be studied independently of the assumptions that are made about them. Instead, the number of mental processes that we assume to exist inherently depends on our theories, in that we accept the ontology of those theories that help us to understand past observations (*explanation*) and correctly forecast future observations (*prediction*).

An important issue in this context is the quest for *parsimony*, which stipulates that researchers should favor theories that involve fewer assumptions to explain a particular empirical finding (Gawronski & Bodenhausen, in press-a). Single-process theorists sometimes appeal to the quest for parsimony, arguing that dual-process theories are less parsimonious than single-process theories, because they postulate two qualitatively distinct processes rather than a single one. However, an often-overlooked aspect of parsimony is that it refers to the *total* number of theoretical assumptions that are required to explain a given finding rather than the number of assumptions of what might be considered the core of a given theory. To explain a particular finding, single-process theories have to rely on a host of additional assumptions over and above the hypothesis that information processing is guided by a single process (e.g., modulation of this process by five conceptually distinct parameters; see Kruglanski et al., 2006). Thus, when evaluating theories on the basis of their parsimony, it does not suffice to count the number of processes they propose. What matters for the criterion of parsimony is the total number of assumptions that is required to explain a given finding.

A final issue concerns the most appropriate level of abstraction in theorizing about mental processes. In some sense, every mental process can be described by the shared feature that they follow if–then rules. Some researchers have interpreted this possibility as an argument for the superiority of single-process theories that attribute all kinds of input–output relations to the same process of rule-based inference (e.g., Kruglanski et al., 2006). However, descriptions of mental processes at such a high level of abstraction do not go far beyond claiming that all mental processes follow some kind of regularity instead of being random (Gawronski & Creighton, 2013). Moreover, to the extent that such if–then conditionals directly refer to inputs as the antecedent and outputs as the consequent, their theoretical claims would be located at Marr's (1982) computational level of analysis. However, computational analysis fails to specify the mental processes and representations that translate inputs into outputs at the algorithmic level, which is a central concern of dual-process theorizing. In this sense, the debate between advocates of single-process and dual-process theories seems at least partly spurious, in that the conflicting claims refer to different levels of analysis (cf. De Houwer & Moors, in press; see also Sherman, 2006).

Similar considerations apply to the debate between dual-process and multiple-process theories. In some sense, every process can be further analyzed for subcomponents that constitute this process. For example, although the distinction between associative and propositional processes may serve as the conceptual foundation of a dual-process theory of evaluation (Gawronski & Bodenhausen, 2006), the functional principles of the two processes may be further divided depending on whether they operate during the formation or the expression of evaluative representations. Moreover, one could argue that the process of propositional validation involves a number of subprocesses, including the default affirmation of validity, the monitoring of consistency, and the resolution of inconsistency (Gawronski & Bodenhausen, 2011). In this sense, every dual-process theory may be regarded as an oversimplification, in that its proposed dualities can always be divided into multiple subordinate processes. In fact, for many theories that have been categorized as *dual-process theories,* the term is actually a misnomer given that the majority of these theories propose more than two processes that are involved in the translation of inputs into outputs.

We argue that the optimal level of theoretical abstraction cannot be determined a priori but has to be decided on the basis of the research question (Sherman, 2006). For many social psychological questions, the conceptual distinctions proposed by dual-process theories have clearly demonstrated their value in explaining and predicting the phenomena of interest. However, for other questions, more fine-grained theories may be needed to account fully for the available evidence. Yet regardless of the chosen level of abstraction, it is important that the proposed process dimensions be clearly defined and their conceptual definitions be distinguished from empirical hypotheses about covariations between different dimensions.

EMERGING THEMES AND FUTURE DIRECTIONS

An interesting line of research that is starting to emerge from dual-process theorizing concerns the mental processes underlying operating conditions. This statement may seem a little puzzling given our strong emphasis on the distinction between operating principles and operating conditions. Yet it is entirely possible to stipulate a clear distinction between operating principles and operating conditions and, at the same time, ask questions about the processes underlying operating conditions.

Traditionally, dual-process theories aimed at identifying the mental processes underlying particular kinds of input–output relations. These processes are conceptually defined by their operating principles, and assumptions about their operating conditions reflect empirical hypotheses about whether they operate (1) when there is no conscious awareness, (2) when there is no goal to start the process, (3) when cognitive resources are reduced, and (4) when there is a goal to alter or stop the process. Operating conditions are typically investigated by means of appropriate manipulations, including supraliminal versus subliminal presentation times (awareness), the presence versus absence of instructions to perform a particular mental operation (intentionality), the relative difficulty of a simultaneously performed secondary task (efficiency), and instructions not to perform a particular mental operation (controllability). Any of these manipulations can be conceptualized as involving contextual inputs (or input characteristics) that may moderate the relation between a primary input and its output (De Houwer & Moors, 2012). In line with this conceptualization, Marr (1982) located operating conditions at the computational rather than the algorithmic level, which is consistent with our emphasis on the distinction between operating principles and operating conditions.

Nevertheless, it is certainly possible to investigate the mental processes by which the inputs of operating conditions influence the input–output relations produced by another process. In this case, the moderating effect of a given input on other input–output relations represents the phenomenon that needs to be explained (*explanandum*), and researchers may develop mental process theories that explain *how* this input moderates input–output relations (*explanans*). For example, researchers may investigate the mental processes by which the affordances of secondary tasks influence the operation of another mental process. Similarly, researchers may be interested in the mental processes by which instructions to inhibit a particular process influence the operation of that process. Such theories differ from traditional dual-process theories, in that they focus on how secondary processes influence the operation of the primary processes postulated by traditional dual-process theories. Applied to the four features of automaticity, potential themes of such theories may include (1) the processes by which subliminal versus supraliminal stimulus presentations moderate the execution of a primary process, (2) the processes by which the presence versus absence of instructions to perform a particular mental operation moderates the execution the primary process, (3) the processes by which secondary task performance moderates the execution of a primary process, and (4) the processes by which instructions not to perform a particular mental operation moderate the execution of the primary process.

What may already be clear from this conceptualization is that research on the mental processes underlying operating conditions requires a sufficient understanding of the input–output relations that are produced by the relevant primary processes. Although such an assumption may seem questionable to critics of dual-process theorizing, cognitive science has a long history of research on similar questions, including the nature of consciousness (Baars, 2002), working memory (Baddeley, 2010), and executive control (Braver, 2012). Of course, the paradigms in this research tend to be much less complex than the ones typically used by social psychologists. Nevertheless, we believe that research under the guidance of dual-process theories has accumulated a sufficiently large body of knowledge to move to the next level of inquiry by studying the interplay between the proposed primary processes and the secondary processes that determine the conditions of their operation. To the extent that the theories inspired by this research adhere to the distinction between operating principles and operating conditions for both primary and secondary processes, they may also provide valuable insights into when and why certain features of automaticity do or do not co-occur (Moors & De Houwer, 2006). Examples of emerging themes in this regard include recent claims about the resource-independence of inhibitory control (e.g., Fujita, 2011) and the resource-dependence of unconscious processing (e.g., Hassin et al., 2009).

CONCLUSION

Emerging in the 1980s, the first generation of dual-process theories has yielded a multiplicity of dualities in theorizing about social information processing. Cumulatively, this work has demonstrated the ability of dual-process theories to be generative and applicable to a broad spectrum of social psychological phenomena. Since the publication of Chaiken and Trope's (1999) seminal volume, *Dual-Process Theories in Social Psychology*, these theories have continued to be highly generative and have further expanded the range of application. At the same time, attempts at integration have shifted the focus to formulating unitary distinctions between different mental processes that cut across multiple domains. Our hope is that future advances will help dual-process theories to further enhance the basic science desiderata of conceptual coherence, precision, generality, and testability without sacrificing their applicability to the problems humans face as members of dyads, groups, and societies.

In this spirit, our main goal in this chapter has been to analyze the explanatory function of dual-process theories, the conceptual nature of their underlying dualities, and the structural features that characterize different types of dual-process theories. Drawing on Marr's (1982) distinction among computational, algorithmic, and implementational levels of analysis, we have argued that a central explanatory function of dual-process theories is to specify the mental mechanisms that translate inputs into outputs. From this perspective, descriptions of a given process as automatic versus nonautomatic simply specify *when* the process is assumed to operate (operating conditions). However, they do not specify *how* the proposed process translates inputs into outputs (operating principles). The latter question requires clear specifications of the underlying mental operations, which are essential for mechanistic explanations at Marr's algorithmic level of analysis. To the extent that dual-process theories include precise and nonoverlapping definitions of the proposed dualities, their hypotheses about covariations between processing dualities are highly falsifiable, in that they prohibit a considerable number of possible events. Yet the explanatory and predictive value of dual-process theories essentially depends on (1) a clear distinction between operating principles and operating conditions, (2) conceptual rigor in the definition of the proposed dualities, (3) precise formulations of empirical hypotheses about covariations between processing dualities, and (4) clearly specified links between the hypothesized mental processes and the causal relations between stimuli and behavior they are supposed to explain.

NOTES

1. Automatic processes are often contrasted with controlled processes. Yet the term *control* has been used to refer to either (1) a particular feature of nonautomatic processing (i.e., controllability) or (2) an umbrella concept subsuming multiple different features of nonautomatic procesing (i.e., awareness, intentionality, resource dependence, controllability). To avoid conceptual confusion, we use the term *nonautomatic* as the semantic antonym of the term *automatic* instead of the more common term *controlled* (see Moors & De Houwer, 2006).
2. Some dual-process theories derive empirical assumptions about operating conditions from their conceptual definitions of operating principles (e.g., inferences about resource dependence from the conceptual distinction between sequential and parallel processing). Although such inferences are theoreticaly valuable to clarify the conceptual basis of the derived hypotheses about operating conditions, it is important to note that operating principles and operating conditions are nevertheless conceptually distinct in these theories, in that the former describe the nature of the mental processes that translate inputs into outputs, whereas the latter refer to the particular conditions under which these processes are assumed to operate.
3. Note that the specification of heuristic attributes as coming more readily to mind does not provide a clear conceptual demarcation, because the accessibility of any given attribute can vary as a function of its salience.

REFERENCES

Baars, B. J. (2002). The conscious access hypothesis: Origins and recent evidence. *Trends in Cognitive Sciences, 6*, 47–52.

Baddeley, A. (2010). Working memory. *Current Biology, 20*, 136–140.

Bargh, J. A. (1992). The ecology of automaticity: Toward establishing the conditions needed to produce automatic processing effects. *American Journal of Psychology, 105*, 181–199.

Bargh, J. A. (1994). The four horsemen of automaticity: Awareness, intention, efficiency, and control in social cognition. In R. S. Wyer & T. K. Srull (Eds.), *Handbook of social cognition* (pp. 1–40). Hillsdale, NJ: Erlbaum.

Bargh, J. A. (2006). What have we been priming all these years?: On the development, mechanisms, and ecology of nonconscious social behavior. *European Journal of Social Psychology, 36*, 147–168.

Baumeister, R. F., Masicampo, E. J., & Vohs, K. D. (2011). Do conscious thoughts cause behavior? *Annual Review of Psychology, 62*, 331–361.

Braver, T. S. (2012). The variable nature of cognitive control: A dual mechanisms framework. *Trends in Cognitive Sciences, 16*, 106–113.

Brewer, M. B. (1988). A dual process model of impression formation. In T. K. Srull & R. S. Wyer (Eds.), *Advances in social cognition* (Vol. 1, pp. 1–36). Hillsdale, NJ: Erlbaum.

Cacioppo, J. T., Berntson, G. G., Sheridan, J. F., & McClintock, M. K. (2000). Multilevel integrative analyses of human behavior: Social neuroscience and the complementing nature of social and biological approaches. *Psychological Bulletin, 126*, 829–843.

Carruthers, P. (2009). An architecture for dual reasoning. In J. St. B. T. Evans & K. Frankish (Eds.), *In two minds: Dual processes and beyond* (pp. 109–127). New York: Oxford University Press.

Cesario, J., Plaks, J. E., & Higgins, E. T. (2006). Automatic social behavior as motivated preparation to interact. *Journal of Personality and Social Psychology, 90*, 893–910.

Chaiken, S. (1987). The heuristic model of persuasion. In M. P. Zanna, J. M. Olson, & C. P. Herman (Eds.), *Social influence: The Ontario Symposium* (Vol. 5, pp. 3–39). Hillsdale, NJ: Erlbaum.

Chaiken, S., & Trope, Y. (Eds.). (1999). *Dual-process theories in social psychology*. New York: Guilford Press.

Conrey, F. R., Sherman, J. W., Gawronski, B., Hugenberg, K., & Groom, C. (2005). Separating multiple processes in implicit social cognition: The Quad-Model of implicit task performance. *Journal of Personality and Social Psychology, 89*, 469–487.

De Houwer, J. (2011). Why the cognitive approach in psychology would profit from a functional approach and vice versa. *Perspectives on Psychological Science, 6*, 202–209.

De Houwer, J., & Moors, A. (2012). How to

define and examine implicit processes? In R. Proctor & J. Capaldi (Eds.), *Implicit and explicit processes in the psychology of science* (pp. 183–198). New York: Oxford University Press.

De Houwer, J., & Moors, A. (in press). Levels of analysis. In B. Gawronski & G. V. Bodenhausen (Eds.), *Theory and explanation in social psychology*. New York: Guilford Press.

Deutsch, R., & Strack, F. (2006). Duality models in social psychology: From dual processes to interacting systems. *Psychological Inquiry, 17,* 166–172.

Devine, P. G. (1989). Stereotypes and prejudice: Their automatic and controlled components. *Journal of Personality and Social Psychology, 56,* 5–18.

Dhar, R., & Gorlin, M. (2013). A dual-system framework to understand preference construction processes in choice. *Journal of Consumer Psychology, 23,* 528–542.

Dijksterhuis, A., & Nordgren, L. F. (2006). A theory of unconscious thought. *Perspectives on Psychological Science, 1,* 95–109.

Epstein, S. (1994). Integration of the cognitive and the psychodynamic unconscious. *American Psychologist, 49,* 709–724.

Evans, J. St. B. T., & Frankish, K. (Eds.). (2009). *In two minds: Dual processes and beyond.* New York: Oxford University Press.

Fazio, R. H. (1990). Multiple processes by which attitudes guide behavior: The MODE model as an integrative framework. *Advances in Experimental Social Psychology, 23,* 75–109.

Fazio, R. H. (2007). Attitudes as object-evaluation associations of varying strength. *Social Cognition, 25,* 603–637.

Fazio, R. H., Jackson, J. R., Dunton, B. C., & Williams, C. J. (1995). Variability in automatic activation as an unobtrusive measure of racial attitudes: A bona fide pipeline? *Journal of Personality and Social Psychology, 69,* 1013–1027.

Fiske, S. T., & Neuberg, S. L. (1990). A continuum of impression formation, from category-based to individuating processes: Influences of information and motivation on attention and interpretation. *Advances in Experimental Social Psychology, 23,* 1–74.

Friese, M., Hofmann, W., & Schmitt, M. (2008). When and why do implicit measures predict behaviour? Empirical evidence for the moderating role of opportunity, motivation, and process reliance. *European Review of Social Psychology, 19,* 285–338.

Fujita, K. (2011). On conceptualizing self-control as more than the effortful inhibition of impulses. *Personality and Social Psychology Review, 15,* 352–366.

Gawronski, B. (2013). What should we expect from a dual-process theory of preference construction in choice? *Journal of Consumer Psychology, 23,* 556–560.

Gawronski, B., & Bodenhausen, G. V. (2006). Associative and propositional processes in evaluation: An integrative review of implicit and explicit attitude change. *Psychological Bulletin, 132,* 692–731.

Gawronski, B., & Bodenhausen, G. V. (2009). Operating principles versus operating conditions in the distinction between associative and propositional processes. *Behavioral and Brain Sciences, 32,* 207–208.

Gawronski, B., & Bodenhausen, G. V. (2011). The associative–propositional evaluation model: Theory, evidence, and open questions. *Advances in Experimental Social Psychology, 44,* 59–127.

Gawronski, B., & Bodenhausen, G. V. (in press-a). Theory evaluation. In B. Gawronski & G. V. Bodenhausen (Eds.), *Theory and explanation in social psychology*. New York: Guilford Press.

Gawronski, B., & Bodenhausen, G. V. (in press-b). Social-cognitive theories. In B. Gawronski & G. V. Bodenhausen (Eds.), *Theory and explanation in social psychology*. New York: Guilford Press.

Gawronski, B., & Creighton, L. A. (2013). Dual-process theories. In D. E. Carlston (Ed.), *The Oxford handbook of social cognition* (pp. 282–312). New York: Oxford University Press.

Gilbert, D. T. (1989). Thinking lightly about others: Automatic components of the social inference process. In J. S. Uleman & J. A. Bargh (Eds.), *Unintended thought* (pp. 189–211). New York: Guilford Press.

Greenwald, A. G., & Banaji, M. R. (1995). Implicit social cognition: Attitudes, self-esteem, and stereotypes. *Psychological Review, 102,* 4–27.

Greenwald, A. G., McGhee, D. E., & Schwartz, J. L. K. (1998). Measuring individual differences in implicit cognition: The Implicit Association Test. *Journal of Personality and Social Psychology, 74,* 1464–1480.

Hassin, R. R., Bargh, J. A., Engell, A. D., & McCulloch, K. C. (2009). Implicit working memory. *Consciousness and Cognition, 18,* 665–678.

Huang, J. Y., & Bargh, J. A. (in press). The Selfish Goal: Autonomously operating motivational structures as the proximate cause of human judgment and behavior. *Behavioral and Brain Sciences.*

Jacoby, L. L. (1991). A process-dissociation framework: Separating automatic from intentional uses of memory. *Journal of Memory and Language, 30,* 513–541.

Johnson-Laird, P. N. (2012). Mental models and consistency. In B. Gawronski & F. Strack (Eds.), *Cognitive consistency: A fundamental principle in social cognition* (pp. 225–244). New York: Guilford Press.

Kahneman, D. (2003). A perspective on judgment and choice: Mapping bounded rationality. *American Psychologist, 58,* 697–720.

Keren, G., & Schul, Y. (2009). Two is not always better than one: A critical evaluation of two-systems theories. *Perspectives on Psychological Science, 4,* 533–550.

Klauer, K. C. (in press). Mathematical modeling. In B. Gawronski & G. V. Bodenhausen (Eds.), *Theory and explanation in social psychology.* New York: Guilford Press.

Klauer, K. C., Voss, A., Schmitz, F., & Teige-Mocigemba, S. (2007). Process components of the Implicit Association Test: A diffusion-model analysis. *Journal of Personality and Social Psychology, 93,* 353–368.

Krieglmeyer, R., & Sherman, J. W. (2012). Disentangling stereotype activation and stereotype application in the Stereotype Misperception Task. *Journal of Personality and Social Psychology, 103,* 205–224.

Kruglanski, A. W., Erb, H.-P., Pierro, A., Mannetti, L., & Chun, W. Y. (2006). On parametric continuities in the world of binary either ors. *Psychological Inquiry, 17,* 153–165.

Kruglanski, A. W., & Gigerenzer, G. (2011). Intuitive and deliberative judgments are based on common principles. *Psychological Review, 118,* 97–109.

Krull, D. S. (1993). Does the grist change the mill?: The effect of the perceiver's inferential goal on the process of social inference. *Personality and Social Psychology Bulletin, 19,* 340–348.

Kunda, Z., & Thagard, P. (1996). Forming impressions from stereotypes, traits, and behaviors: A parallel-constraint satisfaction theory. *Psychological Review, 103,* 284–308.

Lieberman, M. D., Gaunt, R., Gilbert, D. T., & Trope, Y. (2002). Reflexion and reflection: A social cognitive neuroscience approach to attributional inference. *Advances in Experimental Social Psychology, 34,* 199–249.

Loersch, C. & Payne, B. K. (2011). The situated inference model: An integrative account of the effects of primes on perception, behavior, and motivation. *Perspectives on Psychological Science, 6,* 234–252.

Marr, D. (1982). *Vision: A computational investigation into the human representation and processing of visual information.* New York: Freeman.

McGrath, J. E. (1981). Dilemmatics: The study of research choices and dilemmas. *American Behavioral Scientist, 25,* 179–210.

Meissner, F., & Rothermund, K. (2013). Estimating the contributions of associations and recoding in the Implicit Association Test: The ReAL model for the IAT. *Journal of Personality and Social Psychology, 104,* 45–69.

Mitchell, C. J., De Houwer, J., & Lovibond, P. F. (2009). The propositional nature of human associative learning. *Behavioral and Brain Sciences, 32,* 183–198.

Moors, A., & De Houwer, J. (2006). Automaticity: A conceptual and theoretical analysis. *Psychological Bulletin, 132,* 297–326.

Nadarevic, L., & Erdfelder, E. (2011). Cognitive processes in implicit attitude tasks: An experimental validation of the Trip Model. *European Journal of Social Psychology, 41,* 254–268.

Ochsner, K. N., & Lieberman, M. D. (2001). The emergence of social-cognitive neuroscience. *American Psychologist, 56,* 717–734.

Payne, B. K., & Bishara, A. J. (2009). An integrative review of process dissociation and related models in social cognition. *European Review of Social Psychology, 20,* 272–314.

Payne, B. K., & Gawronski, B. (2010). A history of implicit social cognition: Where is it coming from? Where is it now? Where is it going? In B. Gawronski, & B. K. Payne (Eds.), *Handbook of implicit social cognition: Measurement, theory, and applications* (pp. 1–15). New York: Guilford Press.

Payne, B. K., Hall, D. L., Cameron, C. D., & Bishara, A. J. (2010). A process model of affect misattribution. *Personality and Social Psychology Bulletin, 36,* 1397–1408.

Peters, K. R., & Gawronski, B. (2011). Are we puppets on a string?: Comparing the effects of contingency and validity on implicit and explicit evaluations. *Personality and Social Psychology Bulletin, 37,* 557–569.

Petty, R. E., & Cacioppo, J. T. (1986). The Elaboration Likelihood Model of persuasion.

Advances in Experimental Social Psychology, 19, 123–205.

Popper, K. R. (1934). *Logic of scientific discovery.* New York: Basic Books.

Quine, W. V. O. (1960). *Word and object.* Cambridge, MA: MIT Press.

Rydell, R. J., & McConnell, A. R. (2006). Understanding implicit and explicit attitude change: A systems of reasoning analysis. *Journal of Personality and Social Psychology, 91,* 995–1008.

Samuels, R. (2009). The magical number two, plus or minus: Dual-process theory as a theory of cognitive kinds. In J. St. B. T. Evans & K. Frankish (Eds.), *In two minds: Dual processes and beyond* (pp. 129–146). New York: Oxford University Press.

Sherman, J. W. (2006). On building a better process model: It's not only how many, but which ones and by which means. *Psychological Inquiry, 17,* 173–184.

Sherman, J. W., Gawronski, B., Gonsalkorale, K., Hugenberg, K., Allen, T. J., & Groom, C. J. (2008). The self-regulation of automatic associations and behavioral impulses. *Psychological Review, 115,* 314–335.

Sloman, S. A. (1996). The empirical case for two systems of reasoning. *Psychological Bulletin, 119,* 3–22.

Smedslund, G. (2000). A pragmatic basis for judging models and theories in health psychology: The axiomatic method. *Journal of Health Psychology, 5,* 133–149.

Smith, E. R., & DeCoster, J. (2000). Dual-process models in social and cognitive psychology: Conceptual integration and links to underlying memory systems. *Personality and Social Psychology Review, 4,* 108–131.

Stahl, C., & Degner, J. (2007). Assessing automatic activation of valence: A multinomial model of EAST performance. *Experimental Psychology, 54,* 99–112.

Stanovich, K. E., & West, R. F. (2000). Individual differences in reasoning: Implications for the rationality debate? *Behavioral and Brain Sciences, 23,* 645–726.

Strack, F., & Deutsch, R. (2004). Reflective and impulsive determinants of social behavior. *Personality and Social Psychology Review, 8,* 220–247.

Trope, Y. (1986). Identification and inferential processes in dispositional attribution. *Psychological Review, 93,* 239–257.

Trope, Y., & Gaunt, R. (2000). Processing alternative explanations of behavior: Correction or integration? *Journal of Personality and Social Psychology, 79,* 344–354.

Wallach, L., & Wallach, M. A. (1994). Gergen versus the mainstream: Are hypotheses in social psychology subject to empirical test? *Journal of Personality and Social Psychology, 67,* 233–242.

Wheeler, S. C., DeMarree, K. G., & Petty, R. E. (2007). Understanding the role of the self in prime-to-behavior effects: The active-self account. *Personality and Social Psychology Review, 11,* 234–261.

Wilson, T. D., Lindsey, S., & Schooler, T. Y. (2000). A model of dual attitudes. *Psychological Review, 107,* 101–126.

CHAPTER 2

Examining the Mapping Problem in Dual-Process Models

Agnes Moors

Multiprocess models divide the realm of mental processes into two (e.g., Gawronski & Bodenhausen, 2006, 2011; Lieberman, 2003; Sloman, 1996; Smith & DeCoster, 2000; Strack & Deutsch, 2004), three (Leventhal & Scherer, 1987), or four sets of processes (e.g., Conrey, Sherman, Gawronski, Hugenberg, & Groom, 2005; Sherman, 2006). The sets of processes in dual-process models often correspond to dichotomies such as affective versus nonaffective, heuristic versus systematic, automatic versus nonautomatic, associative versus rule-based, perceptual versus conceptual, associative versus propositional, and subcortical versus neocortical. It is perfectly legitimate to create sets on the basis of one or another dichotomy. Most dual-process models, however, take things one step further. They choose two or more dichotomies and make a priori assumptions of overlap among them (Keren & Schul, 2009; Moors & De Houwer, 2006b). A few examples: Associative processes are often said to be automatic, and rule-based processes nonautomatic (e.g., Smith & DeCoster, 2000). Associative processes are often said to operate on perceptual codes, and rule-based processes on conceptual codes (e.g., Leventhal & Scherer, 1987). Heuristic information (e.g., attractiveness of the speaker) is said to exert an automatic influence on decision making, and systematic information (e.g., persuasive arguments of the speaker) a nonautomatic influence (e.g., Chaiken, Liberman, & Eagly, 1989). By mapping various dichotomies onto each other, dual-process models may grow into dual systems models (e.g., Deutsch & Strack, 2006).

The question one may ask is whether it is justified to map dichotomies onto each other. I propose investigating the mapping problem in a stepwise manner. A first step is to engage in the conceptual analysis of various dichotomies to see whether they can be defined independent of each other. If it turns out that they can be so defined, a second step is to investigate empirically whether there is overlap among dichotomies in the real world. To be able to go from the first to the second step, however, an intermediate step is required, in which the definitions proposed in the first step should be translated into methods for diagnosing occurrent processes as belonging to one or the other term of the dichotomy. In this chapter, I engage in a conceptual analysis of the following dichotomies: automatic versus nonautomatic, associative versus rule-based, perceptual versus conceptual, and associative versus propositional (cf. the first step discussed earlier). After that, I examine whether the definitions obtained in the first step lead to criteria for the diagnosis of processes (cf. the intermediate step discussed earlier).

CONCEPTUAL ANALYSIS

Definitions of sets are often of the intensional kind, specifying the necessary and sufficient conditions for something to be an exemplar of a set (i.e., one necessary and sufficient condition, or a collection of necessary conditions that are jointly sufficient). Intensional definitions can be descriptive or prescriptive. Descriptive definitions describe the rules that laypersons (implicitly or explicitly) follow (or seem to follow) when using concepts. Prescriptive definitions stipulate the rules that scientists prescribe for using concepts. The development of prescriptive definitions is often guided by two principles: A first principle is to stay close to natural language or the way in which laypersons use the term (descriptive definitions). As such, it should cover a sufficient number of intuitively clear exemplars (Green, 1992). A second principle stems from the desire to cut nature at its joints or to provide a useful heuristic for future research. These joints are not absolute but context dependent and in this sense involve an element of choice (i.e., they are stipulative). My choice of definitions is explicitly guided by the desire to avoid overlap among dichotomies. The main argument for this is that empirical research can only be carried out with concepts that are logically independent (e.g., Smedslund, 1992). For example, when the dichotomies of automatic versus nonautomatic and associative versus rule-based are defined independently, four combinations are open to investigation: associative and automatic, associative and nonautomatic, rule-based and automatic, and rule-based and nonautomatic. When, by contrast, automatic processes are defined as associative ones, and rule-based processes are defined in terms of nonautomatic features (e.g., conscious), there is no point in empirically investigating any combination. Investigating whether associative processes are automatic, for instance, would be equally absurd as investigating whether bachelors are indeed single and male. By excluding certain combinations from empirical research, we might miss out on relevant findings. Thus, my aim in this section is to examine whether there is a satisfactory way to define each dichotomy without having to make appeal to another dichotomy.

My proposal is to situate the various dichotomies within a levels-of-analysis framework. This framework proposes that any process can be described at (minimally) three levels of analysis (e.g., Anderson, 1987; Marr, 1982; Pylyshyn, 1980). At the functional level, a process is described as the relation between an input and an output. This level includes the content of inputs and outputs, as well as the conditions under which the process operates. For example, affective processing or evaluation can be described as the relation between a stimulus and affective properties (e.g., positive or negative valence). The processing of heuristic information can be described as the relation between a stimulus and heuristic properties (e.g., the attractiveness of the speaker). Conditions include those related to automaticity versus nonautomaticity (e.g., uncontrolled–controlled; unconscious–conscious, efficient–nonefficient, fast–slow). The algorithmic level articulates the mechanisms involved in transforming input into output, as well as the formats of the representations or codes that the mechanisms operate on or produce. For example, evaluation can proceed with an associative mechanism (retrieving stored valence) or a rule-based one (e.g., weighing the implications for various concerns), and both might operate on various types of codes (e.g., conceptual versus perceptual, associative versus propositional). The hardware level is concerned with the physical implementation of processes in the brain. At this level, a process is described in terms of its neurophysiological substrates (e.g., neocortical versus subcortical areas or circuits). For example, evaluation is often linked to circuits involving the amygdala.

The levels-of-analysis framework makes it easy to conceive of the various dichotomies as nonoverlapping. This is because the levels in the framework are only loosely related to each other. For instance, one functional process (e.g., evaluation) can be accounted for by more than one mechanism (e.g., by a rule-based or associative process). Also, presenting automaticity as a matter of conditions provides a natural way to decouple it from processes (described at any level). The next sections include detailed definitions of dichotomies and compare them with alternative definitions, specifically with regard to how successful they are in avoiding overlap with other dichotomies.

Automatic versus Nonautomatic

Contemporary feature-based views of automaticity define it as an umbrella term for a number of features, such as uncontrolled, unintentional, unconscious, efficient, and fast (Bargh, 1992; Moors & De Houwer, 2006a). These features roughly can be defined as follows. An *uncontrolled* process is one that is not influenced by a person's goals about the process. Goals about processes can be either of the promoting kind (e.g., the goal to engage in the process, which can be split into goals to start, continue, and complete the process) or of the counteracting kind (e.g., the goals to avoid, alter, or stop the process). A process is uncontrolled in the promoting sense when it is not caused by the goal to engage in it (or to start, continue, or complete it). Another word for uncontrolled in the promoting sense is *unintentional.* A process is uncontrolled in the counteracting sense when it is not counteracted (avoided, altered, or stopped) by the goal to do so (avoid, alter, or stop). A process is *unconscious* when the person has no awareness of it. I think awareness is possible for processes described at the functional level (i.e., the relation between input and output) but not likely for processes described at the algorithmic or hardware level (Moors & De Houwer, 2006a). People may be aware that they evaluate a person as good or bad, but they probably lack insight into the mechanisms, codes, and brain circuits involved. An *efficient* process is one that makes minimal use of attentional capacity. A *fast* process is one that is completed within a short time interval.

The definitions of automaticity features just given can be reformulated in terms of operating conditions (Bargh, 1992; Moors & De Houwer, 2007; Moors, Spruyt, & De Houwer, 2010). For example, a process is uncontrolled in the promoting sense (unintentional) when the goal to engage in it is not part (or only a redundant part) of the set of conditions that is sufficient for the process to operate. A process is uncontrolled in the counteracting sense when it operates regardless of the presence or absence of a counteracting goal within the set of conditions. A process is unconscious when it operates under the condition of a lack of awareness. A process is efficient when it operates under the condition of minimal available attentional capacity. A process is fast when it can be completed under the condition of minimal available time. In summary, a process is automatic when it operates under suboptimal conditions; a process is nonautomatic when it operates only under optimal conditions.

Logan (1988) proposed to replace feature-based definitions of automaticity with a mechanism-based definition. Specifically, he proposed to define automatic processes as ones that are based on single-step memory retrieval. Single-step memory retrieval is very much akin to what others have called an associative mechanism, that is, the activation of a memory trace leading to previously computed outputs. Such a definition of automaticity is obviously not successful in avoiding conceptual overlap with the associative versus rule-based dichotomy.

Associative versus Rule-Based

The associative versus rule-based dichotomy has a central role in research domains such as problem solving (Anderson, 2005; Mayer, 1992), categorization (Rouder & Ratcliff, 2006; Smith & Sloman, 1994), reasoning (Sloman, 1996), memory (Smith & DeCoster, 2000), and grammar learning (Reber, 1967). It refers to the mechanisms situated at the algorithmic level of analysis. A rule-based mechanism consists of the application of a rule to an input (or a representation of it). Computation of the rule produces an output. An associative mechanism consists of the activation of stored representations of similar past inputs. This activation, in turn, spreads to associated stored representations that determine the output. As an illustration from the domain of problem solving, consider the behavior of two persons paying 4 euros at the counter after having ordered two beers that cost 2 euros each. One person's behavior is caused by the calculation of the rule "$N \times M = 4$," in which N is the number of beers ordered and M is the price of one beer. The other person's behavior is caused by the activation of a memory that she paid 4 euros last time when she ordered the same. As an example from categorization, consider that dolphins are (correctly) categorized as mamals based on the rule that mamals nurse their offspring. Based on similarity with fish exemplars, they can also be (incorrectly) classified as fish. It may be noted that some researchers speak of the similarity-based mechanism instead of the associative mechanism, because the initial activation of stored representations is based on similarity (Hahn & Chater, 1998; Pothos, 2005).

To arrive ultimately at a way to diagnose processes as either rule-based or associative, the previous definitions need to be formalized. What is computation? And in what sense is it different from activation of stored knowledge?[2] I discuss several criteria that have been proposed as capturing the essence of the rule-based versus associative dichotomy. First, it has been suggested that rule-based mechanisms are ones that can be described by an if–then clause. For example, "if $N \times M = p$, then pay p euros." However, several authors have correctly noted that the associative mechanism can be described by an if–then clause as well. For example, "if two beers, then pay 4 euros." In fact, any mechanism that connects an input to an output can be expressed in an if–then format. The if-part specifies the input, and the then-part specifics the output. This has led some authors to conclude that associative and rule-based mechanisms are not qualitatively different, and that an associative mechanism is just a simple type of rule-based mechanism (Kruglanski, Erb, Pierro, Mannetti, & Chun, 2006). Other authors have searched for other criteria to distinguish both types of mechanisms.

A second criterion is that rule-based, but not associative, mechanisms can be described by *abstract* rules (e.g., Sloman, 1996; Smith, Langston, & Nisbett, 1992) in which the premise (the if-part) contains variables. Variables are abstract representations that can be instantiated with more than one constant. In the abstract rule of the beer example (if $N \times M$, then p), the variables N and M can be instantiated with an infinite range of numbers. By contrast, associations can be described with *nonabstract* rules, in which the premise consists of only constants. Constants are representations of concrete instances. The nonabstract rule of the beer example (if two beers, then 4 euros) cannot be applied to novel situations (e.g., ordering five coffees) unless they resemble the situation in the premise (e.g., ordering two soft drinks).

A third criterion is that rule-based mechanisms can operate only if there is a perfect match between the input and the premise, whereas associative mechanisms can also operate if there is a partial match between the input and the premise (or stored representation; Hahn & Chater, 1998). In the beer example, the abstract rule $N \times M$ cannot be computed unless values for N and M are available. The nonabstract rule to pay 4 euros when ordering two beers can be applied to any situation that is similar to this one (the more similarity, the stronger will be the activation of the memory trace). Because of the complementary forces of abstraction and partial matching, both rule-based and associative mechanisms can account for generalization toward new exemplars. Rule-based mechanisms can produce generalization by virtue of abstract variables; the associative mechanism can produce generalization by virtue of partial matching (partial matching compensates for the lack of variables). Nonabstract rules can thus be applied to new input, but only by virtue of similarity among the input and the constants specified in the premise.

A fourth criterion spelled out by some theorists is that rule-based mechanisms are ones that *follow* rules, whereas the associative mechanism merely *conforms* to rules. Rule *following* means that a mental rule sits between the input and the output of a process and causes the output; rule *conforming* means that the relation between input and output merely can be described or summarized according to a rule (Hahn & Chater, 1998; Pylyshyn, 1980; Searle, 1980; Sloman, 1996; Smith et al., 1992). Numerous phenomena can be described with rules without there being actual rule following. Examples are the planetary motions and the dances of honeybees. Planets and bees are unlikely to have internal representations of the rules that describe their behavior. Something similar is assumed to occur with the associative mechanism. However, unlike with planets or bees, associations are internal to the organism (mental) and they do mediate between input and output. Moreover, it has been argued that rules can be implemented by patterns of associations (like the ones proposed in connectionist models; Fodor & Phylyshyn, 1988), or that rules are approximations of such patterns (Smolensky, 1986). These views again suggest no fundamental distinction between associative and rule-based mechanisms: They are the same thing described on different levels of analysis.

A fifth criterion proposed by some theorists is that the rules in rule-based processes must be not only internally represented and causal but also symbolic (e.g., Hahn & Chater, 1998; Smith & DeCoster, 2000). A symbolic representation of a rule has the rule as its content or object (but see Searle, 1980). Because patterns of associations do not represent rules symbolically (they are subsymbolic representations of rules at best), activation of them does not count as rule-based processing. Other theorists (Clark, 1990; Fodor & Pylyshyn, 1988; Pinker & Prince, 1988; Smith et al., 1992) have argued against the view that the rules in rule-based processes must be symbolically represented. They allow rules to be hardwired in the system. Fodor and Pylyshyn (1988, p. 61) maintained that the only things that must be symbolically represented in a computational system are the data on which the rules operate. Patterns of associations are typically not built in but are shaped by the environment. Yet one may wonder why the distinction between innate and learned would be crucial in determining whether something counts as a real rule (i.e., a generator of rule-based processing). In summary, several criteria have been proposed to demarcate rule-based from associative mechanisms: abstract versus nonabstract, perfect versus partial matching of the premise, and rule following versus rule conforming. With regard to the latter criterion, some authors consider internal representations and causal influence as sufficient ingredients for rule following, whereas others also include the ingredient symbolic representation.

An alternative proposal is to define rule-based processes as ones that are conscious, or at least conscious during application (Cleeremans & Destrebecqz, 2004; Zhong, Dijksterhuis, & Galinsky, 2008). Given that consciousness is a feature of nonautomaticity, such a definition is not successful in avoiding overlap with the automatic–nonautomatic dichotomy. As such, it precludes empirical research concerned with whether rule-based mechanisms can be automatic (e.g., Hélie, Roeder, & Asch, 2010; Hélie, Waldschmidt, & Asch, 2010; Van Opstal, Gevers, Osman, & Verguts, 2010).

The next dichotomies to be discussed, perceptual versus conceptual and associative versus propositional, characterize the format of the representations or codes on which mechanisms operate. The terms *conceptual* and *propositional* indicate a resemblance, respectively, with words and sentences in natural language. The resemblance is not physical, but structural or functional (what can be done with it), and various bases for this resemblance have been highlighted.

Perceptual versus Conceptual

The dichotomy of perceptual versus conceptual codes is central in the domain of imagery and has often been referred to as picture-like versus verbal-like (Barsalou, 1999).[3] Conceptual codes are thought to be abstract[4] (e.g., the word *dog* applies to many instances of dogs), context-independent (e.g., the same code for *dog* is activated in all contexts), and amodal (i.e., the same code is activated by a picture of a dog, and the word *dog* in writing or pronounced out loud; Barsalou, 1999). Perceptual (or sensory) codes have perceptual (or sensory) features and are therefore concrete (e.g., an image of a dog cannot be applied to all dogs), context-dependent (e.g., a different *dog* code is activated in the context of a dark alley than in the context of a dog house), and modal (an image of a dog activates a code other than that produced by the word *dog* pronounced out loud). Some authors add motor features to these perceptual codes and call them *embodied* (Barsalou, 1999). Activation of embodied codes leads to partial reenactment or mental simulation of the perceptions and actions that typically occur in the presence of the represented object, which makes them dynamic. This is a further difference with conceptual codes, which are considered static.

Associative versus Propositional

Propositional codes are often said to be *compositional,* which means that they comprise meaningful parts that can be recombined with other parts to form new representations (i.e., productivity; Fodor & Phylyshyn, 1988).[5] In that sense, they are just like sentences in natural language, which also comprise words that can be recombined with other words to form different sentences. An organism that is capable of responding differently to the same stimulus in different contexts must have the capacity to form propositions in the sense that it can isolate parts and reuse them in new combinations.

In addition to being compositional, several authors have proposed that the content of propositional codes also must be truth evaluable (Anderson, 1978). Thus, in addition to comprising (recombinable) parts (e.g., cat–roof), propositional codes also must specify a relation between these parts that can be evaluated as true or false (e.g., the cat is on the roof). In order for a relation to be truth evaluable, it must have a certain quality. These so-called "qualified" relations (e.g., *A* is *B*, *A* is bigger than *B*, *A* is under *B*) are contrasted with unqualified relations, also termed (pure) associations, in which the nature of the relation between the parts is unspecified (e.g., *A*–*B*; De Houwer, Chapter 35, this volume). This aligns with the idea that to hold a proposition (e.g., "the apple is red") is not to hold a list of concepts (apple, is, and red) but to predicate something (redness) onto something (the apple; Soames, 2012). To sum up, *propositional codes* are defined here as complex representations that comprise a qualified relation between elementary representations. *Associations* are defined as complex representations that comprise unqualified relations between elementary representations.

Theorists in the domain of learning (e.g., Gawronski & Bodenhausen, 2011) have used the contrast between associations and propositions as the basis for distinguishing between two types of mechanisms: associative ones and propositional ones.[6] The *associative mechanism* is often defined as the activation of an association in memory, and the *propositional mechanism,* as the validation of a proposition, that is, the evaluation of it as true or false. It may be noted that these definitions comprise two parts: one part is a verb (activation, validation), and the other is a type of representation (association, proposition). Thus, in these definitions, mechanisms are partly defined in terms of formats of representations. Other authors (e.g., De Houwer, Chapter 35, this volume) also define the associative mechanism as the activation of an association, but the propositional mechanism as anything that happens (validation or activation) with a proposition. According to this view, the pure activation of a proposition is also called a *propositional mechanism.* Here too, mechanisms are defined in terms of formats of representations.

One might ask whether it is possible to avoid such overlap between mechanisms and representations. Can associative and propositional mechanisms be defined in such a way that they are allowed to operate on any type of representation? I think this is indeed possible for the associative mechanism but not for the propositional mechanism. The *associative mechanism* can be minimally defined as the activation of a representation in memory, without specifying the format of the representation that is activated. The *propositional mechanism,* on the other hand, if it is defined as validation or the evaluation of something as true or false, can only operate on representations that are truth evaluable. As discussed earlier, only propositions, defined as complex representations comprising a qualified relation between two elementary representations, can be evaluated as true or false. This is not possible for elementary representations (e.g., the concept *cat*), or for associations, defined as complex representations of unqualified relations between two elementary representations (e.g., cat–roof). This being said, some theorists (e.g., Gawronski & Bodenhausen, 2011) seem to suggest that associations give rise to the spontaneous formation of propositions, and that the latter can be validated. For instance, the association "banana–good" gives rise to the proposition "banana is good," which can be evaluated as true or false. But how does the organism know which quality to attribute to an unqualified relation? The banana–good example suggests that the organism follows a default rule, according to which associations suggest a positive or even identity relation (i.e., an "is a" relation). But such a default rule cannot be applied to the cat–roof example. A better solution might be to argue that associations tend to be interpreted in a way that is consistent with existing propositions. But even then, given that people may endorse multiple propositions about the same pair of concepts (the banana is good when I am in a fruit mood, otherwise it is bad; the cat may be under the roof), the question of which proposition is most likely to be chosen as a frame for a given association remains unanswered. In any case, the transition from associations to propositional codes is something that is left largely unspecified.

Theorists have defined the distinction between associative and propositional mechanisms not only in terms of types of representations but also in terms of features of nonautomaticity, in particular the feature *conscious* (e.g., De Houwer, Chapter 35, this volume; Mitchell, De Houwer, & Lovibond, 2009). For example, it has been proposed that the formation of a proposition must be conscious, or at least that the output of this formation process, the proposition itself, must be conscious at some point. In addition, it has been proposed that evaluation of the proposition as true (i.e., belief of the proposition) must be conscious at some point. These theorists accept that once a proposition is stored in memory,[7] it may be retrieved in an unconscious way, and that conscious and unconscious propositions may exert an unconscious (and otherwise automatic) influence on subsequent behavior and thought. Even so, the fact that consciousness of the proposition is put forward as a necessary element in the definition of the propositional mechanism creates overlap with the automatic–nonautomatic dichotomy. Such overlap can be avoided by adopting a minimal definition of the propositional mechanism as validation or truth evaluation irrespective of consciousness.

DIAGNOSIS

The conceptual exercise in the previous section shows that it is possible to define most dichotomies in nonoverlapping ways. A closer look at these nonoverlapping definitions reveals that several of them do not allow one to draw an all-or-none distinction between the two terms of a dichotomy. This has implications for the diagnosis of the mental processes underlying some performance as belonging to either term of a dichotomy.

Automatic versus Nonautomatic

In the former section I defined *automaticity* as an umbrella term for a collection of features. In addition, I favor a gradual approach to automaticity (Logan, 1985; Moors & De Houwer, 2006a; Shiffrin, 1988). This gradualness is manifested in two ways. First, I suggest that a process can be automatic with regard to some but not other features. For example, it seems that some processes are fast and efficient but can be counteracted (Uleman & Moskowitz, 1994). Second, each automaticity feature can itself be considered as gradual. A process more or less can be uncontrolled, unconscious, efficient and/or fast. Although I believe the gradual approach to automaticity is theoretically the most cautious approach, it does not provide an objective criterion for the diagnosis of a process as automatic or nonautomatic. This problem can be dealt with by specifying the sense in which (i.e., the feature according to which) one considers a process to be automatic or nonautomatic, and by making relative conclusions or choosing an intersubjective criterion (i.e., convention) for calling some process controlled or uncontrolled, conscious or unconscious, efficient or nonefficient, and fast or slow (Moors & De Houwer, 2006a).

Researchers have proposed to examine (1) the uncontrolled nature of a process by removing aspects of the procedure (e.g., instructions or other cues) that might induce a processing goal (to engage in or counteract a process), or by blocking implementation of such a goal (e.g., Klauer & Teige-Mocigemba, 2007; Moors, De Houwer, Hermans, & Eelen, 2005; Spruyt, De Houwer, & Hermans, 2009); (2) the unconscious nature of a process by presenting stimuli subliminally (Greenwald, Klinger, & Schuh, 1995); (3) the efficient nature of a process by increasing the load of a secondary task in dual-task studies (e.g., Hermans, Crombez, & Eelen, 2000); and (4) the fast nature of a process by using short stimulus onset asynchronies combined with short response deadlines (Draine & Greenwald, 1998; for a detailed review, see Moors, Spruyt, & De Houwer, 2010).

Associative versus Rule-Based

Assessment of rule-based mechanisms separate from or in addition to the associative mechanism also suffers from the problem that the criteria adduced to distinguish between the two mechanisms not always lead to unequivocal ways to diagnose performance as based on one or the other mechanism. First, as explained earlier, both rule-based and associative mechanisms are able to account for generalization toward new stimuli (abstract rules by virtue of variables, associations by virtue of partial matching).

Second, abstraction is a gradual notion (Hahn & Chater, 1998). The variables in abstract rules and the constants in nonabstract rules occupy two points on a continuum. Variables can be instantiated with a larger set of things than can constants, but the variables in abstract rules often cannot be instatiated by just anything (e.g., in the abstract rule, "if $N \times M = p$, then pay p euros," N and M must be instantiated by the number of beers ordered and the price of one beer, not by the number of words spoken and the color of the curtains). At the extreme abstract end of the continuum are logical rules in which the variables can be substituted by anything (e.g., if [X and Y], then X). Conversely, constants often hold some level of abstraction (e.g., in the nonabstract rule "if two beers, then pay 4 euros" the representation of two beers can itself be instantiated by more than two unique instances of beer). At the extreme nonabstract end of the continuum are constants that represent a unique instance. Given the relative nature of abstraction, no objective line can be drawn between variables and constants. This is reflected in the idea that activation of stored knowledge can be based on concrete as well as abstract similarities (e.g., similar function). Similarity even may pertain to abstract relations among variables (cf. Goldstone, 1994; Redington & Chater, 1996; Hummel & Holyoak, 2003). For instance, dolphins are perceptually similar to fish but they are similar to other mammals in the abstract sense that they nurse their offspring, and the latter type of similarity is indistinguishable from applying the rule that mammals are animals that nurse their offspring. Thus, evidence for generalization toward stimuli that share only abstract features with previously encountered ones (Reber, 1989; Marcus, Vijayan, Bandi Rao, & Vishton, 1999) is equally compatible with rule-based and with associative mechanisms (Redington & Chater, 1996; but see Sloman & Rips, 1998; Smith et al., 1992).

Third, advocates of the idea that rules in rule-based mechanisms must be symbolically represented have proposed to use verbal reports to investigate the content of representations. If a person has a symbolic representation of a rule, there is a possibility that he or she can verbally report the rule. Unfortunately, the criterion of verbal reportability is unsuitable for research concerned with automatic (in the sense of *unconscious*) rule-based processing. It is also not suited for studying nonsymbolic rules, such as subsymbolic patterns of associations or built-in rules.

The research literature contains several other proposals for how to register the operation of rule-based mechanisms independent of the operation of the associative mechanism, but none of the proposed methods seems unequivocal (cf. reviews by Hahn & Chater, 1998; Rouder & Ratcliff, 2006; Sloman, 1996; Smith et al., 1992). One option is to continue searching for a distinction between rule-based and assocative mechanisms that *does* lead to an undisputable empirical test. Another option is to abide by a gradual view of this distinction (e.g., Pothos, 2005) or to specify an intersubjective criterion (i.e., convention) for calling a mechanism rule-based or associative.

Perceptual versus Conceptual

Diagnosing representations as perceptual (picture-like, concrete, modal, dynamic) versus conceptual (verbal-like, abstract, amodal, static) has met with similar difficulties. Various authors (Anderson, 1978; McDowell, 1994; but see Dretske, 1981; Peacocke, 1992) have suggested that the two are informationally equivalent. Any detail of a picture-like representation can be described verbally. Furthermore, activation can spread from amodal and disembodied representations to the sensory and motor systems, and in this way account for modal and embodied effects (Garcia-Marques & Ferreira, 2011; Mahon & Caramazza, 2008). As emphasized by several authors (Anderson, 1978; De Houwer, 2011; Thomas, 1999), it is a fallacy to take the properties of effects as reflecting the properties of the underlying representations. Because of these considerations, it may be difficult, if not impossible, to distinguish empirically between perceptual and conceptual representations (Anderson, 1978; Barsalou, 1992; Garcia-Marques & Ferreira, 2011).

Associative versus Propositional

As argued earlier, it is possible and desirable to (conceptually) distinguish between codes and mechanisms. Propositional codes are different from the propositional mechanism that validates them, and associations are different from the associative mechanism that activates them, and that can also activate propositional codes. According to the definitions presented here, diagnosing whether propositional codes versus associations are involved requires determining whether the information involved is qualified versus unqualified. Diagnosing whether an associative or propositional mechanism is operating on a proposition requires determining whether the proposition was merely activated or also validated. An association can only be activated.

Associations versus Propositional Codes

Dual-process models based on the associative versus propositional dichotomy have assumptions about not only the deployment of associations versus propositional codes but also their formation (cf. Note 6). Associations form gradually by repeated presentation of two elements paired in time and space, whereas propositional codes can form after a single verbal instruction containing the proposition (e.g., Gawronski & Bodenhausen, 2006, 2011; Rydell & McConnell, 2006; Sternberg & McClelland, 2012). To examine associations versus propositional codes, researchers have tried to install them by manipulating the information provided to the participants (two elements related in time and space vs. bound up in a qualified relation) and the way in which the information is presented (repeated pairings vs. a single verbal instruction). There is an important caveat, however. Associations can lead to the spontaneous formation of propositions (cf. supra). For instance, the association banana–good can give rise to the proposition "the banana is good" or even "the banana has a temporospatial relation with good." Propositions, from their part, can also lead to the formation of associations. A qualified relation can be stored partially, without the quality of the relation. Moreover, propositions that were entirely stored can be retrieved partially, leaving the quality of the relation unretrieved (De Houwer, Chapter 35, this volume). These considerations cast doubt on the methods of repeated pairings versus verbally instructing propositions as reliable methods for installing associations versus propositional codes.

Associative versus Propositional Mechanisms

Several researchers (e.g., Gawronski & Bodenhausen, 2006; Rydell & McConnell, 2006; Strack & Deutsch, 2004; Wilson, Lindsey, & Schooler, 2000) have proposed diagnosing the propositional mechanism with direct subjective (i.e., self-report) measures, and the associative mechanism with indirect objective measures such as stimulus–response compatibility (SRC) tasks (e.g., priming task: Fazio, Jackson, Dunton, & Williams, 1995; Implicit Association Test [IAT]: Greenwald, McGhee, & Schwartz, 1998). For instance, the validation of the proposition "the banana is good" can be measured by asking a participant to rate the goodness of the banana on a scale. Activation of the association "banana–good" can be measured by administering a priming task in which it is verified whether *banana* as a prime facilitates responding to positive rather than negative target stimuli. The proposal to measure *propositional mechanisms* (defined here as the validation of a proposition) with self-report is based on the idea that people only report that something is good when they have evaluated this proposition as true. This assumption could be questioned, however. Participants can fill out questionnaires in a mindless manner, that is, without validation or assent, or they may lie. Adding a confidence measure might reduce mindless responding but not lying. The proposal to measure the *associative mechanism* (minimally defined here as the activation of any type of representation) with SRC tasks is based on the assumption that effects on these tasks circumvent validation. This assumption has been challenged by a study of Peters and Gawronski (2001) in which validation information influenced both self-reports and outcomes of indirect measures (the affect misattribution task and the evaluative priming task) and research showing that effects on the IAT can be faked (e.g., De Houwer, Beckers, & Moors, 2007; Steffens, 2004). The mapping of processes onto measurement procedures or outcomes can be considered a different kind of mapping problem, one that should also receive independent empirical testing. As various authors have argued, however, measurement procedures are rarely process pure, and it is therefore problematic to use a measurement outcome as a proxy for a mental process (e.g., De Houwer, Gawronski, & Barnes-Holmes, in press; De Houwer, Teige-Mocigemba, Spruyt, & Moors, 2009; Gawronski, Deutsch, LeBel, & Peters, 2008; Jacoby, 1991; Sherman, 2006).

The use of self-report methods versus SRC tasks for diagnosing propositional versus associative mechanisms is further inspired by the mapping of this dichotomy on the nonautomatic versus automatic dichotomy, as well as the assumption that self-report methods versus SRC tasks uniquely and confidently measure nonautomatic versus automatic processes. Researchers have argued that this assumption, rather than being taken for granted, should be submitted to empirical testing (De Houwer, 2006; De Houwer & Moors, 2007). In addition, as already mentioned, the mapping of dichotomies (propositional vs. associative mechanism onto nonautomatic vs. automatic) does not fit in my plan to avoid overlap between dichotomies.

CONCLUSION

As dual (and multi) process models divide the realm of mental processes, they tend to assume conceptual and/or actual overlap among dichotomies. I argued that such assumptions of overlap may be premature. In fact, they should be investigated empirically. As a preparation to such empirical research, I first examined whether dichotomies can be defined independent of each other and concluded that this is indeed possible for most dichotomies. I then considered whether the definitions resulting from this exercise allow researchers to distinguish empirically between the two terms in each dichotomy. In this respect, I pointed out the difficulty in finding unequivocal empirical criteria to classify processes as automatic versus nonautomatic, associative versus rule-based, associative versus propositional, and as operating on perceptual versus conceptual codes and associations versus propositional codes.

In particular, the gradual views proposed for the dichotomy of automatic versus nonautomatic (Moors & De Houwer, 2006a; Shiffrin, 1988) and associative versus rule-based (Pothos, 2005) obstructs the creation of sharply delineated sets. This is not problematic for research concerned with automaticity and mechanisms as such; it remains valuable to examine the degree to which a process is rule-based, and the degree to which it possesses individual features of automaticity. But it is problematic for dual-process models that rely on a sharp, principled, distinction between sets of automatic and sets of nonautomatic processes and between sets of associative and sets of rule-based processes (cf. Moors & De Houwer, 2006b).

One solution might be to revert to a reformulation of dual-process models in gradual terms, including their assumptions of overlap among dichotomies. For instance, a dual-process model might distinguish between more associative versus more rule-based processes (e.g., defined as more concrete vs. more abstract) and might assume that more associative processes are more automatic than more rule-based ones. The latter assumption could be put to an empirical test. One could, for instance, examine whether a process applied to a set of stimuli generalizes to untrained stimuli that are similar in a more or less abstract sense, and whether this generalization takes place under less or more optimal conditions (e.g., Van Opstal et al., 2010).

Not all dichotomies seem amenable to a gradual definition, however. The dichotomy of associations versus propositional codes seems to be of a matter of all or nothing: A relation is either qualified or unqualified. Once a relation is *somewhat* qualified, it is already qualified. The same can be said of the dichotomy of associative versus propositional mechanisms: A person either does or does not evaluate a proposition as true or false. On closer scrutiny, however, it may not be mandatory to consider truth ascription as a discrete mental act. As Hume (1739–1740, Part 3, Book 1) suggested, people do not decide about the truth of a statement; a statement imposes itself as more or less true, based on features such as salience and the degree of coherence with other propositions (cf. Gawronski & Bodenhausen, 2011). Or consider the scenario that the truth value of a proposition is stored together with the proposition and is activated to varying degrees (Petty et al., 2007). Such a scenario depicts the dichotomy of associative versus propositional mechanisms as gradual. Thus, one could investigate whether propositions that receive a higher truth value operate under more or less optimal conditions than propositions that receive a lower truth value. The dichotomy of perceptual versus conceptual also can be framed in categorical terms (when the features modal–amodal, and embodied–disembodied are emphasized), as well as gradual terms (when the features abstraction and context dependence are emphasized). It may be noted that dual-process models relying on a gradual definition of mechanisms actually are unimodels, unless they also rely on other distinctions (e.g., associations vs. propositional codes) that are of a categorical nature.

A related solution for dichotomies that are of a gradual nature is to install intersubjective dividing lines between the two terms of the dichotomy. Rather than calling a process more or less automatic, more or less rule-based, or more or less propositional, the community of researchers may come to an agreement about a set of operational criteria that determines when they consider a process as automatic, rule-based, or propositional.[8]

Dichotomies that resist a gradual definition (associations vs. propositional codes) or that researchers do not accept as being gradual (e.g., some researchers insist on a categorical distinction between associative and rule-based mechanisms) may not escape a gradual treatment. A dichotomy may be categorical on a conceptual level, but conclusions about the presence of the terms often can be only gradual: One often cannot identify with certainty which code or mechanism is at stake, at least not with behavioral methods (although I do not exclude that corroborating evidence can be obtained with neurophysiological methods). To conclude, the fate of dual-process models may be gradual and/or a matter of convention.

ACKNOWLEDGMENTS

Preparation of this chapter was supported by Ghent University Methusalem Grant No. BOF09/01M00209.

NOTES

1. Full-blown dual-systems models assume not only that various dichotomies map onto each other but also that the two systems thus created are isolatable (i.e., that each system can operate without the other; Keren & Schul, 2009). In addition, systems often comprise several correlated processes (e.g., the slow vs. fast learning systems each comprise processes for learning and deployment).
2. Rule-based mechanisms often operate on stored representations that themselves are activated with the associative mechanism (although they may also operate on newly formed ones). So the associative mechanism is often embedded in the rule-based mechanism (e.g., Smith & DeCoster, 2000).
3. The dichotomy of perceptual versus conceptual *codes* discussed here differs from the dichotomy of perceptual versus conceptual *processing* in the memory literature, which refers to encoding and retrieval of semantic versus physical information (e.g., Weldon, Roediger, Beitel, & Johnston, 1995). The former dichotomy is situated at the algorithmic level, the latter at the functional level.
4. At first sight, the abstract nature of propositional codes evoked in this definition overlaps with the abstract nature of rule-based mechanisms in one of the definitions discussed earlier. On second thought, however, abstract rules contain variables that can be instantiated with both concrete and abstract codes.

5. It may be noted that if formats of representations are defined in terms of aspects of their content, then the previously drawn distinction between formats and contents of representations is somewhat blurred.
6. It is important to keep in mind the distinctions between mechanisms involved in learning or encoding (i.e., the formation of propositions and associations) and mechanisms involved in deployment. Here I discuss the mechanisms involved in deployment.
7. An issue of debate is whether in addition to the content of the proposition, the person's evaluation of the proposition as true is itself stored in memory (e.g., Petty, Briñol, & DeMarree, 2007) or not (e.g., Gawronski & Bodenhausen, 2007).
8. This is already the case in some research domains. For instance, in search tasks, a process is called efficient if slope ß of the linear function $y = ßx + \alpha$ (where y is the reaction time, x is the set size, and α is a constant) is smaller than 10 milliseconds (Hansen & Hansen, 1988).

REFERENCES

Anderson, J. R. (1978). Arguments concerning representations for mental imagery. *Psychological Review, 85*, 249–277.

Anderson, J. R. (1987). Methodologies for studying human knowledge. *Behavioral and Brain Sciences, 10*, 467–505.

Anderson, J. R. (2005). *Cognitive psychology and its implications* (6th ed.). New York: Worth.

Bargh, J. A. (1992). The ecology of automaticity. Toward establishing the conditions needed to produce automatic processing effects. *American Journal of Psychology, 105*, 181–199.

Barsalou, L. W. (1990). On the indistinguishability of exemplar memory and abstraction in category representation. In T. K. Wyer & S. R. Srull (Eds.), *Advances in social cognition III: Content and process specificity in the effects of prior experiences* (pp. 61–88). Hillsdale, NJ: Erlbaum.

Barsalou, L. W. (1999). Perceptual symbol systems. *Behavioral and Brain Sciences, 22*, 577–660.

Chaiken, S., Liberman, A., & Eagly, A. H. (1989). Heuristic and systematic information processing within and beyond the persuasion context. In J. S. Uleman & J. A. Bargh (Eds.), *Unintended thought* (pp. 212–252). New York: Guilford Press.

Clark, A. (1990). Connectionism, competence, and explanation. *British Journal for the Philosophy of Science, 41*, 195–222.

Cleeremans, A., & Destrebecqz, A. (2004). Real rules are conscious. *Behavioral and Brain Sciences, 28*, 19–20.

Conrey, F. R., Sherman, J. W., Gawronski, B., Hugenberg, K., & Groom, C. (2005). Separating multiple processes in implicit social cognition: The quad model of implicit task performance. *Journal of Personality and Social Psychology, 89*, 469–487.

De Houwer, J. (2006). What are implicit measures and why are we using them? In R. W. Wiers & A. W. Stacy (Eds.), *The handbook of implicit cognition and addiction* (pp. 11–28). Thousand Oaks, CA: Sage.

De Houwer, J. (2011). Why the cognitive approach in psychology would profit from a functional approach and vice versa. *Perspectives on Psychological Science, 6*, 202–209.

De Houwer, J., Beckers, T., & Moors, A. (2007). Novel attitudes can be faked on the Implicit Association Test. *Journal of Experimental Social Psychology, 43*, 972–978.

De Houwer, J., Gawronski, B., & Barnes-Holmes, D. (in press). A functional-cognitive framework for attitude research. *European Review of Social Psychology.*

De Houwer, J., & Moors, A. (2007). How to define and examine the implicitness of implicit measures. In B. Wittenbrink & N. Schwarz (Eds.), Implicit measures of attitudes: Procedures and controversies (pp. 179–194). New York: Guilford Press.

De Houwer, J., Teige-Mocigemba, S., Spruyt, A., & Moors, A. (2009). Implicit measures: A normative analysis and review. *Psychological Bulletin, 135*, 347–368.

Deutsch, R., & Strack, F. (2006). Duality-models in social psychology: From opposing processes to interacting systems. *Psychological Inquiry, 17*, 166–172.

Draine, S. C., & Greenwald, A. G. (1998). Replicable unconscious semantic priming. *Journal of Experimental Psychology: General, 127*, 286–303.

Dretske, F. (1981). *Knowledge and the flow of information.* Cambridge, MA: MIT Press.

Fazio, R. H., Jackson, J. R., Dunton, B. C., & Williams, C. J. (1995). Variability in automatic activation as an unobtrusive measure of racial attitudes: A bona fide pipeline? *Journal of Personality and Social Psychology, 69,* 1013–1027.

Fodor, J. A., & Pylyshyn, Z. (1988). Connectionism and cognitive architecture: A critical analysis. *Cognition, 28,* 3–71.

Garcia-Marques, L., & Ferreira, M. B. (2011). Friends and foes of theory construction in psychological science: Vague dichotomies, unified theories of cognition, and the next experimentalism. *Perspectives on Psychological Science, 6,* 192–201.

Gawronski, B., & Bodenhausen, G. V. (2006). Associative and propositional processes in evaluation: An integrative review of implicit and explicit attitude change. *Psychological Bulletin, 132,* 692–731.

Gawronski, B., & Bodenhausen, G. V. (2007). Unraveling the processes underlying evaluation: Attitudes from the perspective of the APE Model. *Social Cognition, 25,* 687–717.

Gawronski, B., & Bodenhausen, G. V. (2011). The associative–propositional evaluation model: Theory, evidence, and open questions. In (J. M. Olson & M. P. Zanna (Eds.), *Advances in experimental social psychology* (Vol. 44, pp. 59–127). Amsterdam: Elsevier.

Gawronski, B., Deutsch, R., LeBel, E. P., & Peters, K. R. (2008). Response interference as a mechanism underlying implicit measures: Some traps and gaps in the assessment of mental associations with experimental paradigms. *European Journal of Psychological Assessment, 24,* 218–225.

Goldstone, R. L. (1994). The role of similarity in categorization—Providing a groundwork. *Cognition, 52,* 125–157.

Green, O. H. (1992). *The emotions: A philosophical theory.* Dordrecht: Kluwer.

Greenwald, A. G., Klinger, M. R., & Schuh, E. S. (1995). Activation by marginally perceptible ("subliminal") stimuli: Dissociation of unconscious from conscious cognition. *Journal of Experimental Psychology: General, 124,* 22–42.

Greenwald, A. G., McGhee, D. E., & Schwartz, J. L. K. (1998). Measuring individual differences in implicit cognition: The Implicit Association Test. *Journal of Personality and Social Psychology, 74,* 1464–1480.

Hahn, U., & Chater, N. (1998). Similarity and rules: Distinct? Exhaustive? Empirically distinguishable? *Cognition, 65,* 197–230.

Hansen, C. H., & Hansen, R. D. (1988). Finding the face in the crowd: An anger superiority effect. *Journal of Personality and Social Psychology, 54,* 917–924.

Hélie, S., Roeder, J. L., & Ash, F. G. (2010). Evidence for cortical automaticity in rule-based categorization. *Journal of Neuroscience, 30,* 14225–14234.

Hélie, S., Waldschmidt, J. G., & Ash, F. G. (2010). Automaticity in rule-based and information-integration categorization. *Attention, Perception, and Psychophysics, 72,* 1013–1031.

Hermans, D., Crombez, G., & Eelen, P. (2000). Automatic attitude activation and efficiency: The fourth horseman of automaticity. *Psychologica Belgica, 40,* 3–22.

Hume, D. (1739–1740). *A treatise of human nature.* London, UK: John Noon.

Hummel, J. E., & Holyoak, K. J. (2003). A symbolic-connectionist theory of relational inference and generalization. *Psychological Review, 110,* 220–264.

Jacoby, L. L. (1991). A process dissociation framework: Separating automatic from intentional uses of memory. *Journal of Memory and Language, 30,* 513–541.

Keren, G., & Schul, Y. (2009). Two is not always better than one: A critical evaluation of two-system theories. *Perspectives on Psychological Science, 4,* 533–550.

Klauer, K. C., & Teige-Mocigemba, S. (2007). Controllability and resource dependence in automatic evaluation. *Journal of Experimental Social Psychology, 43,* 648–655.

Kruglanski, A. W., Erb, H.-P., Pierro, A., Mannetti, L., & Chung, W. Y. (2006). On parametric continuities in the world of binary either ors. *Psychological Inquiry, 17,* 53–165.

Leventhal, H., & Scherer, K. R. (1987). The relationship of emotion to cognition: A functional approach to a semantic controversy. *Cognition and Emotion, 1,* 3–28.

Lieberman, M. D. (2003). Reflective and reflexive judgment processes: A social cognitive neuroscience approach. In J. P. Forgas, K. R. Williams, & W. von Hippel (Eds.), *Social judgments: Implicit and explicit processes* (pp. 44–67). New York: Cambridge University Press.

Logan, G. D. (1985). Skill and automaticity: Relations, implications, and future directions. *Canadian Journal of Psychology, 39,* 367–386.

Logan, G. D. (1988). Toward an instance theory of automatization. *Psychological Review, 95,* 492–527.

Mahon, B. Z., & Caramazza, A. (2008). A critical look at the Embodied Cognition Hypothesis and a new proposal for grounding conceptual content. *Journal of Physiology—Paris, 102*, 59–70.

Marcus, G. F., Vijayan, S., Bandi Rao, S., & Vishton, P. M. (1999). Rule learning by seven-month-old infants. *Science, 283*, 77–80.

Marr, D. (1982). Vision: The philosophy and the approach. In *Vision: A computational investigation into the human representation and processing of visual information* (pp. 103–126). New York: Freeman.

Mayer, R. E. (1992). *Thinking, problem solving, cognition*. New York: Freeman.

McDowell, J. (1994). *Mind and world*. Cambridge, MA: Harvard University Press.

Mitchell, C. J., De Houwer, J., & Lovibond, P. F. (2009). The propositional nature of human associative learning. *Behavioral and Brain Sciences, 32*, 183–198.

Moors, A., & De Houwer, J. (2006a). Automaticity: A theoretical and conceptual analysis. *Psychological Bulletin, 132*, 297–326.

Moors, A., & De Houwer, J. (2006b). Problems with dividing the realm of cognitive processes. *Psychological Inquiry, 17*, 199–204.

Moors, A., & De Houwer, J. (2007). What is automaticity?: An analysis of its component features and their interrelations. In J. A. Bargh (Ed.), *Social psychology and the unconscious: The automaticity of higher mental processes* (pp. 11–50). New York: Psychology Press.

Moors, A., De Houwer, J., Hermans, D., & Eelen, P. (2005). Unintentional processing of motivational valence. *Quarterly Journal of Experimental Psychology: A, 58*, 1043–1063.

Moors, A., Spruyt, A., & De Houwer, J. (2010). In search of a measure that qualifies as implicit: Recommendations based on a decompositional view of automaticity. In B. Gawronski & K. B. Payne (Eds.), *Handbook of implicit social cognition: Measurement, theory, and application* (pp. 19–37). New York: Guilford Press.

Peacocke, C. (1992). *A study of concepts*. Cambridge, MA: MIT Press.

Peters, K. R., & Gawronski, B. (2011). Are we puppets on a string?: Comparing the impact of contingency and validity on implicit and explicit evaluations. *Personality and Social Psychology Bulletin, 37*, 557–569.

Petty, R. E., Briñol, P., & DeMarree, K. G. (2007). The meta-cognitive model (MCM) of attitudes: Implications for attitude measurement, change, and strength. *Social Cognition, 25*, 657–686.

Pinker, S., & Prince, A. (1988). On language and connectionism: Analysis of a parallel distributed processing model of language acquisition. *Cognition, 28*, 73–193.

Pothos, E. M. (2005). The rules versus similarity distinction. *Behavioral and Brain Sciences, 28*, 1–14.

Pylyshyn, Z. W. (1980). Computation and cognition: Issues in the foundations of cognitive science. *Behavioral and Brain Sciences, 3*, 111–132.

Reber, A. S. (1967). Implicit learning of artificial grammars. *Journal of Verbal Learning and Verbal Behavior, 6*, 855–863.

Reber, A. S. (1989). Implicit learning and tacit knowledge. *Journal of Experimental Psychology: General, 125*, 123–138.

Redington, M., & Chater, N. (1996). Transfer in artificial grammar learning: a re-evaluation. *Journal of Experimental Psychology: General, 125*, 123–138.

Rouder, J. N., & Ratcliff, R. (2006). Comparing exemplar- and rule-based theories of categorization. *Current Directions in Psychological Science, 15*, 9–13.

Rydell, R. J., & McConnell, A. R. (2006). Understanding implicit and explicit attitude change: A systems of reasoning analysis. *Journal of Personality and Social Psychology, 91*, 995–1008.

Searle, J. R. (1980). Minds, brains, and programs. *Behavioral and Brain Sciences, 3*, 93–94.

Sherman, J. W. (2006). On building a better process model: It's not only how many, but which ones and by which means? *Psychological Inquiry, 3*, 173–184.

Shiffrin, R. M. (1988). Attention. In R. C. Atkinson, R. J. Hernstein, G. Lindzey, & R. D. Luce (Eds.), *Stevens' handbook of experimental psychology* (Vol. 2, pp. 739–811). New York: Wiley.

Sloman, S. A. (1996). The empirical case for two systems of reasoning. *Psychological Bulletin, 119*, 3–22.

Sloman, S. A., & Rips, L. J. (1998). Similarity as an explanatory construct. *Cognition, 65*, 87–101.

Smedslund, J. (1992). Are Frijda's laws of emotion empirical? *Cognition and Emotion, 6*, 435–456.

Smith, E. E., Langston, C., & Nisbett, R. (1992). The case for rules in reasoning. *Cognitive Science, 16*, 1–40.

Smith, E. E., & Sloman, S. A. (1994). Similarity

versus rule-based categorization. *Memory and Cognition, 22,* 377–386.

Smith, E. R., & DeCoster, J. (2000). Dual-process models in social and cognitive psychology: Conceptual integration and links to underlying memory systems. *Personality and Social Psychology Review, 4,* 108–131.

Smolensky, P. (1986). Information processing in dynamical systems: Foundations of harmony theory. In D. E. Rumelhart, J. L. McClelland, & the PDP Research Group (Eds.), *Parallel distributed processing: Explorations in the microstructure of cognition. Vol. 2, Psychological and biological models* (pp. 194–281). Cambridge, MA: The MIT Press.

Soames, S. (2012). Propositions. In D. Graff Fara & G. Russell (Eds.), *The Routledge companion to the philosophy of language* (pp. 209–220). Abingdon, UK: Routledge.

Spruyt, A., De Houwer, J., & Hermans, D. (2009). Modulation of semantic priming by feature-specific attention allocation. *Journal of Memory and Language, 61,* 37–54.

Steffens, M. (2004). Is the Implicit Association Test immune to faking? *Experimental Psychology, 51,* 165–179.

Sternberg, D. A., & McClelland, J. L. (2012). Two mechanisms of human contingency learning. *Psychological Science, 23,* 59–68.

Strack, F., & Deutsch, R. (2004). Reflective and impulsive determinants of human behavior. *Personality and Social Psychology Review, 8,* 220–247.

Thomas, N. J. T. (1999). Are theories of imagery theories of imagination?: An active perception approach to conscious mental content. *Cognitive Science, 23,* 207–245.

Uleman, J. S., & Moskowitz, G. B. (1994). Unintended effects of goals on unintended inferences. *Journal of Personality and Social Psychology, 66,* 490–501.

Van Opstal, F., Gevers, W., Osman, M., & Verguts, T. (2010). Unconscious task application. *Consciousness and Cognition 19,* 999–1006.

Weldon, M. S., Roediger, H. L., Beitel, D. A., & Johnston, T. R. (1995). Perceptual and conceptual processes in implicit and explicit tests with picture fragment and word fragment cues. *Journal of Memory and Language, 34,* 268–285.

Wilson, T. D., Lindsey, S., & Schooler, T. Y. (2000). A model of dual attitudes. *Psychological Review, 107,* 101–126.

Zhong, C.-B., Dijksterhuis, A., & Galinsky, A. D. (2008). The merits of unconscious thought in creativity. *Psychological Science, 19,* 912–918.

CHAPTER 3

Conscious and Unconscious

Toward an Integrative Understanding of Human Mental Life and Action

Roy F. Baumeister and John A. Bargh

Human consciousness is one of the wonders of the world. It integrates sensation, perception, emotion, and interpretation, often understanding events in sequences that include causal analyses and extended narrative structures. How inert bits of lifeless physical matter, such as protons, neutrons, and electrons, combine and organize so as to make conscious experience possible remains one of the most unassailable mysteries in the scientific understanding of the universe. Yet consciousness itself is, of course, no mystery for the billions of human beings who have and use it all day, every day.

We, the authors of this chapter, have found ourselves on opposite sides of debates about several important questions, including the efficacy of conscious thought and the scientific viability of free will. Still, we have followed each other's work over the years with interest, respect, and admiration, and this has enabled our programs of research to benefit and to be informed by each other's work. Moreover, we actually agree on far more than our periodic debates might suggest. Our purpose in this chapter is to explore and elucidate these areas of agreement.

POSSIBLE ROLES OF CONSCIOUSNESS

The relation of conscious thoughts to behavior has been depicted in multiple ways, running the full spectrum from complete control to complete irrelevance. Here we briefly delineate the range of possible views.

At one extreme is the commonsense impression that consciousness is in full control of behavior. People know they are conscious. They experience their actions as stemming from conscious choices. Almost by definition, they are unaware of unconscious influences on their behavior. (To borrow a metaphor from Jaynes, 1976, a flashlight in a dark room would mistakenly conclude that all the lights are on, because whichever way it turns to look, everything is illuminated!)

Concerning definitions, *conscious* and *unconscious processes* have been distinguished historically in terms of several different features (e.g., Bargh, 1994)—awareness, intentionality, efficiency, and controllability, with the former two at the heart of the terms in common usage. However, because of mounting evidence that motivations and goal pursuits (roughly speaking, intentionality) operate unconsciously in much the same way as they operate consciously (e.g., Marien, Custers, Hassin, & Aarts, 2012; McCulloch, Ferguson, Kawada, & Bargh, 2008), the intentionality (purposive, goal-oriented) quality no longer differentiates conscious and unconscious processes. Thus, it is the awareness and reportability of a mental process that most clearly distinguish between what is considered a conscious versus an unconscious mental process or experience. Indeed, the most recent distinctions between conscious and unconscious processes have focused exclusively on the various forms of awareness people have about their mental content (Schooler, Mrazek, Baird, & Winkielman, in press).

The view that consciousness enjoys full control over behavior has mainly intuitive appeal these days. Few serious researchers endorse it, because the case for unconscious causation of behavior is overwhelming. Years ago, Freud (1933/1965) made a persuasive and extensive argument for the position that people are not fully aware of many causes of their behavior, including ones originating in their own unconscious mind. Modern social psychology has repeatedly shown that people are not aware of many situational cues and stimuli that can influence behavior. Nisbett and Wilson (1977) showed that introspection is often unable to furnish accurate accounts of the causation of behavior. Wegner (2002) showed that people's subjective experiences of initiating and controlling behavior can be mistaken in both directions; that is, sometimes people believe they have done something when they have not, and sometimes they believe they have not done something when they have. And, of course, one of us has devoted much of his career to demonstrating a great many ways in which situations cause behavior by means of unconscious, automatic processes, thus bypassing or circumventing any conscious control (Bargh, 1994, 1997, 2005).

A watered-down version of the theory of full conscious control holds that people are at least conscious of what they are doing, and that unconscious processes influence behavior by way of influencing conscious thoughts.

Opposite to the theory of full conscious control is the view that conscious processes have effectively zero impact on actual behavior. The view that consciousness is an *epiphenomenon,* which is to say a side effect of other processes and itself does not have true causal impact, has a long history. Thomas Huxley (1874) articulated the so-called "steam whistle hypothesis" that compared consciousness to the steam whistle on a train locomotive. The steam whistle's activity is caused by what is happening in the engine and may also reveal something about the inner state of the engine, but it does not move or steer the train. By analogy, consciousness may be a rich subjective experience of one's own life that derives from unconscious processes and reveals something about these inner states, but it does not have any influence on behavior.

More recent writers have continued to question the efficacy of conscious thoughts. Wegner (2002) wrote of the "illusion of conscious will," proposing that people's subjective awareness of deciding, controlling, and initiating actions is liberally subject to distortion and error. Dijksterhuis and Nordgren (2006) proposed that unconscious thought is generally superior to conscious thought, and although they conceded that conscious thinking can sometimes cause behavior, its effects are not very helpful, and people would be well advised to minimize its influence. Wilson (2002) likewise provided evidence of the fallibility of conscious thinking and recommended that people rely on unconscious processes rather than conscious ones (see also Gladwell, 2004).

In between the two extremes of seeing behavior as mainly conscious versus mainly unconscious, there are emerging new models that seek to regard conscious and unconscious processes as complementary instead of competing systems. One approach would accept that conscious thoughts are highly influential in guiding behavior, but that unconscious and automatic processes can have considerable influence by means of shaping the content of consciousness. This position is amenable to the commonsense view that conscious thoughts are ultimately in charge of action, but it assigns an important role to unconscious processes as providing support and input.

The other compromise view, which both of us currently advocate, is that behavior is normally carried out by unconscious, automatic processes, while consciousness can occasionally intervene to override, regulate, redirect, and otherwise alter the stream of behavior—often at a distance, with unconscious processes filling in. As Baumeister and Masicampo (2010) proposed, the idea that consciousness plays a supporting (but nonetheless powerful) role in human functioning has lacked traditional advocacy, intuitive appeal, and other advantages of the rival theoretical views, but it may provide the best fit to the currently available evidence. In the next section we spell out this view.

CONSCIOUSNESS AS NAVIGATIONAL SYSTEM

In the 1990s, the two of us engaged in a public exchange of views that we have come to remember as "the steering wheel debate." At this time Bargh, emboldened by early findings to move into what he later characterized as his "feisty period" (e.g., 1997), had shrugged off his initial, cautious view (e.g., 1989) that all effects of automatic and unconscious processes depended on influencing conscious processes in order to reach behavior. He began to speculate that the majority of behavior, and perhaps close to all of it, was the produce of unconscious processes rather than conscious ones.

At the same time, Baumeister had been emboldened in a different direction by his first findings about the importance of conscious control in self-regulation. Although his thinking about conscious control was in a sense the opposite of Bargh's thinking on automatic, unconscious control, both were largely in sympathy with the view that the majority of causes of behavior are in the latter category. Baumeister and Sommer (1997) proposed, however, that even if conscious control were directly responsible for only 5% of behavior, that 5% could make all the difference in long-term behavioral outcomes. By analogy, they suggested that although cars may be driven straight ahead 95% of the time, the 5% of the time that the steering wheel is used to change directions is inordinately important in enabling the car to reach the driver's preferred destination.

Contemplating the importance of a steering wheel dodges a couple of vital questions, including the extent to which conscious processes are themselves the product of unconscious ones. We find it hard to imagine where conscious thought could come from if not from unconscious processes (see Morsella & Bargh, 2010). For example, a person may read a poem or story and be transported into vividly imagined, emotionally rich responses. In order for these to happen, however, the unconscious must accomplish considerable work, including the transformation of the visual stimuli into meaningful words, the evocation of associated knowledge, and initiation of evaluative, emotional responses, perhaps complete with bodily arousal.

To revisit the car metaphor, therefore, we can ask what is the appropriate metaphor for conscious thoughts. The full conscious control metaphor would suggest that consciousness is the car's driver, who works the controls so as to direct the car toward his or her intended destination. The steam whistle view would depict consciousness as a passenger, perhaps in the back seat. The passenger may have a rich subjective experience of the journey but is simply seeing what happens, without having any influence on where the car goes.

In that context, our preferred metaphor would be that consciousness is akin to a fancy navigational system. Unconscious processes mostly drive the car, but occasionally they do not know how to get where they want to go, so they consult the navigational system, which can perform calculations that the driver cannot (see Bongers & Dijksterhuis, 2009). The driver is thus better off, and more likely to reach the destination, because of having used the navigational system, although the navigational system does not directly move or steer the car. Its influence is purely advisory—but quite adaptive and valuable.

In that view, consciousness is not needed for perceiving and understanding the immediate environment, nor is it responsible for the direct execution of action. But (among other things) consciousness can mentally simulate various possible courses of action and their likely, anticipated consequences. The unconscious can use these simulations in deciding what to do and in carrying out these plans for action. The result may well be superior outcomes that are more adaptive and successful than what would have happened had the person simply responded unconsciously to the situation, without consciously imagining various courses of action.

HOW DOES BEHAVIOR ORIGINATE?

The question of how behavior starts has been a perennial bugaboo for action theory (see Morsella, 2009). Most theorists today accept that cognitions can cause behavior, but many cognitions occur without initiating any behavior, so the step from thinking to doing remains difficult to explain. (And thoughts, too, may be merely an intermediate step between the original causes and behavior.)

The approach emphasized by Bargh and his colleagues has been to see the origins of behavior as they occur in the social situation. External cues may activate automatic, often unconscious processes that produce behavioral responses, for example, in the automatic tendency to mimic or imitate what others in that situation are currently doing (Chartrand & Bargh, 1999). Conscious thoughts may be entirely irrelevant, or they may possibly play a mediating role. This view gets past the problem of how to leap from cognition to behavior, because the cognitions are mainly active in mediating between stimulus and response. The stimulus–response (S-R) link remains paramount, although the responses are driven by the particular mental representations activated by that stimulus, and these representations—the meaning of the stimulus for the individual—may vary from person to person, and from culture to culture.

Situational influences can be perceived consciously or unconsciously. They can initiate behavior. Along the way, many unconscious processes are indispensable, including the coordination of muscle movements that execute walking or speech or writing. Consciousness might possibly be entirely bypassed, but probably in the majority of cases it must at least cooperate with the unconscious execution. For example, walking to the corner store may be executed largely by unconscious processes—or *productions* (Wyer, Xu, & Chen, 2012) —that move first one foot and then the other. But consciousness must at least be sympathetic to the project of walking to the store, to support the unconscious operation of the production of walking. It seems implausible that a person would walk to the store by entirely unconscious causation even while his or her conscious mind was screaming at the feet to turn around.

To be sure, often extensive inner processing mediates between the stimulus and the response (Bargh & Ferguson, 2000). Automatic stereotype effects on judgment and behavior depend on the particular content of the stereotype; different stereotypes of the same social group produce automatic different effects (cf. Devine, 1989; Lepore & Brown, 1997). Perhaps even more important, motivational tendencies within the individual may moderate the impact of stimulus on response. The simple formula that the stimulus causes the response glosses over the fact that the organism's attitudes and values dictate whether any response is called for in the first place. If the person has no relevant motivation—if one really does not care a fig either way—then the situation or event is unlikely to spark action. Insofar as the situation is relevant to the goals, values, fears, and desires of the individual, it will stimulate behavioral responses.

This *asymptote*—apparently unreachable limit—of unconscious effects of stimuli on behavior and other higher mental processes was recognized early on, first by Koestler (1967) and Neisser (1967), then by Bargh (1989) and Srull and Wyer (1986): Although automatic stimulus effects could influence perceptual interpretation, orienting of attention, and other early-stage processes, they could not directly drive responses to the environment, because those were the purview of the particular goal active at that moment. Responses back to the environment, loosely defined to include judgments, as well as behaviors, were determined by the person's current purposes. The classic examples of automatic processes such as typing and driving were, of course, dependent on the person wanting to type something or to drive somewhere in the first place; once that goal was active, then the movement of the fingers to type or the complicated attentional–motoric processes involved in driving operated automatically. Traveling a bit too fast around a curve and suddenly seeing a stop sign ahead causes one's right foot to kick out and slam on the brakes without need for any conscious intention or decision. But viewing that same stop sign while meandering on a pleasant walk along the sidewalk does not cause one's leg suddenly to kick out, fortunately for any fellow pedestrians nearby. The same stimulus (stop sign) has dramatically different effects depending on one's currently active goals.

Faced with this situation, Bargh (1989) was ready to pack up shop and call it quits regarding the extent of automatic influences of the environment. They seemed, as Neisser (1967) had originally argued, to be limited to early attentional and perceptual processes (pattern detection, figural synthesis) with an asymptotic limit at directly controlling any actual responses. But one last chance of direct environmental control had to be examined before he closed the books on the potential automaticity of higher mental processes: What if the goals themselves could be triggered and put into motion directly by environmental stimuli?

This idea was the heart of the "automotive model" of unconscious motivation, which Bargh (1990) originally presented as just a hypothesis with no supporting data. Soon, however, in collaboration with motivational psychologist Peter Gollwitzer and then-graduate student Tanya Chartrand, a series of studies showed that goals such as achievement and cooperation, activated (primed) outside of awareness by goal-relevant environmental stimuli, produced the same effects on judgment and behavior as when they were consciously pursued (Bargh & Gollwitzer, 1994; Bargh, Gollwitzer, Lee-Chai, Barndollar, & Troetschel, 2001; Chartrand & Bargh, 1996). Yes, the goal in place did determine the effects of stimuli on responses, but the goal in place—akin to the steering wheel in the earlier analogy itself could be automatically activated, and put into motion, by external environmental stimuli. This automatic goal activation was argued to occur in the same way as for other mental representations, such as stereotypes (Bargh, 1990). Conscious intent and awareness of the goal pursuit were not necessary to produce goal-directed behavior, extended over time, a conclusion borne out by much subsequent research (Aarts, Custers, & Marien, 2008; Custers & Aarts, 2010; Dijksterhuis & Aarts, 2010).

So far, so good—and no need for consciousness. Consciousness is entirely dispensable, except perhaps as route of input for situational influences. Remember, behavior happens all the time in animals, without needing anything approaching the sophistication of human conscious control, without requiring our whole, big human frontal cortex. Consciousness is not needed to originate behavior. It can perhaps intervene to change the course of action, to steer it, as it were, but there is no reason at all to assume that actional impulses originate in consciousness. (Note, however, that consciousness *is* needed to understand sentences [but not single words or concepts], so all meanings that come in by sentences require consciousness first to parse them for meaning in order to influence behavior.)

But this is hardly the extent of conscious activity, to enable the unconscious to receive complex messages from the world. (Though it is extremely important given the use of culture as human biological strategy.) The demonstrations of environmental priming effects on higher mental processes such as social perception (including stereotyping), judgment, behavior (as in imitation or emotional contagion), as well as goal pursuit (see reviews in Bargh, 2007), all focus on just one priming effect at a time. This is the nature of laboratory research in which a single phenomenon is isolated for study. But in the buzzing, booming real world out there, multiple primes are constantly present. People are arguably constantly barraged by potential priming influences. Although this huge set of potentials is winnowed down somewhat by the currently active goal, which directs attention toward goal-relevant stimuli and away from others (Neuberg, Kenrick, Maner, & Schaller, 2004), people still face a surplus of riches regarding the prediction of priming effects in busy, real-world environments (see Bargh, 2006). Note that this is the same problem of ecological validity that Skinner and his behaviorist colleagues faced when attempting to generalize the S-R model from the extremely simple rat laboratory environments to the complex social world of human beings (see, especially, Koestler, 1967).

Not only that, but a given stimulus can have multiple priming effects, be relevant to competing goals, and have multiple features triggering conflicting responses. Here is where consciousness, and especially the consciousness bottleneck, comes in very handy. A prominent idea that is gaining consensus today regarding the purpose of consciousness is that it alone is capable of integrating and managing the different response outputs generated by the variety of sensory, information-processing, and motivationally relevant systems housed within the human skin (Morsella, 2005). Take as an example the classic Stroop task, in which words are presented in a variety of colors and one's task as experimental participant is just to name the color of the word as quickly as possible. The single stimulus word *red* presented in blue ink has two task-relevant features (the word meaning and the word color), both processed automatically (one does not consciously have to figure out the meaning of the word *red*, and one immediately recognizes without any deliberation that its color is blue). So to make the correct response "blue," one has to manage the competing responses, select "blue" and inhibit "red." We can all do this (there are very few errors typically made on this task), though it takes a bit longer here (compared, e.g., to the word *five* presented in blue) because of the additional effort to inhibit the competing response.

Now, what if the experimenter comes into your cubicle and tells you from now on you are to say the word itself out loud, and not its color. Again, you can do this at a near perfect level, making few if any mistakes. It might again take you longer to say "red" when that word is presented in blue color, but you still manage to stifle the competing response and make the correct answers. The telling point here is that the stimulus—the word *red* in blue color—is identical in the two versions of the task. The stimulus alone did not drive the response. Moreover, this single stimulus generated two different, competing, task-relevant responses, "red" and "blue," yet you were able to get it right. And even more than that, the task instructions were given to you verbally by the experimenter, not by some internal goal or motivation you had internal and private to yourself. Even for such a simple experimental task as the Stroop effect, there is a whole lot for which consciousness is absolutely necessary and that could not be done without it.

Without consciousness the experimenter could not tell you what to do (see Dennett, 1991). You might have learned the correct responses if there were feedback after each trial (as there often is in the dangerous, real world in which you quickly learn not to touch a hot stove), but this would likely take some floundering around to learn the rule; if someone tells you the rule instead, performance is nearly perfect from the get-go (Dulany, 1968). This illustrates one huge domain of consciousness—that people can share information with each other about the correct responses to make, and that they can thus hand down this information generation by generation. Other animals have to reinvent the wheel during each lifetime and cannot, as humans do, build on the hard-won gains of their ancestors and stand on their shoulders. That consciousness is needed to parse sentences is thus no small potatoes.

In what might be a telling example of ontogeny recapitulating phylogeny, young children first "think aloud" before thinking silently to themselves (Vygotsky, 1934/1986). They use their emerging skills of communicating with others to begin to communicate with themselves; after a few months they can do this silently. Thus, internal conscious thought is born out of social communication, taking oneself as the object or target of the communication instead of another person. The phylogentic implications are transparent, suggesting again that conscious thought processes emerged as a functional outgrowth of members of our species' ability to communicate (especially verbally) with each other.

WHAT ABOUT FREE WILL?

At a 2009 conference, the two of us staged a lively debate about whether the notion of free will is scientifically viable. Although some in the audience seemed to have gotten the impression that our views were miles apart (and even that we disliked each other!), our respective positions were probably much closer than it appeared. It is perhaps unfortunate that terms such as "free will" and "determinism" have acquired multiple meanings and connotations. Although these help to attract multidisciplinary attention, they can mislead and confuse, because different theorists use different definitions and therefore argue past each other.

One traditional understanding of free will is an exemption from causality. Neither of us thinks that that view is promising, particularly for a scientific theory. Indeed, scientific theories are causal theories. Hence, we both assume that all behavior is caused. Baumeister thinks free will is simply a different kind of causation, as compared to physical or billiard-ball causation. There are many forms of causation, so having one more is hardly a major concession or adjustment, especially given that the behavior of humans, unlike the deportment of inanimate physical objects, may be influenced by contemplation of moral principles, legal constraints, anticipated future consequences, socially shared understandings, and other factors not easily reducible to Newtonian physics.

Bargh thinks similarly, that the will is caused and not "free" from causation, and that different answers are given to the question of whether free will exists mainly because of where people choose to cut off the causal chain. For political scientists, external constraints on the individual will, such as use of force or coercion (as in totalitarian regimes), are what matter, and when those are not in play, free will (free from external constraint) is said to exist. (Indeed, as Hannah Arendt, 1978, once said, without the existence of free will in this sense the field of political science itself could not exist.) The causal chain is not traced any farther back than this. For psychologists, however, internal constraints are fair game, so behavior is considered less free, for example, in the case of strong addictions, or difficult-to-overcome compulsions such as hoarding or hand washing. Provocations, too, are understood as mitigating circumstances, such as when angry behavior produced by a strong insult is considered as partially outside the person's control or free will.

The key distinction seems not to be free will per se but the role of conscious processes in producing the behavior. Conscious processes are just as causal as unconscious processes. But for many, especially in the field of psychology, conscious causation is equated with free will and unconscious causation, with the lack of same. This is a longstanding historical position dating back to Watson (1912) and the rise of behaviorism; not for nothing was B. F. Skinner's 1971 book titled *Beyond Freedom and Dignity*. Bargh believes that conscious processes are just as caused as are unconscious processes (see especially Bargh & Ferguson, 2000), so both are equally "free" or "not free" depending on how one defines *freedom*; yet psychologists are not really as interested in the "freedom" question as much as they are interested in the question of whether conscious states themselves are causal (see Bargh, 2013).

Baumeister is interested in the social reality of free will, which includes how behaviors such as self-control, rational choice, and initiative are executed. The implications of belief in free will are also important; as a growing body of work has documented, differences in beliefs about free will contribute to various behavioral outcomes. He thinks that humans do have some traits that differentiate them from other animals—and that most of these, including whatever inner processes commonly go by the name of free will, are adaptations to facilitate culture (see Baumeister, 2005). Hence, his interest is in whether the behaviors associated with free will and beliefs about free will are largely conducive to the effective operation of cultural systems (and helpful to the individuals who seek to survive, reproduce, and otherwise flourish in them).

In any case, we agree that human action is best explained in causal terms. For Baumeister, the issue of free will is whether humans actually make choices from among multiple options that are genuinely possible, which strict Laplacian determinism rules out. (Laplace insisted that there is only one possible future, which is precisely the same as what will actually happen, so there cannot be multiple alternative possibilities.) For Bargh, who believes that these choices, as well as the will itself (goal pursuits), are driven mainly by unconsciously operating processes, the particular flavor of "free will" that matters to psychologists and laypeople alike (but seemingly not to philosophers) is whether choices and behaviors are influenced by what is "now playing" in the conscious Cartesian theater of the mind.

Regardless of the philosophical niceties and the unfortunately emotional connotations of terms such as *free will*, we agree on key issues. The production of action in humans differs in some fundamental ways from the production of action in other animals. Human action takes into account many factors, such as man-made laws, moral principles, symbolism, expressive meaning, and other factors that are generally presumed to be absent from the causation of animal behavior. Humans are in crucial ways able to conceptualize alternatives to current reality and alternative scenarios in which their own various possible courses of action lead to different (and differentially appealing) consequences, and to use these conscious simulations to inform their own behavior. The challenge for psychology is to elucidate the processes that produce those actions.

DOES CONSCIOUSNESS CAUSE BEHAVIOR?

As we have said, psychology's dominant views about how conscious thoughts influence behavior have ranged and oscillated widely. At some points, the reigning assumption has been that conscious thoughts enjoy extensive control over behavior, and unconscious thoughts have at best indirect effects that depend on influencing the conscious thoughts. At other points, conscious thought has been regarded as a dubious side effect of other processes, lacking scientific viability and pragmatic efficacy.

In recent decades, one of the most influential but also controversial lines of work to impugn conscious control was provided by Libet (1985, 2004). The experiments instructed people to decide arbitrarily when to make a meaningless physical movement and to record the moment of that decision. Findings indicated that brain activity showed an uptick about half a second before the movement and (more important) about 300 milliseconds before the conscious decision. Skeptics of conscious control have used those findings to argue that a conscious decision is not a cause of behavior, because the response is already in motion before the conscious event.

To respond to that interpretation of Libet's findings, Baumeister, Masicampo, and Vohs (2011) conducted a literature search for evidence of conscious causation of behavior. Specifically, they sought experimental work in which the (manipulated) independent variable was a conscious event or state, and the dependent variable was genuine behavior (as opposed to a cognition or emotion). By the logic of experimental design, such findings would generally be regarded as evidence that conscious thoughts cause behavior.

That search yielded a broad variety of findings. The efficacy of conscious states for causing behavior is difficult to dispute in light of that evidence. The patterns of findings reviewed in that work include the following (for full review, see Baumeister et al., 2011). When people consciously imagine future actions, they become more likely to perform them. Mentally practicing difficult or skillful actions improves the quality of subsequent performance. Making specific plans improves likelihood and efficacy of behavior. Rehearsing, ruminating about, or reinterpreting recent events alters how one responds subsequently. Performance on logical reasoning tests is heavily dependent on conscious thought. Taking other people's perspective and empathizing with their feelings or desires alters how one treats them, as does imagining the constraints, pressures, and stereotypes that may impinge on their behavior. Trying to override specific automatic or habitual responses is sometimes effective in altering behavior. Altering views of self can alter how one reacts to subsequent challenges and opportunities. Setting particular goals or interpretively framing issues in a particular way can alter how one deals with them.

None of this evidence contradicts the findings of Libet (2004)—only the (mis)interpretation that Libet's findings disprove the efficacy of conscious thoughts. Baumeister et al. (2011) reported no findings that indicated direct control of muscle movements, independent of unconscious processes, which is perhaps what Libet was searching for. Indeed, Libet's (1985) experimental participants were specifically instructed not to plan when to respond, which arguably eliminated the only role that conscious thought could play in that situation.

The findings are also consistent with Bargh's (1997) assertion that the direct, immediate causes of behavior are almost always unconscious and automatic. They suggest a view in which the unconscious carries out the moment-to-moment execution of behavior, with conscious operating at a remove but offering helpful guidance and insights (akin to the navigational system model we outlined earlier). Baumeister et al. (2011) pointed out that none of the findings they reviewed indicated causation by conscious thoughts alone. Rather, they depict conscious and unconscious processes working together. Indeed, they speculated that almost every human behavior is the result of both conscious and unconscious processes.

There was also no evidence in all the work reviewed by Baumeister et al. (2011) that behaviors originate in consciousness. They cited a great deal of work, but it was all congenial to the auto-motive theory's account that action begins when external cues activate unconscious motivations and tendencies. Thus, behavior starts with an interaction between the external situation and the internal but unconscious motivational tendencies. Still, it makes a difference whether the possible action is first contemplated and simulated consciously.

Unconscious processes may accomplish the specific execution of specific behaviors in the here and now. Indeed, unconscious processes seem to correspond to "old brain" systems of dealing constantly with present-time dangers and needs, just in order to survive to the next present moment. The various automatic processes discovered in social cognition research over the past quarter-century or so have all been found to lead directly, and unconsciously, to overt behavioral responses (Bargh & Morsella, 2010)—exactly what would be expected if these processes were selected by evolutionary processes because of their adaptive value, because natural selection can only operate on overt behavioral responses. This is why, for example, internal automatic processes, such as automatic attitude activation, have been found to produce immediate muscular, behavioral predispositions to approach versus avoid the attitude object (Chen & Bargh, 1999), and automatic social perceptual activity such as trait concept and stereotype activation have also been found unconsciously to produce behavioral tendencies to act in line with the content of the trait concept or stereotype.

Unconscious processes therefore evolved to guide behavior in adaptive ways in the present moment, and this has the happy advantage of freeing conscious processes to "time-travel" into the past or future, comparing present events to past occurrences through memory processes, and making plans for future circumstances (Bargh, 1997). This would not be a safe thing to do unless unconscious processes were home "minding the store" while consciousness was away in time. Conscious thoughts are therefore very useful in coordinating past, present, and future, such as when contemplation of future goals influences present selection of actions (Trope & Liberman, 2003), or when interpretation or reinterpretation of past events alters how one will respond to a similar situation in the future. The literature review by Baumeister et al. (2011) concluded that one major pattern of conscious causation was indeed the integration of past, present, and future.

Planning is a useful example. Behavior does not originate with a plan, because the very making of a plan is occasioned by some combination of inner motivation and external constraint or opportunity. One only makes a plan because one wants to reach a goal, and reaching it is not guaranteed. For all its powers and merits, the unconscious is probably not capable of making a complex plan itself, so it uses consciousness in order to make the plan. This is probably why people are often kept awake at night, against their will and their strong desire to get back to sleep, thinking about their uncompleted tasks or the yet-unsolved major problems in their life (Morsella, Ben-Zeev, Lanska, & Bargh, 2010). When the conscious mind does form a plan to take care of these unresolved issues, the unconscious stops nagging consciousness about them (Masicampo & Baumeister, 2011).

Once again, in the case of planning, however, conscious and unconscious processes are found to work most effectively together. When consciousness does make a plan, it turns out that the most effective and reliable plan in terms of probability of success at reaching the desired goal is to form "strategically automatic" mental associations concerning future behavior. Gollwitzer (1999) described the most effective type of plan (at least in terms of what has been proven), implementation intentions, as delegation of control to the environment. Plans are, in essence, specification in advance of what one wants to do given a reliable future event or situation. Implementation intentions work by specifying in concrete detail those future circumstances and linking one's intended course of action to them, so that when the future event occurs, the intended behavior is triggered automatically.

Note in both of these scenarios, in which consciousness sets a goal and the unconscious works to find a path to it (as occurs in incubation or tip-of-the-tongue effects, in which the sought-for answer pops into consciousness only much later; Koriat, 1993; or a future situation–behavior contingency that then unfolds unconsciously upon the future event), that conscious and unconscious processes are working together. Implementation intentions require conscious processes to set them in the first place but, once established, produce the intended behavior efficiently, reliably, and automatically. Plans require conscious work to establish the desired end state and then allow unconscious processes to work out a way to that goal.

Another, related way that conscious and unconscious processes work together is demonstrated by how conscious attentional processes are automatically directed to unusual, unexpected, or (to a lesser extent) novel events, as noted early on by Mandler (1975) in his model of emotion and by Taylor and Fiske (1978) in their work on attentional salience effects in social cognition, and perhaps especially in Shiffrin and Schneider's (1977) pioneering work on the interaction of controlled (i.e., conscious) and automatic (i.e., unconscious) information processing. The unconscious is continually building a model of the world, using mechanisms such as priming and concept accessibility (both chronic and temporary) with fluent processing (low attentional demand) given to events that fit that model (Higgins & Bargh, 1987); this leaves more of one's limited attentional capacity for those events that do not fit the current model. Given these limits, the unconscious monitoring of the world that generates expectancies, explicit and implicit alike, helps conscious resources to be automatically directed where they are most needed and can be the most helpful.

FUNCTIONS OF CONSCIOUSNESS IN AN AUTOMATICALLY DRIVEN PERSON

Thus far we have argued that automatic, unconscious processes are the direct and original causes of most actions—yet conscious thoughts do play a causal role. If behavior starts with impulses originating in the unconscious, and if it is executed by unconscious processes that control movement, what does consciousness do? The answer suggests that conscious thoughts work closely with unconscious ones to produce the optimal behavioral outcomes.

Conscious thoughts can facilitate decision making in several ways. Conscious thoughts are mentally constructed simulations, and as such they can simulate various courses of action and their probable outcomes. These imagined future events are constructed with the help of extensive unconscious work, including retrieval of relevant knowledge from similar past experiences. Also, crucially, the selection among the various options is informed by comparing the affective reactions to each scenario, and these depend on automatic activation of affective associations. People learn from experience partly by having emotional responses to how things turn out, and these leave emotional traces that are activated when they encounter or imagine similar experiences later (see Damasio, 1994, on somatic markers; also see Baumeister, Vohs, DeWall, & Zhang, 2007, on how emotion guides behavior).

Conscious self-regulation (aka self-control) is another possible mechanism by which conscious thoughts can influence behavior. Morsella (2005) argued persuasively that inner response conflicts that involve skeletomotor muscles—thus, ones about physical action—prompt conscious awareness. This suggests that consciousness is important for mediating between conflicting motivations. Several common types of motivational conflict pit a so-called "lower impulse," such as that stemming from animalistic needs and desires, against higher ones, such as moral principles and long-range goals. Self-control typically operates in service of the higher impulse.

Self-control is typically understood as a conscious process, though there are undoubtedly some unconscious forms of self-regulation (e.g., for maintaining bodily and even social and emotional homeostasis; see Bargh & Shalev, 2012, and, of course, we continue to think and insist that conscious processes are themselves constructed by unconscious ones. One way that consciousness can benefit self-control is by simulating the long-term outcome, which can then exert a motivational pull to compete with the more immediately tempting stimulus for the short-term impulse. Thus, the person is tempted by the cake, the drug, the drink, the insulting provocateur, or whatever, any one of which could lead to impulsive action that might be briefly satisfying but regretted in the long run. To enable the higher impulse to prevail, it is helpful to imagine future outcomes that would be thwarted by indulging, such as the fashionably slim self, the nonaddicted self, the nonhungover self, or the nonjailed self. A vivid conscious thought of these desired outcomes can bolster the otherwise feeble wish to do the right thing.

CONSCIOUS THINKING IS FOR TALKING

Our views about the role of consciousness in the genesis of action have changed several times and no doubt may evolve further. But a different approach to the question of what consciousness is for was proposed by Baumeister and Masicampo (2010). One crucial function of human conscious thought may be for communicating (see also Dennett, 1991). Although many things can be done while conscious thought is directed elsewhere, talking does not appear to be one of them (nor does writing!).

Cognitive psychologists and others have long used reportability as a methodological indicator of consciousness. That is, to establish whether some thought is conscious, one ascertains whether the participant can report on it. But few researchers seem to have seriously contemplated the possibility that reportability may be far more than a handy methodological tool—that it may be precisely the central purpose of consciousness in the first place.

The assumption that communication is one central purpose of conscious thought offers a useful solution to several thorny dilemmas. The question of why humans would have evolved their advanced capacity for conscious thought is vexing if one seeks to use it to explain improved control over behavior. As we have said, we both think automatic and unconscious processes do a fine job of executing almost all behavior. There is no evidence that consciousness can dispense with unconscious processes in action. There is no reason to think that natural selection would have favored early humans who were able to be more conscious of their own actions than were their rivals.

In contrast, the adaptive benefits of communication seem uncontroversial. Sharing information is something humans do extensively and deliberately, far more frequently, more extensively, and more effectively than any other species. Early human kin-based groups that could communicate better than others could well have enjoyed profound advantages, so that natural selection might relatively quickly have favored communicative abilities. The idea that communication was the basic human trait that set our ancestors off on their uniquely human evolutionary past can integrate much of what is known. This includes the fact that upright posture (freeing the hands for gestural communication, which preceded speech) preceded the increase in brain size, contrary to early views that the emergence of the large brain was the original basis for distinctively human evolution. Our ancestors began to share information by gesturing, and the gradual but huge increase in information available in the social environment would certainly have created a selection factor favoring increases in intelligence and brain size.

Earlier we noted evidence (e.g., DeWall, Baumeister, & Masicampo, 2008) that logical reasoning seems to require conscious thought (though, as always, in conjunction with automatic and unconscious processes). The presumptive advantages of reasoning would seemingly constitute a possible explanation for why consciousness evolved. With reasoning, too, however, there is a strong case that the driving force has been interpersonal communication and interaction rather than solitary or solipsistic ratiocination. Mercier and Sperber (2011) reviewed the evidence about common lapses, errors, and flaws in human reasoning, and pointed out that these are only flaws if one assumes that the purpose of reasoning is a solitary, dispassionate search for the truth. Instead, they proposed that reasoning evolved primarily for the sake of arguing, in which case many of those seeming flaws appear instead as helpful to the cause of survival.

For example, the *confirmation bias* is a tendency to attend more to evidence supporting one's hypothesis than to evidence contradicting it. Many writers have deplored this as a sad lapse, and an invitation to bias and error. And, of course, scientists who ignore contrary evidence will likely end up with mistaken theories. But people are not intuitive scientists so much as they are intuitive lawyers who want to argue for their position (see Tetlock, 2002). In that case, supportive evidence is much more useful than contrary evidence. A defense lawyer who brought up evidence of her client's guilt would be less successful than one who focused on the facts that supported his innocence. Mercier and Sperber have also suggested that reasoning is for evaluating the arguments made by others—in which case people have a *disconfirmation bias,* which is to say they look eagerly for flaws in the reasoning used by their adversaries in an argument.

There would seem to be clear adaptive advantages in being able to argue in one's own defense within one's social group, as argued in Tetlock's (2002) model of evolved social mindsets. Take as a starting point Gazzaniga's (1985) prescient idea based on hypnosis, as well as early neuroscience research, that impulses to action arise unconsciously and are then interpreted consciously to form a coherent narrative account of what one is doing and why. He noted that people's behavior under posthypnotic suggestion, in which they found themselves down on the floor on all fours because of the hypnotist's command, or getting up from the chair and leaving the room, found immediate rational explanations and justifications ("I lost an earring down here"; "I'm thirsty and want to get some water"). One can imagine how helpful to maintaining one's good graces with one's group, back in the day when ostracism was a certain death sentence, it would be to have readily at hand a positive spin for whatever one was doing or had just done. Without this ready explanation and ability to communicate it effectively, one could be seen as personally responsible and as having intended all of the accidental mishaps (spilling the jar of water on the long walk back from the well, falling asleep and letting the sheep wander away, picking some poisonous berries on a foraging run) that can occur to any of us given the vagaries and uncertainties of life. Indeed, given the strong evidence of the correspondence bias or fundamental attribution error, each of us would be likely to be seen as intending each of these bad outcomes, and situational or circumstantial causes would tend to be dismissed by the group. Thus, we can see a clear case for the adaptive, survival value of being able to give quickly and argue effectively for a positive, pro-group version of whatever one has just done.

Logical reasoning and planning can also be helpful in guiding behavior toward optimal, desired outcomes, and these appear to require conscious thought. As one example, most travelers engage in calculating simulations so as to get to the airport with sufficient time to make their plane (but without so much lead time as to require sitting for many hours in the airport). Knowing one has a 1:35 P.M. flight departure time might dictate arriving at the airport by 12:35 (earlier for big, busy airports), which in turn may require being in the taxi by 12:15, which requires being at the taxi stand by 12:05, which requires being checked out of the hotel room and into the elevator by noon, which requires being fully packed by 11:45 in time to check the room again for potentially forgotten items, which means having an early lunch, and so forth.

CONCLUSIONS

Whatever we may have thought and seemed to say in the past, at present we both think that most human behavior comes from a blend of conscious and unconscious processes working together to meet the person's critical needs and facilitate important goal pursuits. Baumeister et al.'s (2011) survey of the literature turned up no convincing evidence that any action is caused entirely by conscious processes, and it is doubtful that this would even be possible. In principle, a few behaviors could be produced entirely independently of consciousness, and the direct execution of behavior is probably the result of unconscious and automatic processes, but in most cases, consciousness may have some say in the matter, especially with regard to upstream influences such as planning, logical reasoning, interpreting, and communicating.

The unconscious evolved primarily to produce adaptive responses in the immediate present. Conscious processes evolved to do other things. They are necessary for people to time-travel away from the immediate present, especially to anticipate, simulate, and plan for the future. They are necessary to communicate verbally with others, thus gaining a huge competitive advantage for our species in the capacity to share knowledge with others and coordinate individual efforts effectively. One prime adaptive advantage of being able to communicate with others seems to have been the production of good arguments, both to persuade others to help one pursue one's own important goals (or at least not hinder one's pursuits) and perhaps especially to defend one's sometimes deleterious behaviors to one's social group, to avoid retribution and ostracism. Insofar as consciousness evolved to facilitate communication, and human communication continues to take new forms and present new challenges and opportunities, it is tempting to speculate that human consciousness itself may continue to evolve. The mental state that defines human waking activity may be a work in progress.

The two of us have worked separately for many years to emphasize the positive benefits and utility of conscious processes on the one hand, and unconscious processes on the other. We have managed to convince each other of our respective positions, so that we have come to share the view today that both conscious and unconscious processes are important in their own right and in their own domains, but more than that, they need each other to work at all. Neither conscious nor unconscious processes can do it all by themselves: They must rely on each other in much the same way that individual humans do.

REFERENCES

Aarts, H., Custers, R., & Marien, H. (2008). Preparing and motivating behavior outside of awareness. *Science*, *319*, 1639.

Arendt, H. (1978). *The life of the mind*. New York: Harcourt.

Bargh, J. A. (1989). Conditional automaticity: Varieties of automatic influence on social perception and cognition. In J. Uleman & J. Bargh (Eds.), *Unintended thought* (pp. 3–51). New York: Guilford Press.

Bargh, J. A. (1990). Auto-motives: Preconscious determinants of social interaction. In E. T. Higgins & R. M. Sorrentino (Eds.), *Handbook of motivation and cognition* (Vol. 2, pp. 93–130). New York: Guilford Press.

Bargh, J. A. (1994). The four horsemen of automaticity: Awareness, intention, efficiency, and control in social cognition. In R. S. Wyer, Jr., & T. K. Srull (Eds.), *Handbook of social cognition* (2nd ed., Vol., 3, pp. 1–40). Hillsdale, NJ: Erlbaum.

Bargh, J. A. (1997). The automaticity of everyday life. In R. S. Wyer, Jr. (Ed.), *Advances in social cognition* (Vol. 10, pp. 1–63). Mahwah, NJ: Erlbaum.

Bargh, J. A. (2005). Bypassing the will: Towards demystifying behavioral priming effects. In R. Hassin, J. Uleman, & J. Bargh (Eds.), *The new unconscious* (pp. 37–58). Oxford, UK: Oxford University Press.

Bargh, J. A. (Ed.). (2007). *The unconscious in social psychology: The automaticity of higher mental processes*. Philadelphia: Psychology Press.

Bargh, J. A. (2013). Social psychology cares about causal conscious thought, not free will *per se*. *British Journal of Social Psychology, 52*(2), 228–230.

Bargh, J. A., & Ferguson, M. J. (2000). Beyond behaviorism: The automaticity of higher mental processes. *Psychological Bulletin, 126*, 925–945.

Bargh, J. A., & Gollwitzer, P. M. (1994). Environmental control of goal-directed action: Automatic and strategic contingencies between situations and behavior. In W. D. Spaulding (Ed.), *Nebraska Symposium on Motivation: Vol. 41. Integrative views of motivation, cognition, and emotion* (pp. 71–124). Lincoln: University of Nebraska Press.

Bargh, J. A., Gollwitzer, P. M., Lee-Chai, A., Barndollar, K., & Troetschel, R. (2001). The automated will: Nonconscious activation and pursuit of behavioral goals. *Journal of Personality and Social Psychology, 81*, 1014–1027.

Bargh, J. A., & Morsella, E. (2010). Unconscious behavioral guidance systems. In C. Agnew, D. Carlston, W. Graziano, & J. Kelly (Eds.), *Then a miracle occurs: Focusing on behavior in social psychological theory and research* (pp. 89–118). New York: Oxford University Press.

Bargh, J. A., & Shalev, I. (2012). The substitutibility of physical and social warmth in everyday life. *Emotion, 12,* 154–162.

Baumeister, R. F. (2005). *The cultural animal: Human nature, meaning, and social life.* New York: Oxford University Press.

Baumeister, R. F., & Masicampo, E. J. (2010). Conscious thought is for facilitating social and cultural interactions: How mental simulations serve the animal–culture interface. *Psychological Review, 117,* 945–971.

Baumeister, R. F., Masicampo, E. J., & Vohs, K. D. (2011). Do conscious thoughts cause behavior? *Annual Review of Psychology, 62,* 331–361.

Baumeister, R. F., & Sommer, K. L. (1997). Consciousness, free choice, and automaticity. In R. S. Wyer (Ed.), *Advances in social cognition* (Vol. 10, pp. 75–81). Mahwah, NJ: Erlbaum.

Baumeister, R. F., Vohs, K. D., DeWall, C. N., & Zhang, L. (2007). How emotion shapes behavior: Feedback, anticipation, and reflection, rather than direct causation. *Personality and Social Psychology Review, 11,* 167–203.

Bongers, K. C. A., & Dijksterhuis, A. (2009). Consciousness as a trouble shooting device?: The role of consciousness in goal-pursuit. In E. Morsella, J. A. Bargh, & P. Gollwitzer (Eds.), *The Oxford handbook of human action* (pp. 589–604). New York: Oxford University Press.

Chartrand, T. L., & Bargh, J. A. (1996). Automaticity of impression formation and memorization goals. *Journal of Personality and Social Psychology, 71,* 464–478.

Chartrand, T. L., & Bargh, J. A. (1999). The chameleon effect: The perception-behavior link and social interaction. *Journal of Personality and Social Psychology, 76,* 893–910.

Chen, M., & Bargh, J. A. (1999). Consequences of automatic evaluation: Immediate behavioral predispositions to approach or avoid the stimulus. *Personality and Social Psychology Bulletin, 25,* 215–224.

Custers, R., & Aarts, H. (2010). The unconscious will: How the pursuit of goals operates outside of conscious awareness. *Science, 329,* 47–50.

Damasio, A. (1994). *Descartes' error: Emotion, reason, and the human brain.* New York: Grosset/Putnam.

Dennett, D. (1991). *Consciousness explained.* Boston: Little, Brown.

Devine, P. G. (1989). Stereotypes and prejudice: Their automatic and controlled components. *Journal of Personality and Social Psychology, 56,* 5–18.

DeWall, C. N., Baumeister, R. F., & Masicampo, E. J. (2008). Evidence that logical reasoning depends on conscious processing. *Consciousness and Cognition. 17,* 628–645.

Dijksterhuis, A., & Aarts, H. (2010). Goals, attention and (un)consciousness. *Annual Review of Psychology, 61,* 467–490.

Dijksterhuis, A., & Nordgren, L. F. (2006). A theory of unconscious thought. *Perspectives on Psychological Science, 1,* 95–109.

Dulany, D. E. (1968). Awareness, rules, and propositional control: A confrontation with S-R behavior theory. In T. Dixon & D. Horton (Eds.), *Verbal behavior and general behavior theory* (pp. 340–387). New York: Prentice Hall.

Freud, S. (1965). *New introductory lectures on psychoanalysis* (J. Strachey, Trans.). New York: Norton. (Original work published 1933)

Gazzaniga, M. S. (1985). *The social brain.* New York, Basic Books.

Gladwell, M. (2004). *Blink: The power of thinking without thinking.* Boston: Little, Brown.

Gollwitzer, P. M. (1999). Implementation intentions: Strong effects of simple plans. *American Psychologist, 54,* 493–503.

Higgins, E. T., & Bargh, J. A. (1987). Social cognition and social perception. *Annual Review of Psychology, 38,* 369–425.

Huxley T. (1874). On the hypothesis that animals are automata, and its history. *Nature, 10,* 362–366.

Jaynes, J. (1976). *The origin of consciousness in the breakdown of the bicameral mind.* Boston: Houghton Mifflin.

Koestler, A. (1967). *The ghost in the machine.* New York: Macmillan.

Koriat, A. (1993). How do we know that we know?: The accessibility model of the feeling of knowing. *Psychological Review, 100,* 609–639.

Lepore, L., & Brown, R. (1997). Category and stereotype activation: Is prejudice inevitable? *Journal of Personality and Social Psychology, 72,* 275–287.

Libet, B. (1985). Unconscious cerebral initiative and the role of conscious will in voluntary action. *Behavioral and Brain Sciences, 8,* 529–566.

Libet, B. (2004). *Mind time: The temporal factor in consciousness.* Cambridge, MA: Harvard University Press.

Mandler, G. (1975). *Mind and emotion.* New York: Wiley.

Marien, H., Custers, R., Hassin, R. R., & Aarts, H. (2012). Unconscious goal activation and the hijacking of the executive function. *Journal of Personality and Social Psychology, 103*(3), 399–415.

Masicampo, E. J., & Baumeister, R. F. (2011). Consider it done!: Plan making can eliminate the cognitive effects of unfulfilled goals. *Journal of Personality and Social Psychology, 101,* 667–683.

McCulloch, K. C., Ferguson, M. J., Kawada, C. C. K., & Bargh, J. A. (2008). Taking a closer look: On the operation of nonconscious impression formation. *Journal of Experimental Social Psychology, 44,* 614–623.

Mercier, H., & Sperber, D. (2011). Why do humans reason?: Arguments for an argumentative theory. *Behavioral and Brain Sciences, 34,* 57–111.

Morsella, E. (2005). The function of phenomenal states: Supramodular interaction theory. *Psychological Review, 112,* 1000–1021.

Morsella, E. (2009). The mechanisms of human action. In E. Morsella, J. A. Bargh, & P. Gollwitzer (Eds.), *The Oxford handbook of human action* (pp. 1–32). New York: Oxford University Press.

Morsella, E., & Bargh, J. A. (2010). What is an output? *Psychological Inquiry, 21,* 354–370.

Morsella, E., Ben-Zeev, A., Lanska, M., & Bargh, J. A. (2010). The spontaneous thoughts of the night: How future tasks breed intrusive cognitions. *Social Cognition, 28,* 640–649.

Neisser, U. (1967). *Cognitive psychology.* New York: Appleton-Century-Crofts.

Neuberg, S. L., Kenrick, D. T., Maner, J. K., & Schaller, M. (2004). From evolved motives to everyday mentation: Evolution, goals, and cognition. In J. P. Forgas & K. D. Williams (Eds.), *Social motivation: Conscious and unconscious processes* (pp. 133–152). New York: Cambridge University Press.

Nisbett, R. E., & Wilson, T. D. (1977). Telling more than we can know: Verbal reports on mental processes. *Psychological Review, 84,* 231–259.

Schooler, J. W., Mrazek, M. D., Baird, B., & Winkielman, P. (in press). The value of distinguishing between unconscious, conscious, and meta-conscious processes. In G. Borgida & J. Bargh (Eds.), *Handbook of personality and social psychology.* Washington, DC: American Psychological Association.

Shiffrin, R. M., & Schneider, W. (1977). Controlled and automatic human information processing: II. Perceptual learning, automatic attending, and a general theory. *Psychological Review, 84,* 127–190.

Skinner, B. F. (1971). *Beyond freedom and dignity.* New York: Knopf.

Srull, T. K., & Wyer, R. S. (1986). The role of chronic and temporary goals in social information processing. In R. M. Sorrentino & E. T. Higgins (Eds.), *Handbook of motivation and cognition* (pp. 503–549). New York: Guilford Press.

Taylor, S. E., & Fiske, S. T. (1978). Salience, attention, and attribution: Top-of-the-head phenomena. In L. Berkowitz (Ed.), *Advances in experimental social psychology* (Vol. 11, pp. 249–288). New York: Academic Press.

Tetlock, P. E. (2002). Social-functionalist frameworks for judgment and choice: The intuitive politician, theologian, and prosecutor. *Psychological Review, 109,* 451–472.

Trope, Y., & Liberman, N. (2003). Temporal construal. *Psychological Review, 110,* 403–421.

Vygotsky, L. (1986). *Thought and language.* Cambridge, MA: MIT Press. (Original work published 1934)

Watson, J. B. (1912). Psychology as the behaviorist views it. *Psychological Review, 20,* 158–177.

Wegner, D. M. (2002). *The illusion of conscious will.* Cambridge, MA: MIT Press.

Wilson, T. D. (2002). *Strangers to ourselves.* Cambridge, MA: Belknap Press.

Wyer, R. S., Jr., Xu, A. J., & Chen, H. (2012). The effects of past behavior on future goal-directed activity. *Advances in Experimental Social Psychology, 46,* 237–283.

CHAPTER 4

What Is Control?

A Conceptual Analysis

Kentaro Fujita, Yaacov Trope, William A. Cunningham, and Nira Liberman

The emergence of dual-process and dual-systems theories represents one of the most significant scientific advances in psychology. As this volume attests, numerous formulations of these models continue to be developed. Most postulate a distinction between some psychological processes that are "automatic" and others that are "controlled." Much of the conceptual and theoretical development of this distinction has focused on defining what constitutes an automatic process, with comparably less attention invested in examining what constitutes a controlled process.

In this chapter, we critically examine what is meant by the term *control,* and suggest that there are actually two meanings. One meaning of control, as suggested by numerous dual-process and dual-systems theories, refers to whether a process can be characterized by one or more of the features associated with automatic processes (i.e., the absence of conscious intention, the absence of conscious awareness, the inability to disrupt, and/or the efficiency of operation; Bargh, 1994). In short, a controlled process is one that is not automatic. There is, however, a second meaning of control—one that refers instead to the extent to which a process helps to attain a desired goal or end. This sense of control refers not to some specific feature of an isolated process but rather to its relation to other processes from the perspective of the whole. Key to this second meaning of control is the notion of structure—the top-down organization of thoughts, feelings, and behavior to promote a given end. When a process operates in harmony with and sustains the goal-directed structure of the whole, that process can be described as "controlled." When a process, however, is discordant with and undermines the goal-directed structure of the whole, that process can be described as "out-of-control" or "lacking control." Our central thesis is that the conflating of these two meanings of control—as something that is not automatic and something that is goal-directed—has led many to make erroneous conclusions about the nature of controlled processing and its relationship to automaticity. We review empirical evidence that highlights the conceptual independence of these two meanings of control, and argue that it is time to recognize that "control" is not necessarily the opposite of "automatic."

WHAT IS AUTOMATIC?

In an influential review of the literature, Bargh (1994) noted that despite decades of scientific scrutiny, there is a surprising lack of consensus on what is meant by the term *automatic.* He noted instead that researchers tend to label a process as automatic to the extent that it has one or more of the following features: (1) It operates without conscious awareness; (2) it can be initiated without conscious intention; (3) it cannot be interrupted or controlled; and (4) it operates efficiently without consuming too many cognitive resources. Bargh (1996) and others (e.g., Bargh & Chartrand, 1999; Wegner & Bargh, 1998) have suggested that although these features are conceptually independent, one of two clusters or combinations have traditionally attracted research scrutiny. One major strain of research focuses on intentional processes that after repeated practice operate more efficiently and require less effort. Thus, what began as a consciously intended, effortful process that required active initiation and monitoring may, after repeated practice, become routinized and no longer require the same conscious intention and effort. The key emphasis of this line of research, the efficient use of limited cognitive resources, is exemplified by processes such as skills acquisition and habits. A second strain of research focuses on processes that operate not only effortlessly but also with little conscious intention or awareness that it has taken place. Research, for example, reveals that people attend to, encode, and are influenced by stimuli presented outside of conscious awareness (e.g., Bargh, 1996; Bargh & Chartrand, 1999; Wegner & Bargh, 1998). The key emphasis of this strain of research is not necessarily on efficiency, but rather on consciousness. That people can process and respond to their environments without conscious intention or awareness has led many to question assumptions about the function and centrality of consciousness in the operation of the mind. Collectively, this work on automatic processes has suggested that a lot of information processing appears to occur "behind the scenes." That automatic processes can operate efficiently and with minimal conscious guidance leads to the possibility that they may promote thoughts, feelings, and behaviors that are inconsistent with people's conscious intentions and desires. The efficiency and people's lack of awareness of such processes may render people unable to intervene and to disrupt such undesired processing. Specifically, people may not be aware that these automatic processes are undermining their conscious intentions; and even when they are aware, these processes may operate so efficiently that they are initiated and completed before comparatively less efficient conscious processing can intervene. These implications have led many to propose automatic processing as an anathema to control.

WHAT IS CONTROL?

As stated earlier, we propose that there are actually two meanings of the term *control.* Most dual-process and dual-systems models tend to use the term to refer to any process that lacks those features generally associated with automaticity—a controlled process is one that is not automatic. The second meaning of *control,* however, is independent of issues of automaticity. We argue that the use of the same term to refer to two distinct phenomena has caused conceptual confusion and erroneous conclusions. We focus our subsequent discussion of control on the second of these two meanings.

When entities such as children, people, organizations, and societies are described as "out of control," they are generally characterized by two related features: (1) a lack of governance, and (2) a lack of direction or purpose. By *governance,* we refer to a set of mechanisms or principles that organize and structure thoughts, feelings, and behaviors. Consider the metaphor of a senate. A senate without mechanisms about how legislation gets introduced, discussed, and voted upon would be out of control. Senators at their own whim could pursue actions that maximize their self-interest and the interests of their constituents to the detriment of others. What one senator might do may contradict or undermine the actions of another. The lack of governance would in turn render engaging in any goal-directed purpose impossible. The chaos caused by a lack of structure or order would allow for the pursuit of too many contradictory ends, leading the senate to be pushed and pulled by the loudest, most forceful voices at any given moment. Thus, the lack of rules and principles with which to organize discussion and action would lead to an inability to decide at a collective level what is most desired and how best to achieve those ends.

We might draw a similar parallel to the operation of the mind. When various signals within the mind operate without some structure or organization, they can push and pull the organism in contradictory directions. For example, consider dieters presented with an opportunity to indulge in eating a piece of chocolate cake. Whereas the elements of the mind concerned about immediate hedonics might clamor and urge dieters to eat the cake, those elements concerned about weight-loss concerns would encourage restraint. Left unimpeded, whether dieters choose to eat versus not eat cake would depend on the relative strength of those two opposing voices. The dieters' affective, cognitive, and behavioral responses would consequently appear chaotic, and would depend on a variety of factors that may vary from situation to situation. What should be clear is that this lack of organization and structure may frequently lead dieters to behave in a manner contrary to their valued goals, eating the cake despite their goal to lose weight. Thus, their thoughts, feelings, and behavior vis-à-vis weight-loss goals would appear "out of control."

Following others (Carver & Scheier, 1982, 1990; Hebb, 1949; Kruglanski et al., 2002; Shannon & Weaver, 1949), we define *control* as both a state and the act of producing that state in which thoughts, feelings, and behaviors are organized and prioritized around a desired end. What defines control is structure. By *structure,* we refer to the top-down reductive process of creating coherence from more fragmented and disorganized elemental components. Structure requires the perspective of the whole rather than the individual perspective of the parts. Constituent elements are arranged and integrated in a manner that allows them to work together to support and sustain the whole. When something is highly structured, its constituent elements are relationally organized, such that knowledge of one element allows one to deduce logically or predict the other elements. Thus, valuing weight loss should be associated with negative rather than positive thoughts about cake, and positive rather than negative thoughts about eating fruit salad. The resonance and coherence that structure provides among elemental units produces systemic order to one's thoughts, feelings, and behaviors, thus enhancing organized action (i.e., control).

Inherent to creating structure is also the process of constructing hierarchies (e.g., Carver & Scheier, 1982, 1990; Hebb, 1949; Kruglanski et al., 2002; Shannon & Weaver, 1949). By *hierarchies,* we refer to the appreciation that some elements are nested or embedded within others. To create meaningful structure from the elements "weight loss," "jogging," and "eating celery," one must recognize that "jogging" and "eating celery" are embedded within the broader element of "weight loss" as two means to the same end. This understanding of embeddedness allows one to better recognize goal-relevant opportunities and to coordinate thoughts, feelings, and behaviors appropriately. The construction of hierarchies, however, is not limited to means–ends relationships. Through structure, people may also come to appreciate relationships between specific behaviors (e.g., stealing money) and more general traits (e.g., dishonesty), as well as how subcategories (e.g., poodles) may exemplify broader superordinate categories (e.g., pets). Thus, hierarchies help people appreciate the relational links between more elemental units, promoting integration and the creation of structure.

Through structure, rather than reflect fragmentation and chaos, thoughts, feelings, and behaviors become organized and ends-directed (i.e., controlled). To create structure, people must engage in *subordination,* which entails the identification and categorization of inputs as relevant or irrelevant to a given end. Information that is relevant to a desired end is "foregrounded," preferentially weighted and attended to; information that is irrelevant is "backgrounded," preferentially deweighted and ignored (see Zelazo & Cunningham, 2007). The flavor of the icing on a piece of cake is irrelevant to one's weight-loss goal and is therefore subordinated in favor of information about the cake's calorie count. Similarly, behaviors relevant to eating cake are irrelevant with respect to weight-loss goals, and are therefore subordinated in favor of restraint and other behaviors directed toward losing weight (e.g., exercise or eating alternative foods). Note that by contrast, the hedonist—one who is not committed to weight-loss goals and instead is primarily concerned with the enjoyment of food—should evidence a different pattern of subordination: Calorie count would be subordinated in favor of a cake's icing, and restraint behaviors would be subordinated in favor of eating behaviors. Thus, irrespective of the content of the desired end state, it is through this process of subordination that thoughts, feelings, and behavior are structured to form a coherent whole.

A psychological process can therefore be considered "controlled" to the extent that it operates in a manner that is consistent with and sustains the larger integrated, goal-directed whole. Control, however, does not necessitate that all processes actively promote the goal-directed end. Returning to our senate metaphor, senators can agree to disagree and vote against any legislation. However, when a senate is operating in a controlled manner, all senators agree to follow certain rules. When overruled by the majority, senators must comply with the passed legislation and the collective will of the senate. Similarly, there can be discord and inconsistencies in a "controlled mind." Dieters' minds may still be characterized as "controlled" when debating the merits of eating cake versus weight-loss goals, as long as there are in place structures and principles that promote the resolution of this debate in a systematic, goal-directed manner. For dieters, given the importance and value of their long-term weight-loss goals over their more short-term hedonic desires, control might constitute subordinating thoughts, feelings, and behavior around the former rather than the latter. Thus, discord and dissonance have their place in a controlled mind; their impact, however, is limited and does not co-opt the structured, organized pursuit of desired ends.

THE ROLE OF ABSTRACTION IN CONTROL

Given that we define *control* as state in which people's thoughts, feelings, and behaviors are integrated and prioritized toward a given end, some mechanism is necessary for identifying which of the many ends they can possibly pursue is to be the one around which they create structure, and having created structure, how they maintain that prioritization and organization. This is a particularly vexing problem when goals conflict (dieters who want to eat cake but also want to lose weight). How do people appropriately select one goal over another? We propose that abstraction serves as the means by which this identification of goals and maintenance of structure takes place.[1,2]

Abstraction is the cognitive process of integrating inputs and extracting from them emergent commonalities that may not be evident in any one signal. Abstraction may promote control in two ways. First, it may facilitate the recognition of emerging patterns from lower-level inputs, which may help to determine what goals should be pursued. By analogy, the will of the senate is determined not by inquiring about the demands of a single senator but by querying the many that form the broader collective. Some senators may be particularly partisan and support one cause at the expense of others. Other senators may be more neutral but can still consider the available information and throw their support behind one cause or another. It is the systematic voting process that allows the will of the senate to emerge and become evident. Abstraction may similarly promote a bottom-up, emergent organization of thought, feeling, and behavior toward a single end. In the simplest case, bottom-up processing converges around a single desired end state, and abstraction merely promotes the emergent pattern. In more complicated situations, as is the case when goals conflict, people may have to engage in abstraction to integrate the two competing concerns. Abstraction promotes the ability to compare proverbial "apples and oranges" (i.e., inputs with features that may not align for direct comparison). Instead, it may facilitate the comparison of competing concerns on some common abstract dimension (e.g., utility or value) and promote the ability to determine which should be considered primary to the other (e.g., Malkoc, Zauberman, & Ulu, 2005).

The second way that abstraction may promote control is by promoting the ability to recognize discrepancies from coherent organization after thought, feelings, and behavior have been integrated and structured. Metaphorically, an individual senator may fail to recognize that his or her actions are inconsistent with the will of the senate after a vote has passed. It may be easier for the senate leader charged with maintaining order in the senate, who has the broader perspective of the senate as a collective body, to see that senator's actions as being problematic. Abstraction, in a similar way, may promote awareness of inconsistencies and promote top-down efforts to maintain and sustain structured organization. Thus, abstraction may have roles in both detecting emergent patterns that form the consensual goal in a bottom-up construction process and imposing structure and order to promote and protect that in a top-down fashion.

ON THE FLEXIBILITY AND STABILITY OF GOAL-DIRECTED BEHAVIOR

One should also not assume that the notion of structure (and the corresponding notion of control) necessitates rigidity or lack of flexibility. Creating structure is a dynamic process that can be sensitive to changes in both internal and external environments. One can create and re-create structure. The structure that one forms through abstraction fundamentally depends on the constituent elemental inputs. When those elemental units change, the corresponding structure generated from such elements (along with the goals that are pursued) may also change. Note, however, that although not entirely inflexible, one of the benefits of structure, at least with respect to the notion of control, is that it is relatively more stable than any individual constituent element. Small changes in incidental or peripheral elements within a structure are not likely to generate much change in the overall structure. This in turn promotes consistent goal-directed action across diverse contexts and circumstances. Thus, whether the icing on a piece of cake is chocolate or vanilla, for example, should have little impact on one's striving toward weight-loss goals. Large changes to more central elements, however, may cause more fundamental changes in the structure that is created and to the goals such structure promotes. When one's dieting has led to life-threatening health conditions, one might expect to see a shift in structure to support health over weight-loss goals. Thus, structure within the mind can provide stability yet be sensitive to changing circumstances.

Similarly, structure does not mean that people become insensitive to context. Context provides some of the bottom-up input around which structure is created, thus allowing people to pursue those goals that are best afforded by a given context. As an example, consider the working mother. When at home, the working mother might note that not much work can be done out of the office, and that child care concerns are pressing. Although part of her might be tempted to work, the perspective of the whole would suggest prioritizing the needs of her child over responding to the off-hour e-mails that her colleagues send. Creating coherent structure in this context would entail prioritizing child care over work. Thus, whereas work-related responses would be "out-of-control," child care-related responses would be "controlled." When she is at work and her child is at school, however, the "senate" of her mind may note that her child is already well cared for and that she now has the ability to address her to-do list. Although part of her might be tempted to daydream about her child, the perspective of the whole would suggest prioritizing the demands of her colleagues. Creating coherent structure for the working mother in this context would entail prioritizing work over child care. Thus, work-related responses would be "controlled," whereas child care-related responses would be "out of control." Although parenting and career goals may initially appear at odds, the creation of structure can organize the pursuit of these goals in a manner that allows the working mother to pursue each in its respective context. Creating structure through abstraction is therefore a dynamic process that provides both stability and flexibility in the ends that are pursued, and control is defined by the structure created.

INTERIM SUMMARY

Whereas dual-process and dual-systems models use the term *control* to denote a process that operates without conscious awareness and intention, is impervious to disruption, and is efficient, we highlight instead an alternative meaning that refers to the extent to which a process operates within an ordered whole to promote a given end. That researchers can use the same term (i.e., *control*) to refer to very different constructs may promote conceptual confusion. Our concern is that many researchers have conflated the two meanings, and have mistakenly drawn premature and problematic conclusions about the nature of control and its relationship to automaticity.

To support our argument, we explore three implications that the alternative meaning of control advances. First, it suggests that, in an apparent contrast to the predictions of many dual-process and dual-systems models, it is conceptually possible to have processes that are automatic (i.e., lack conscious intention, lack conscious awareness, cannot be disrupted, and/or are efficient) and controlled at the same time (i.e., operate within and promote goal-directed structure). That is, rather than positing a strict dichotomy in which a process is either automatic *or* controlled, we propose that, depending on one's definition of control, it is possible to describe processes as automatic *and* controlled. Second, given the central role of abstraction in goal-directed structure, one might expect that promoting abstraction should promote greater control (at least, when control is defined as structured goal pursuit). Third, the alternative meaning of *control* suggests the possibility that effortful, conscious (i.e., "not automatic") processing may under some circumstances impair effective goal-directed thought, feelings, and behavior. In what follows, we review empirical evidence for each of these assertions.

EVIDENCE OF AUTOMATIC *AND* CONTROLLED IMPLEMENTATION INTENTIONS

Research on implementation intentions highlights goal-directed (i.e., "controlled") processes that are consciously intended yet operate efficiently. *Implementation intentions* are behavioral plans that detail a specific behavior cued by a specific cue (e.g., Gollwitzer, 1999). These plans are structured in an "if–then" format, such that if the cue is encountered, then the behavior is to be enacted. A dieter with the goal of losing weight, for example, might generate the implementation intention: "If I see dessert on the table, then I will avert my gaze." By specifying a goal-directed behavior in response to a critical cue, implementation intentions preferentially background other potentially goal-irrelevant responses in that specific context. Thus, rather than attend to the cake, by generating an implementation intention, the dieter in the earlier example has subordinated that response in service of his or her dieting goals. Research indeed demonstrates that implementation intentions can help promote the pursuit of desired ends. For example, students who intended to complete a homework assignment over a holiday break were more likely to do so if they had generated implementations intentions (Gollwitzer & Brandstätter, 1997). Implementation intentions not only promote goal-directed behavioral responses, but they also appear to aid in the control of cognitive and emotional responses (e.g., Achtziger, Gollwitzer, & Sheeran, 2008; Bayer, Gollwitzer, & Achtziger, 2010; Cohen, Bayer, Jaudas, & Gollwitzer, 2008; Schweiger Gallo, Keil, McCulloch, Rockstroh, & Gollwitzer, 2009).[3]

Like habits and acquired skills, implementation intentions begin as consciously intended cognitive processes. What is remarkable about implementation intentions, however, is that unlike habits and acquired skills, they do not appear to require repeated practice to automate. Indeed, simply repeating an implementation intention several times ("If I see the number 5 on the computer screen, then I will type in my response particularly fast!") is sufficient to prompt cognitively efficient goal-directed behavior when the context specified by the plan is later encountered (Brandstätter, Lengfelder, & Gollwitzer, 2001). These goal-directed behaviors are not only more efficient (i.e., apparent under conditions of cognitive load), but they also do not appear to require conscious awareness of the critical cue. Research suggests that once an implementation intention is formed, even when the cues specified in the "if" component, are presented subliminally, outside of conscious awareness, participants still evidence goal-directed responding consistent with the "then" component (Bayer, Achtziger, Gollwitzer, & Moskowitz, 2009). Thus, implementation intentions represent controlled responses (i.e., subordinating some responses in favor of others in service of one's goals) that are automatic in that once formed, they appear to prompt goal-directed behavior efficiently and in the absence of conscious intention.

Goal Shielding

Research on goal shielding has also illuminated cognitive processes that are automatic (in that they operate outside of conscious awareness) yet represent a means of maintaining subordination and structure to promote control. *Goal shielding* refers to the inhibition of goal-irrelevant inputs when a person is engaged in goal-directed behavior, preventing competing desires and goals from interfering with ongoing goal-directed action. As a concrete example, consider an individual who wishes to mail a letter. On her way to the post office, this individual might encounter a number of stimuli that cue alternative courses of action, such as the bakery, which suggests stopping for a snack, or a television, which suggests watching cartoons instead. Ignoring these alternative goals (i.e., through cognitive inhibition) prevents them from distracting the individual from her focal goal: mailing the letter. Goal shielding is therefore a critical mechanism by which structure is created and maintained.

Supporting the existence of goal-shielding mechanisms is research that indicates identifying and thinking about one goal makes it more difficult to remember and to think about alternative competing goals (e.g., McCulloch, Aarts, Fujita, & Bargh, 2008; Shah, Friedman, & Kruglanski, 2002). Not only do people indeed engage in goal shielding, but they may also be able to do so without conscious intention or awareness. To test this, Shah and colleagues asked participants to list several personal goals, summarized in one-word phrases (e.g., "diet," "church," "grades"). They then embedded these goals into a lexical-decision task that capitalized on subliminal priming procedures. In critical trials, each participant was subliminally primed with one of his or her goals, then presented with another of his or her goals as a target and asked to identify it as word or nonword. Participants' lexical judgments were slower when one goal primed a second goal. This suggests that the activation of one goal (the primed goal) interfered with the activation of the second goal (i.e., the target goal). That activation of one goal outside of awareness leads to the inhibition of competing goals may suggest that goal shielding represents a controlled process (i.e., maintains structure and subordination) that also happens to be automatic (i.e., initiated and operates without conscious intention).

Asymmetrical Temptation–Goal Associations

As noted earlier, self-control dilemmas are a prototypical context in which to understand the operation of controlled processes. People must subordinate the temptation to pursue immediate rewards in favor of pursuing more valuable yet distal rewards. Research has highlighted a number of automatic processes—those that are initiated without conscious awareness or intention—that help people in this subordination process and therefore enhance self-control. One such mechanism may be asymmetrical cognitive associations between immediate temptation and distal goal concepts (Fishbach, Friedman, & Kruglanski, 2003; see also Papies, Stroebe, & Aarts, 2008). Specifically, self-control is enhanced to the extent that the activation of temptation concepts promotes the activation of goal concepts, but the activation of goal concepts does not reciprocally promote activation of temptation concepts. This asymmetrical pattern of associations subordinates the activation of temptations in favor their distal goals when they encounter salient proximal temptations, thus increasing the likelihood of self-control success.

Research not only highlights the operation of asymmetrical temptation–goal associations but also suggests that such operations may occur efficiently and outside of conscious awareness (Fishbach et al., 2003; see also Papies et al., 2008). Fishbach and colleagues (2003), for example, demonstrated that whereas the subliminal presentation of temptation-related concepts (e.g., cake) facilitated the lexical identification of goal-related concepts (e.g., diet), the subliminal presentation of goal-related concepts interfered with the identification of temptation-related concepts. Not only do these asymmetrical associations appear to operate outside of awareness, they also appear to be cognitively efficient: They are evident even when people are under cognitive load. Supporting the functional role of these associations in promoting control are findings that individual differences in these associations reliably distinguish those who report being successful versus unsuccessful in overcoming temptation in favor of their goals. Moreover, exposure to temptation cues can ironically promote rather than impair goal-directed behavior, as would be expected by the operation of these asymmetrical temptation–goal associations. Thus, research has documented the existence of asymmetrical temptation–goal associations as a controlled process that operates efficiently and in the absence of conscious intention and awareness.

Goal-Directed Evaluative Associations

Beyond semantic networks, there also appear to be control processes operating on people's evaluative networks that are automatic in the sense that they operate efficiently. People's attitudes appear to be sensitive to their goals, and these goal-directed changes in evaluation can be detected even on measures that do not require participants to deliberate consciously (i.e., implicit measures). Thus, goal-directed changes in evaluation appear to be supported by processes that require little conscious intention or effort. For example, Ferguson and Bargh (2004) had participants complete an implicit measure of attitudes toward goal relevant objects—namely, an evaluative priming task—either during the active pursuit of a goal or shortly after successful completion of that goal. Those actively pursuing the goal evidenced greater ease of associating positivity to goal-related concepts relative to those who had successfully completed the goal. Note that the parameters of the evaluative priming task that Ferguson and Bargh used—a stimulus-onset asynchrony of less than 350 milliseconds between prime and target—suggest that participants' behavioral responses were not the result of conscious reflection but rather the operation of more cognitively efficient processes. Thus, people's attitudes and evaluations can shift to promote control (i.e., goal-directed structure), yet these processes may still operate in a manner that can be characterized as automatic (see also Fishbach & Shah, 2006).

More recent research suggests that such goal-directed changes in evaluation may occur outside of conscious awareness as well. Fishbach, Zhang, and Trope (2010) presented participants with an evaluative priming task that presented prime stimuli subliminally. Results indicated that participants evaluated goal-directed concepts more positively and goal-undermining concepts (those relevant to short-term temptations to detract from successful goal attainment) more negatively, even when they were consciously unaware of the stimuli they were evaluating. Goal-directed evaluations, then, can also be characterized as processes that are controlled and automatic.

Goal-Directed Early Attention

Even more compelling evidence for processes that are both automatic and controlled comes from psychophysiological experiments examining how goals can modulate even the very earliest levels of attentional processing. Research has suggested that people differentiate own-race and other-race faces within 100–150 milliseconds of stimulus presentation (e.g., Ito & Urland, 2003). Specifically, people appear to allocate greater attentional resources to faces of their own race than to those of other races. Early unsuccessful efforts to modulate this difference in race-based attention has led Ito, Willadsen-Jensen, and Correll (2007, p. 410) to conclude that "automatic attentional allocation cannot be inhibited" except under conditions of perceptual load or during subsequent conscious, effortful processing (e.g., Devine, 1989). Yet more recent research suggests that even these very early attentional processes are malleable and sensitive to one's motivational states. Cunningham, Van Bavel, Arbuckle, Packer, and Waggoner (2012), for example, collected electrophysiological recordings of participants engaged in approach versus avoidance behaviors using a joystick in response to black and white faces. They reasoned that a social target that one approaches is more motivationally relevant than a social target that one avoids, and that this approach behavior would promote individuation rather than processing in terms of category membership (e.g., Neuberg & Fiske, 1987). Replicating past research, when participants were given the goal to avoid black faces and approach white faces, they evidenced early attentional bias as indexed by the P100 component of participants' event-related potential waveforms. Yet adopting the alternative goal to approach black and avoid white faces attenuated this difference in early attention. This suggests that even automatic processes that occur within the first 100–150 milliseconds of encountering a stimulus are sensitive to one's goals and can be considered "controlled."

EVIDENCE THAT ABSTRACTION PROMOTES CONTROL

As noted earlier, our analysis of the alternative meaning of control suggests that abstraction plays a critical role in promoting the creation and maintenance of structure that advances desired ends. Empirical research supports this assertion. Cognitive neuroscience research, for example, highlights the central role of abstraction in cognitive control and working memory (e.g., Badre, 2008; Hazy, Frank, & O'Reilly, 2007; O'Reilly, Noelle, Braver, & Cohen, 2002). Bottom-up processing of inputs is stimulus-driven and may or may not promote a single desired end state. To ensure that these bottom-up inputs are goal-consistent, computational models of cognitive control suggest that areas in the cortex are responsible for the abstraction processes necessary to identify and maintain desired goals. Mechanistically, these cortical areas are hypothesized to promote some cognitive associations preferentially over others. In this way, people are able to maintain cognitive activation patterns that sustain their goals. This promotes two important control functions. First, it maintains goal activation in the absence of direct sensory inputs, allowing one to keep goals in mind even when the immediate environment does not provide concrete cues. Second, it helps facilitate the processing of inputs in a goal-relevant manner. For example, holding in mind the abstract goal to lose weight may preferentially facilitate associations that promote attention to a cake's calorie content at the expense of other associations that might promote processing of its taste (Zelazo & Cunningham, 2007; Fishbach et al., 2003; Fujita & Sasota, 2011; Todd, Cunningham, Anderson, & Thompson, 2012; Fishbach, Zhang, & Trope, 2010). Thus, by biasing some cognitive associations over others, regions of the brain responsible for high-level abstraction promote control by maintaining patterns of cognitive activation that sustain goal-directed processing.

Behavioral research has also suggested that abstraction promotes subordination and structure, and therefore control. Much of this work relies on the technique of priming abstraction as a procedural mindset. Specifically, research suggests that inducing people to engage in cognitive abstraction in one task leads them to use similar abstraction processes to represent subsequent unrelated tasks. For example, having participants generate superordinate category labels rather than subordinate exemplars for a series of 40 disparate objects (e.g., "pet" vs. "poodle" for the target "dog") leads them to be more likely in an unrelated task to identify actions in terms of the superordinate ends achieved rather than by the subordinate behaviors necessary to execute them (e.g., "caring for the environment" vs. "bagging paper, glass, and cans" for the action "recycling"; Fujita, Trope, Liberman, & Levin-Sagi, 2006). Such findings suggest that getting people to engage in abstraction in one task procedurally primes the tendency to use abstraction in later tasks.

Using such procedural priming procedures, Torelli and Kaikati (2009; see also Eyal, Sagristano, Trope, Liberman, & Chaiken, 2009; Giancomantonio, de Dreu, Shalvi, Sligte, & Leder, 2010) demonstrated that when engaged in greater cognitive abstraction, people demonstrate greater *value-behavior consistency,* the correspondence between people's expressed values and their actual behavior. In one study, participants first completed a measure of *universalism*, a value that promotes protecting the welfare of all (Sagiv & Schwartz, 1995). Some time later, following a manipulation of abstraction as described earlier, participants were given an opportunity to participate in a volunteer program designed to provide tutoring for the youth of underserved populations. Inducing abstraction led to greater correspondence between participants' endorsement of universalism and how much time they were willing to volunteer in this tutoring program. This suggests that abstraction helps people align their current judgments, decisions, and behavior in line with their more global values, an indication of enhanced subordination and control.

Research on self-control may be most relevant to documenting the role of abstraction in subordination and control (e.g., Fujita, 2008; Fujita & Carnevale, 2012; Fujita, Trope, & Liberman, 2006; Rachlin, 1995). In a self-control conflict, immediately available rewards tempt people to abandon more distal and more valued ends (Ainslie, 1975; Fujita, 2011; Mischel, Shoda, & Rodriguez, 1989; Strotz, 1955). The conflict is structured such that the two choice options are mutually exclusive. For example, the ability to indulge in eating a piece of chocolate cake now may tempt dieters to sacrifice their more long-term weight-loss goal. As dieters cannot engage in both behaviors simultaneously (eating cake necessitates deviation from one's weight-loss goal), they must choose one option or the other. To maintain control and adherence to the more valued yet imperiled end of weight loss, dieters must subordinate eating chocolate cake in favor of the dieting goal. Research suggests that abstraction enhances this subordination process. For example, inducing cognitive abstraction via the procedural priming procedures described earlier enhanced preferences to eat an apple over a candy in members of a population concerned about watching their weight (i.e., female undergraduate students; Fujita & Han, 2009). This suggests that cognitive abstraction promoted the subordination of the immediate rewards of eating chocolate in favor of the more distal rewards of weight loss. Similarly, abstraction reduces *temporal discounting*, the tendency to prefer smaller yet more immediate rewards in favor of larger yet delayed rewards (Fujita et al., 2006; Malkoc, Zauberman, & Bettman, 2010). Abstraction in this instance appears to have enhanced the ability to subordinate the pursuit of smaller, immediate rewards in favor of larger, delayed rewards.

These behavioral changes in control as a function of abstraction may be supported and sustained by some of the goal-directed automatic processes reviewed earlier, such as asymmetrical temptation–goal associations and goal-directed evaluation associations. That is, abstraction may initiate those goal-directed automatic processes to create and sustain the structure necessary for behavioral control. For example, Fujita and Sasota (2011) manipulated abstraction using the procedural priming techniques described earlier, and found evidence for goal-directed asymmetries in temptation–goal associations only among those who were engaged (vs. not engaged) in abstraction. Similarly, research by Fujita and Han (2009) suggests that abstraction promotes goal-directed evaluative associations, making it easier to associate positivity with goal-promoting stimuli and negativity with goal-undermining stimuli. These data further support the notion that abstraction is a critical component to subordination and control, helping to determine what end to pursue and setting into motion those processes necessary to create and maintain structure around that end.

EFFORTFUL PROCESSING CAN IMPAIR CONTROL

Conflating the two meanings of control that we have distinguished may lead some to conclude that conscious effortful processing is beneficial (particularly when it operates in opposition to "out-of-control" automatic processes). Understanding that control has two distinct meanings, however, leads to an alternative possibility: Conscious, effortful processes may at times impair rather than enhance control. This is especially likely to be the case when effortful processing interferes with the structure and organization created by more automatic processes.

Some evidence for this assertion comes from research examining the effect of effortful processing on preferences and decisions (e.g., Dijksterhuis, 2004; Dijksterhuis, Bos, Nordgren, & van Baaren, 2006; Wilson et al., 1993; Wilson & Schooler, 1991). This work suggests that, under some circumstances, consciously and effortfully working through a decision problem can lead to poorer decisions, whether measured according to some objective criteria or by postdecisional satisfaction. For example, verbalizing one's reasons for choosing one jam over another led research participants to prefer jams that were objectively of lesser quality (Wilson & Schooler, 1991). Similarly, when asked to choose among posters, those who consciously weighed their decision by elaborating reasons why they should select one over the other were later less satisfied with their choice than were those who did not elaborate reasons (Wilson et al., 1993). To the extent that one's goal is to select the best jam or poster, these examples suggest that conscious, effortful processing can impair control. Note, too, that researchers suggest that these phenomena occur because people's effortful processing interferes with the structure that more automatic processes create. Conscious elaboration of a decision problem can lead people to attend and overweight features that are incidental or secondary to the choice (Wilson et al., 1993; Wilson & Schooler, 1991). Similarly, effortful processing may interfere with the integration and abstraction mechanisms set into motion by more automatic processes, making it more difficult to attend to and parse decision information in a goal-directed manner (e.g., Dijksterhuis, 2004). Thus, effortful processes can at times impair control, and this is particularly likely when such processing runs afoul of the structure created by more automatic processes. Such findings further highlight the conceptual independence between conscious effortful processing and control.

REACTIVE VERSUS PROACTIVE CONTROL

That the term *control* has two meanings that are often not distinguished from one another may not only create conceptual confusion but also obstruct research progress, as it carries implicit assumptions about the nature of control as being something that is necessarily slow, effortful, and reactive. That is, influenced by the dual-process and dual-motive automatic versus controlled dichotomies, many researchers have explicitly modeled control as a corrective response that is initiated only after a problem has already begun to develop. By contrast, we might propose that control is not necessarily retroactive, and need not be limited solely to addressing deviations from structured organization as they occur. Instead, we might propose that control can be directed prospectively, with people proactively preparing for anticipated problems and setting up anticipatory mechanisms that address them before they occur. The distinction between retroactive and proactive control is applicable at both cognitive and behavioral levels.

Research on the control of racial bias provides evidence for proactive control at the cognitive level. Much research has shown that racial cues can facilitate the activation of stereotypical associations. For example, exposure to black versus white faces facilitates the identification of objects such as guns versus tools, respectively, presumably because people stereotypically tend to associate lack individuals with guns (e.g., Payne, 2001). Control of this racial bias by nonprejudiced individuals may occur in a reactive manner, as suggested by various dual-process models (e.g., Devine, 1989; Macrae, Bodenhausen, Milne, & Jetten, 1994). Specifically, in performing a sequential priming paradigm in which the presentation of black and white faces immediately precedes the identification of guns and tools, participants may notice the influence of the faces on their responses. Concerned about racial bias, they may engage in corrective attempts to limit this unwanted influence of the primed faces, imposing control during the identification of guns and tools to ensure high accuracy. Noting the initiation of a stereotypical response (misidentifying a tool as a gun following the presentation of a black face), they may attempt to alter this response before it affects their behavior.[4] More recent research, however, has suggested the possibility of proactive mechanisms as well. Rather than engage in corrective control during the presentation of the critical targets (guns vs. tools), electrophysiological recordings suggest that low-prejudice individuals initiate anticipatory or proactive control during the presentation of the primes (black vs. white faces; Amodio, 2010). Rather than inhibit an undesired response after activation, it appears that low-prejudice individuals use the presentation of the prime as a cue that a potential problem may occur and engage in processing to prevent the problematic activation in the first place. This provides some evidence that cognitive control need not be a reactive or corrective process; instead, control can be directed forward in an anticipatory manner.

Like Odysseus, who had himself tied to the mast of his ship so that he could listen to the song of the Sirens without endangering his men, people also engage in a number of behavioral forms of proactive control, structuring and organizing their social environments in ways to promote desired ends. That is, rather than trying to correct and inhibit a response after it has been initiated in a particular context, people adopt a variety of behavioral precommitment or counteractive control strategies to reduce or eliminate their ability to engage in the undesired behavior in the first place. Research suggests, for example, that people will deposit their money into "Christmas club accounts," savings accounts that pay little interest yet entail steep early withdrawal fees (Thaler & Shefrin, 1981). This financially counternormative behavior promotes savings behavior by prospectively making it difficult to withdraw one's money to squander impulsively. Similarly, people will make "side bets" with themselves, imposing penalties for goal-inconsistent behavior (e.g., Ainslie, 1975; Trope & Fishbach, 2000). For example, when faced with the prospect of a diagnostic yet uncomfortable health assessment, people will willingly impose steeper cancellation fees to motivate successful completion of the assessment (e.g., Trope & Fishbach, 2000). They will similarly engineer their environments to reward themselves when they have successfully engaged in goal-directed behavior. When given a choice between being paid before or after a diagnostic yet uncomfortable health assessment, people prefer to be paid after in order to make payment contingent on (and thus provide greater motivation for) successful completion of the assessment (e.g., Trope & Fishbach, 2000). Moreover, people will restrict exposure to and availability of goal-undermining alternatives. For example, smokers will purchase cigarettes by the pack rather by cheaper bulk cartons to limit the ability to smoke freely (Wertenbroch, 1998). Learning to implement these behavioral forms of proactive control appears to explain age-related differences in delay of gratification. Whereas 4-year-old children mistakenly believe that exposure to goal-undermining temptation promotes control, 7- and 8-year-old children understand that occluding or removing these cues is a more effective goal-promoting strategy (e.g., Mischel & Mischel, 1983). Thus, research suggests that control need not be a reaction to an undesired response to an environmental stimulus. Instead, people can anticipate these situations and take proactive steps to create social environments that prevent disruption of goal-directed behavior.

We discussed earlier the role of abstraction in control, and how promoting abstraction promotes not only promotes goal-consistent behavior but also automatic forms of controlled processing (namely, asymmetrical temptation–goal associations and goal-directed evaluative associations). We might add here that research also highlights the role of abstraction in proactive forms of control. Specifically, research suggests that inducing abstraction promotes the likelihood that people will adopt strategies such as self-imposed punishment to forestall the possibility of future goal failures (Fujita & Roberts, 2010). In one study, for example, participants were presented an opportunity to participate in a psychology study that would assess their cognitive skills at night. They were led to believe that this feedback would be diagnostic and useful, yet assessing these skills would entail uncomfortable procedures (i.e., appearing for the study in the middle of the night). Participants were asked how much they would pay as a cancellation fee if they failed to appear for their scheduled session. Those induced to engage in abstraction via a procedural priming manipulation similar to the ones discussed earlier were willing to pay 50% more in cancellation fees, presumably as a deterrent to failing to appear. Thus, abstraction appears to promote both automatic and proactive forms of control.

Although earlier we reviewed examples of proactive control, we note that the overwhelming emphasis on control in psychology has focused on corrective or reactive mechanisms. We might speculate that such lack of attention to proactive forms of control in psychology may have resulted from the underlying assumptions that control must be the opposite of automatic. That is, to the extent that controlled processing is slower and more effortful than automatic processing, one might reasonably assume that control must be a reaction to undesired situations prompted by automatic processes. We might instead suggest that it is time to question this assumption that control is necessarily a reaction to automatic processing, and instead recognize that there are two meanings to the term *control.* Researchers must appreciate that some forms of control are not only automatic but also proactive.

SUMMARY AND CONCLUSIONS

In this chapter, we have examined what is meant by the term *control* and explored the implications of this conceptual analysis for our understanding of the distinction between automatic versus controlled. We have suggested that there are two meanings to the term *control.* One meaning highlights the absence of features that are emblematic of automatic processes: lack of conscious intention, lack of conscious awareness, inability to be disrupted, and cognitive efficiency. A second meaning ignores whether a process is automatic or not and instead focuses on the degree to which a process sustains and promotes structured goal pursuit. To have control, thoughts, feelings, and behaviors must be prioritized and organized around desired ends. Therefore, the target of analysis from the perspective of this second meaning of *control* is not the conditions under which a process operates, but rather the relationship of that process to others around it. A process can be considered controlled to the extent that it promotes and operates within this top-down structure to promote a given goal.

We have argued that abstraction promotes the creation and maintenance of this structure, helping to identify those ends around which processing must be organized. Abstraction may also help to detect processing that deviates from this structured organization, and to activate the subordination processes necessary to promote or foreground goal-directed over goal-irrelevant processing. To understand control as structured goal pursuit, then, we suggest that more needs to be understood about the mechanisms of abstraction and its role in structuring thought, feeling, and behavior to promote the attainment of desired ends.

We might further suggest that whether a process is automatic or not may at times be irrelevant to understanding control. At minimum, researchers need to take greater care in distinguishing and explicitly explaining the meaning of the term to which they are referring. We, however, might go a step further and recommend that researchers abandon altogether the use of the term *control* when referring to processes that are not automatic. Greater clarity might be gained instead by labeling the opposite of *automatic* as *not automatic.* This would allow researchers to reserve the term *control* to refer to structured goal pursuit and prevent any potential conceptual confusion. Thus, we argue that rather than representing two extremes of a dichotomy, the labels "automatic" and "controlled" should be conceptualized as independent concepts. The opposite of *control* is not *automatic,* but rather *lack of control* or *out of control.* Similarly, the opposite of *automatic* is not *control,* but rather *not automatic.* Although to some this may seem like semantic squabbling, we have highlighted in this chapter some of the conceptual confusion and erroneous conclusions that semantics can create.

Although we have reviewed supporting evidence for independence of the two meanings of control, we recognize that more work is needed to appreciate control more fully as structured goal pursuit. We hope researchers will follow our lead and question whether the latent assumptions that underlie the distinction between automatic and controlled processing are necessary, appreciating instead that control is a phenomenon independent of automaticity. We look forward to the insights that future research may have with this heightened conceptual clarity.

NOTES

1. We use the term *goal* to describe the desired end state to which thoughts, feelings, and behavior are directed. Goals do not necessarily need to be adopted consciously, nor do people need to be consciously aware that they are pursuing a particular end state (for reviews, see Bargh, 1990; McClelland, Koestner, & Weinberger, 1989; Schultheiss & Brunstein, 2010). Moreover, what goal people are pursuing in a given situation may shift dynamically, as we detail in the next section.
2. An important point is that although enhanced control via structure may promote goal pursuit, it says nothing about the worthiness of the goal being pursued. People may pursue harmful or dangerous goals with great con-

trol. Whether a goal is worthy of attainment is independent of the efficiency and efficacy of the goal pursuit (i.e., issues of control).

3. We note that implementation intentions do not universally promote control. Under some conditions (i.e., negation of an undesired behavior), implementation intentions may impair rather than promote control (e.g., Adriaanse, van Oosten, de Ridder, de Wit, & Catharine Evers, 2011).
4. Parenthetically, although research suggests that people attempt to control biased responses through reactive control, some attempts may ironically enhance the biased responses (e.g., Payne, Lambert, & Jacoby, 2002).

REFERENCES

Achtziger, A., Gollwitzer, P. M., & Sheeran, P. (2008). Implementation intentions and shielding goal striving from unwanted thoughts and feelings. *Personality and Social Psychology Bulletin, 34*, 381–393.

Adriaanse, M. A., van Oosten, J. M. F., de Ridder, D. T. D., de Wit, J. B. F., & Evers, C. (2011). Planning what not to eat: Ironic effects of implementation intentions negating unhealthy habits. *Personality and Social Psychology Bulletin, 37*, 69–81.

Ainslie, G. (1975). Specious reward: A behavioral theory of impulsiveness and impulse control. *Psychological Bulletin, 82*, 463–496.

Amodio, D. M. (2010). Coordinated roles of motivation and perception in the regulation of intergroup responses: Frontal cortical asymmetry effects on the P2 event-related potential and behavior. *Journal of Cognitive Neuroscience, 22*, 2609–2617.

Badre, D. (2008). Cognitive control, hierarchy, and the rostro-caudal organization of the frontal lobes. *Trends in Cognitive Sciences, 12(5)*, 193–220.

Bargh, J. A. (1990). Auto-motives: Preconscious determinants of social interaction. In E. T. Higgins & R. M. Sorrentino (Eds.), *Handbook of motivation and cognition: Foundations of social behavior* (Vol. 2, pp. 93–130). New York: Guilford Press.

Bargh, J. A. (1994). The four horsemen of automaticity: Awareness, intention, efficiency, and control in social cognition. In R. S. Wyer & T. K. Srull (Eds.), *Handbook of social cognition* (2nd ed., pp. 1–40). Hillsdale, NJ: Erlbaum.

Bargh, J. A. (1996). Principles of automaticity. In E. T. Higgins & A. Kruglanski (Eds.), *Social psychology: Handbook of basic principles* (pp. 169–183). New York: Guilford Press.

Bargh, J. A., & Chartrand, T. L. (1999). The unbearable automaticity of being. *American Psychologist, 54*, 462–479.

Bayer, U. C., Achtziger, A., Gollwitzer, P. M., & Moskowitz, G. (2009). Responding to subliminal cues: Do if-then plans facilitate action preparation and initiation without conscious intent? *Social Cognition, 27*, 183–201.

Bayer, U. C., Gollwitzer, P. M., & Achtziger, A. (2010). Staying on track: Planned goal striving is protected from disruptive internal states. *Journal of Experimental Social Psychology, 46*, 505–514.

Brandstätter, V., Lengfelder, A., & Gollwitzer, P. M. (2001). Implementation intentions and efficient action initiation. *Journal of Personality and Social Psychology, 81*, 946–960.

Carver, C. S., & Scheier, M. F. (1982). Control theory: A useful conceptual framework for personality–social, clinical, and health psychology. *Psychological Bulletin, 92*(1), 111–135.

Carver, C. S., & Scheier, M. F. (1990). Origins and functions of positive and negative affect: A control-process view. *Psychological Review, 97*(1), 19–35.

Cohen, A.-L., Bayer, U. C., Jaudas, A., & Gollwitzer, P. M. (2008). Self-regulatory strategy and executive control: Implementation intentions modulate task switching and Simon task performance. *Psychological Research, 72*, 12–26.

Cunningham, W. A., Van Bavel, J. J., Arbuckle, N. L., Packer, D. J., & Waggoner, A. S. (2012). Rapid social perception is flexible: Approach and avoidance motivational states shape P100 responses to other-race faces. *Frontiers in Human Neuroscience, 6*, 1–7.

Devine, P. G. (1989). Stereotypes and prejudice: Their automatic and controlled components. *Journal of Personality and Social Psychology, 56*, 5–18.

Dijksterhuis, A. (2004). Think different: The merits of unconscious thought in preference development and decision-making. *Journal of Personality and Social Psychology, 87*, 586–598.

Dijksterhuis, A., Bos, M. W., Nordgren, L. F. & van Baaren, R. B. (2006). On making the right choice: The deliberation-without-attention effect. *Science, 311*, 1005–1007.

Eyal, T., Sagristano, M. D., Trope, Y., Liberman, N., & Chaiken, S. (2009). When values matter: Expressing values in behavioral intentions for the near vs. distant future. *Journal of Experimental Social Psychology, 45*, 35–43.

Ferguson, M. J., & Bargh, J. A. (2004). Liking is for doing: The effects of goal pursuit on automatic evaluation. *Journal of Personality and Social Psychology, 87*, 557–572.

Fishbach, A., Friedman, R. S., & Kruglanski, A. W. (2003). Leading us not into temptation: Momentary allurements elicit overriding goal activation. *Journal of Personality and Social Psychology, 84*, 296–309.

Fishbach, A., & Shah, J. Y. (2006). Self-control in action: Implicit dispositions toward goals and away from temptations. *Journal of Personality and Social Psychology, 90*(5), 820–832.

Fishbach, A., Zhang, Y., & Trope, Y. (2010). Counteractive evaluation: Asymmetric shifts in the implicit value of conflicting motivations. *Journal of Experimental Social Psychology, 46*, 29–38.

Fujita, K. (2011). On conceptualizing self-control as more than the effortful inhibition of impulses. *Personality and Social Psychology Review, 15*, 352–366.

Fujita, K. (2008). Seeing the forest beyond the trees: A construal-level approach to self-control. *Social and Personality Psychology Compass, 2*, 1475–1496.

Fujita, K., & Carnevale, J. J. (2012). Transcending temptation through abstraction: The role of construal level in self-control. *Current Directions in Psychological Science, 21*, 248–252.

Fujita, K., & Han, H. A. (2009). Moving beyond deliberative control of impulses: The effect of construal levels on evaluative associations in self-control conflicts. *Psychological Science, 20*, 799–804.

Fujita, K., & Roberts, J. C. (2010). Promoting prospective self-control through abstraction. *Journal of Experimental Social Psychology, 46*, 1049–1054.

Fujita, K., & Sasota, J. A. (2011). The effect of construal levels on asymmetric temptation–goal cognitive associations. *Social Cognition, 29*, 125–146.

Fujita, K., Trope, Y., & Liberman, N. (2006). The role of mental construal in self-control. In D. DeCremer, M. Zeelenberg, & J. K. Murnighan (Eds.), *Social psychology and economics* (pp. 193–211). New York: Sage.

Fujita, K., Trope, Y., Liberman, N., & Levin-Sagi, M. (2006). Construal levels and self-control. *Journal of Personality and Social Psychology, 90*, 351–367.

Giancomantonio, M., de Dreu, C. K. W., Shalvi, S., Sligte, D., & Leder, S. (2010). Psychological distance boosts value–behavior correspondence in ultimatum bargaining and integrative negotiation. *Journal of Experimental Social Psychology, 16*, 824–829.

Gollwitzer, P. M. (1999). Implementation intentions: Strong effects of simple plans. *American Psychologist, 54*, 493–503.

Gollwitzer, P. M., & Brandstätter, V. (1997). Implementation intentions and effective goal pursuit. *Journal of Personality and Social Psychology, 73*, 186–199.

Hazy, T. E., Frank, M. J., & O'Reilly, R. C. (2007). Toward an executive without a homunculus: Computational models of the prefrontal cortex/basal ganglia system. *Philosophical Transactions of the Royal Society B: Biological Sciences, 362*, 1601–1613.

Hebb, D. O. (1949). *The organization of behaviour.* Hoboken, NJ: Wiley.

Ito, T. A., & Urland, G. R. (2003). Race and gender on the brain: Electrocortical measures of attention to the race and gender of multiply categorizable individuals. *Journal of Personality and Social Psychology, 85*, 616–626.

Ito, T. A., Willadsen-Jensen, E. C., & Correll, J. (2007). Social neuroscience and social perception: New perspectives on categorization, prejudice, and stereotyping. In E. Harmon-Jones & P. Winkielman (Eds.), *Social neuroscience: Integrating biological and psychological explanations of social behavior* (pp. 401–421). New York: Guilford Press.

Kruglanski, A. W., Shah, J. Y., Fishbach, A., Friedman, R., Chun, W. Y., & Sleeth-Keppler, D. (2002). *Advances in experimental social psychology: Vol. 34. A theory of goal systems* (pp. 331–378). San Diego: Academic Press.

Macrae, C. N., Bodenhausen, G. V., Milne, A. B., & Jetten, J. (1994). Out of mind but back in sight: Stereotypes on the rebound. *Journal of Personality and Social Psychology, 67*, 808–817.

Malkoc, S., Zauberman, G., & Bettman, J. (2010). Unstuck from the concrete: Carryover effects of abstract mindsets in intertemporal preferences. *Organization Behavior and Human Decision Processes, 113*, 112–126.

Malkoc, S. A., Zauberman, G., & Ulu, C. (2005). Consuming now or later? The interactive effect of timing and attribute alignability. *Psychological Science, 16*(5), 411–417

McClelland, D. C., Koestner, R., & Weinberger, J. (1989). How do self-attributed and implicit motives differ? *Psychological Review, 96*, 690–702.

McCulloch, K. C., Aarts, H., Fujita, K., & Bargh, J. A. (2008). Inhibition in goal systems: A retrieval-induced forgetting account. *Journal of Experimental Social Psychology, 44*, 857–865.

Mischel, H. N., & Mischel, W. (1983). The development of children's knowledge of self-control strategies. *Child Development, 54*, 603–619.

Mischel, W., Shoda, Y., & Rodriguez, M. L. (1989). Delay of gratification in children. *Science, 244*, 933–938.

Neuberg, S. L., & Fiske, S. T. (1987). Motivational influences on impression formation: Outcome dependency, accuracy-driven attention, and individuating processes. *Journal of Personality and Social Psychology, 53*, 431–444.

O'Reilly, R. C., Noelle, D. C., Braver, T. S., & Cohen, J. D. (2002). Prefrontal cortex and dynamic categorization tasks: Representational organization and neuromodulatory control. *Cerebral Cortex, 12*, 246–257.

Papies, E., Stroebe, W., & Aarts, H. (2008). Healthy cognition: Processes of self-regulatory success in restrained eating. *Personality and Social Psychology Bulletin, 34*, 1290–1300.

Payne, B. K. (2001). Prejudice and perception: The role of automatic and controlled processes in misperceiving a weapon. *Journal of Personality and Social Psychology, 81*(2), 181–192.

Payne, B. K., Lambert, A. J., & Jacoby, L. L. (2002). Best laid plans: Effects of goals on accessibility bias and cognitive control in race-based misperceptions of weapons. *Journal of Experimental Social Psychology, 38*, 384–396.

Rachlin, H. (1995). Self control: Beyond commitment. *Behavior and Brain Sciences, 18*, 109–159.

Sagiv, L., & Schwartz, S. H. (1995). Value priorities and readiness for out-group social contact. *Journal of Personality and Social Psychology, 69*, 437–448.

Schultheiss, O. C., & Brunstein, J. C. (2010). *Implicit motives*. New York: Oxford University Press.

Schweiger Gallo, I., Keil, A., McCulloch, K. C., Rockstroh, B., & Gollwitzer, P. M. (2009). Strategic automation of emotion regulation. *Journal of Personality and Social Psychology, 96*, 11–31.

Shah, J. Y., Friedman, R., & Kruglanski, A. W. (2002). Forgetting all else: On the antecedents and consequences of goal shielding. *Journal of Personality and Social Psychology, 83*, 1261–1280.

Shannon, C. E., & Weaver, W. (1949). *The mathematical theory of communication*. Urbana: University of Illinois Press.

Strotz, R. H. (1955). Myopia and inconsistency in dynamic utility maximization. *The Review of Economic Studies, 23*, 165–180.

Thaler, R. H., & Shefrin, H. M. (1981). An economic theory of self-control. *Journal of Political Economy, 89*, 392–406.

Todd, R. M., Cunningham, W. A., Anderson, A. K., & Thompson, E. (2012). Affect-biased attention as emotion regulation. *Trends in Cognitive Sciences, 16*, 365–372.

Torelli, C. J., & Kaikati, A. M. (2009). Values as predictors of judgments and behaviors: The role of abstract and concrete mindsets. *Journal of Personality and Social Psychology, 96*, 231–247.

Trope, Y., & Fishbach, A. (2000). Counteractive self-control in overcoming temptation. *Journal of Personality and Social Psychology, 79*, 493–506.

Wegner, D. M., & Bargh, J. A. (1998). Control and automaticity in social life. In D. Gilbert, S. Fiske, & G. Lindzey (Eds.), *Handbook of social psychology* (4th ed., pp. 446–496). Boston: McGraw-Hill.

Wertenbroch, K. (1998). Consumption self-control by rationing purchase quantities of virtue and vice. *Marketing Science, 17*, 317–337.

Wilson, T. D., Lisle, D. J., Schooler, J. W., Hodges, S. D., Klaaren, K. J., & LaFleur, S. J. (1993). Introspecting about reasons can reduce post-choice satisfaction. *Personality and Social Psychology Bulletin, 19*, 331–359.

Wilson, T. D., & Schooler, J. W. (1991). Thinking too much: Introspection can reduce the quality of preferences and decision. *Journal of Personality and Social Psychology*, 60, 181–192.

Zelazo, P. D., & Cunningham, W. A. (2007). Executive function: Mechanisms underlying emotion regulation. In J. J. Gross (Ed.), *Handbook of emotion regulation* (pp. 135–158). New York: Guilford Press.

PART II

DUAL-SYSTEMS MODELS

CHAPTER 5

Two Systems of Reasoning

An Update

Steven Sloman

In 1996, I published a paper in which I argued that *high-level cognition*—reasoning, categorization, judgment, and decision making—involves the interaction of two systems that are distinct in terms of their operating principles, their representations and processes, and their sources of information (Sloman, 1996). Many theorists before me had proposed dual systems (e.g., James, 1890/1950; Freud, 1913) and others made related proposals at about the same time (Epstein, 1994; Evans & Over, 1996; Stanovich & West, 2000). A lot of relevant research has been done since then. I still believe that the evidence suggests that the mind consists of two systems, although my view of the systems and their interaction has changed in the intervening years. In this chapter, I recount the developments that suggest revisions to my earlier view and offer an updated framework. To foreshadow, my view of the intuitive system has evolved: It is now apparent, on one hand, that it is capable of sophisticated causal reasoning and, on the other, that its processing supports and is influenced by certain affective, somatic states. I have also revised my conception of how the systems interact at the lowest level: Deliberation attenuates intuitive processing via a leaky inhibitory mechanism.

In my 1996 paper I labeled one system "associative," because I claimed that it operated on the basis of similarity and contiguity; it represented statistical structure of one kind or another, the currency of all associative models; and its processing involved relatively fast spreading of activation along associative pathways. It was well known at the time that associative processing could be highly sophisticated, that associative machinery could engage in complex pattern recognition and pattern completion (Rumelhart & McClelland, 1986). So I considered the associative system the workhorse of everyday cognition. A hallmark example of associative thought is identifying the affordances associated with an object (e.g., using a lamppost to lean on), what is really a form of categorization, an extremely sophisticated ability that depends on a variety of tacit knowledge. Yet it is a skill beyond the capabilities of the most modern artificial intelligence that people take advantage of thousands of times per day in a blink of an eye, generally with no perceived effort.

The second system, the "rule-based" system, I considered more specialized. It was intended to capture the fact that a substantial portion of thought has certain attributes in common with those of a traditional computer: It is sequential and therefore slower than associative thought, and also abstract and symbolic. The form of thought I described enforces strict constraints on how we manipulate mental symbols and draw conclusions, the kind of constraints that come with well-defined procedures or algorithms. A canonical example of this kind of processing is long division, a skill I retain, although implementing it involves multiple steps of applying rules to transform symbols. It takes time and, in my case, a huge amount of effort. Other examples include forms of categorization that require deliberation, such as deciding on the legal status of a harmful act.

The dual systems I proposed were never simply between conscious and unconscious thought. The products of both systems are available to conscious introspection; they differ in whether the process is also open. Here is how I expressed it then:

> When a response is produced solely by the associative system, a person is conscious only of the result of the computation, not the process. Consider an anagram such as *involnutray* for which the correct answer likely pops to mind associatively (involuntary). The result is accessible, but the process is not. In contrast, a person is aware of both the result and the process in a rule-based computation. Consider a harder anagram such as *uersoippv*. If you figured out the answer (purposive), and even if you did not, you likely applied various rules (like put different letters in the first position) which were consciously accessible. If you did get the answer, you were aware not only of the process but also of the result. (Sloman, 1996, p. 6)

Neither was the distinction between rational and irrational processes. Rule-based thought can lead to rational conclusions—conclusions justified by a normative system—as it does when a long division problem is solved correctly. But it can also lead to irrational conclusions when the wrong set of rules is systematically applied. For instance, it is irrational to use long division as a method to determine the sum of two numbers. Similarly, intuitive thought can be rational (it usually is), as exemplified by its use to identify what is food and what is not food at the dinner table. And, of course, numerous instances exist of irrationality arising from intuition, such as the conjunction fallacy and many other cognitive illusions.

NEW DEVELOPMENTS

Since 1996, issues and problems with dual-systems formulations have emerged. These include the labels used to make the distinction, whether the use of rules is limited to a single system, the number of systems, the role of affect, whether intuition represents causal structure, and how the systems interact. I discuss each in turn.

Proliferation of Terms

Stanovich and West's (2000) review of dual-system theories pointed out that dual systems had been proposed under many labels (associative–rule-based, tacit–explicit thought, implicit–explicit, experiential–rational, intuitive–analytical, etc.). This led them to conclude that the safest route is to refer to the systems as System 1 (including my associative system) and System 2 (including my rule-based system). The appeal of generic terms is that they do not require a commitment to a particular theoretical view. This nomenclature became standard when it was adopted by Kahneman and Frederick (2002) in their highly influential paper.

I find these labels not only unhelpful but also misleading. They are unhelpful because they are not descriptive; they say nothing about the function or role of the systems, relying instead on the audience's fallible memory to achieve reference. They are misleading if taken as a generic description of all dual-systems theories in that they imply a single distinction when, in fact, different theorists have made different (if related) distinctions (as noted by, for instance, Evans, 2009, and Stanovich, 2011).

While I believe there are good reasons to abandon the terms *associative* and *rule-based,* I also believe there are perfectly good English words that capture the common essence of the dual-systems distinction without requiring strong theoretical commitments: *intuition* and *deliberation*. These terms do require some commitment because, in English, an intuition is a thought whose source one is not conscious of, and deliberation involves sequential consideration of symbolic strings in some form. To be a viable theoretical framework, dual-systems theory must require some commitment.

And the distinction between intuition and deliberation is precisely the minimum commitment the theory requires. I therefore use these terms in what follows to refer to the dual-systems theory that I now consider most valid.

Intuitive Rules

Osman and Stavy (2006) review abundant evidence that some rules in science and mathematics are deployed intuitively. Heuristic rules such as "if one thing is bigger than another on one dimension, then it is bigger on a second dimension," are available to relatively young children and likely responsible for the conservation biases discussed by Piaget and Inhelder (1974). Based primarily on earlier work by Stavy (reviewed in Stavy & Tirosh, 2000), Osman and Stavy (2006) argue that such rules are applied rapidly and independently of problem solvers' goals. They are also counternormative and hence not learned in school. It takes years for students to gain the insight required to see the errors they produce. They are rules in the sense that they are abstract and analytic. But they do not appear to be objects of deliberation; they share key properties with other intuitive objects. They are elicited in context-specific ways that depend on the focus of attention and the existence of competing rules. The existence of such rules is a reason not to describe either system as *rule-based,* because the term does not distinguish the deliberative and intuitive systems in a clear way. They suggest that intuitions are not always driven by gross superficial similarity but can involve relatively abstract relations.

Proliferation of Systems

Some have argued that—while the deliberative–intuitive distinction is sensible and plausible—two systems are not enough. This argument comes in two forms. One view is hierarchical: Each system should be broken down into subsystems (especially intuition; see Evans [2009] or Stanovich [2004, 2011], who substitutes the "autonomous set of systems" for System 1). I do not see this as a winning strategy for understanding the architecture of cognition. To be a "system," a set of cognitive processes and representations must have some individual autonomy; they must operate and compute independently enough that they can be held responsible for critical aspects of behavior. While there has been much discussion of the modules responsible for thought (Fodor, 1983), few would argue that intuition and deliberation can be divided up into truly autonomous systems.

A more likely possibility is that the components of intuition are not systems but rather elemental processes (e.g., Newell & Simon, 1972) that operate through interaction with one another to achieve an intuitive output synergistically. And, in fact, this is where Stanovich (2011) ends up, arguing that System 1 does not refer to a single system in the brain but rather to a set of autonomous processes (see also Evans, 2009). Thus, he now prefers the terms Type 1 and 2 processing rather than the language of systems. For instance, he classifies elicitation of a conditioned response as a Type 1 process, because it is autonomous in the sense that its execution is mandatory given that its triggering condition has been encountered and it does not depend on input from high-level control systems.

I believe these theorists are casting their nets too wide. The vast majority of what goes on in the body and the brain meet this defintion of Type 1 processing including (say) laughing when being tickled. This is not necessarily a behavior that a theory of high-level cognition needs to explain.

Another argument in favor of the proliferation of systems is that a third reflective system is needed to examine the output of intuition and deliberation, weigh them, and decide what to do: to respond intuitively or deliberatively when the systems provide conflicting responses, or opt to continue reasoning (Stanovich, 2011). There is no doubt that a decision process to determine which response to emit must be present, and that individuals differ in whether they tend to appeal to intuition or deliberation (Frederick, 2005). But that decision process does not require its own hardware. It could be implemented via simple propensities to rely on one or the other system, through some form of winner-take-all strategy that depends on the relative strengths of the systems' outputs along with mutual inhibition, or the decision process could be implemented within the deliberative system, or through some combination of these mechanisms.

The Importance of Affect

I have focused on dual systems as supporting two different kinds of cognition, deliberation versus intuition. Much of the evidential base for this distinction comes from work on reasoning and other high-level tasks. But some dual-system theories, especially those focused on risk perception and decision making, make a different distinction, between deliberation and affect (Epstein, 1994; Slovic, Finucane, Peters, & MacGregor, 2007). Since Freud's (1913) discussion of primary process thought, it has been apparent that unconscious mental processes are affectively laden in the sense of being associated with valence and arousal. The "gut feeling" associated with intuition can manifest amorphously as generalized anxiety, or an affective state can be appraised cognitively and be classified as an emotion such as fear, disgust (LeDoux, 1996), or craving. Deliberative processes are associated with their own range of emotions, including regret and frustration.

The importance of affect has been discussed most carefully with regard to moral judgment. Haidt (2001, 2012) argues that deliberation can at best serve as a corrective on judgments that are determined by affective reactions. Relatedly, Prinz (2007) claims that emotions are necessary and sufficient for moral judgment. Nichols (2008) offers a richer view positing that people apply a normative theory to their affective reactions to determine what is and is not moral. Although there is some controversy about the role of disgust in moral judgment (cf. Pizarro, Inbar, & Helion, 2011), there is some consensus that affective responses play a significant role in most individual moral reactions (e.g., Hutcherson & Gross, 2011).

It is not terribly controversial to say that emotional responses incorporate a cognitive component (Lazarus, 1984). What we feel is somehow bound to what we are thinking, either because cognitive construal determines physiological responses or because physiology elicits a cognitive appraisal, or both. I propose that the cognitive component in this case is almost always intuitive, not deliberative. The kind of cognitive appraisal that is associated with our physiological responses is automatic and outside conscious awareness, not a sequential, deliberative act. It is indeed cognitive, as Lazarus argues, but it is only under special circumstances that most people deliberate about the nature of their feelings (e.g., psychotherapy). So a complete theory of the systems involved in human thought will need to include both a deliberative component on one hand and an affective component that is tied to our intuitions on the other.

Causal Structure in Intuition

In my 1996 paper I argued that the intuitive system is purely associative and that causal reasoning is a matter of deliberation. What I meant was that intuitions are based on some sort of co-occurrence information ("statistical structure"), not on an analysis of any other kind of logical structure. Causal reasoning does depend on a different kind of structure (see Pearl [2000] for a thorough analysis and Sloman [2005] for an introduction to those concepts). For instance, a simple correlation between two variables, *A* and *B* can reflect an infinite number of causal structures (*A* causes *B*, *B* causes *A*, *C* causes *A* and *B*, *C* causes *D*, which causes *A*, and *C* causes B, etc.). And to say "A causes *B*" is to say more than "*A* predicts *B*"; it is also to say, all else being equal, an intervention that makes a sufficiently large change to the value of *A* will also change the value of *B* (Woodward, 2003). This could be true of an associative relation, but not necessarily as associations have been defined in a variety of ways. I might associate knife and fork, but removing my knife does not affect the presence of my fork. So causal reasoning is not merely associative but implies logical elements such as support for intervention, as well as diagnostic reasoning.

I now believe that I was wrong that intuition does not represent causal structure. There are several forms of evidence that it does. For instance, we use causal structure when we resolve pronouns. Consider the following two sentences:

Steven admires Daniel because he is so candid.

Steven annoys Daniel because he is so candid.

The sentences have identical syntax; indeed they differ by only one word. Yet in the first sentence, "he" refers to Daniel and in the second, to Steven. And any native English speaker knows this immediately and automatically. The best evidence (Rudolph & Försterling, 1997) is that "he" refers to the causal agent and that the sentences differ in whether the causal agent is the subject of the main clause (Steven) or the object (Daniel). In both cases, "he" causes the state described by the main verb, Daniel is the cause of admiration, but Steven is the cause of annoyance. This suggests that causal structure is buried deep in our processing systems.

A second example was inspired by Meek and Glymour (1994): Having yellow teeth is correlated with lung cancer. Therefore, you should whiten your teeth to lower the probability of getting lung cancer. True or false? Obviously this is false, and we know it immediately and automatically (Hagmayer & Sloman [2009] offer experimental data). Yet the conclusion rests on quite a sophisticated causal analysis, one that distinguishes observation from intervention. If you observed someone with white teeth, that person would be less likely to get lung cancer than someone you observed with yellow teeth, because the first person is less likely to be a smoker. But the act of whitening your teeth is an intervention, and it renders the color of your teeth independent of whether or not you smoke (Spirtes, Glymour, & Scheines, 1993). So there is no advantage to whitening. This is a lot of causal analysis, and it all seems to take place intuitively.

More evidence that intuition is sensitive to causal structure comes from cases of experts making decisions in the context of complex causal systems (e.g., Klein, 1998). A doctor, mechanic, or electrician who can quickly and accurately diagnose and treat a problem within his or her field of expertise must be using more than correlational information, because the conclusions he or she comes to often require causal analysis of the specific problem at hand. Data suggest that experienced physicians are intutive in their decision making, generally failing to use causal knowledge (Patel & Kaufman, 2000) except in difficult cases (Norman, Trott, Brooks, & Smith, 1994). But those intuitions have to take advantage of causal structure in order to be effective. Medical students must have more conscious access to pathophysiology as they recently learned it and they have no other basis to make decisions, and experienced physicians must have access in the sense that causal structure has to inform their assessments even if they cannot express it explicitly.

We are all experts in this sense with regard to moral judgments. We immediately and automatically classify some actions as immoral in a way that depends on an analysis of causal antecedents such as intention and causal consequences such as harm (e.g., Sloman, Fernbach, & Ewing, 2009).

Even apparent violations of causal logic imply that intuition is sensitive to causal structure. Our hesitation to tempt fate (Risen & Gilovich, 2008) depends on (magical) causal beliefs about how actions lead to consequences (Swirsky, Fernbach, & Sloman, 2011). Our willingness to deceive ourselves by acting in a way that produces self-serving evidence (Quattrone & Tversky, 1984) depends on an understanding of how our personal characteristics are causally related to performance (Sloman, Fernbach, & Hagmayer, 2010). For instance, to the extent that we deceive ourselves that we exercise to be healthy when in fact we do it to improve our appearance, we require a causal model specifying that exercise improves health and appearance. Similarly, we suffer from "illusory correlations" (Chapman & Chapman, 1969), beliefs that variables are correlated when in fact they are independent (e.g., that paranoid people are more likely to see eyes in abstract drawings). These illusory beliefs rest on prior causal commitments (e.g., that watching somebody is a prerequisite to judging or hurting them).

The apparent evidence against the presence of causal structure in intuition is not compelling. We do learn correlations among arbitrary variables implicitly (Seger, 1994). But that implicit knowledge could be structured causally.

How the Systems Cooperate

All dual-system theorists suppose that the two systems cooperate to perform most tasks. One critical form of cooperation occurs at an exclusively functional level. Since the era of Newell and Simon (1972), it has been clear that solving insight problems involves the following cycle:

1. A representation of a problem space is formed.
2. The representation is examined to see if a solution falls out.
3. If it does, the problem is solved.
4. If it does not, go back to Step 1.

Indeed, much of thought can be described this way. For instance, making a decision involves finding a representation that affords a satisfactory comparison among options. Once the correct representation is found, the most preferred option falls out. Similarly, object categorization involves choosing a representation of the object that highlights the attributes of the object that are most relevant for current purposes. Once this representation is available, the category is obvious: It is the set of objects with the relevant attributes.

Whenever the cognitive act (problem solving, decision making, etc.) is novel, so that the required representation in Step 1 is not immediately available, constructing that representation is an act of deliberation. Only through deliberation can we do the analysis required to extract a set of relevant features and construct a symbolic structure out of them. Step 2, on the other hand, involves pattern recognition and pattern completion. It demands precisely the strengths of intuition. So the cycle described earlier is essentially a cycle of deliberation followed by intuition. This could well be the two systems' primary form of functional interaction.

Does Deliberation Dominate?

In 1996, I proposed that whenever people have access to both an intuitive and deliberative response, they go with the deliberative one; deliberation dominates. Under certain conditions, this must be right. If intuition says that the cashier owes you about $11 in change but you deliberate by doing some arithmetic and determine you are owed $10, then presumably you will only demand $10 back. More generally, when the deliberative response is compelling and the conflicting intuitive one can be ignored with little personal cost, the deliberative response will dominate.

But it does not always. For instance, people are unwilling to tempt fate even in the face of conscious beliefs that the actions could not have the feared consequence. For instance, people will avoid wearing a Stanford sweatshirt if they have applied to Stanford and not yet heard the result (Risen & Gilovich, 2008), though they do not actually believe that wearing a sweatshirt will affect their likelihood of admittance. The willingness to let an intuition that is obviously faulty dominate decision making may be licensed in this case by the fact that the negative consequences of doing so are negligible. After all, our intuitions can be vehement spokespeople for their cause and not easily ignored. Even in fairly open-and-shut cases such as the conjunction fallacy, a certain percentage of respondents maintain that their responses are valid in the face of an obvious contradiction (Tversky & Kahneman, 1983). This can be seen directly in the Ratio Bias phenomenon (Denes-Raj & Epstein, 1994). Given a choice between two lotteries, people tend to choose the lottery with more opportunities to win, even when it offers a smaller probability of success (because it also offers more opportunities to lose).

More commonly, our deliberations do not lead to conclusions that we can be certain of, and this opens the door to intuition. There is often uncertainty associated with political, moral, risky, and even consumer decisions, and when deliberation is not delivering a knock-down argument, there is little to silence the powerful voice of intuition. Sometimes we do not even bother to deliberate because we are not sufficiently motivated, or because we are doing something else. In fact, Gilbert (1991) argues that failure to deliberate is the norm. We tend to believe what we are told; rejection requires an additional effortful process.

Finally, people rely on their gut feelings when failure to do so has real costs. The hallmark case of this is addiction. One might be fully aware of the strong arguments against drinking, smoking, gambling, and so forth, but the craving compelled by the affective system may be too strong to ignore (Loewenstein, 1996). At a more cognitive level, it may be deemed too costly not to obey a strong intuition, because it is so central to our belief system. The costs of not following our religious or political beliefs, or beliefs that are wrapped up with our identity, might appear so large that we stick with their prescriptions even in the face of compelling arguments otherwise.

TWO SYSTEMS OF REASONING: THE SEQUEL

On the basis of these considerations, I would like to update my view of the dual-process architecture of higher-level thought. My revised view does not increase the number of systems. The concept of a *system* needs to be constrained to maintain its explanatory power. If systems are identified with any type of cognitive function, they will come to be treated in the same way as modules: They will proliferate and lose their theoretical force. Of course, there are many cognitive processes that are not supported by either intuition or deliberation but serve quite different functions (e.g., parsing language, gauging the depth one must reach to grasp an object). I take deliberation to serve the function of thoughtful reflection implemented via a symbolic medium. Intuition serves the function of sophisticated pattern recognition implemented via a representational medium that integrates knowledge structures with physical processes and that produces symbolic outputs as well as certain affective states.

I also do not propose a separate reflective process that determines which system dominates behavior at a given point in time. Instead I assume this function is served in part by inhibitory relations between systems and in part by the deliberative process itself. The architecture that supports the interaction between systems has been hinted at in the cognitive neuroscience literature. Anatomically, the brain includes multiple parallel frontal corticobasal ganglia loops (Alexander, DeLong, & Strick, 1986). The interactions among these loops can be interpreted as a set of gating mechanisms (Frank, Cohen, & Sanfey, 2009). My proposal is that one such loop is the intuitive loop, though it is best characterized as jointly intuitive and affective. Deliberation, in contrast, involves a more anterior prefrontal corticobasal ganglia loop. One critical function of deliberation is to serve to gate or at least modulate the intuitive–affective loop.

Lieberman (2007) proposes a dual-system theory of social cognition and offers perhaps the most complete analysis of the neural underpinnings of intuition and deliberation (or what he calls "reflexive" and "reflective" systems, respectively). According to his analysis, the intuitive network includes both areas normally associated with intuitive cognitive processes, including lateral temporal cortex and ventromedial prefrontal cortex, as well as areas more strongly associated with aspects of affect such as pain, disgust, and fear, including the dorsal anterior cingulate cortex and the amygdala, as well as an area associated with both, namely, the basal ganglia. Lieberman associates deliberation with anterior cingulate cortex, lateral prefrontal cortex, posterior parietal cortex, and the hippocampus and surrounding medial temporal lobe region.

On this view, one form of interaction between deliberation and intuition is that deliberation attempts, sometimes successfully and sometimes not, to inhibit intuitive processing. The proposed interaction in the domain of thought parallels Libet's (2004) notion of "Free Won't" in the domain of motor control: that conscious control does not anticipate motor events but can inhibit those we become aware of.

How the Systems Interact

At a purely functional level, the picture is that a fairly autonomous system operates through positive feedback between intuitive and affective components to relate the body to pattern recognition processes. A second deliberative system operates independently and in parallel, and serves to modulate the intuitive–affective loop via inhibition. But the inhibition is not always successful, so deliberation does not always dominate. Inhibition is likely to be successful to the degree that deliberation is compelling. That is, the greater the coherence and importance of the representation arrived at in the deliberative system, the greater its inhibitory strength over intuition. Inhibition is unlikely to be successful to the degree that the intuitive–affective system is active, coherent, and relaying important information. For instance, if the affective system is responding strongly to temptation, the intuitive–affective loop will be harder to inhibit. Also, if the intuitive system is converging strongly on a pattern, then the loop will be harder to inhibit.

It is clear that there are individual differences in the strength of this inhibitory link. This is what Frederick's (2005) Cognitive Reflection Test (CRT) measures, the likelihood that an individual will suppress intuitive responding to respond deliberatively. Such differences could reflect differences in the strength of intuitive signals, in the ability and willingness to deliberate, in the strength of the inhibitory link, or some combination of these three (cf. Conrey, Sherman, Gawronski, Hugenberg, & Groom, 2005). The fact that the CRT is highly predictive of performance across a wide variety of tasks (Fernbach, Sloman, St. Louis, & Shube, 2013; Frederick, 2005; Toplak, West, & Stanovich, 2011) suggests some stability within individuals in the behavior of the systems and their interaction, which in turn provides support for the claim that the architecture described here has some psychological reality.

More support for this architecture comes from the evidence in favor of a very similar proposal to explain obsessive–compulsive disorder (OCD). Boyer and Liénard (2006) propose that OCD arises from hyperactive error-detecting networks, such that the urge to engage in compulsions becomes excessively strong and the systems that usually inhibit these urges are too weak. Their error-detection system is responsible for obsessive thoughts and their second system functions to inhibit it. On this view, OCD could reflect failure in the mechanism by which deliberation inhibits the intuitive–affective system (Goldin, van't Wout, Sloman, Evans, Greenberg, et al., in press).

De Neys (2012) has amassed a large amount of data suggesting that performance on tasks that induce cognitive illusions is affected by deliberative knowledge even in cases in which responses are governed by intuition and fail to respect deliberative considerations. For instance, when the base rate of an event is extreme and thus highly salient, reaction times are slower when responses are inconsistent with base rates than when they are consistent. This suggests that deliberative knowledge can be available even when intuitive knowledge is dominating a response. This is exactly what one would expect if the function of deliberative knowledge were to attenuate but not eliminate intuitive responses.

What Intuition Represents

I also propose that intuition is not merely associative but encodes rich causal structure. Causal structure often takes the form of narrative (Pennington & Hastie, 1992; Kahneman, 2011). People are formidable storytellers, finding patterns in events that assign causal roles so that deviations from normality can be discussed and explained, costs and benefits can be predicted, and credit and blame can be attributed. As phenomena such as illusory correlation and the hot hand (Gilovich, Vallone, & Tversky, 1985) demonstrate, intuition imposes causal structure even when it is not present in nature.

Causal knowledge can be thought of as an extension of the contingent stimulus–response rules that support action. Like those rules, causal knowledge indicates the conditions under which states and actions will lead to consequences. An organism sophisticated enough to know that pressing a button that turns on a brand new type of appliance is safe even when immersed in water, as long as there is no source of electricity, must represent more than just correlations in the environment, even higher-order correlations. They have to know something about the underlying causal structures that produce those contingencies. The fact that we can recognize these causal patterns quickly and automatically suggests that this information is encoded in intuition.

Other kinds of structure may also become encoded intuitively as people develop expertise. For instance, extended practice with arithmetic or chess turns aspects of those activities into intuitive pattern recognition.

CONCLUSION

The thrust of my argument in 1996 was that the world presents itself with different kinds of structure to reason about: statistical structure that allows us to make educated guesses and more formal relations that have a syntactic structure. The human mind takes advantage of these different structures, I argued, by devoting a system of reasoning to each, an associative system that represents and reasons about statistical structure, and a rule-based system that reasons about formal structure using symbolic language.

I still believe there are two systems with different operating principles, but my view of what structure is represented has changed in part. Rather than representing statistical structure directly, I now believe that the intuitive system is generative: It represents the causal structure that produces statistical facts rather than representing the statistical facts themselves as associations. I also believe it cues us to action through tight links to affect. Despite the change in label, my view of deliberation remains the same: It can reason from any learned formal representation.

I have proposed that the two systems differ in other ways as well. In terms of awareness, we are aware of both the process and products of our deliberations but only the products of our intuitive inferences. Both systems are intentional in the sense of being goal-driven, though the deliberative system can be more directly controlled through force of will. The intuitive system responds automatically to environmental input. It can be inhibited by the deliberative system, though the control system is leaky; it sometimes fails. In that sense, we have only indirect control of our intuitions. Being sequential, deliberation is slower than the parallel processing that the intuitive system engages in, and it requires more energy. In that sense, intuition is more efficient. However, conclusions reached through deliberation tend to be more certain.

A weak view on the dual-systems framework—that it is a useful tool for understanding higher-level cognitive processes—has gained widespread if not universal acceptance. The stronger claim that there are two distinct systems in the brain that serve complementary functions (and that interact strongly) has not been as widely accepted. Although my thinking about the architecture of cognition has changed considerably since 1996, it has not changed so much that I am willing to let go of this stronger view. The distinction is intuitively compelling by virtue of its explanatory value in every domain of cognition and it is also compelled by a slow, deliberative analysis of the available evidence.

ACKNOWLEDGMENTS

I would like to thank Fiery Cushman, Adam Darlow, and Michael Frank for penetrating comments on an earlier draft of this chapter.

REFERENCES

Alexander, G. E., DeLong, M. R., & Strick, P. L. (1986). Parallel organization of functionally segregated circuits linking basal ganglia cortex. *Annual Review of Neuroscience, 9*, 357–381.

Boyer, P., & Liénard, P. (2006). Why ritualized behavior?: Precaution systems and action parsing in developmental, pathological and cultural rituals. *Behavioral and Brain Sciences, 29*, 595–612.

Chapman, L. J., & Chapman, J. P. (1969). Illusory correlation as an obstacle to the use of valid psychodiagnostic signs. *Journal of Abnormal Psychology, 74*, 271–280.

Conrey, F. R., Sherman, J. W., Gawronski, B., Hugenberg, K., & Groom, C. (2005). Separating multiple processes in implicit social cognition: The Quad Model of implicit task performance. *Journal of Personality and Social Psychology, 89*, 469–487.

Denes-Raj, V., & Epstein, S. (1994). Con?ict between intuitive and rational processing: When people behave against their better judgement. *Journal of Personality and Social Psychology, 66*, 819–829.

De Neys, W. (2012). Bias and conflict: A case for logical intuitions. *Perspectives on Psychological Science, 7*, 28–38

Epstein, S. (1994). Integration of the cognitive and the psychodynamic unconscious. *American Psychologist, 49*(8), 709–724.

Evans, J. St. B. T. (2009). How many dual-process theories do we need: One, two or many? In J. St. B. T. Evans & K. Frankish (Eds.), *In two minds: Dual processes and beyond* (pp. 31–54). Oxford, UK: Oxford University Press.

Evans, J. St. B. T., & Over, D. E. (1996). *Rationality and reasoning*. Hove, UK: Psychology Press.

Fernbach, P. M., Sloman, S. A., St. Louis, R., & Shube, J. N. (2013). Explanation fiends and foes: How mechanistic detail determines understanding and preference. *Journal of Consumer Research, 39*(5), 1115–1131.

Fodor, J. (1983). *The modularity of mind*. Cambridge, MA: MIT Press.

Frank, M. J., Cohen, M. X., & Sanfey, A. G. (2009). Multiple systems in decision making: A neurocomputational perspective. *Current Directions in Psychological Science, 18*, 73–77.

Frederick, S. (2005). Cognitive reflection and decision making. *Journal of Economic Perspectives, 19*(4), 25–42.

Freud, S. (1913). *The interpretation of dreams*. London: Allen & Unwin.

Gilbert, D. T. (1991). How mental systems believe. *American Psychologist, 46*, 107–119.

Gilovich, T., Vallone, R., & Tversky, A. (1985). The hot hand in basketball: On the misperception of random sequences. *Cognitive Psychology*, 17, 295–314.

Goldin, G., van't Wout, M., Sloman, S. A., Evans, D. W., Greenberg, B. D., & Rasmussen, S. A. (in press). Two systems of risk judgment in obsessive–compulsive disorder. *Journal of Obsessive–Compulsive and Related Disorders*.

Hagmayer, Y., & Sloman, S. A. (2009). Decision makers conceive of themselves as interveners, not observers. *Journal of Experimental Psychology: General, 138*, 22–38.

Haidt, J. (2001). The emotional dog and its rational tail: A social intuitionist approach to moral judgment. *Psychological Review, 108*, 814–834.

Haidt, J. (2012). *The righteous mind: Why good people are divided by politics and religion*. New York: Random House.

Hutcherson, C. A., & Gross, J. J. (2011). The moral emotions: A social-functionalist account of anger, disgust, and contempt. *Journal of Personality and Social Psychology, 100*, 719–737.

James, W. (1950). *The principles of psychology*. New York: Dover. (Original work published 1890)

Kahneman, D. (2011). *Thinking fast and slow*. New York: Farrar, Straus & Giroux.

Kahneman, D., & Frederick, S. (2002). Representative revisited: Attribute substitution in intuitive judgment. In T. Gilovich, D. Griffin, & D. Kahneman (Eds.), *Heuristics and biases: The psychology of intuitive judgment*. New York: Cambridge University Press.

Klein, G. (1998). *Sources of power: How people make decisions*. Cambridge, MA: MIT Press.

Lazarus, R. S. (1984). On the primacy of cognition. *American Psychologist, 39*(2), 124–129.

LeDoux, J. (1996). *The emotional brain: The mysterious underpinnings of emotional life*. New York: Simon & Schuster.

Libet, B. (2004). *Mind time: The temporal factor in consciousness*, Cambridge, MA: Harvard University Press.

Lieberman, M. D. (2007). The X- and C-systems: The neural basis of automatic and controlled social cognition. In E. Harmon-Jones & P. Winkelman (Eds.), *Fundamentals of social neuroscience* (pp. 290–315). New York: Guilford Press.

Loewenstein, G. (1996). Out of control: Visceral influences on behavior. *Organizational Behavior and Human Decision Processes, 65* (3), 272–292.

Meek, C., & Glymour, C. (1994). Conditioning and intervening. *British Journal for the Philosophy of Science, 45*, 1001–1021.

Newell, A., & Simon, H. (1972). *Human problem solving*. Englewood Cliffs, NJ: Prentice Hall.

Nichols, S. (2008). Moral rationalism and empirical immunity. In W. Sinnott-Armstrong (Ed.), *Moral psychology, Vol. 2* (pp. 395–407). Cambridge, MA: MIT Press.

Norman, G. R., Trott, A. D., Brooks, L. R., & Smith, E. K. (1994). Cognitive differences in clinical reasoning related to postgraduate training. *Teaching and Learning in Medicine*, 6, 114–120.

Osman, M., & Stavy, R. (2006). Intuitive rules: From formative to developed reasoning. *Psychonomic Bulletin and Review, 13*, 935–953.

Patel, V. L., & Kaufman, D. R. (2000). Clinical reasoning and biomedical knowledge: Implications for teaching. In J. Higgs & M. Jones (Eds.), *Clinical reasoning in the health professions* (pp. 117–128). Oxford, UK: Butterworth-Heinemann.

Pearl, J. (2000). *Causality*. Cambridge, UK: Cambridge University Press.

Pennington, N., & Hastie, R. (1992). Reasoning in explanation-based decision making. *Cognition, 49*, 123–163.

Piaget, J., & Inhelder, B. (1974). *The construction of quantity*. London: Routledge & Kegan Paul.

Pizarro, D., Inbar, Y., & Helion, C. (2011). On disgust and moral judgment. *Emotion Review, 3,* 267–268.

Prinz, J. J. (2007). *The emotional construction of morals.* Oxford, UK: Oxford University Press.

Quattrone, G., & Tversky A. (1984). Causal versus diagnostic contingencies: On self-deception and on the voter's illusion. *Journal of Personality and Social Psychology, 46,* 237–248.

Risen, J. L., & Gilovich, T. (2008). Why people are reluctant to tempt fate. *Journal of Personality and Social Psychology, 95*(2), 293–307.

Rudolph, U., & Försterling, F. (1997). The psychological causality implicit in verbs: A review. *Psychological Bulletin, 121,* 192–218.

Rumelhart, D. E., & McClelland, J. L. (1986). *Parallel distributed processing, Vols. 1 and 2.* Cambridge, MA: MIT Press.

Seger, C. A. (1994). Implicit learning. *Psychological Bulletin, 115,* 163–196.

Sloman, S. A. (1996). The empirical case for two systems of reasoning. *Psychological Bulletin, 119*(1), 3–22.

Sloman, S. A. (2005). *Causal models: How we think about the world and its alternatives.* New York: Oxford University Press.

Sloman, S. A., Fernbach, P., Ewing, S. (2009). Causal models: The representational infrastructure for moral judgment. In B. H. Ross (Series Ed.) & D. M. Bartels, C. W. Bauman, L. J. Skitka, & D. L. Medin (Eds.), *Psychology of learning and motivation: Vol. 50. Moral judgment and decision making* (1–26). San Diego: Academic Press.

Sloman, S. A., Fernbach, P. M., & Hagmayer, Y. (2010). Self deception requires vagueness. *Cognition, 115,* 268–281.

Slovic, P., Finucane, M. L., Peters, E., & MacGregor, D. G. (2007). The affect heuristic. *European Journal of Operational Research, 177*(3), 1333–1352.

Spirtes, P., Glymour, C., & Scheines, R. (1993). *Causation, prediction, and search.* New York: Springer-Verlag.

Stanovich, K. E. (2004). *The robot's rebellion: Finding meaning in the age of Darwin.* Chicago: Chicago University Press.

Stanovich, K. E. (2011). *Rationality and the reflective mind.* New York: Oxford University Press.

Stanovich, K. E., & West, R. F. (2000). Individual differences in reasoning: Implications for the rationality debate. *Behavioral and Brain Sciences, 23,* 645–726.

Stavy, R., & Tirosh, D. (2000). *How students (mis-)understand science and mathematics: Intuitive rules.* New York: Teachers College Press.

Swirsky, C. L., Fernbach, P. M., & Sloman, S. A. (2011). An illusion of control modulates the reluctance to tempt fate. *Judgment and Decision Making, 6,* 688–696.

Toplak, M. E., West, R. F., & Stanovich, K. E. (2011). The Cognitive Reflection Test as a predictor of performance on heuristics-and-biases tasks. *Memory and Cognition, 39,* 1275–1289.

Tversky, A., & Kahneman, D. (1983). Extensional versus intuitive reasoning: The conjunction fallacy in probability judgment. *Psychological Review, 90,* 293–315.

Woodward, J. (2003). *Making things happen: A theory of causal explanation.* New York: Oxford University Press.

CHAPTER 6

Rationality, Intelligence, and the Defining Features of Type 1 and Type 2 Processing

Keith E. Stanovich, Richard F. West, and Maggie E. Toplak

The idea that the brain comprises many different subsystems has recurred in conceptualizations in many different disciplines—from the society of minds view in artificial intelligence (Minsky, 1985) to Freudian analogies (Ainslie, 1982) to discussions of the concept of multiple selves in philosophy, economics, and decision science (Ainslie, 2001). Just how ubiquitous dual-process models are in psychology and related fields is illustrated in Table 6.1, which lists a variety of such theories that have appeared during the last couple of decades.

Some common terms for the dual processes are listed in Table 6.1. The terms *heuristic* and *analytic* are two of the oldest and most popular terms for the two processes. However, in order to attenuate the proliferation of nearly identical theories, Stanovich (1999) suggested the more generic terms *System 1* and *System 2*. Although these terms have become popular (see Kahneman, 2011), there is an infelicitousness to the System 1–System 2 terminology. Such terminology seems to connote that the two processes in dual-process theory map explicitly to two distinct brain systems. This is a stronger assumption than most theorists wish to make. For similar reasons, Evans (2008, 2009) has suggested a terminology of Type 1 processing versus Type 2 processing. The Type 1–Type 2 terminology captures better than previous terminology that a dual-process theory is not necessarily a dual-*systems* theory (see Evans & Stanovich, 2013, for an extensive discussion). Thus, we adopt the Type 1–Type 2 terminology here, as it more accurately characterizes how each refers to sets of systems rather than single systems.

DEFINING VERSUS INCIDENTAL FEATURES OF DUAL-PROCESS MODELS

In the same book where the System 1–System 2 terminology was introduced, Stanovich (1999) attempted to bring together some of the pairs of properties that had been posited in the literature to indicate the differences between the two processes. We have reproduced a slightly updated version of the property list in Table 6.2. The purpose of this original table in Stanovich (1999) was simply to bring together the many properties assigned to the two processes in the proliferation of dual-process theories of the 1990s. The list was not intended as a strict theoretical statement of necessary and defining features. As Stanovich noted in his discussion, he was searching for "family resemblances" among the various theories. The

TABLE 6.1. Some Alternative Terms for Type 1 and Type 2 Processing Used by Various Theorists

Theorist	Type 1	Type 2
Bargh & Chartrand (1999)	Automatic processing	Conscious processing
Bazerman, Tenbrunsel, & Wade-Benzoni (1998)	Want self	Should self
Bickerton (1995)	Online thinking	Offline thinking
Brainerd & Reyna (2001)	Gist processing	Analytic processing
Chaiken et al. (1989)	Heuristic processing	Systematic processing
Evans (1984)	Heuristic processing	Analytic processing
Evans & Over (1996)	Tacit thought processes	Explicit thought processes
Evans & Wason (1976); Wason & Evans (1975)	Type 1 processes	Type 2 processes
Fodor (1983)	Modular processes	Central processes
Gawronski & Bodenhausen (2006)	Associative processes	Propositional processes
Haidt (2001)	Intuitive system	Reasoning system
Johnson-Laird (1983)	Implicit inferences	Explicit inferences
Kahneman & Frederick (2002, 2005)	Intuition	Reasoning
Lieberman (2003)	Reflexive system	Reflective system
Loewenstein (1996)	Visceral factors	Tastes
Metcalfe & Mischel (1999)	Hot system	Cool system
Norman & Shallice (1986)	Contention scheduling	Supervisory attentional system
Pollock (1991)	Quick and inflexible modules	Intellection
Posner & Snyder (1975)	Automatic activation	Conscious processing
Reber (1993)	Implicit cognition	Explicit learning
Shiffrin & Schneider (1977)	Automatic processing	Controlled processing
Sloman (1996)	Associative system	Rule-based system
Smith & DeCoster (2000)	Associative processing	Rule-based processing
Stanovich (2004)	Autonomous processes	Decoupled simulation
Strack & Deutsch (2004)	Impulsive system	Reflective system
Thaler & Shefrin (1981)	Doer	Planner
Toates (2006)	Stimulus-bound	Higher order
Wilson (2002)	Adaptive unconscious	Conscious

list was descriptive of distinctions drawn in the literature—not a full-blown theory of necessarily co-occurring properties. No one at the time could have made such a list of necessarily co-occurring properties, because the unsystematic and non-cross-referenced work of the 1990s meant that no one could have known such a thing. In the past decade however, several investigators have made an attempt to zero in on the crucial defining features of the two types of processing—and by inference make a statement about which properties are incidental correlates. We sketch out our own theoretical attempt below, but first we indicate how Table 6.2 has been misused in the literature in an effort to discredit dual-process theory.

The main misuse of such tables is to treat them as strong statements about necessary co-occurring features—in short, to aid in the creation of a straw man. The longer the list of properties in any one table, the easier it is to create the complete straw man claim that if all of these features do not always co-occur, then the dual-process view is incorrect. Kruglanski and Gigerenzer (2011) most recently created such a straw man with their claim that dual-process views fail because "these dimensions are unaligned rather than aligned" (p. 98). They explicitly construct their straw man by considering six dichotomies to carry the assumption that all are defining and must therefore co-occur: "Assuming six dichotomies, one would end up with a $2^6 = 64$ cell matrix of which only two cells (those representing the conjunction of all six dichotomies) had entries. Again, such logical implication of the alignment assumption has never been considered seriously or tested empirically" (p. 98).

But the so-called "alignment assumption" here is not attributed to a specific dual-process theorist in their article. This is not surprising, because dual-process theory does not stand or fall on the full set of properties necessarily co-occurring. Tables of properties such as those seen in Table 6.2 appeared in publications over a decade ago (see Stanovich, 1999) and were meant to organize a nascent theoretical literature, not to lay out an absurdly specific prediction about the co-occurrence of features that had been generated from over two-dozen different dual-process conceptions. *All* of these dichotomies were *never* necessary to establish the two types of processing (which itself suggests that this was not the purpose of such lists)—the only thing needed is *one* fairly

TABLE 6.2. Commonly Listed Properties of Type 1 and Type 2 Processing

Type 1 processes	Type 2 processes
Holistic	Analytic
Automatic	Controlled
Relatively undemanding of cognitive capacity	Capacity demanding
Relatively fast	Relatively slow
Acquisition by biology, exposure, and personal experience	Acquisition by culture and formal tuition
Parallel	Sequential
Evolutionarily old	Evolutionarily recent
Implicit	Explicit
Often unconscious or preconscious	Often conscious
Lower correlations with intelligence	Higher correlations with intelligence
Short-leashed genetic goals	Long-leashed goals that tend toward personal utility maximization

dichotomous property that is necessary and sufficient. As argued previously, the whole pedantic "2 out of 64" exercise collapses if the each of the dichotomous characteristics were never viewed as essential characteristics in the first place—that is, if it was never assumed that each of the properties listed was necessary in order to define qualitatively different types of processing.

In our model (Stanovich, 2004, 2009, 2011), the defining feature of Type 1 processing is its autonomy: The execution of Type 1 processes is mandatory when their triggering stimuli are encountered, and they are not dependent on input from high-level control systems. Autonomous processes have other correlated features: Their execution tends to be rapid, they do not put a heavy load on central processing capacity, and they tend to be associative—but these other correlated features are not defining. Into the category of autonomous processes would go some processes of emotional regulation; the encapsulated modules for solving specific adaptive problems that have been posited by evolutionary psychologists; processes of implicit learning; and the automatic firing of overlearned associations (see Evans, 2008, 2009; Shiffrin & Schneider, 1977).

These disparate categories make clear that Type 1 processing is a grab bag—encompassing *both* innately specified processing modules/procedures and experiential associations that have been learned to automaticity. Their only uniform commonality is their autonomy. The point that Type 1 processing does not arise from a singular system is stressed by both Evans (2008, 2009) and Stanovich (2004, 2011; see Evans & Stanovich, 2013). The many kinds of Type 1 processing have in common the property of autonomy, but otherwise, their neurophysiology and etiology might be considerably different.

All of the different kinds of Type 1 processing (processes of emotional regulation, Darwinian modules, associative and implicit learning processes) can produce responses that are nonoptimal in a particular context if not overridden. For example, humans often act like cognitive misers (an old theme in cognitive–social psychology) by engaging in *attribute substitution*—the substitution of an easy-to-evaluate characteristic for a harder one, even if the easier one is less accurate (Kahneman, 2011). For example, the cognitive miser will substitute the less effortful attributes of vividness or affect for the more effortful retrieval of relevant facts. Most times, such Type 1 processing will be adequate for the situation, but it is not designed for the type of fine-grained analysis called for in situations of unusual importance (financial decisions, fairness judgments, employment). When we are evaluating important risks—such as the risk of certain activities and environments for our children—we do not want to substitute vividness for careful thought about the situation. In such situations, we want to employ Type 2 override processing to block the attribute substitution of the cognitive miser.

In order to override Type 1 processing, Type 2 processing must display at least two related capabilities. One is the capability of interrupting Type 1 processing and suppressing its response tendencies. Thus, Type 2 processing involves inhibitory mechanisms of the type that have been the focus of work on executive functioning (Miyake & Friedman, 2012). But the ability to suppress Type 1 processing gets the job only half done. Suppressing one response is not helpful unless there is a better response available to substitute for it. Where do these better responses come from? One answer is that they come from processes of hypothetical reasoning and cognitive simulation (Evans, 2007, 2010). When we reason hypothetically, we create temporary models of the world and test out actions (or alternative causes) in that simulated world. In order to reason hypothetically we must, however, have one critical cognitive capability—we must be able to prevent our representations of the real world from becoming confused with representations of imaginary situations. These cognitive decoupling operations are the central feature of Type 2 processing that make this possible (Stanovich, 2004, 2009, 2011). In an article much-cited in developmental psychology, Leslie (1987) modeled pretense by positing a secondary representation (see Perner, 1991) that was a copy of the primary representation but decoupled from the world, so that it could be manipulated—that is, be a mechanism for simulation. Nichols and Stich (2003) model this cognitive decoupling as a separate "possible world box" (PWB) in which the simulations are carried out without contaminating the relationship between the world and primary representation.

The important issue for our purposes is that decoupling secondary representations from the world, then maintaining the decoupling while simulation is carried out is the defining feature of Type 2 processing. To engage in exercises of hypotheticality and high-level cognitive control, one has to represent explicitly a psychological attitude toward the state of affairs, as well as the state of affairs itself. Thus, decoupled representations of actions about to be taken become representations of potential actions, but the latter must not infect the former while the mental simulation is being carried out. However, dealing with secondary representations—keeping them decoupled—is costly in terms of cognitive capacity. Evolution has guaranteed the high cost of decoupling for a very good reason. As we were becoming the first creatures to rely strongly on cognitive simulation, it was especially important that we not become "unhooked" from the world too much of the time. Thus, dealing with primary representations of the world always has a special salience that may feel aversive to overcome.

Nevertheless, decoupling operations must be continually in force during any ongoing simulations. Stanovich (2004, 2009, 2011) has conjectured that the raw ability to sustain such mental simulations while keeping the relevant representations decoupled is likely the key aspect of the brain's computational power that is being assessed by measures of fluid intelligence. Decoupling—outside of certain domains such as behavioral prediction (so-called "theory of mind")—is a cognitively demanding operation. Decoupling and autonomy are antagonistic in our view: Autonomous processes do not have the capacity to decouple, and decoupling requires central processing capacity and is hence nonautonomous, except for a few exceptions (e.g., the theory of mind module).

FROM DUAL-PROCESS THEORY TO A TRIPARTITE MODEL OF MIND

Figure 6.1 represents a preliminary model of mind, based on what has been outlined thus far, with one important addition. The addition stems from the fact that instructions to

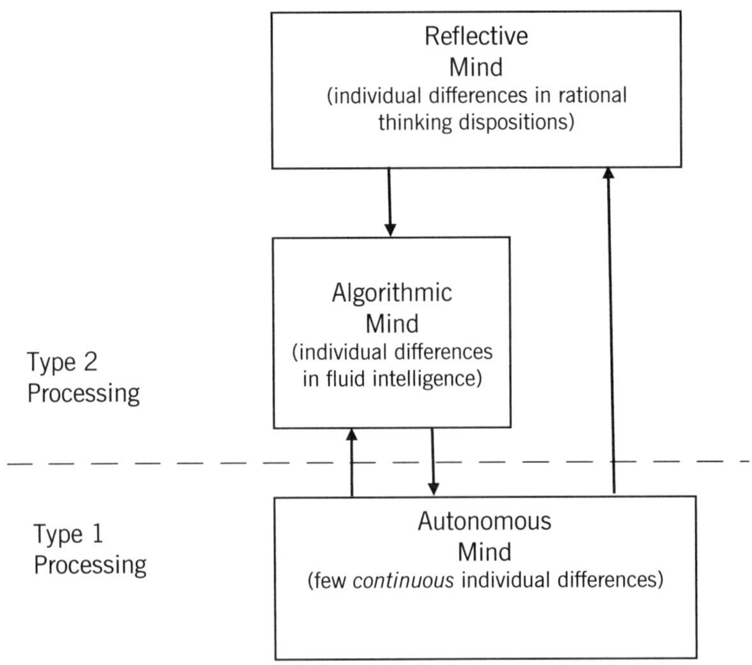

FIGURE 6.1. The tripartite structure and the locus of individual differences.

initiate override of Type 1 processing (and to initiate simulation activities) must be controlled by cognitive machinery at a higher-level than the decoupling machinery itself. Type 2 processing needs to be understood in terms of two levels of cognitive control—what are termed in Figure 6.1 the algorithmic level and the reflective level. There, we have presented the tripartite proposal in the spirit of Dan Dennett's (1996) book *Kinds of Minds*. He used that title to suggest that within the brain of humans are control systems of very different types—different kinds of minds. We have labeled the traditional source of Type 1 processing as the autonomous mind but differentiated Type 2 processing into the algorithmic mind and the reflective mind. The autonomous mind can be overridden by algorithmic-level mechanisms, but override itself is initiated by higher-level control. That is, the algorithmic level is conceptualized as subordinate to the higher-level goal states and epistemic thinking dispositions of the reflective mind.

Work on individual differences in psychological function supports the distinction between the algorithmic and reflective levels of cognition that support Type 2 processing. Psychometricians have long distinguished typical performance situations from optimal (sometimes termed *maximal*) performance situations. Typical performance situations are unconstrained, in that no overt instructions to maximize performance are given, and the task interpretation is determined to some extent by the participant. The goals to be pursued in the task are left somewhat open. The issue is what a person would typically do in such a situation given few constraints. Typical performance measures are measures of the reflective mind—they assess in part goal prioritization and epistemic regulation. In contrast, optimal performance situations are those in which the task interpretation is determined externally. The person performing the task is instructed to maximize performance. Thus, optimal performance measures examine questions of the efficiency of goal pursuit—they capture the processing efficiency of the algorithmic mind. All tests of intelligence or cognitive aptitude are optimal performance assessments, whereas measures of critical or rational thinking are often assessed under typical performance conditions.

The difference between the algorithmic mind and the reflective mind is captured in another well-established distinction in the measurement of individual differences—the distinction between cognitive ability and thinking dispositions. The former are, as just mentioned, measures of the efficiency of the algorithmic mind. The latter travel under a variety of names in psychology—thinking dispositions or cognitive styles being the two most popular ones. Many thinking dispositions concern beliefs, belief structure and, importantly, attitudes toward forming and changing beliefs. Other thinking dispositions that have been identified concern a person's goals and goal hierarchy. Examples of some thinking dispositions that have been investigated by psychologists include actively open-minded thinking, need for cognition, consideration of future consequences, need for closure, superstitious thinking, and dogmatism.

The types of cognitive propensities that these thinking disposition measures reflect include the tendency to collect information before making up one's mind, the tendency to seek various points of view before coming to a conclusion, the disposition to think extensively about a problem before responding, the tendency to calibrate the degree of strength of one's opinion to the degree of evidence available, the tendency to think about future consequences before taking action, the tendency to explicitly weigh pluses and minuses of situations before making a decision, and the tendency to seek nuance and avoid absolutism. In short, individual differences in thinking dispositions are assessing variation in people's goal management, epistemic values, and epistemic self-regulation—differences in the operation of the reflective mind. They are psychological characteristics that underpin rational thought and action.

The cognitive abilities assessed on intelligence tests are not of this type. They are not about high-level personal goals and their regulation, or the tendency to change beliefs in the face of contrary evidence, or about how knowledge acquisition is internally regulated when not externally directed. People have indeed come up with *definitions* of intelligence that encompass such things. Theorists often define intelligence in ways that encompass rational action and belief; nevertheless, *the actual measures of intel-*

ligence in use assess only algorithmic-level cognitive capacity. No current intelligence test that is even moderately used in practice assesses rational thought or behavior (Stanovich, 2009).

Figure 6.1 represents the classification of individual differences according to the tripartite view. The broken horizontal line represents the location of the key distinction in older, dual-process views. Figure 6.1 identifies variation in fluid intelligence (Gf) with individual differences in the efficiency of processing of the algorithmic mind. Individual differences in rational thinking dispositions indicate variation in the properties of the reflective mind. Whereas the reflective and algorithmic minds are characterized by continuous individual differences and substantial variability, there are fewer continuous individual differences in the autonomous mind and less variability. Disruptions to the autonomous mind often reflect damage to cognitive modules that result in very discontinuous cognitive dysfunction, such as autism or the agnosias and alexias.

RATIONALITY AND THE TRIPARTITE STRUCTURE

When a cognitive scientist terms a behavior *irrational,* he or she means that the behavior departs from the optimum prescribed by a particular normative model. The scientist is not implying that no thought or reason was behind the behavior (see Stanovich, 2012). Cognitive scientists recognize two types of rationality: epistemic and instrumental. *Epistemic rationality* concerns how well beliefs map onto the actual structure of the world. The simplest definition of *instrumental rationality* is behaving in the world so that one gets exactly what one most wants given the resources (physical and mental) available. Somewhat more technically, we could characterize *instrumental rationality* as the optimization of the individual's goal fulfillment. Economists and cognitive scientists have refined the notion of optimization of goal fulfillment into the technical notion of expected utility. The model of rational judgment used by decision scientists is one in which a person chooses options based on which option has the largest expected utility (see Baron, 2008). One of the fundamental advances in the history of modern decision science was the demonstration that if people's preferences follow certain patterns (the so-called "axioms of choice"—things such as transitivity and freedom from certain kinds of context effects), then they are behaving as if they are maximizing utility—they are acting to get what they most want (Luce & Raiffa, 1957). This is what makes people's degrees of rationality measurable by the experimental methods of cognitive science.

Figure 6.1 highlights an important sense in which rationality is a more encompassing construct than intelligence. To be rational, a person must have well-calibrated beliefs and must act appropriately on those beliefs to achieve goals—both properties of the reflective mind. The person must, of course, have the algorithmic-level machinery that enables him or her to carry out the actions and to process the environment in a way that enables the correct beliefs to be fixed and the correct actions to be taken. Thus, individual differences in rational thought and action can arise because of individual differences in fluid intelligence (the algorithmic mind), or because of individual differences in thinking dispositions (the reflective mind).

The conceptualization in Figure 6.1 has several advantages. First, it conceptualizes intelligence in terms of what intelligence tests actually measure. IQ tests do not attempt to measure directly any aspects of epistemic or instrumental rationality, nor do they examine any thinking dispositions that relate to rationality. It is also clear from Figure 6.1 why rationality and intelligence can become dissociated. Rational thinking depends on thinking dispositions, as well as algorithmic efficiency. Thus, as long as variation in thinking dispositions is not perfectly correlated with fluid intelligence, there is the statistical possibility of dissociations between rationality and intelligence.

In fact, substantial empirical evidence indicates that individual differences in thinking dispositions and intelligence are far from perfectly correlated. Many different studies involving thousands of subjects (Stanovich, 2011) have indicated that measures of intelligence display only moderate to weak correlations (usually less than .30) with some thinking dispositions (e.g., actively open-minded thinking, need for cognition) and near-zero correlations with others (e.g., conscientiousness, curiosity, diligence). Other important evidence supports the conceptual distinction made here between algorithmic cognitive capacity and thinking dispositions. For example, across a variety of tasks from the heuristics and biases literature, it has consistently been found that rational thinking dispositions predict variance after the effects of general intelligence have been controlled (Bruine de Bruin, Parker, & Fischoff, 2007; Finucane & Gullion, 2010; Kokis, Macpherson, Toplak, West, & Stanovich, 2002; Parker & Fischhoff, 2005; Stanovich & West, 1997, 1998, 2000; Toplak, Liu, Macpherson, Toneatto, & Stanovich, 2007; Toplak & Stanovich, 2002; Toplak et al., 2011; West, Toplak, & Stanovich, 2008). The model we have outlined predicts that both rational thinking dispositions and fluid intelligence are necessary for rational performance—an interactive relationship.

The functions of the different levels of control in the tripartite theory are illustrated more completely in Figure 6.2, in which it is clear that the override capacity itself is a property of the algorithmic mind and it is indicated by the arrow labeled A. However, previous dual-process theories have tended to ignore the higher-level cognitive function that initiates the override function in the first place. This is a dispositional property of the reflective mind that is related to rationality. In the model in Figure 6.2, it corresponds to arrow B, which represents (in machine intelligence terms) the call to the algorithmic mind to override the Type 1 response by taking it offline. This is a different mental function than the override function itself (arrow A). The evidence cited earlier indicates that the two functions are indexed by different types of individual differences (rational thinking dispositions and fluid intelligence).

Figure 6.2 represents another aspect of cognition that has been somewhat neglected by previous dual-process theories. Specifically, the override function has loomed large in dual-process theory but less so has the

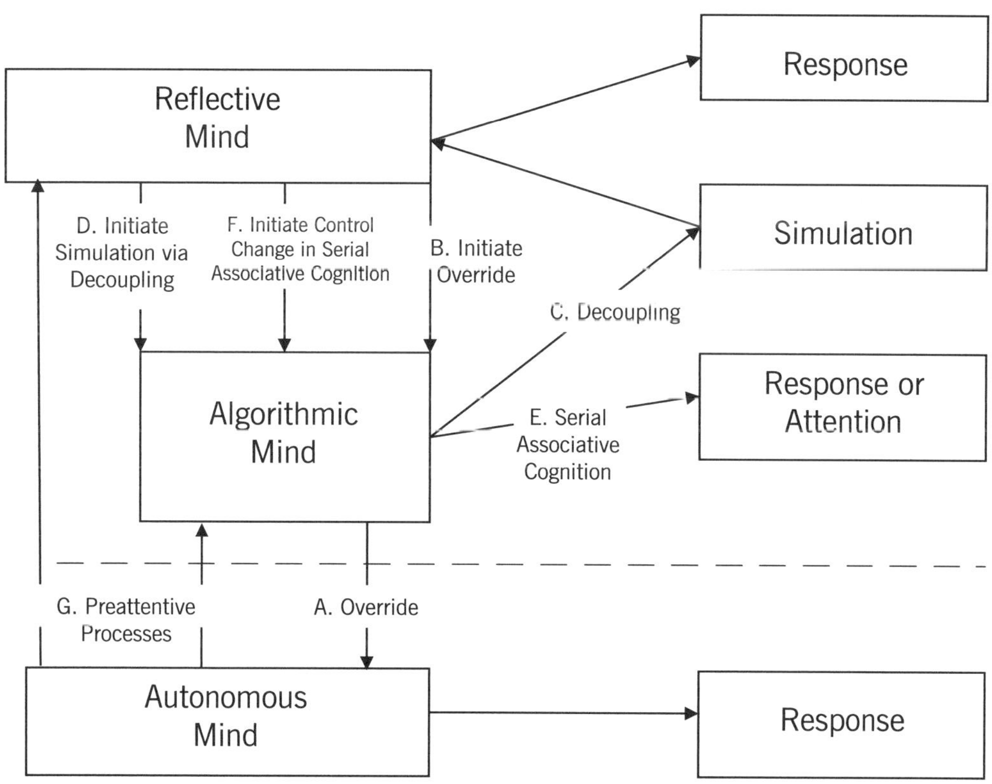

FIGURE 6.2. A more complete model of the tripartite structure.

simulation process that computes the alternative response that makes the override worthwhile. Figure 6.2 explicitly represents the simulation function, as well as the fact that the call to initiate simulation originates in the reflective mind. The decoupling operation (indicated by arrow C) itself is carried out by the algorithmic mind, and the call to initiate simulation (indicated by arrow D) by the reflective mind. Again, two different types of individual differences are associated with the initiation call and the decoupling operator—specifically, rational thinking dispositions with the former, and fluid intelligence with the latter. The arrows labeled E and F reflect the decoupling and higher-level control of a kind of Type 2 processing (serial associative cognition) that does not involve fully explicit cognitive simulation (see Stanovich, 2011, for a much more detailed description of this framework). Also represented is the fact that the higher levels of control receive inputs from the computations of the autonomous mind (arrow G) via so-called preattentive processes (Evans, 2008, 2009). These preattentive processes include Thompson's (2009) feeling of rightness mechanism, which the reflective level uses in part to determine whether an override will be triggered.

Within the tripartite framework, rationality requires mental characteristics of three different types. Problems in rational thinking arise when cognitive capacity is insufficient to sustain autonomous system override, when the necessity of override is not recognized, or when simulation processes do not have access to the knowledge necessary for the synthesis of a better response. The source of these problems, and their relation to intelligence, help to explain one data trend that has been uncovered—that some rational thinking problems show surprising degrees of dissociation from cognitive ability (Stanovich, 2009, 2011; Stanovich & West, 2007, 2008a, 2008b; West et al., 2008). Myside bias, for example, is virtually independent of intelligence (Stanovich & West, 2007, 2008a, 2008b; Toplak & Stanovich, 2003). Individuals with higher IQs in a university sample are no less likely to process information from an egocentric perspective than are individuals with relatively lower IQs.

CONCLUSIONS AND IMPLICATIONS

Many critics of dual-process models have mistaken long lists of descriptive terms in the literature for a full-blown theory of necessarily co-occurring properties. These critiques have distracted attention from the cumulative progress being made in identifying the much smaller set of properties that truly do define Type 1 and Type 2 processing. Our view of the literature is that autonomous processing is the defining feature of Type 1 processing.

Even more convincing is the converging evidence that the key feature of Type 2 processing is the ability to sustain the decoupling of secondary representations. The latter is a foundational cognitive requirement for hypothetical thinking. Through the process of cognitive decoupling, we are able to create temporary models of the world and test the outcomes of imaginary actions. By taking early representations triggered by Type 1 processing offline and substituting better responses that have survived the cognitive selection process of simulation, Type 2 processing exemplifies activities often labeled as executive or inhibitory control. Decoupling for the purpose of offline simulation is a cognitively demanding operation. The raw ability to sustain such simulations while keeping the relevant representations decoupled is one key aspect of the brain's computational power that is being assessed by measures of fluid intelligence. The high degree of overlap in individual differences in working memory and other executive functioning tasks and individual differences in fluid intelligence is probably due to the necessity for sustained decoupling operations on all the tasks involved (Kane, Hambrick, & Conway, 2005).

Our studies of individual differences have led us to the important conclusion that Type 2 processing needs to be understood in terms of two levels of processing—the algorithmic level and the reflective level. We can see this if we consider the logic of autonomous system override. Type 1 processing will determine the response unless overridden by the algorithmic mechanisms of the analytic system. But override itself is initiated by higher-level control. That is, the algorithmic level of the analytic system is conceptualized as subordinate to higher-level goal states and epistemic thinking dispositions. These goal states and epistemic dispositions exist at what might be termed the *reflective level of processing*—a level containing control states that regulate behavior at a high level of generality. Efficient functioning at both levels is necessary to sustain rational behavior.

ACKNOWLEDGMENTS

Preparation of this chapter was supported by a grant from the John Templeton Foundation. The opinions expressed in this chapter are those of the authors and do not necessarily reflect the views of the John Templeton Foundation. We thank Paula J. Stanovich for her technical assistance.

REFERENCES

Ainslie, G. (1982). A behavioral economic approach to the defence mechanisms: Freud's energy theory revisited. *Social Science Information, 21*, 735–780.

Ainslie, G. (2001). *Breakdown of will*. Cambridge, UK: Cambridge University Press.

Bargh, J. A., & Chartrand, T. L. (1999). The unbearable automaticity of being. *American Psychologist, 54*, 462–479.

Baron, J. (2008). *Thinking and deciding* (4th ed.). New York: Cambridge University Press.

Bazerman, M., Tenbrunsel, A., & Wade-Benzoni, K. (1998). Negotiating with yourself and losing: Understanding and managing conflicting internal preferences. *Academy of Management Review, 23*, 225–241.

Bickerton, D. (1995). *Language and human behavior*. Seattle: University of Washington Press.

Brainerd, C. J., & Reyna, V. F. (2001). Fuzzy-trace theory: Dual processes in memory, reasoning, and cognitive neuroscience. In H. W. Reese & R. Kail (Eds.), *Advances in child development and behavior* (Vol. 28, pp. 41–100). San Diego: Academic Press.

Bruine de Bruin, W., Parker, A. M., & Fischhoff, B. (2007). Individual differences in adult decision-making competence. *Journal of Personality and Social Psychology, 92*, 938–956.

Chaiken, S., Liberman, A., & Eagly, A. H. (1989). Heuristic and systematic information within and beyond the persuasion context. In J. S. Uleman & J. A. Bargh (Eds.), *Unintended thought* (pp. 212–252). New York: Guilford Press.

Dennett, D. C. (1996). *Kinds of minds: Toward an understanding of consciousness*. New York: Basic Books.

Evans, J. St. B. T. (1984). Heuristic and analytic processes in reasoning. *British Journal of Psychology, 75*, 451–468.

Evans, J. St. B. T. (2007). *Hypothetical thinking: Dual processes in reasoning and judgment*. New York: Psychology Press.

Evans, J. St. B. T. (2008). Dual-processing accounts of reasoning, judgment and social cognition. *Annual Review of Psychology, 59*, 255–278.

Evans, J. St. B. T. (2009). How many dual-process theories do we need? One, two, or many? In J. Evans & K. Frankish (Eds.), *In two minds: Dual processes and beyond* (pp. 33–54). Oxford, UK: Oxford University Press.

Evans, J. St. B. T. (2010). *Thinking twice: Two minds in one brain*. Oxford, UK: Oxford University Press.

Evans, J. St. B. T., & Over, D. E. (1996). *Rationality and reasoning*. Hove, UK: Psychology Press.

Evans, J. St. B. T., & Stanovich, K. E. (2013). Dual-process theories of higher cognition: Advancing the debate. *Perspectives on Psychological Science, 8*(3), 223–241.

Evans, J. St. B. T., & Wason, P. C. (1976). Rationalization in a reasoning task. *British Journal of Psychology, 67*, 479–486.

Finucane, M. L., & Gullion, C. M. (2010). Developing a tool for measuring the decision-making competence of older adults. *Psychology and Aging, 25*, 271–288.

Fodor, J. A. (1983). *The modularity of mind*. Cambridge, MA: MIT Press.

Gawronski, B., & Bodenhausen, G. V. (2006). Associative and propositional processes in evaluation: An integrative review of implicit and explicit attitude change. *Psychological Bulletin, 132*, 692–731.

Haidt, J. (2001). The emotional dog and its rational tail: A social intuitionist approach to moral judgment. *Psychological Review, 108*, 814–834.

Johnson-Laird, P. N. (1983). *Mental models*. Cambridge, MA: Harvard University Press.

Kahneman, D. (2011). *Thinking, fast and slow*. New York: Farrar, Straus & Giroux.

Kahneman, D., & Frederick, S. (2002). Representativeness revisited: Attribute substitution in intuitive judgment. In T. Gilovich, D. Griffin, & D. Kahneman (Eds.), *Heuristics and biases: The psychology of intuitive judgment* (pp. 49–81). New York: Cambridge University Press.

Kahneman, D., & Frederick, S. (2005). A model of heuristic judgment. In K. J. Holyoak & R. G. Morrison (Eds.), *The Cambridge handbook of thinking and reasoning* (pp. 267–293). New York: Cambridge University Press.

Kane, M. J., Hambrick, D. Z., & Conway, A. R. A. (2005). Working memory capacity and fluid intelligence are strongly related constructs: Comment on Ackerman, Beier, and Boyle (2005). *Psychological Bulletin, 131*, 66–71.

Kokis, J., Macpherson, R., Toplak, M., West, R. F., & Stanovich, K. E. (2002). Heuristic and analytic processing: Age trends and associations with cognitive ability and cognitive styles. *Journal of Experimental Child Psychology, 83*, 26–52.

Kruglanski, A., & Gigerenzer, G. (2011). Intuitive and deliberate judgments are based on common principles. *Psychological Review, 118*, 97–109.

Leslie, A. M. (1987). Pretense and representation: The origins of "theory of mind." *Psychological Review, 94*, 412–426.

Lieberman, M. D. (2003). Reflexive and reflective judgment processes: A social cognitive neuroscience approach. In J. P. Forgas, K. R. Williams, & W. von Hippel (Eds.), *Social judgments: Implicit and explicit processes* (pp. 44–67). New York: Cambridge University Press.

Loewenstein, G. F. (1996). Out of control: Visceral influences on behavior. *Organizational Behavior and Human Decision Processes, 65*, 272–292.

Luce, R. D., & Raiffa, H. (1957). *Games and decisions*. New York: Wiley.

Metcalfe, J., & Mischel, W. (1999). A hot/cool-system analysis of delay of gratification: Dynamics of will power. *Psychological Review, 106*, 3–19.

Minsky, M. L. (1985). *The society of mind*. New York: Simon & Schuster.

Miyake, A., & Friedman, N. P. (2012). The nature and organization of individual differences in executive functions: Four general conclusions. *Current Directions in Psychological Science, 21*, 8–14.

Nichols, S., & Stich, S. P. (2003). *Mindreading: An integrated account of pretence, self-awareness, and understanding other minds*. Oxford, UK: Oxford University Press.

Norman, D. A., & Shallice, T. (1986). Attention to action: Willed and automatic control of behavior. In R. J. Davidson, G. E. Scwartz, & D. Shapiro (Eds.), *Consciousness and self-regulation* (pp. 1–18). New York: Plenum.

Parker, A. M., & Fischhoff, B. (2005). Decision-making competence: External validation through an individual differences approach. *Journal of Behavioral Decision Making, 18*, 1–27.

Perner, J. (1991). *Understanding the representational mind*. Cambridge, MA: MIT Press.

Pollock, J. L. (1991). OSCAR: A general theory of rationality. In J. Cummins & J. L. Pollock (Eds.), *Philosophy and AI: Essays at the interface* (pp. 189–213). Cambridge, MA: MIT Press.

Posner, M. I., & Snyder, C. R. R. (1975). Attention and cognitive control. In R. L. Solso (Ed.), *Information processing and cognition: The Loyola Symposium* (pp. 55–85). New York: Wiley.

Reber, A. S. (1993). *Implicit learning and tacit knowledge*. New York: Oxford University Press.

Shiffrin, R. M., & Schneider, W. (1977). Controlled and automatic human information processing: II. Perceptual learning, automatic attending, and a general theory. *Psychological Review, 84*, 127–190.

Sloman, S. A. (1996). The empirical case for two systems of reasoning. *Psychological Bulletin, 119*, 3–22.

Smith, E. R., & DeCoster, J. (2000). Dual-process models in social and cognitive psychology: Conceptual integration and links to underlying memory systems. *Personality and Social Psychology Review, 4*, 108–131.

Stanovich, K. E. (1999). *Who is rational?: Studies of individual differences in reasoning*. Mahwah, NJ: Erlbaum.

Stanovich, K. E. (2004). *The robot's rebellion: Finding meaning in the age of Darwin*. Chicago: University of Chicago Press.

Stanovich, K. E. (2009). *What intelligence tests miss: The psychology of rational thought*. New Haven, CT: Yale University Press.

Stanovich, K. E. (2011). *Rationality and the reflective mind*. New York: Oxford University Press.

Stanovich, K. E. (2012). On the distinction

between rationality and intelligence: Implications for understanding individual differences in reasoning. In K. Holyoak & R. Morrison (Eds.), *The Oxford handbook of thinking and reasoning* (pp. 343–365). New York: Oxford University Press.

Stanovich, K. E., & West, R. F. (1997). Reasoning independently of prior belief and individual differences in actively open-minded thinking. *Journal of Educational Psychology, 89*, 342–357.

Stanovich, K. E., & West, R. F. (1998). Individual differences in rational thought. *Journal of Experimental Psychology: General, 127*, 161–188.

Stanovich, K. E., & West, R. F. (2000). Individual differences in reasoning: Implications for the rationality debate? *Behavioral and Brain Sciences, 23*, 645–726.

Stanovich, K. E., & West, R. F. (2007). Natural myside bias is independent of cognitive ability. *Thinking and Reasoning, 13*, 225–247.

Stanovich, K. E., & West, R. F. (2008a). On the failure of intelligence to predict myside bias and one-sided bias. *Thinking and Reasoning, 14*, 129–167.

Stanovich, K. E., & West, R. F. (2008b). On the relative independence of thinking biases and cognitive ability. *Journal of Personality and Social Psychology, 94*, 672–695.

Strack, F., & Deutsch, R. (2004). Reflective and impulsive determinants of social behavior. *Personality and Social Psychology Review, 8*, 220–247.

Thaler, R. H., & Shefrin, H. M. (1981). An economic theory of self-control. *Journal of Political Economy, 89*, 392–406.

Thompson, V. A. (2009). Dual-process theories: A metacognitive perspective. In J. Evans & K. Frankish (Eds.), *In two minds: Dual processes and beyond* (pp. 171–195). Oxford, UK: Oxford University Press.

Toates, F. (2006). A model of the hierarchy of behavior, cognition, and consciousness. *Consciousness and Cognition, 15*, 75–118.

Toplak, M., Liu, E., Macpherson, R., Toneatto, T., & Stanovich, K. E. (2007). The reasoning skills and thinking dispositions of problem gamblers: A dual-process taxonomy. *Journal of Behavioral Decision Making, 20*, 103–124.

Toplak, M. E., & Stanovich, K. E. (2002). The domain specificity and generality of disjunctive reasoning: Searching for a generalizable critical thinking skill. *Journal of Educational Psychology, 94*, 197–209.

Toplak, M. E., & Stanovich, K. E. (2003). Associations between myside bias on an informal reasoning task and amount of post-secondary education. *Applied Cognitive Psychology, 17*, 851–860.

Toplak, M. E., West, R. F., & Stanovich, K. E. (2011). The Cognitive Reflection Test as a predictor of performance on heuristics and biases tasks. *Memory and Cognition, 39*, 1275–1289.

Wason, P. C., & Evans, J. St. B. T. (1975). Dual processes in reasoning? *Cognition, 3*, 141–154.

West, R. F., Toplak, M. E., & Stanovich, K. E. (2008). Heuristics and biases as measures of critical thinking: Associations with cognitive ability and thinking dispositions. *Journal of Educational Psychology, 100*, 930–941.

Wilson, T. D. (2002). *Strangers to ourselves*. Cambridge, MA: Harvard University Press.

CHAPTER 7

The Reflective–Impulsive Model

Fritz Strack and Roland Deutsch

In this chapter we describe the core tenets of a general theory of social cognition and behavior, the reflective–impulsive model (RIM; Strack & Deutsch, 2004). The model suggests that social cognition and behavior are the outcome of two broad systems of information processing, the reflective system and the impulsive system (see Figure 7.1). The two systems differ in (1) how information is represented, (2) what kind of psychological processes govern their operation, and (3) the degree of automaticity of processing. As such, the RIM belongs to the family of duality models in social psychology and beyond (for reviews, see Deutsch & Strack, 2006; Evans, 2008; Gawronski & Creighton, 2013; Kruglanski & Orehek, 2007; Strack & Deutsch, in press).

The RIM shares many characteristics with other duality models. However, it differs from other approaches in a number of important aspects. First, it uses the standard sequence of information processing as an organizing temporal structure. Second, it specifies the interaction of two systems at various points in the sequence of information processing. Third, and most important, it attempts to integrate cognitive, motivational, and emotional influences with a focus on behavior. Before we explain how the systems interact, we describe the two systems in terms of their representation, processes, and automaticity. In conclusion, we discuss the model's potential at solving problems in applied domains.

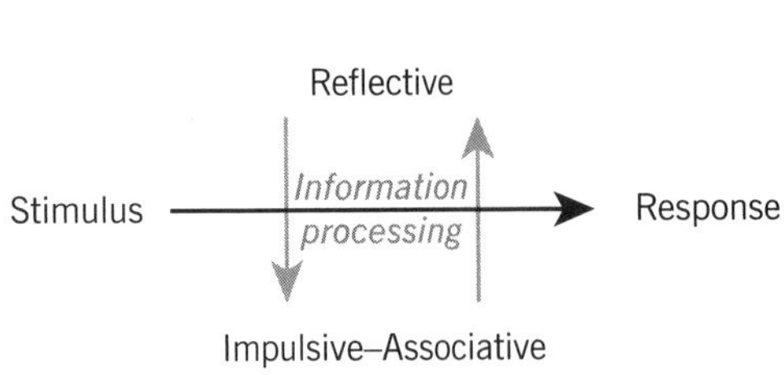

FIGURE 7.1. Dual systems and information processing.

THE TWO SYSTEMS

The Reflective System

Representations

The building blocks of the reflective system are propositional representations. Such representations contain one or more elements and relational schemas that are applied to the element(s). For example, the elements *lightning* and *thunder* might be linked with a causal relation (e.g., Waldmann, Hagmayer, & Blaisdell, 2006). As another example, the elements *Joanna* and *Female* might be linked with an *is-a* relation. Crucially, propositional representations come with a truth value attached to the relation. In other words, the reflective system is made of propositions about state of affairs that people believe to be true or false. As we discuss below, subjective truth is a necessary precondition for the types of processes that generate the dynamics of the system. It is important to note that propositional representations may be factual and evaluative. That is, the subjective truth may equally refer to what is the case, or to what is good or bad. In the latter case, a truth value would be assigned to the relation between an element and valence (e.g., *health is good*). Through its flexibility in reducing the lack of knowledge or in resolving inconsistencies, the reflective system can learn fast and without practice. Specifically, the reflective one-trial learning affords efficient adaptation to new situations.

Processes

The reflective system is specialized in creating and transforming subjective knowledge, in that it describes how perceptual input is being transformed into beliefs and how these beliefs are transformed into ensuing judgments or decisions. The reflective system operates like a working memory that flexibly encodes, maintains, and updates information, and is limited in its capacity (cf. Engle, 2002; Miyake & Shah, 1999). Specifically, it retrieves information from the associative store and keeps it for a limited time to afford propositional transformations and syllogistic operations. The RIM assumes that that the prototypical sequence of decisions begins with a "propositional categorization." At this early stage, a perceptual or experiential input must be linked to a semantic category, and this assignment of the category must be qualified by an affirmative truth value. For example, the perception of a particular stimulus may result in a propositional categorization, such as "This is a box of pralines," which means that it is true that the characteristics of the designated target fulfill this description.

The second step on the reflective path from stimulus to response is the "noetic decision." Specifically, the previously assigned category affords assignment of further characteristics that go beyond perceivable features. If the object has been categorized as a "box of pralines," it may be assumed that the content is edible, tasty but highly calorie, it might make a nice gift, it costs a certain amount, and so forth. The noetic decisions may be factual and evaluative in nature, and include explicit attitudes.

Positive or negative evaluations provide the bases of "means–ends decisions" that serve as links to behavior. That is, the transition from liking to wanting in the reflective system is mediated by a decision about a goal and the ways to attain it. For example, the person might decide to own this box of pralines. Of course, setting such a goal will only occur if the positively evaluated end state has not yet been reached, that is, if the actor does not yet possess the same product. For this purpose, the current state has to be assessed and attention is directed to the self. In addition, the actor has to identify an appropriate behavior and assess its feasibility and effectiveness with respect to the goal. For example, the necessary funds need to available, and the pros and cons of buying it at a local store versus ordering it through the Internet have to be weighed. Finally, the temporal gap between the goal and its realization has to be closed and the "behavioral schema" has to be activated to execute the behavior. In general, these representations of the reflective system are assumed to be accompanied by a "noetic" state of awareness, which consists of knowledge that something is or is not the case (Tulving, 1985).

The RIM assumes that three psychological processes operate in the reflective system. To transform the perceptual experience into propositional knowledge the RIM proposes a deictic procedure that can be metaphorically described as *pointing and referring*. That is, an experience or its referent is identified and related to a category. The resulting truth value can then enter into the second and most important type of mechanism, namely, *syllogistic reasoning*, which the RIM proposes to be a process that involves drawing an inference from two premises, with at least one of them representing a general rule (cf. Chater & Oaksford, 1999; Kruglanski & Thompson, 1999; Sloman, 1996). A typical type of syllogistic inference in social cognition connects the categorization of a person with stereotypical knowledge, which includes a number of category–feature links. For example, the belief that an old person may be gentle, live on a pension, and need occasional help may be generated by an inference based on the premise that the target belongs to the category *old* and the premise that old people are typically gentle and live on a pension (Kruglanski et al., 2003).

The third mechanism creates the cognitive link between the behavioral decision and the execution of the behavior, and is modeled after the concept of implementation intentions (Gollwitzer, 1999). It is named *intending,* and it forms a predisposition to behave in a way that will achieve the goal under the appropriate conditions. The RIM assumes that intending temporarily activates behavioral schemas that are relevant for the goal at hand. After the goal has been achieved, the mechanism is turned off.

In summary, the path from perception to behavior is structured by decisions that involve semantic categorizations, evaluations, and behavioral commitments. Reflective interventions must focus on any of these decisions and attempt to influence their outcome by challenging their validity. For example, relative to the box of pralines, one may remind actors of the negative implication for their health or about the recent increase in price to reduce the likelihood of the behavior.

Automaticity

Modern views (e.g., Bargh, 1994; Moors & De Houwer, 2006) suggest differentiating between multiple, potentially independent components of automaticity, such as awareness, intentionality, controllability, and efficiency. The RIM contains several hypotheses on how these automaticity features relate to processes in the two systems. Importantly, the RIM refrains from boldly assigning full automaticity to the impulsive system and full nonautomaticity to the reflective system. For example, representations and processes in both systems are assumed to have the potential to come along with (albeit different types of) awareness.

The processes of the reflective system are assumed to adhere to a specific pattern of automaticity features that makes them distinct from those of the impulsive system. First, processes in the reflective system are relatively inefficient and therefore require high cognitive resources. As a consequence, distraction, cognitive load, low effort, time pressure, or insufficient energy (Muraven & Baumeister, 2000) may diminish its operation. For example, processing even simple propositions (i.e., negations) was shown to be compromised under time pressure or distraction (Deutsch, Kordts-Freudinger, Gawronski, & Strack, 2009; Gilbert, Tafarodi, & Malone, 1993). Second, processes in the reflective system may be accompanied by noetic awareness (i.e., the state of awareness of whether something is or is not the case). Third, the reflective system is in charge of generating and executing intentions, and provides the starting point of intentional processes. Intentions, however, can affect impulsive processes, too (see section on interaction), such that intentions may start impulsive processes, which then continue to run autonomously (e.g., preactivating a motor schema and pushing it above the threshold of execution). Also, intentions may stop impulsive processes, as in the case of self-control (cf. Hofmann, Friese, & Strack, 2009). In other words, intentions can be the starting point of reflective top-down control of impulsive processes. Because of the required cognitive capacity, the execution of a behavior may be slow and maladaptive in situations that require an immediate response. Thus, a second, complementary system may increase the adaptation of the organism, and some features of the impulsive system serve this goal. Although intentionality, inefficiency, and noetic awareness are attributed to reflective processes, this does not imply that each and every reflective process has all of these qualities. Under certain conditions, intending was demonstrated to be relatively efficient (Gollwitzer, Bayer, & McCulloch, 2005). Likewise, evidence suggests that negations may also be processed without a specific intention to negate (Deutsch et al., 2009). Investigating the scope of nonautomaticity for reflective processes is an important avenue for future research.

The Impulsive System

Representations

The basis of the impulsive system is an associative memory that contains multimodal concepts representing correlations between external stimuli and affective and behavioral responses. It is assumed that, other than the temporary working memory of the reflective system, the associative store contains all the information that may be retrieved and transformed into temporary propositional knowledge. In accordance with most associative network models (Smith, 1998), the RIM suggests that contents in the impulsive system are connected through links of varying strength. It is further assumed that the links extend to behavioral representations. A special type of behavioral representation in the impulsive system, behavioral schemas are abstractions of reoccurring behaviors that contain typical situational conditions, typical consequences, and the motoric aspects.

Processes

Two core mechanisms of the impulsive system are spreading activation and associative learning. They imply that activation may spread among the contents, and that the amount of activation depends on the strength of the links between them, while the strength is a function of the frequency and recency of joint activation. For example, activating the concept "old" may spread activation to the concept "slow," which in turn may spread activation to specific behavioral schemas (Bargh, Chen, & Burrows, 1996). One-trial learning is the exception (e.g., Öhman, Eriksson, & Olofsson, 1975), and learning is a function of the frequency of joint activation in temporal and spatial proximity. The nature of the simple associative processes suggested to operate in the impulsive system can be expected to result in cognitive limitations. Specifically, the RIM suggests that the impulsive system cannot flexibly combine multiple elements by means of abstract concepts such as causality, time, or truth (Strack & Deutsch, 2004). As a consequence, abstract concepts of this kind are predicted not to effect purely impulsive responses (e.g., Deutsch, Gawronski, & Strack, 2006). For example, the impulsive system is predicted not to be able to distinguish between causation and correlation, but to treat covariations of all kinds alike. Similarly, contents tagged as false are predicted to have the same effects as contents tagged as true in the impulsive system (e.g., Deutsch et al., 2006; Gilbert et al., 1993).

While these paths are semantically determined, the RIM posits that valence may modify the semantic links to behavior. Specifically, the module named "motivational orientation" (Cacioppo, Priester, & Berntson, 1993) may facilitate activation spread along links that are motivationally compatible with the valence of the content. In detail, positive information is assumed to be compatible with behavioral tendencies toward approach and negative information, toward avoidance (e.g., Krieglmeyer, Deutsch, De Houwer, & De Raedt, 2010). It is important to note that the described compatibility is bidirectional. That is, valence may facilitate the execution of compatible behavior, and behavior may facilitate the processing of compatible valence (Neumann, Förster, & Strack, 2003). Moreover, the dysregulation of vital needs is predicted to affect behavioral schemas. Specifically, those schemas that helped in overcoming the need in the past will receive activation, along with relevant semantic and evaluative schemas (e.g., Aarts, Dijksterhuis, & De Vries, 2001; Höfling et al., 2009; Seibt, Häfner, & Deutsch, 2007). Thus, a purely impulsive transition from evaluation to motivation and behavior is not mediated by a means–ends decision. Instead, automatic facilitation of approach versus avoidance, along with effects of homeostatic dysregulation, will elicit the appropriate behaviors. Moreover, the representation of value in the impulsive system is not noetic but experiential, such that a stimulus is not accompanied by the knowledge of goodness but by the feeling of pleasantness. However, as both systems always interact (see section on interactions), a purely anoetic determination of behavior is unlikely to occur.

Automaticity

Compared to the reflective system, the mechanisms of its impulsive counterpart operate on a higher level of automaticity. First, given that impulsive processes are theorized to be based on activation processes in associative memory, they are predicted not to require cognitive resources, resulting in an efficient execution of cognitive and behavioral action. That is, despite distractions, load, or low effort, impulsive mechanisms continue to operate. In fact, associative learning may even occur during sleep (Arzi et al., 2012). Second, impulsive processes may generate an experiential awareness possessing a positive or negative valence. That is, just like reflective processes, impulsive processes are not conceptualized as necessarily being fully unaware. Third, impulsive processes are unintentional in the sense that intentions are solely generated in the reflective system, and impulsive processes may operate autonomously and independently of the reflective system. However, impulsive processes can be controlled by intentions, such that they can be activated, modified, or inhibited by the reflective system.

INTERACTIONS BETWEEN THE SYSTEMS

An important part of the RIM is the interaction between the systems (see Figure 7.2). To make this interaction possible, it is necessary that the systems operate in parallel. However, based on the differences in the absorption of attention, the activity of the reflective system is moderated by the available cognitive capacity, whereas the impulsive system is assumed always to be active. As we already mentioned, interactions may occur at different stages of the processing and are described later in this chapter. They concern the relation between syllogistic inferences and the accessibility of associative contents, the two types of emotional influences, and decisions and synergistic versus antagonistic influences on behavior.

The Interaction between Propositions and Associations

Most important, we propose that the mechanisms of syllogistic reasoning depend on the accessibility of associative contents from the impulsive system.

Specifically, the use of categories depends on their accessibility (Higgins, 1996), which does not obey the principles of syllogistic reasoning. Rather, the described mechanisms of associative processing determine the categories' accessibility, that is, the frequency and recency of their prior use. As a consequence, the first step of reflective processing hinges on associative mechanisms. That is, concepts that have previously been used have a greater chance to serve as categories for propositional processes, particularly if the temporal distance from their previous activation was short and its use has occurred in a repeated fashion.

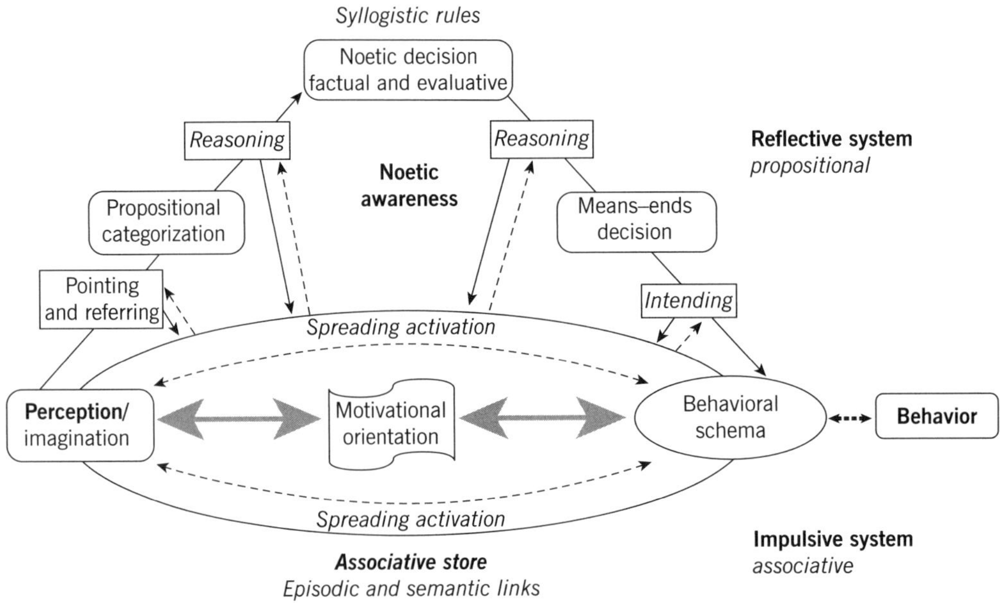

FIGURE 7.2. The reflective–impulsive model (RIM).

For example, having been exposed to information about older adults may increase the likelihood that that a person is being categorized as being old, particularly if the target is ambiguous (Higgins, Rholes, & Jones, 1977).

This impact of associative processing is matched by the reverse influence of reflective operations. That is, any act of reflective reasoning uses concepts whose accessibility will then be increased. For example, if someone ponders about the age of another person, the *old* category becomes more accessible for a subsequent judgment. As a consequence, two reflective operations influence one another in an automatic fashion that can hardly be corrected.

As a general rule, each of these reflective operations is influenced by the accessibility of associative contents. In reverse, the activation potential is increased by reflective operations that are based on the retrieval of a certain type of information. As a consequence, reflective operations may influence each other through associative mechanisms in an automatic fashion that is difficult to control.

This has been demonstrated by Mussweiler and Strack (Mussweiler, Förster, & Strack, 1997; Strack & Mussweiler, 1997) in their selective-accessibility account of judgmental anchoring, in which preceding comparative judgments were found to assimilate subsequent absolute judgments. In a number of studies, it was demonstrated that comparative judgments trigger a search for information that is consistent with the standard (Klayman & Ha, 1987). As a result, this selectively activated information is more accessible and therefore more likely to enter into subsequent absolute judgments that are generated. Thus, the anchoring effect was shown to be produced not by insufficient adjustments from different starting points but by a selective accessibility of information that comes to mind. It is this interaction between automatic associative mechanisms that operates outside of awareness and intentional reflective processes that makes controlling for unwanted influences difficult. In fact, explicitly requesting participants to avoid being influenced by the anchoring task or even offering them money did not result in a substantial reduction of the bias (Wilson, Houston, Etling, & Brekke, 1996). For the domain of attitudes, this interaction has been aptly described in the associative–propositional evaluation (APE) model (Gawronski & Bodenhausen, 2006, 2011). This has led to new predictions about differential inconsistency for implicit versus explicit attitudes (Gawronski, Strack, & Bodenhausen, 2009). Specifically, it was found that dissonance-induced attitude change was limited to explicit attitudes, while implicit evaluations were left unaffected (Gawronski & Strack, 2004). This suggests that dissonance is based on noetic inconsistencies that imply propositional incompatibilities. The lack of concomitant associative consequences provides additional evidence for the different operating principles.

The Interaction between Propositions and Experiences

A second example for the interaction of the two systems is the propositionalization of experiences. That is, subjective experiences that have emerged in the impulsive system may be categorized and enter into syllogistic reasoning. Thus, feelings may serve "as information" (Schwarz & Clore, 1983) and turn complicated judgments into intuitive ones. At the same time, even if they are experienced, their reflective use may be prevented if they are not representative for the judgment at hand (Strack, 1992). In a more recent set of studies, Topolinski and Strack (2009a) used people's tendency to judge semantic coherence on the basis of experienced fluency (cf. Topolinski & Strack, 2009b) and found that when provided with an irrelevant source for their feeling, they did not use it to decide about the coherence of the triads. Like previous results (e.g., Schwarz et al., 1991) this finding shows that subjective experiences may enter syllogistic reasoning and may be used, or not used, for inferences. For this purpose, however, subjective experiences need to be propositionally categorized like perceptual input from outside. This use of feelings in judgments suggests a psychological mechanism that is responsible for intuition (e.g., Deutsch & Strack, 2008). To have "a good feeling about something" means that a positive experience is categorized and attributed to a particular source. In other words, intuitive judgments do not imply the operation of a special system. Instead, intuitive judgments can be understood as a special case of reflective reasoning in which subjective experiences become the bases of inferences.

DIFFERENT ROUTES TO BEHAVIOR

A further important feature is that the RIM contains different routes to behavior. In the reflective system, behavior is a function of the expected value of the anticipated outcome that is inferred on the basis of the generated knowledge. The resulting behavioral decision (goal) serves as an immediate precursor of the behavior. The fulfillment of the goal is rewarding and a source of positive affect. In contrast, the impulsive system generates behavioral responses as a function of preexisting, habit-like behavioral schemas (cf. Wood & Neal, 2007). In addition, behavioral responses are influenced by motivational orientation and homeostatic dysregulation.

Through mechanisms of associative learning, reflective acquired and controlled behaviors are gradually transformed into habits. As a consequence, their execution requires less cognitive capacity. Because the operations of the reflective system require this limited resource, impulsive components are useful to facilitate the execution of reflective operations. In return, habitually emitted behaviors may be suppressed, overruled, or modified by goal-directed reflective intervention. The increase of fluency in the execution of the behavior may generate positive affect and therefore become a source of intrinsic motivation (Custers & Aarts, 2005). Moreover, a target that elicits a positive valence facilitates the reduction of the distance between the actor and the source, whereas a negative valence increases it (Cacioppo et al., 1993; Krieglmeyer, De Houwer, & Deutsch, 2011; Neumann et al., 2003). Going beyond their mere valence, full-blown emotions have their own action tendencies that are more specific than approach and avoidance (Frijda, Kuipers, & Terschure, 1989). Finally, the deprivation of basic needs is predicted to increase the accessibility of behavioral schemas that were previously associated with need fulfillment. As a consequence, deprivation automatically facilitates behavioral tendencies toward its termination.

Whenever these impulsive mechanisms generate responses that serve or are compatible with the decisions of the reflective system, the execution of the behavior is synergistically supported. However, if impulsive tendencies are incompatible with the goals of the reflective system, conflicts may emerge, and strategies of self-regulation are necessary to ensure that the goals exert the ultimate influence.

CONFLICT BETWEEN THE SYSTEMS

The two systems are in conflict if the cognitive, affective, or behavioral tendencies generated by the impulsive system are incompatible with the reflective judgments or goals. In the case of cognitive conflict, knowledge that is activated in the impulsive system is incompatible with noetic decisions made in the reflective system. One example of such a conflict is the activation of stereotypical associations upon perception of a member of a stereotyped group, while the social perceiver at the same time concludes that these associations are invalid (Devine, 1989). As another example, the processing of social stimuli may activate evaluative associations in the form of prejudice, while the reflective system generates incompatible, egalitarian evaluations of the same targets (Dovidio, Kawakami, & Gaertner, 2002).

Because there exist cognitive and motor bottlenecks (cf. Ulrich et al., 2006) limiting the number of behaviors that can be executed at a given time, the two systems may compete in pushing different behavioral schemas above execution threshold. In the case of behavioral conflict, behavioral schemas activated in the impulsive system are incommensurable with behavioral decisions held in the reflective system. Under such circumstances, the person experiences the facilitation or inhibition that is triggered by the stimulus and feels "tempted" to give in to the impulsive force. Alternatively, the person may overcome the impulsive tendencies and enforce the behavioral decisions. This, however, requires those preconditions that are necessary for reflective processes to operate. An example for behavioral conflict is the situation in which one's perception of a member of a stigmatized group induces a tendency to avoid this person, whereas one's egalitarian goals create a tendency to approach or at least not to avoid (e.g., Dotsch & Wigboldus, 2008).

The RIM can readily explain a wide range of cognitive and behavioral conflicts. Specifically, because they differ in their operating principles, the two systems can be predicted to generate diverging responses under specific conditions. As such, the RIM helps in understanding basic phenomena relating to conflict (for a more detailed discussion, see Strack & Deutsch, in press). Moreover, cognitive and behavioral conflicts that regularly occur in situations of self-regulation are part of some mental disorders and also influence economic decision making. As we describe in the next section, the RIM has been successfully applied to these situations.

APPLICATIONS OF THE RIM

The RIM has served as a conceptual framework to achieve a better understanding of various applied phenomena. In the domain of health-destructive behaviors, it has contributed to a better understanding of the role of automatic processes (Marteau, Hollands, & Fletcher, 2012). Perhaps more important, the RIM has helped identify conditions that promote rather than prevent self-control (Hofmann, Friese, & Strack, 2009), especially for health-related behavior that is often in conflict with unhealthy alternatives (Hofmann, Friese, & Wiers, 2008). Also, various clinical phenomena, such as addictive behaviors (Deutsch & Strack, 2005), eating disorders, phobias, and compulsions (Roefs et al., 2011; Wiers, Teachman, & De Houwer, 2007) involve self-inflicted injurious behaviors that occur against people's better judgment and may therefore be interpreted as and behavioral conflicts. Another field of application is consumer behavior and decision making, in which impulse buying is an example of a behavior occurring against rational considerations (Hofmann, Strack, & Deutsch, 2008; Strack, Werth, & Deutsch, 2006).

Self-control typically involves the change of an ongoing or prepotent behavior (e.g., Hofmann et al., 2009; Muraven & Baumeister, 2000). Prototypical forms of self-control involve tradeoffs between consequences that occur at different points in time (Loewenstein, Read, & Baumeister, 2003): trading relatively positive short-term consequences for even better long-term consequences. Both, short- and long-term consequences may involve nourishing or harming end-states (Higgins, 1997). For example, one may accept a negative short-term event (e.g., visiting a dentist) to avoid the occurrence of an even more negative long-term event (e.g., toothache). As another example, one may forego a relatively positive short-term consequence (e.g., eating a high-calorie desert) to avoid the occurrence of a negative long-term event (e.g., being socially rejected because of being obese). The RIM contributes to understanding a great number of phenomena in the realm of self-control by identifying the two systems as sources of diverging behavioral tendencies. It can predict situations in which such dissociations are likely to occur, as well as conditions under which behavior will be more likely to be guided by rational considerations of short- and long-term utility or by behavioral tendencies based on different motivational principles (for reviews and extensions, see Hofmann, Friese, Müller, & Strack, 2011; Hofmann et al., 2009).

Theoretical concepts of the RIM also contribute to the understanding of mental disorders (e.g., Deutsch & Strack, 2005; Stacy & Wiers, 2010). Some core concepts of the RIM have been established in clinical theory, research, and practice for a long time, such as automaticity (e.g., Tiffany, 1990), habits (Everitt, Dickinson, & Robbins, 2001), approach and avoidance motivation (Fowles, 1994), or associative processes (e.g., Teachman & Woody, 2003). On a very general level, the RIM may aid in recognition of interrelations between these concepts in the realm of addiction and provide a framework for integrating these concepts into a larger-scale theory.

On a more specific level, theoretical assumptions of the RIM have a particular potential to be fruitfully applied to clinical phenomena. Some mental disorders involve consistent behavioral conflicts and attempts at self-control. For example, addictive behaviors often occur in the face of knowledge about hazardous long-term consequences (Stacy & Wiers, 2010; Tiffany, 1990). Likewise, compulsive behaviors and phobic responses involve simultaneous dissociations between belief that a certain behavior is irrational or that a situation is not objectively dangerous and intense behavioral tendencies and affective responses (cf. Wiers et al., 2007). From the perspective of the RIM, such knowledge–behavior dissociations represent a special case of behavioral conflicts, that is, the simultaneous operation of beliefs and behavioral schemas in the reflective system that have diverging behavioral implications. Therefore, knowledge about the operating dynamics of the two systems may help us to better understand such conflicts in the clinical realm. Another example is the notion of approach–avoidance motivation, which in itself is not unique to the RIM. But the model specifies in detail how such motivation may interact with evaluative associations, deprivation, and reflective processes. For example, principles of the RIM were applied to develop approach–avoidance training to reduce the motivational pull of drugs (Wiers, Rinck, Kordts, Houben, & Strack, 2010).

While traditional models of decision making in psychology (e.g., Edwards, 1961) and economy (e.g., Becker, 1976) had a strong focus on a rational expected-utility calculus, a plethora of studies suggest systematic deviations from optimal decision making (e.g., Kahneman, 2003; Loewenstein, 2001). For example, decision making was demonstrated to be influenced by current affective states of the decision maker (e.g., Han, Lerner, & Keltner, 2007; Loewenstein, Weber, Hsee, & Welch, 2001; Slovic, Finucane, Peters, & MacGregor, 2002). Apparently, decision-makers use affective feelings as cues that are deemed informative about the options at hand. Likewise, feelings of cognitive or perceptual fluency were demonstrated to influence a wide range of decisions (Novemsky, Dhar, Schwarz, & Simonson, 2007; Song & Schwarz, 2009; Topolinski & Strack, 2010). Within the RIM such effects are seen as interactions between the reflective and the impulsive system. More specifically, judgments generated in the reflective system may be based on various inputs from the impulsive system, including affective and cognitive feelings (for a detailed discussion, see Deutsch & Strack, 2008). This has led to therapeutic interventions that focus not on people's goals but on the impulsive components that contribute to heath damage (Veling, Aarts, & Stroebe, 2013; Wiers et al., 2010).

A second challenge for duality models lies in the domain of consumer behavior (e.g., Samson & Voyer, 2012). The RIM may serve as a unified framework that accounts for different methods of economic exchange. On the one hand, it describes the cognitive determinants of choices that are driven by the evaluation of the anticipated outcome. Of course, the mechanisms of the reflective system with its heuristic simplifications can be invoked to explain such decisions. In particular, the use of affect in consumer judgments (Pham, 2004) fits well into the mechanisms of the reflective system. More important, perhaps, is the conceptual integration of a phenomenon known as "impulse buying" (Beatty & Ferrell, 1998; Faber & Vohs, 2004; Kalla & Arora, 2011), whereby consumers acquire goods in an unplanned fashion and also report strong urges and little control over these occurrences. From the perspective of the RIM, impulse buying resembles situations of self-regulation in which resources that are necessary for reflective system are depleted or undermined. As a consequence, the behavioral dispositions in the impulsive system become dominant, along with behavioral orientations that are affectively elicited (Hofmann, Strack, et al., 2008; Strack et al., 2006).

CONCLUSION

In summary, the RIM describes the interaction among cognitive, motivational, and emotional processes, along with the accruing behavioral consequences. Although the model cannot be tested as a whole, its component mechanisms can be, and have been examined empirically. The cited research provides substantial corroboration. Moreover, the RIM has proved to possess a remarkable applied potential. On the cognitive level, the model has helped to account for the interaction between explicit and implicit attitudes. On the behavioral dimension, the RIM has identified conditions under which people's actions are not determined by the long-term goals or their anticipated consequences. Finally, the RIM has stimulated interventions that proved successful in modifying problematic behaviors. These examples suggest that the RIM has become an integrative tool that affords a better understanding of the mutual influence of thoughts, feelings, and actions under specified conditions.

REFERENCES

Aarts, H., Dijksterhuis, A., & De Vries, P. (2001). On the psychology of drinking: Being thirsty and perceptually ready. *British Journal of Psychology, 92*, 631–642.

Arzi, A., Shedlesky, L., Ben-Shaul, M., Nasser, K., Oksenberg, A., Hairston, I. S., et al. (2012). Humans can learn new information during sleep. *Nature Neuroscience, 15*(10), 1460–1465.

Bargh, J. A. (1994). The four horsemen of automaticity: Awareness, intention, efficiency, and control in social cognition. In R. S. Wyer & T. K. Srull (Eds.), *Handbook of social cognition* (Vol. 1, pp. 1–40). Hillsdale, NJ: Erlbaum.

Bargh, J. A., Chen, M., & Burrows, L. (1996). Automaticity of social behavior: Direct effects of trait construct and stereotype activation on action. *Journal of Personality and Social Psychology, 71*, 230–244.

Beatty, S. E., & Ferrell, M. E. (1998). Impulse buying: Modeling its precursors. *Journal of Retailing, 74*, 169–191.

Becker, G. (1976). *The economic approach to human behavior.* Chicago: University of Chicago Press.

Cacioppo, J. T., Priester, J. R., & Berntson, G. G. (1993). Rudimentary determinants of attitudes: II. Arm flexion and extension have differential effects on attitudes. *Journal of Personality and Social Psychology, 65*, 5–17.

Chater, N., & Oaksford, M. (1999). The probability heuristics model of syllogistic reasoning. *Cognitive Psychology, 38*, 191–258.

Custers, R., & Aarts, H. (2005). Beyond priming effects: The role of positive affect and discrepancies in implicit processes of motivation and goal pursuit. *European Review of Social Psychology, 16*, 257–300.

Deutsch, R., Gawronski, B., & Strack, F. (2006). At the boundaries of automaticity: Negation as reflective operation. *Journal of Personality and Social Psychology, 91*, 385–405.

Deutsch, R., Kordts-Freudinger, R., Gawronski, B., & Strack, F. (2009). Fast and fragile: A new look at the automaticity of negation processing. *Experimental Psychology, 56*, 434–446.

Deutsch, R., & Strack, F. (2005). Reflective and impulsive determinants of addictive behaviors. In R. W. Wiers & A. W. Stacy (Eds.), *Handbook of implicit cognition and addiction* (pp. 45–57). Thousand Oaks, CA: Sage.

Deutsch, R., & Strack, F. (2006). Duality models in social psychology: From dual processes to interacting systems. *Psychological Inquiry, 17*, 166–172.

Deutsch, R., & Strack, F. (2008). Variants of judgment and decision making: The perspective of the reflective–impulsive model. In H. Plessner, C. Betsch, & T. Betsch (Eds.), *Intuition in judgment and decision making* (pp. 39–53). Mahwah, NJ: Erlbaum.

Devine, P. G. (1989). Stereotypes and prejudice: Their automatic and controlled components. *Journal of Personality and Social Psychology, 56*, 5–18.

Dotsch, R., & Wigboldus, D. H. J. (2008). Virtual prejudice. *Journal of Experimental Social Psychology, 44*, 1194–1198.

Dovidio, J. F., Kawakami, K., & Gaertner, S. L. (2002). Implicit and explicit prejudice and interracial interaction. *Journal of Personality and Social Psychology, 82*, 62–68.

Edwards, W. (1961). Behavioral decision theory. *Annual Review of Psychology, 12*, 473–498.

Engle, R. W. (2002). Working memory capacity as executive attention. *Current Directions in Psychological Science, 11*, 19–23.

Evans, J. S. B. T. (2008). Dual-processing accounts of reasoning, judgment, and social cognition. *Annual Review of Psychology, 59*, 255–278.

Everitt, B. J., Dickinson, A., & Robbins, T. W. (2001). The neuropsychological basis of addictive behaviour. *Brain Research Reviews, 36*, 129–138.

Faber, R. J., & Vohs, K. D. (2004). To buy or not to buy?: Self-control and self-regulatory failure in purchase behavior. In R. F. Baumeister & K. D. Vohs (Eds.), *Handbook of self-regulation: Research, theory, and applications* (pp. 509–524). New York: Guilford Press.

Fowles, D. C. (1994). A motivational theory of psychopathology. In W. D. Spaulding (Ed.), *Integrative views of motivation, cognition, and emotion* (pp. 181–238). Lincoln: University of Nebraska Press.

Frijda, N. H., Kuipers, P., & Terschure, E. (1989). Relations among emotion, appraisal, and emotional action readiness. *Journal of Personality and Social Psychology, 57*, 212–228.

Gawronski, B., & Bodenhausen, G. V. (2006). Associative and propositional processes in evaluation: An integrative review of implicit and explicit attitude change. *Psychological Bulletin, 132*, 692–731.

Gawronski, B., & Bodenhausen, G. (2011). The associative–propositional evaluation model: Theory, evidence, and open questions. *Advances in Experimental Social Psychology, 44*, 59–127.

Gawronski, B., & Creighton, L. A. (2013). Dual-process theories. In D. A. Carlston (Ed.), *The Oxford handbook of social cognition.* (pp. 282–321). New York: Oxford University Press.

Gawronski, B., & Strack, F. (2004). On the propositional nature of cognitive consistency: Dissonance changes explicit, but not implicit attitudes. *Journal of Experimental Social Psychology, 40,* 535–542.

Gawronski, B., Strack, F., & Bodenhausen, G. V. (2009). Attitudes and cognitive consistency: The role of associative and propositional processes. In R. E. Petty, R. H. Fazio, & P. Briñol (Eds.), *Attitudes: Insights from the new implicit measures* (pp. 85–117). New York: Psychology Press.

Gilbert, D. T., Tafarodi, R. W., & Malone, P. S. (1993). You can't not believe everything you read. *Journal of Personality and Social Psychology, 65,* 221–233.

Gollwitzer, P. M. (1999). Implementation intentions: Strong effects of simple plans. *American Psychologist, 54,* 493–503.

Gollwitzer, P. M., Bayer, U. C., McCulloch, K. C. (2005). The Control of the unwanted. In R. R. Hassin, J. S. Uleman, & J. A. Bargh (Eds.), *The new unconscious* (pp. 485–515). Oxford, UK: Oxford University Press.

Han, S., Lerner, J. S., & Keltner, D. (2007). Feelings and consumer decision making: The appraisal-tendency framework. *Journal of Consumer Psychology, 17,* 158–168.

Higgins, E. T. (1996). Knowledge activation: Accessibility, applicability, and salience. In E. T. Higgins & A. W. Kruglanski (Eds.), *Social psychology: Handbook of basic principles* (pp. 133–168). New York: Guilford Press.

Higgins, E. T. (1997). Beyond pleasure and pain. *American Psychologist, 52,* 1280–1300.

Higgins, E. T., Rholes, W. S., & Jones, C. R. (1977). Category accessibility and impression formation. *Journal of Experimental Social Psychology, 13,* 141–154.

Höfling, A., Likowski, K. U., Deutsch, R., Häfner, M., Seibt, B., Mühlberger, A., et al. (2009). When hunger finds no fault with moldy corn: Food deprivation reduces food-related disgust. *Emotion, 9,* 50–58.

Hofmann, W., Friese, M., Müller, J., & Strack, F. (2011). Two souls live in my breast: Psychological and philosophical considerations concerning the conflict between impulses and self-control. *Psychologische Rundschau, 62,* 147–166.

Hofmann, W., Friese, M., & Strack, F. (2009). Impulse and self-control from a dual-systems perspective. *Perspectives on Psychological Science, 4,* 162–176.

Hofmann, W., Friese, M., & Wiers, R. W. (2008). Impulsive versus reflective influences on health behavior: A theoretical framework and empirical review. *Health Psychology Review, 2,* 111–137.

Hofmann, W., Strack, F., & Deutsch, R. (2008). Free to buy?: Explaining self-control and impulse in consumer behavior. *Journal of Consumer Psychology, 18,* 22–26.

Kahneman, D. (2003). Maps of bounded rationality: Psychology for behavioral economics. *American Economic Review, 93,* 1449–1475.

Kalla, S. M., & Arora, A. P. (2011). Impulse buying: A literature review. *Global Business Review, 12,* 145–157.

Klayman, R. B., & Ha, Y. W. (1987). Confirmation, disconfirmation, and information in hypothesis testing. *Psychological Review, 94,* 211–228.

Krieglmeyer, R., De Houwer, J., & Deutsch, R. (2011). How farsighted are behavioral tendencies of approach and avoidance?: The effect of stimulus valence on immediate vs. ultimate distance change. *Journal of Experimental Social Psychology, 47,* 622–627.

Krieglmeyer, R., Deutsch, R., De Houwer, J., & De Raedt, R. (2010). Being moved: Valence activates approach–avoidance behavior independently of evaluation and approach–avoidance intentions. *Psychological Science, 21,* 607–613.

Kruglanski, A., & Orehek, E. (2007). Partitioning the domain of social inference: Dual mode and systems models and their alternatives. *Annual Review of Psychology, 58,* 291–316.

Kruglanski, A. W., Chun, W. Y., Erb, H. P., Pierro, A., Mannetti, L., & Spiegel, S. (2003). A parametric unimodel of human judgment: Integrating dual-process frameworks in social cognition from a single-mode perspective. In J. P. Forgas, K. D. Williams, & W. von Hippel (Eds.), *Social judgments: Implicit and explicit processes* (pp. 137–161). New York: Cambridge University Press.

Kruglanski, A. W., & Thompson, E. P. (1999). Persuasion by a single route: A view from the unimodel. *Psychological Inquiry, 10,* 83–109.

Loewenstein, G. F. (2001). The creative destruction of decision research. *Journal of Consumer Research, 28,* 499–505.

Loewenstein, G. F., Read, D., & Baumeister, R. (2003). *Time and decision: Economic and psychological perspectives on intertemporal choice*. New York: Russell Sage Foundation.

Loewenstein, G. F., Weber, E. U., Hsee, C. K., & Welch, N. (2001). Risk as feelings. *Psychological Bulletin, 127*, 267–286.

Marteau, T. M., Hollands, G. J., & Fletcher, P. C. (2012). Changing human behavior to prevent disease: The importance of targeting automatic processes. *Science, 337*, 1492–1495.

Miyake, A., & Shah, P. (1999). *Models of working memory: Mechanisms of active maintenance and executive control*. Cambridge, UK: Cambridge University Press.

Moors, A., & De Houwer, J. (2006). Automaticity: A theoretical and conceptual analysis. *Psychological Bulletin, 132*, 297–326.

Muraven, M., & Baumeister, R. F. (2000). Self-regulation and depletion of limited resources: Does self-control resemble a muscle? *Psychological Bulletin, 126*, 247–259.

Mussweiler, T., Förster, J., & Strack, F. (1997). Anchoring effects and the applicability of anchor-consistent information: A selective accessibility model. *Zeitschrift für Experimentelle Psychologie, 44*, 589–615.

Neumann, R., Förster, J., & Strack, F. (2003). Motor compatibility: The bidirectional link between behavior and evaluation. In J. Musch & K. C. Klauer (Eds.), *The psychology of evaluation* (pp. 371–391). London: Erlbaum.

Novemsky, N., Dhar, R., Schwarz, N., & Simonson, T. (2007). Preference fluency in choice. *Journal of Marketing Research, 44*, 347–356.

Öhman, A., Eriksson, A., Olofsson, C. (1975). One-trial learning and superior resistance to extinction of autonomic responses conditioned to potentially phobic stimuli. *Journal of Comparative and Physiological Psychology, 88*, 619–627.

Pham, M. T. (2004). The logic of feeling. *Journal of Conmsumer Psychology, 14*, 360–369.

Roefs, A., Huijding, J., Smulders, F. T. Y., MacLeod, C. M., de Jong, P. J., Wiers, R. W., et al. (2011). Implicit measures of association in psychopathology research. *Psychological Bulletin, 137*, 149–193.

Samson, A., & Voyer, B. G. (2012). Two minds, three ways: Dual system and dual process models in consumer psychology. *AMS Review, 2*, 48–71.

Schwarz, N., Bless, H., Strack, F., Klumpp, G., Rittenauerschatka, H., & Simons, A. (1991). Ease of retrieval as information—another look at the availability heuristic. *Journal of Personality and Social Psychology, 61*, 195–202.

Schwarz, N., & Clore, G. L. (1983). Mood, misattribution, and judgments of well-being: Informative and directive functions of affective states. *Journal of Personality and Social Psychology, 45*, 513–523.

Seibt, B., Häfner, M., & Deutsch, R. (2007). Prepared to eat: How immediate affective and motivational responses to food cues are influenced by food deprivation. *European Journal of Social Psychology, 37*, 359–379.

Sloman, S. A. (1996). The empirical case for two systems of reasoning. *Psychological Bulletin, 119*, 3–22.

Slovic, P., Finucane, M., Peters, E., & MacGregor, D. G. (2002). The affect heuristic. In T. Gilovich, D. Griffin, & D. Kahneman (Eds.), *Heuristics and biases: The psychology of intuitive judgment* (pp. 397–420). New York: Cambridge University Press.

Smith, E. R. (1998). Mental representation and memory. In D. T. Gilbert, S. T. Fiske, & G. Lindzey (Eds.), *Handbook of social psychology* (4th ed., Vol. 1, pp. 391–445). New York: Oxford University Press.

Song, H. J., & Schwarz, N. (2009). If it's difficult to pronounce, it must be risky. *Psychological Science, 20*, 135–138.

Stacy, A. W., & Wiers, R. W. (2010). Implicit cognition and addiction: A tool for explaining paradoxical behavior. *Annual Review of Clinical Psychology, 6*, 551–575.

Strack, F. (1992). The different routes to social judgments: Experiential versus informational strategies. In L. L. Martin & A. Tesser (Eds.), *The construction of social judgment* (pp. 249–275). Hillsdale, NJ: Erlbaum.

Strack, F., & Deutsch, R. (2004). Reflective and impulsive determinants of social behavior. *Personality and Social Psychology Review, 8*, 220–247

Strack, F., & Deutsch, R. (in press). The duality of everyday life: Dual-process and dual-system models in social psychology. In M. Mikulincer & P. Shaver (Eds.), E. Borgida & J. Bargh (Assoc. Eds.), *APA handbook of personality and social psychology: Vol. 1. Attitudes and social cognition*. Washington, DC: American Psychological Association.

Strack, F., & Mussweiler, T. (1997). Explaining the enigmatic anchoring effect: Mechanisms of selective accessibility. *Journal of Personality and Social Psychology, 73*, 437–446.

Strack, F., Werth, L., & Deutsch, R. (2006). Reflective and impulsive determinants of consumer behavior. *Journal of Consumer Psychology, 16*, 205–216.

Teachman, B. A., & Woody, S. (2003). Automatic processing among individuals with spider phobia: Change in implicit fear associations following treatment. *Journal of Abnormal Psychology, 112*, 100–109.

Tiffany, S. T. (1990). A cognitive model of drug urges and drug-use behavior: Role of automatic and nonautomatic processes. *Psychological Review, 97*, 147–168.

Topolinski, S., & Strack, F. (2009a). The analysis of intuition: Processing fluency and affect in judgements of semantic coherence. *Cognition and Emotion, 23*, 1465–1503.

Topolinski, S., & Strack, F. (2009b). The architecture of intuition: Fluency and affect determine intuitive judgments of semantic and visual coherence and judgments of grammaticality in artificial grammar learning. *Journal of Experimental Psychology: General, 138*, 39–63.

Topolinski, S., & Strack, F. (2010). False fame prevented: Avoiding fluency effects without judgmental correction. *Journal of Personality and Social Psychology, 98*, 721–733.

Tulving, E. (1985). How many memory systems are there? *American Psychologist, 40*, 385–398.

Ulrich, R., Fernandez, S. R., Jentzsch, I., Rolke, B., Schröter, H., & Leuthold, H. (2006). Motor limitation in dual-task processing under ballistic movement conditions. *Psychological Science, 17*, 788–793.

Veling, H., Aarts, H. & Stroebe, W. (2013). Using stop signals to reduce impulsive choices for palatable unhealthy foods. *British Journal of Health Psychology, 18*, 354–368.

Waldmann, M. R., Hagmayer, Y., & Blaisdell, A. P. (2006). Beyond the information given: Causal models in learning and reasoning. *Current Directions in Psychological Science, 15*, 307–311.

Wiers, R. W., Rinck, M., Kordts, R., Houben, K., & Strack, F. (2010). Retraining automatic action-tendencies to approach alcohol in hazardous drinkers. *Addiction, 105*, 279–287.

Wiers, R. W., Teachman, B. A., & De Houwer, J. (2007). Implicit cognitive processes in psychopathology: An introduction. *Journal of Behavior Therapy and Experimental Psychiatry, 38*, 95–104.

Wilson, T. D., Houston, C. E., Etling, K. M., & Brekke, N. (1996). A new look at anchoring effects: Basic anchoring and its antecedents. *Journal of Experimental Psychology: General, 125*, 387–402.

Wood, W., & Neal, D. T. (2007). A new look at habits and the habit–goal interface. *Psychological Review*, 843–863.

PART III

MEASUREMENT AND FORMAL MODELING

CHAPTER 8

Dual-Process Theory from a Process Dissociation Perspective

B. Keith Payne and C. Daryl Cameron

When Shelly Chaiken and Yaacov Trope's *Dual-Process Theories in Social Psychology* was published in 1999, I (Payne) had begun my first year in graduate school. The book became my bible for graduate school, my field guide for social psychology, and quite literally my reading list for comprehensive oral exams. Nearly 15 years later, it is humbling to have the opportunity to contribute a chapter to this volume from my perspective on dual process theories. The only question I remember from "comps" is when Larry Jacoby said he imagined that the editors had aimed to uncover some fundamental duality behind the diversity of dual-process theories collected in the book, and he asked me what the fundamental duality might be. I don't remember what kind of answer I managed to cobble together. But in this chapter we would like to take another stab at that question.

The fundamental duality on which we want to focus is that sometimes people do things intentionally, sometimes they do things unintentionally, and usually they do both at the same time. In other words, any behavior that is complicated enough to be socially interesting is likely to be a blend of intentional (controlled) and unintentional (automatic) processes. What counts as a "process" will, of course, depend on what one is doing. Taking a driving test and running a three-legged race involve different operations, to be sure; nonetheless, some aspects of each are intended and others are not. A useful way to decompose those blends is to arrange situations in which intended and unintended processes lead to the same response, as well as situations in which they compete to drive opposing responses (Jacoby, 1991). With a few assumptions and some arithmetic, this approach provides a way to study the interactions between intentionally controlled and unintended components of behavior. The approach is fundamental in the sense that this distinction between intended and unintended components can apply across a huge variety of specific topic areas, yet stay focused on the distinctions between processes that are meaningful and important for dual-process theories in psychological science.

There is always a tradeoff between the generality of a psychological theory and how well it can explain the details of specific behavioral effects. One solution to this problem is to circumscribe the boundaries of the model to deal with one specific topic. So for example, whereas some dual-process models aim to explain attitudes, others deal with social perception, and still others, emotion, self-regulation, and so on. This approach makes it easier to specify what *process* means by dealing only with a narrow set of options. However, this approach is vulnerable to slippage between the specifics studied in an experiment and the notion of systems or processing architectures that underpin the theory. For example, many theorists have invoked a "System 1" that is intuitive, associative, experiential, or affective, and a "System 2" that is reflective, propositional, rule-based, or cognitive. As critics have pointed out, demonstrating that some effect is intuitive does not imply that it is also associative, experiential, or affective (Gigerenzer & Regier, 1996; Keren & Schul, 2009). Moreover, this approach leads to a proliferation of theories, in which each phenomenon is explained by one set of systems or processes, and it is not clear when each system or process refers to the same thing as the system or process invoked in another theory.

These problems result from specifying the dual-process theory at a rather high level of analysis (e.g., System 1, System 2) and applying it at a lower level of analysis where variables are operationalized in an experiment (e.g., How does cognitive load affect performance in a three-legged race?). Conclusions can be drawn about the specific topic, but inferences back to the nature of automatic and controlled processes become difficult, because the findings are specific to the phenomenon.

Suppose that cognitive load improves performance at three-legged racing. We might conclude that cooperative racing is automatic, and that "overthinking" leads people to "choke." We have not learned anything about that nature of Systems 1 and 2, only about three-legged racing. We have not learned much about that either, because we do not know whether cognitive load had its effects by reducing controlled processes (thereby relieving participants of their overthinking problem), or by increasing the contribution of automatic processes (perhaps by releasing subjects' spontaneous cooperation instinct), or both.

An alternative approach is to define study variables at the same level of analysis as the duality is defined. Process dissociation takes this approach. They key idea behind most process dissociation research is that the fundamental duality is based on intention. *Control* is defined as behaving in accord with intentions. *Automatic processes,* in contrast, are defined by how people behave in the absence of control.

DEFINING AUTOMATICITY

From a process dissociation perspective, understanding the intentional and unintentional components underpinning behavior requires answering three questions. First, *What does a person intend to do*? That is, what does he or she do when in perfect control? Second, *To what extent does the person actually do what is intended*? The difference between those two questions assesses how much control a person has. The third question is *What does a person do when control fails*? A pattern of systematic errors is revealing about what kinds of automatic processes are at play. If we know what a person intends to do, how well he or she actually does it, and also what kinds of unintended errors he or she makes, we can draw conclusions about both intended and unintended components of behavior.

As this discussion makes clear, the conceptual definition of the two process dissociation parameters is rooted in intention, within the context of the task goal. We have said nothing up to this point about consciousness or cognitive resources, for instance. These other features that are sometimes used as defining characteristics of automatic and controlled behavior can be addressed in two ways. One is to arrange the experimental paradigm such that a particular feature is necessary to carry out intentional responses. For example, as described in detail below, memory experiments are sometimes arranged so that completing the memory test as instructed requires conscious awareness in the form of recollecting past events. In paradigms where conscious awareness is necessary and sufficient for responding as intended, the process dissociation parameters can be used to study the conscious–unconscious distinction. A second way to study other aspects of automaticity is to treat them as empirical questions to be tested rather than as defining characteristics. For example, we might manipulate cognitive load to test whether it selectively affects intentional responding. To the extent that cognitive efficiency and intentionality are related, manipulations of resources should affect estimates based on intent, but this does not have to be the case.

But we are getting ahead of ourselves. In the next sections we explain how process dissociation can be applied to quantify these components of behavior, beginning with the procedure's development as a tool in memory research. Next we discuss some of the ways it has been employed in social psychology to answer important questions about attitudes, stereotypes, and other aspects of social cognition. In the final section we consider the relevance of process dissociation within the broader context of dual-process theories.

THEORETICAL BACKGROUND: SEPARATING CONSCIOUS AND UNCONSCIOUS USES OF MEMORY

Jacoby (1991) developed the process dissociation procedure in response to the observation that implicit and explicit memory tests were not "process-pure." That is, implicit tests do not purely reflect implicit memory processes, and explicit tests do not purely reflect explicit memory processes. As an example, in an implicit memory test, subjects might be instructed to complete a word fragment with the first word that comes to mind. Conscious memory could contaminate the test if a subject thinks back to a studied list for cues to the completion. In an explicit test, subjects might be instructed to think back intentionally to the studied list to complete the word fragment. In this case, unconscious memory could contaminate the test, if a person cannot remember the item but guesses, based on the first item that comes to mind (Jacoby, Toth, & Yonelinas, 1993; Schacter, 1987).

Jacoby's first innovation was to separate intentional and unintentional influences by placing them in opposition. One study asked subjects to study a list of nonfamous names, and either a few minutes or a full day later, to discriminate between famous and nonfamous names (Jacoby, Kelley, Brown, & Jasechko, 1989). Critically, subjects were told that none of the names on the studied list were famous. If they consciously remembered studying a name, then they could reject it as nonfamous. But studying the names made them more familiar, an influence that could easily be misattributed to the name being famous. As a result, subjects were more likely to call nonfamous names famous when they had been previously studied, but only after a day's delay, when recollection for the list was poor. Conscious recollection for studying a name enabled subjects to respond as intended by rejecting it as nonfamous. But familiarity created systematic errors when recollection failed. Placing conscious memory and automatic influences of memory in opposition allowed them to be clearly separated.

Opposition procedures such as the false fame study tend to underestimate unintended memory influences, because conscious memory works against detecting the unintended influence. When unintended influences are demonstrated, researchers can have confidence that they are unlikely to be contaminated by intentionally controlled memory. But opposition procedures may miss unintended influences if intentionally controlled influences are strong. Jacoby's solution was to correct for this underestimation by comparing conditions in which unintended and intended influences were opposed to conditions in which they worked in concert.

In one experiment (Jacoby et al., 1993), words were presented for study with full or divided attention, then later tested with word stems (e.g., *table; ta– – –*). In the inclusion test subjects were instructed to use the stem as a cue for recall of a studied word or, if they could not remember the item, to complete the stem with the first word that came to mind. Subjects could complete a stem with a studied word either because they consciously recollected the word, with a probability R, or because the studied word came automatically to mind (A) as a completion even when they did not recollect ($1 - R$). The probability of correctly completing the item with a studied word in the inclusion condition can be described by the equation

$$P(\text{correct in inclusion}) = R + A \cdot (1 - R) \quad (8.1)$$

In the exclusion test, subjects were instructed to complete the stem with the first word that came to mind, but to not use a recalled word. That is, they were told to exclude old words and use only new words. In this condition, a stem would be completed incorrectly with a studied word only if recollection failed and the word came automatically to mind:

$$P(\text{incorrect in exclusion}) = A \cdot (1 - R) \quad (8.2)$$

Assuming that automatic and controlled uses of memory are independent, researchers can then solve for estimates of automatic and controlled memory processes. The difference between the inclusion (trying to use old words) and exclusion (trying not to use old words) provides a measure of recollection:

$$R = [R + A \cdot (1 - R)] - [A \cdot (1 - R)] \quad (8.3)$$

Note how this equation maps on the three questions discusses earlier. Intent is defined by the test instructions to include or exclude studied words. Recollection then reflects how well subjects are able to carry out their intention (based on conscious experience in this case). Given that estimate, one can compute the probability of an automatic influence of old words. Automatic influences are reflected by incorrectly producing a studied word in the exclusion condition, but this is an underestimate of automatic influence, because it is opposed by recollection. To correct for this underestimation we divide by the probability that recollection has failed:

$$A = P(\text{incorrect in exclusion})/(1 - R) \quad (8.4)$$

Results of the experiment showed that divided, as compared to full, attention during the study significantly decreased recollection but had no effect on automatic influences.

Memory studies with inclusion and exclusion conditions allow automatic and controlled responses to be separated, because they answer all three of the questions outlined earlier. First, the inclusion and exclusion instructions define subjects' intentions, so the researcher knows how subjects intend to respond. Second, the difference between performance on inclusion and exclusion conditions provides an estimate of how much control subjects have over their memory performance; it is the difference between how they intend to respond and how they actually respond. And third, the automatic estimate measures the errors subjects make when control fails. Across many studies, these procedures have shown that controlled use of memory is strongly affected by variables such as cognitive load, depth of processing, speeded responding, and aging. In contrast, automatic influences of memory tend to be affected by variables that influence how easily an item comes to mind, such as perceptual fluency, conceptual fluency, and habitual responses (for a review see Yonelinas, 2002).

BEYOND MEMORY: PROCESS DISSOCIATION STUDIES IN SOCIAL PSYCHOLOGY

Although process dissociation was developed to separate memory processes, it represents a general theoretical approach to automatic and controlled processes that can be applied in virtually any field. As the distinction between automatic and controlled processes has become important across many areas of psychology, the process dissociation procedure has been applied more broadly. In recent years it has been increasingly applied in social psychology, especially in studies of implicit attitudes, prejudice, and stereotypes.

Attitudes and Stereotyping

The steep decline in racial prejudice over the last half-century has been so dramatic that in the 1980s some observers began to suspect that it was too good to be true. In nationally representative surveys, for example, the proportion of white Americans supporting racially integrated schools rose from 32% in 1942 to 90% by 1982; the proportion saying that they would vote for a qualified black presidential candidate rose from 37% in 1958 to 81% in 1983 (Schumann, Steeh, & Bobo, 1985). But while survey responses were becoming more egalitarian, studies using subtle, unobtrusive measures continued to show evidence of racial bias (Crosby, Bromley, & Saxe, 1980). An influential explanation holds that white Americans' consciously controlled responses have become more egalitarian in response to changing social norms, while their automatic responses have remained relatively negative (Devine, 1989).

Studies pursuing this idea have flourished in the last two decades with the development of implicit tests, whose aim is to measure automatically activated attitudes. Implicit tests measure attitudes indirectly, often using reaction times or behavioral responses rather than relying on self-report (e.g., Fazio, Jackson, & Dunton, 1995; Greenwald, McGhee, & Schwartz, 1998; Payne, Jacoby, & Lambert, 2005; Wittenbrink, Judd, & Park, 1997). Across hundreds of studies using various implicit attitude tests, there is one clear commonality: Implicit tests of race attitudes and stereotypes tend to show different results than explicit tests. They tend to be only modestly correlated (Hofmann, Gawronski, Gschwendner, Le, & Schmitt, 2005; Cameron, Brown-Iannuzzi, & Payne, 2012), and they sometimes predict different behaviors or behaviors under different conditions (e.g., Cameron, Brown-Iannuzzi, & Payne, 2012).

Many researchers have concluded from these findings that implicit cognitions are very different than explicit cognitions. In some theories, the divergence results because implicit tests tap automatic responses, whereas explicit tests tap strategically edited responses (Fazio et al., 1995). In other theories, it is because implicit tests tap unconscious attitudes, whereas explicit tests tap conscious attitudes (Greenwald & Banaji, 1995; Wilson, Lindsey, & Schooler, 2000). Both kinds of theories, however, have relied on a task dissociation approach that equates automatic processes with implicit tests and consciously controlled processes with explicit tests. That is, these theories assume the tests are process-pure, in that implicit tests exclusively reflect automatic processes and explicit tests reflect consciously controlled processes. In many cases the assumption may be unrealistic.

Consider all the ways that implicit and explicit tests differ. Explicit attitude tests are usually surveys in which subjects read sentences, decide how they feel about items, and formulate their answers on a numerical scale. The items are sometimes as abstract as policies such as affirmative action or busing. In an implicit test such as affective priming, subjects see a picture or word flashed briefly as a prime, followed by a pleasant or unpleasant word, and they must classify the word as good or bad (Fazio et al., 1995). The metric is the reaction time to classify the word, depending on the prime. In the Implicit Association Test (IAT), subjects sort two sets of items into four combined categories (Greenwald et al., 1998). For example, they may see pictures of black and white faces, and good and bad words, and sort each into the categories "black or good," "white or bad," "black or bad," and "white or good." Again, the measure of interest is reaction time.

To be sure, people can control their responses on a questionnaire more easily than they can control their reaction times on these implicit tests. But this is only one of many differences between the tests. They also differ in the concreteness of the items that subjects evaluate, the ways that attitude objects are represented (e.g., sentences vs. pictures), the complexity of the tasks, the metric (e.g., Likert scales vs. reaction times), and more. If an implicit test and an explicit test show different results, or if they fail to correlate strongly, is it because of differences between implicit and explicit cognition? Or is it because of any of these other differences? It is impossible to tell, because a task dissociation approach confounds these features with the implicit–explicit distinction (Payne, Burkley, & Stokes, 2008).

In contrast to the task dissociation approach, the process dissociation approach overcomes this problem by separating processes within the same task rather than comparing two different tasks. Consider a study conducted soon after the highly publicized death of Amadou Diallo, mistakenly shot by New York City police officers who mistook the wallet in his hand for a gun (Payne, 2001). Because Diallo was unarmed and black, some critics alleged that race biased the officers' use of force. The question in this 2001 study was whether this kind of error systematically mistaking a harmless object for a weapon—reveals unintended influences of racial stereotypes. Subjects distinguished between guns and harmless hand tools that were flashed briefly but perceptibly on a computer screen. Immediately preceding each object was a black or white male face that served as a prime.

This 2 × 2 design creates conditions in which intentional responding to the target items and automatic (i.e., unintended) influences of racial stereotypes are in concert (an inclusion condition), and in opposition (an exclusion condition). For example, when the prime was black and the target was a gun, subjects could correctly respond "gun" either by intentionally controlled (C) detection of the gun, or by an automatic stereotypical response (A) when control failed ($1 - C$); with $C + A(1 - C)$ representing the likelihood of a correct "gun" response. In contrast, when the prime was black and the target was a tool, subjects would incorrectly respond "gun" when controlled detection failed, but automatic stereotyping favored the gun response: $A(1 - C)$. The degree of intentional control can be solved by taking the difference between "gun" responses in the inclusion and exclusion conditions. Given that estimate, the degree of automatic bias can be solved by dividing stereotypical false "gun" responses by failures of control ($1 - C$).

What do the process estimates mean in this context? This experiment controlled subjects' intentions via the task requirements to distinguish guns from tools. For that reason, the ability to discriminate between target items accurately provides an index of how much control subjects have over their responses. The control estimate indexes how well subjects carried out their intentions by distinguishing between target objects. In contrast, subjects do not intend to be influenced by the racial primes. The automatic estimate indexes how much these unintended influences biased their responses. Automatic and controlled processes can be estimated within the same task, avoiding all the problems involved in equating processes with tasks.

The results of the study showed that the race primes biased responses, as a tool was more likely to be mistaken for a gun when it was primed with a black face than with a white face. But more importantly for present concerns, the process estimates successfully separated automatic and controlled components of responses. Requiring subjects to respond quickly sharply reduced the controlled component, a well-established characteristic of controlled processing. But the race primes did not affect the controlled component. In contrast, the race primes affected the automatic component, but response speed did not.

The automatic component also correlated in systematic ways with other measures of racial attitudes, increasing confidence in the validity of the estimate as an index of automatic racial bias. These findings have been replicated and extended in a number of subsequent studies. In one study, depleting self-regulation resources by having subjects complete hundreds of trials of a difficult cognitive task reduced the controlled component in the weapon bias, but not the automatic component (Govorun & Payne, 2006). This suggests that even though the estimate was based on intended versus unintended responding, the process underlying it also required cognitive resources. In another study, the automatic component correlated with implicit measures of race bias, whereas the controlled component correlated with other measures of cognitive control, such as an antisaccade task, in which subjects must effortfully direct attention away from a character flashing on the screen that would automatically attract attention (Payne, 2005).

These studies depict automatic and controlled processes very differently than would a task dissociation approach. By identifying processes with tasks, the task dissociation approach assumes any variable that affects an implicit test affects automatic processing, and variables that affect an explicit task affect controlled processing. Given all of the differences between tasks that are confounded with the automatic–controlled distinction, this mapping creates a number of problems. The studies described here show that both automatic and controlled components of responses can be affected in different ways within the same task, overcoming these confounds.

Given that in several studies process dissociation estimates have been validated as useful measures of automatic and controlled components of responses, they can also be used to explain findings that would otherwise be puzzling. For instance, Lambert and colleagues (2003) found that subjects ironically made more stereotypical errors in a weapon identification task when they anticipated that their responses would be public, as compared to private. Process dissociation analyses helped shed light on why. Subjects who anticipated having to share their responses showed poorer control over their responses but no difference in automatic influences of stereotypes. In the anticipated public setting, subjects had the same degree of automatic influence, but it was less opposed by controlled responding, thus producing a net increase in stereotypical errors. Impairments in control were most pronounced for subjects who were anxious about the impending discussion. Together, these findings show how process dissociation analyses can be used to explain a counterintuitive finding that would otherwise be puzzling.

The process dissociation approach also helps link concepts of automatic and controlled processing in social cognition to the ways that the terms are understood in cognitive and neuroscientific studies. Cognitive control in these fields is measured using tasks such as the antisaccade task or the Stroop task, in which subjects see color words written in colored fonts and must name the font color and ignore the word meaning. According to a neurocognitive model, control requires monitoring for conflict between goals and responses, and directing attention to prevent or overcome automatic responses (e.g., Botvinick, Braver, Barch, Carter, & Cohen, 2001). These processes are associated with specific patterns of neural activity and with specific brain regions. They do not map well to the type of "control" measured by self-report attitude questionnaires, but they map onto cognitive control as assessed by process dissociation. In a series of studies, Amodio and colleagues (2004; Amodio, Devine, & Harmon-Jones, 2008) studied event-related brain potentials that have previously been linked to conflict monitoring and cognitive control. They found that the same potentials were associated with process dissociation estimates of control in a weapons task, and that they were related to individual differences in motivations to control prejudice.

These studies help integrate control processes as studied in implicit social cognition with the kinds of control studied widely in other fields. More generally, process dissociation advances a broad construal of "control" as acting in line with intentions, and "automatic influences" as those that drive behavior when control fails (Bishara & Payne, 2009; Payne & Bishara, 2009). The automatic and controlled influences estimated in the crucible of the weapons task have been linked to other meaningful behaviors. For instance, in one study, after completing the weapons task, subjects formed an impression of a new black person from a vignette about a typical day in this person's life (Payne, 2005; see Srull & Wyer, 1989). Although the facts and behaviors in the vignette were identical for all subjects, the kinds of impressions they formed varied widely and depended on the kinds of automatic and controlled processes each subject displayed in the weapons task. Subjects who showed the most stereotypical automatic biases in the weapons task liked the black character less. This correlation is consistent with dozens of studies showing that automatic racial attitudes and stereotypes can color social perception.

But the process dissociation analyses also revealed another pattern that is more striking. The impact of automatic bias depended on how much control subjects exerted over their behaviors. Subjects who were good at controlling their responses in the weapons task were also good at controlling the influence of automatic stereotyping in their social perceptions. For these subjects, automatic stereotyping was not associated with more negative impressions. But for subjects who were poor at controlling their responses in the weapons task, the correlation between automatic bias and social impression was much stronger.

This pattern, in which the amount of intentional control determines whether automatic biases translate into overt behaviors, is consistent with verbally described dual-process theories. One example is Strack and Deutsch's (2004) model that distinguishes between reflective and impulsive determinants of behavior. Consistent with such models, several studies have shown that individual differences in cognitive control are important in moderating the relationship between implicit attitudes and behavior. For example, Hofmann, Gshwendner, Friese, Wiers, and Schmitt (2008) examined behaviors that can be jointly driven by automatic impulses and self-control efforts, including eating sweets. They measured cognitive control using tests of working memory—the ability to mentally maintain and manipulate multiple pieces of information at the same time. Individuals with greater working memory are believed to have greater cognitive capacity to engage in controlled processing. Hofmann and colleagues measured automatic impulses toward sweets using the IAT (Greenwald et al., 1998), and explicit attitudes and beliefs about sweets using self-report measures. As predicted by dual-process models, consciously reported attitudes and beliefs were better predictors of behavior among subjects with high working memory. In contrast, automatic impulses were better predictors among subjects with low working memory (see also Hofmann, Friese, & Roefs, 2009). The same pattern was replicated for other tempting behaviors, including responding with anger to a provocation and time spent viewing erotic pictures. This relationship is similar to the pattern assumed by process dissociation: Deliberate intentions drive behavior when control is high, but automatic impulses drive behavior when control is low.

These studies provide converging evidence, across several topics and several measures, for the systematic relationship between conscious intentions–beliefs, automatic impulses, and cognitive control abilities. Some of these studies relied on three different tests to measure intentions, automatic impulses, and control processes. But the process dissociation procedure provides an advantage by capturing dual processes within the same task. Rather than equating automatic and controlled processes with different tasks, the components can then be modeled as they contribute to the same behavior.

This ability to model different components within the same task provides the opportunity to study processes underlying varieties of prejudice well beyond the weapon bias. For example, many studies have shown that older adults tend to display greater prejudice than younger adults. There are competing explanations for why this happens. A common assumption is that older adults are more prejudiced because they grew up in an era in which prejudice was more widespread and more acceptable. By this account, older adults simply have more prejudiced thought patterns that have stayed with them over the years. In contrast, older adults might display more prejudice because they are poorer at exerting control over their responses. By this account, older and younger adults may have similar levels of prejudice in their automatic responses, but younger adults are better able to control its expression (von Hippel, Silver, & Lynch, 2000).

Stewart, von Hippel, and Radvansky (2009) measured the racial attitudes of older and younger adults using the IAT and replicated the finding that older adults showed greater bias then their younger counterparts. Although the IAT is often considered a measure of solely implicit processes (i.e., the process-pure assumption) the process dissociation approach assumes instead that behavior in any task reflect the joint operation of both automatic and controlled processes. The IAT includes "compatible" trials (e.g., white–good, black–bad) in which automatic stereotypes and the correct task-appropriate response share a response key, and "incompatible" trials (e.g., white–bad, black–good) in which automatic stereotypes and the correct response are in conflict. Although response time is typically used to score the IAT, errors and correct responses can also be used, because respondents make more errors in incompatible conditions than compatible conditions. These compatible and incompatible trials are analogous to "inclusion" and "exclusion" conditions or "in concert" and "in opposition" conditions of the process dissociation procedure. Thus, Stewart et al. applied the process dissociation procedure to examine whether the difference was driven by automatic or controlled aspects of responses. Consistent with the control-deficit hypothesis, older adults showed lower control estimates than younger adults, but the groups did not differ in their automatic biases.

Another common observation is that white Americans display greater anti-black prejudice than do black Americans. This difference, too, could be explained by differences in either automatic responses or control over responses. Black Americans might be more favorable to blacks in their automatic responses for the same reasons that most any other group shows ingroup preferences. On the other hand, some theorists argue that black people internalize the prejudices and stereotypes that are dominant in society and may therefore have the same automatic associations as whites do. If so, then blacks may have to work harder to exert control over their responses. Stewart et al. (2009) also compared process dissociation components of IAT performance between white and black respondents. Only the automatic component of responses distinguished the racial groups. So, both race and age influenced the amount of bias displayed on the IAT, but they did so through different processes. White Americans showed more bias because they had more biased automatic impulses. Older adults showed more bias because they lacked control.

The studies reviewed here illustrate that the automatic and controlled components estimated by process dissociation have different meanings when applied to different tasks or different contexts. Unlike approaches that define automaticity using lists of inherent features (e.g., intentionality, efficiency, controllability, and awareness), process dissociation requires that the researcher specify what it means to exert control in any given task. *Automaticity* is then defined as those influences that drive responses when control fails. As an example, in the weapons task, *control* is defined by respondents' task-relevant intentions to discriminate between guns and tools. This intention is what defines experimental conditions as "inclusion" or "exclusion," that is, whether putative automatic influences such as stereotyping are congruent or incongruent with intended responses. To the extent that subjects successfully carry out their task goal, they are considered to have control over their responses. But to the extent that stereotypical reactions to black faces influence responses independent of that goal, those stereotypes are driving behavior automatically. It then becomes an empirical question how control and automatic influences, defined in terms of intent, relate to features such as efficiency, controllability, and awareness.

As the reviewed studies illustrate, there has been a good deal of convergence between process dissociation analyses and feature-based definitions of automatic and controlled processes. In the weapons task, *C* estimates were reduced under speeded responding (Payne, 2001) and self-control depletion (Govorun & Payne, 2006), providing evidence that controlled processes estimated by *C* were resource demanding. In contrast, *A* estimates were unaffected by these variables, suggesting efficiency.

Yet the two approaches do not always converge. Consider, for example, the study by Stewart and Payne (2008) in which implementation intentions to think counterstereotypical thoughts reduced automatic bias, and did so under speeded responding. This effect has qualities of both automatic and controlled processes. Implementation intentions altered the (automatic) influence of racial stereotypes, but did so intentionally. An advantage of defining automatic and controlled influences in terms of specific task requirements or goals is that this approach can naturally accommodate cases that seem puzzling from a feature-based perspective. For instance, when an initially unconscious process becomes conscious through introspection, it gains some features of controlled processing (awareness) but may lack others (e.g., efficiency, controllability). And when an initially controlled process becomes automatized through practice, it gains some "automatic" features, such as efficiency, but may retain features such as intentionality and controllability. As in the case of implementation intentions, the process dissociation framework handles these cases by defining control and automaticity based on one set of criteria, and considering the others as empirical questions rather than defining assumptions.

In measures such as the weapons task or the IAT, the criterion that defines control and automaticity is intent. Respondents intend to respond according to task instructions despite the presence of interfering information that may unintentionally influence responses. But in other tasks different criteria may be used. For example, in Jacoby's (1991; Jacoby et al., 1993) early memory studies, it was conscious memory (recollection) that allowed participants to respond as intended. To respond correctly in the exclusion condition, respondents had to remember not simply that a word was familiar but also the context in which they experienced the word. Thus, the *C* estimate can be used to measure conscious memory for the studied item, and the *A* estimate can measure unconscious memory—influences of past experience despite the subject's inability to recollect the experience consciously. Notice that the equations stay the same across these tasks even though the interpretation of the parameters changes. This is because the equations do not define the nature of the processes. It is the experimental design that difines what the equations mean. In an experiment that pits intentional and unintentional influences, the estimates reflect this. And in a design that pits conscious and unconscious processes, the equations reflect this. Keeping the experimental conditions in mind helps to prevent confusion about the meaning of the process dissociation estimates, because the equations can only estimate whatever processes are isolated by experimental comparisons.

Moral Judgments and Decisions

Many of the most contentious and consequential judgments that we make in everyday life are about deciding whether actions are morally right or wrong. For centuries, philosophers have debated whether these moral judgments are, and should be, guided by deliberative reasoning or emotional intuitions. Whereas rationalists, such as Immanuel Kant, argued that moral judgment is essentially about deliberation over duty and principle, others, such as David Hume, claimed that moral judgment is like aesthetic taste, deeply shaped by emotional reactions (Haidt & Kesebir, 2010). Philosophers continue to debate how moral judgment *should* operate (Kennett & Fine, 2009; Prinz, 2007). Empirical psychologists have tackled the more tractable question of which processes underpin everyday moral decisions (for reviews, see Payne & Cameron, 2010; Doris & the Moral Psychology Research Group, 2012).

Over the past decade, social psychological theories of moral judgment have started to incorporate insights from dual-process models of social cognition. For instance, Haidt's (2001) social intuitionist model gives central importance to moral intuitions: "the sudden appearance in consciousness, or at the fringe of consciousness, of an evaluative feeling (like–dislike, good–bad) about the character or actions of a person, without any conscious awareness of having gone through steps of search, weighing evidence, or inferring a conclusion" (Haidt & Kesebir, 2010, p. 802). Moral intuitions are typically characterized as automatic processes (Haidt & Kesebir, 2010).

Although most social psychologists agree that automatic intuitions are influential, they disagree over how these intuitions interact with deliberative reasoning to shape moral judgment (Haidt & Kesebir, 2010; Kennett & Fine, 2009; Paxton & Greene, 2010). According to the social intuitionist model, deliberative reasoning usually seeks to confirm automatic intuitions rather than provide an independent test of their validity (Haidt, 2001). In support of this view, people are often unable to articulate the basis of their moral intuitions (Haidt & Bjorklund, 2008) and are influenced by incidental emotions while making moral judgments (Horberg, Oveis, Keltner, & Cohen, 2009; Schnall, Haidt, Clore, & Jordan, 2008; Wheatley & Haidt, 2005).

By contrast, others have argued that deliberative reasoning can sometimes override automatic intuitions. According to Greene's (2008) dual-process model, automatic intuitions lead to deontological moral judgments that it can never be acceptable to harm one person for a greater good (e.g., helping many people), whereas deliberative reasoning leads to utilitarian moral judgments that such a tradeoff is acceptable. In support of this view, moral judgment is modulated by working memory capacity (Moore, Clark, & Kane, 2008), cognitive reflection (Paxton & Greene, 2010), and emotion regulation (Feinberg, Willer, Antonenko, & John, 2012).

In a recent review of moral psychology, Haidt and Kesebir (2010) declared a theoretical stalemate between these positions: "The precise roles played by intuition and reasoning in moral judgment cannot yet be established based on the existing empirical evidence" (p. 807). We agree. Even if emotion inductions or cognitive load manipulations change the content of moral judgments, it is not necessarily clear which processes are being changed. Emotion inductions may change automatic intuitions, but they may also change whether people are motivated and able to engage in deliberative reasoning; similarly, cognitive load may interfere with deliberative reasoning, but it may also intensify automatic intuitions. Because different theorists use different moral stimuli (vignettes vs. dilemmas), it is also unclear whether processes have been confounded with measures (Monin, Pizarro, & Beer, 2007; also see Payne et al., 2008).

Process dissociation is ideally situated to address these questions and provide a more refined process model of moral judgment. By quantifying how automatic and controlled processes each contribute to a single behavior—moral judgment—the procedure unconfounds processes with stimuli, and allows for the independent verification of whether automatic and controlled moral judgments have the features they are commonly assigned.

In a series of studies, we utilized a sequential priming task to capture automatic and controlled moral judgment within a single paradigm (Cameron, Payne, & Sinnott-Armstrong, 2013). On each trial of the priming task, people saw two words in quick succession. The prime and target words were either noncontroversially morally wrong (*murder, rape*) or noncontroversially morally neutral (*baking, golf*). People were instructed to judge whether the target words were morally wrong, without being influenced by the prime words. The task was designed so that, in some conditions, intentional responding to the target words and automatic influences of the prime words would act in concert (inclusion condition), and in other conditions they would act in opposition (exclusion condition). For example, when the prime word was morally wrong (*murder*) and the target word was morally wrong (*rape*), subjects could correctly respond with the judgment "wrong" either by intentionally controlled (C) moral judgment of the target word, or by an unintended influence of the prime (A) when control failed ($1 - C$). By contrast, when the prime word was morally wrong (*murder*) and the target word was morally neutral (*baking*), subjects would incorrectly respond "wrong" when intentional moral judgment failed but the automatic tendency favored the "wrong" response: $A(1 - C)$.

In this paradigm, subjects are intentionally trying to make a moral judgment of the target word but not the distracting prime word. Yet, to the extent that people cannot help having a moral evaluation activated when a word such as "murder" or "rape" is presented, this unintentional influence can be detected by the automatic estimate. This paradigm differs from other implicit social cognition paradigms we have discussed because the primes and the targets come from the same set of stimuli (i.e., words denoting morally wrong or neutral actions). Because of this feature, we can examine intentional and unintentional moral evaluations of the same items.

The automatic estimate captures some aspects of the moral intuition described by Haidt (2001)—the quick influence of a morally wrong action—while modeling it more precisely as a response that operates without intention. Importantly, these process estimates cleanly separated intentional and unintentional moral judgment based on theoretically predicted manipulations. Imposing time pressure on responding reduced the controlled moral judgment estimate, but not the automatic estimate. On the other hand, type of prime word (morally wrong vs. morally neutral) influenced automatic moral judgment but not the controlled estimate. This double dissociation suggests that automatic and controlled moral judgment (based on intent) are separable processes with other features (e.g., efficiency) commonly ascribed to automatic and controlled processes.

Another way to validate these process estimates is to relate them to morally relevant individual differences and behaviors. In one study, we adapted our priming task to assess automatic and controlled moral judgments toward a controversial moral issue: gay marriage (Cameron, Payne, & Sinnott-Armstrong, 2013). Prime and target words referred to either gay marriage or morally neutral actions, and accuracy was defined idiosyncratically based on subjects' prior self-reports of whether gay marriage was morally wrong or not. Estimates of intentionally controlled moral judgment reflected the ability to judge gay marriage accurately as morally wrong based on the subject-specific criterion, and unintentional moral judgment reflected the tendency to judge gay marriage as morally wrong when control failed. We collected data in the form of an exit poll during a referendum on a North Carolina state amendment to define marriage as being between one man and one woman. Voters who unintentionally evaluated gay marriage as wrong were more likely to vote in favor of the amendment (i.e., to forbid same-sex marriage in the state constitution).

In another study with noncontroversially morally wrong items (e.g., *murder* and *rape*), we found that subjects who scored high on a self-report measure of psychopathic tendencies—including the willingness to manipulate and harm others for personal gain—showed deficits in both unintentionally and intentionally controlled moral judgment estimates (Cameron, Payne, & Sinnott-Armstrong, 2013). Not only did subjects with psychopathic tendencies have more difficulty intentionally judging actions as morally wrong, but they also lacked the automatic moral impulses toward morally wrong actions that most people share. Process dissociation could be especially useful for assessing automatic and controlled moral judgments in incarcerated psychopaths, who are often motivated to appear moral but may lack the automatic impulses to act morally (Hare, 1999; Kiehl, 2008).

THE FUNDAMENTALS

The process dissociation approach to dual-process theories shares with many other dual-process theories the conceptual distinction between automatic and intentionally controlled processes. But from there, the approach diverges in important ways. First, process dissociation does not assume separate systems, one responsible for automatic processes and the other for control. Second, it does not assume different modes of processing, such that people are sometimes in control and at other times skate by as if on autopilot. Most importantly, process dissociation does not assume that some tasks are automatic, whereas others are controlled. It assumes instead that any task, even a single response within a task, is the culmination of both automatic and controlled processes. They operate simultaneously and in parallel, although control processes generally come online more slowly than automatic ones.

The model is focused on processes rather than content. In fact, the it is content-free in the sense that automatic and controlled components can be studied with respect to any given task or behavior. This is why there not a "process dissociation model of attitudes," and a "process dissociation model of memory," and so on. Automatic and controlled processes, from this perspective, are not systems in the brain or properties of tasks. They are things that people do. Some aspects of them are done intentionally, and other aspects occur regardless of whether we intend them or not. This duality seems to apply to just about any activity one can think of. That is what makes it fundamental.

REFERENCES

Amodio, D. M., Devine, P. G., & Harmon-Jones, E. (2008). Individual differences in the regulation of intergroup bias: the role of conflict monitoring and neural signals for control. *Journal of Personality and Social Psychology, 94*, 60.

Amodio, D. M., Harmon-Jones, E., Devine, P. G., Curtin, J. J., Hartley, S. L., & Covert, A. E. (2004). Neural signals for the detection of unintentional race bias. *Psychological Science, 15*, 88–93.

Bishara, A. J., & Payne, B. K. (2009). Multinomial process tree models of control and automaticity in weapon misidentification. *Journal of Experimental Social Psychology, 45*, 524–534.

Botvinick, M. M., Braver, T. S., Barch, D. M., Carter, C. S., & Cohen, J. D. (2001). Conflict monitoring and cognitive control. *Psychological Review, 108*, 624–652.

Cameron, C. D., Brown-Iannuzzi, J. L., & Payne, B. K. (2012). Sequential priming measures of implicit social cognition: A meta-analysis of associations with behavior and explicit attitudes. *Personality and Social Psychology Review, 16*(4), 330–350.

Cameron, C. D., Payne, B. K., Sinnott-Armstrong, W., Scheffer, J., & Inzlicht, M. (2014). *Modeling moral intuitions: Using process dissociation to separate automatic and controlled moral judgment.* Unpublished manuscript, University of Iowa, Iowa City.

Chaiken, S., & Trope, Y. (Eds.). (1999). *Dual-process theories in social psychology.* New York: Guilford Press.

Crosby, F., Bromley, S., & Saxe, L. (1980). Recent unobtrusive studies of Black and White discrimination and prejudice: A literature review. *Psychological Bulletin, 87*, 546–563.

Devine, P. G. (1989). Stereotypes and prejudice: Their automatic and controlled components. *Journal of Personality and Social Psychology, 56*, 5–18.

Doris, J. M., & the Moral Psychology Research Group. (2012). *The moral psychology handbook.* New York: Oxford University Press.

Fazio, R. H., Jackson, J. R., & Dunton, B. C. (1995). Variability in automatic activation as an unobtrusive measure of racial attitudes: A bona fide pipeline? *Journal of Personality and Social Psychology, 69*, 1013–1027.

Feinberg, M., Willer, R., Antonenko, O., & John, O. P. (2012). Liberating reason from the passions: Overriding intuitionist moral judgments through emotion reappraisal. *Psychological Science, 23*(7), 788–795.

Gigerenzer, G., & Regier, T. (1996). How do we tell an association from a rule? Comment on Sloman (1996). *Psychological Bulletin, 119*, 23–26.

Govorun, O., & Payne, B. K. (2006). Ego depletion and prejudice: Separating automatic and controlled components. *Social Cognition, 24*, 111–136.

Greene, J. D. (2008). The secret joke of Kant's soul. In W. Sinnott-Armstrong (Ed.), *Moral psychology: Vol. 3. The neuroscience of morality: Emotion, disease, and development* (pp. 35–79). Cambridge, MA: MIT Press.

Greenwald, A. G., & Banaji, M. R. (1995). Implicit social cognition: Attitudes, self-esteem, and stereotypes. *Psychological Review, 102*, 4–27.

Greenwald, A. G., McGhee, D. E., & Schwartz, J. L. K. (1998). Measuring individual differences in implicit cognition: The Implicit Association Test. *Journal of Personality and Social Psychology, 74*, 1464–1480.

Haidt, J. (2001). The emotional dog and its rational tail: A social intuitionist approach to moral judgment. *Psychological Review, 108*, 814–834.

Haidt, J., & Bjorklund, F. (2008). Social intuitionists answer six questions about moral psychology. In W. Sinnott-Armstrong (Ed.), *Moral psychology: Vol. 2. The cognitive science of morality: Intuition and diversity* (pp. 181–218). Cambridge, MA: MIT Press.

Haidt, J., & Kesebir, S. (2010). Morality. In S. T. Fiske, D. T. Gilbert, & G. Lindzey (Eds.), *The handbook of social psychology* (5th ed., pp. 797–832). Hoboken, NJ: Wiley.

Hare, R. M. (1999). *Without conscience: The disturbing world of the psychopaths among us*. New York: Guilford Press.

Hofmann, W., Friese, M., & Roefs, A. (2009). Three ways to resist temptation: The independent contributions of executive attention, inhibitory control, and affect regulation to the impulse control of eating behavior. *Journal of Experimental Social Psychology, 45*, 431–435.

Hofmann, W., Gawronski, B., Gschwendner, T., Le, H., & Schmitt, M. (2005). A meta-analysis on the correlation between the Implicit Association Test and explicit self-report measures. *Personality and Social Psychology Bulletin, 31*, 1369–1385.

Hofmann, W., Gschwendner, T., Friese, M., Wiers, R. W., & Schmitt, M. (2008). Working memory capacity and self-regulatory behavior: Towards an individual differences perspective on behavior determination by automatic versus controlled processes. *Journal of Personality and Social Psychology, 95*, 962–977.

Horberg, E. J., Oveis, C., Keltner, D., & Cohen, A. B. (2009). Disgust and the moralization of purity. *Journal of Personality and Social Psychology, 97*, 963–976.

Jacoby, L. L. (1991). A process dissociation framework: Separating automatic from intentional uses of memory. *Journal of Memory and Language, 30*, 513–541.

Jacoby, L. L. (1998). Invariance in automatic influences of memory: Toward a user's guide for the process-dissociation procedure. *Journal of Experimental Psychology: Learning, Memory, and Cognition, 24*, 3–26.

Jacoby, L. L., Kelley, C., Brown, J., & Jasechko, J. (1989). Becoming famous overnight: Limits on the ability to avoid unconscious influences of the past. *Journal of Personality and Social Psychology, 56*, 326–338.

Jacoby, L., Toth, J., & Yonelinas, A. (1993). Separating conscious and unconscious influences of memory: Measuring recollection. *Journal of Experimental Psychology: General, 122*, 139–154.

Kennett, J., & Fine, C. (2009). Will the real moral judgment please stand up?: The implications of social intuitionist models of cognition for meta ethics and moral psychology. *Ethical Theory and Moral Practice, 12*, 77–96

Keren G., & Schul, Y. (2009). Two is not always better than one: A critical evaluation of two-system theories. *Perspectives on Psychological Science, 4*, 533–550.

Kiehl, K. A. (2008). Without morals: The cognitive neuroscience of criminal psychopaths. In W. Sinnott-Armstrong (Ed.), *Moral psychology: Vol. 3. The neuroscience of morality: Emotion, disease, and development* (pp. 119–149). Cambridge, MA: MIT Press.

Lambert, A. J., Payne, B. K., Shaffer, L. M, Jacoby, L. L., Chasteen, A., & Khan, S. (2003). Stereotypes as dominant responses: On the "social facilitation" of prejudice in anticipated public contexts. *Journal of Personality and Social Psychology, 84*, 277–295.

Monin, B., Pizarro, D. A., & Beer, J. (2007). Deciding vs. reacting: Conceptions of moral judgment and the reason–affect debate. *Review of General Psychology, 11*, 99–111.

Moore, A., Clark, B., & Kane, M. (2008). Who shalt not kill?: Individual differences in working memory capacity, executive control, and moral judgment. *Psychological Science, 19*, 549–557.

Paxton, J. M., & Greene, J. D. (2010). Moral reasoning: Hints and allegations. *Topics in Cognitive Science, 2*, 511–527.

Payne, B. K. (2001). Prejudice and perception: The role of automatic and controlled processes in misperceiving a weapon. *Journal of Personality and Social Psychology, 81*, 181–192.

Payne, B. K. (2005). Conceptualizing control in social cognition: How executive functioning modulates the expression of automatic stereotyping. *Journal of Personality and Social Psychology, 89*, 488–503.

Payne, B. K., & Bishara, A. J. (2009). An integrative review of process dissociation and related models in social cognition. *European Review of Social Psychology, 20*, 272–314.

Payne, B. K., Burkley, M., & Stokes, M. B. (2008). Why do implicit and explicit attitude tests diverge?: The role of structural fit. *Journal of Personality and Social Psychology, 94*, 16–31.

Payne, B. K., & Cameron, C. D. (2010). Divided minds, divided morals: How implicit social cognition underpins and undermines our sense of social justice. In B. Gawronski & B. K. Payne (Eds.), *Handbook of implicit social cognition: Measurement, theory, and applications* (pp. 445–460). New York: Guilford Press.

Payne, B. K., Jacoby, L. L., & Lambert, A. J. (2005). Attitudes as accessibility bias: Dissociating automatic and controlled components. In R. Hassin, J. Bargh, & J. Uleman (Eds.), *The new unconscious* (pp. 393–420). Oxford, UK: Oxford University Press.

Prinz, J. J. (2007). *The emotional construction of morals*. Oxford, UK: Oxford University Press.

Schacter, D. L. (1987). Implicit memory: History and current status. *Journal of Experimental Psychology: Learning, Memory, and Cognition, 13*, 501–518.

Schnall, S., Haidt, J., Clore, G., & Jordan, A. (2008). Disgust as embodied moral judgment. *Personality and Social Psychology Bulletin, 34*, 1096–1109.

Schumann, H., Steeh, C., & Bobo, L. (1985). *Racial attitudes in America*. Cambridge, MA: Harvard University Press.

Srull, T. K., & Wyer, R. S. (1989). Person memory and judgment. *Psychological Review, 96*, 58–83.

Stewart, B., & Payne, B. (2008). Bringing automatic stereotyping under control: Implementation intentions as efficient means of thought control. *Personality and Social Psychology Bulletin, 34*, 1332–1345.

Stewart, B., von Hippel, W., & Radvansky, G. (2009). Age, race, and implicit prejudice: Using process dissociation to separate the underlying components. *Psychological Science, 20*, 164–188.

Strack, F., & Deutsch, R. (2004). Reflective and impulsive determinants of social behavior. *Personality and Social Psychology Review, 8*, 220–247.

Von Hippel, W., Silver, L. A., & Lynch, M. E. (2000). Stereotyping against your will: The role of inhibitory ability in stereotyping and prejudice among the elderly. *Personality and Social Psychology Bulletin, 26*, 523–532.

Wheatley, T., & Haidt, J. (2005). Hypnotic disgust makes moral judgments more severe. *Psychological Science, 16*, 780–784.

Wilson, T. D., Lindsey, S., & Schooler, T. Y. (2000). A model of dual attitudes. *Psychological Review, 107*, 101–126.

Wittenbrink, B., Judd, C. M., & Park, B. (1997). Evidence for racial prejudice at the implicit level and its relationship with questionnaire measures. *Journal of Personality and Social Psychology, 72*, 262–274.

Yonelinas. A. P. (2002). The nature of recollection and familiarity: A review of 30 years of research. *Journal of Memory and Language, 46*, 441–517.

CHAPTER 9

Process Models Require Process Measures

Jeffrey W. Sherman, Regina Krieglmeyer, and Jimmy Calanchini

The goal of dual-process models (DPMs) is to describe the contributions of two distinct classes of cognitive processes to judgments and behavior. One of the major challenges to achieving this goal is the need for a comprehensive measurement strategy that provides clear indicators of the dual processes, the conditions under which they operate, and the manner in which they interact to transform input into behavior. In this chapter, we review the most common measurement strategies applied to DPMs and some of the difficulties associated with those strategies. Many problems for DPMs result from the confounding of the qualitative nature of the dual processes in the models with the distinction between automaticity and control. Other problems arise from the use of behavioral measure outcomes as proxies for unmeasured cognitive processes and their operating conditions. We detail the advantages of a formal modeling approach and highlight some of the uses to which this approach has been applied in our own research with the Quadruple Process (Quad) model (Sherman et al., 2008). Finally, we describe theoretical insights related to DPMs that have been gleaned from this research.

MEASUREMENT CHALLENGES IN DPMs

Operating Principles versus Operating Conditions

Common measurement strategies developed for DPMs and some of their attendant problems can be traced to the historical origins of DPMs. Specifically, many DPMs arose in the wake of the long-standing dispute between two competing views of human information processing. The naive scientist view proposes that people try to understand their world much as scientists try to understand their topic of study—via careful, rational attempts to discover the true state of the world (e.g., Heider, 1958; Kelley, 1967). In contrast, the cognitive miser view holds that people have limited processing capacity and, as a result, rely on cognitively efficient mental shortcuts and heuristics that provide sufficiently accurate information for little effort (e.g., March & Simon, 1958; Tversky & Kahneman, 1974). Throughout the 1970s and 1980s, it became apparent that the distinction between effortful, optimizing processes and effortless, satisficing processes was not an either–or proposition. Rather, it is clear that people engage in both kinds of processes, depending on their motivation to think carefully about a problem and the availability of the cognitive resources required to do so (e.g., Fiske & Taylor, 1984).

Broadly speaking, DPMs represent the field's attempts to characterize the moderators of when people behave like a naive scientist or a cognitive miser, and the processing mechanisms that guide these actions. In pursuit of this goal, the operations of the two types of processes proposed in many DPMs were mapped onto the distinction between automatic and controlled processes (e.g., Bargh, 1994; Schneider & Shiffrin, 1977; Shiffrin & Schneider, 1977). Whereas a process is considered to be *automatic* if it is initiated unintentionally, operates efficiently, cannot be terminated once started, and operates outside of conscious awareness, a process is considered to be *controlled* if it is initiated intentionally, dependent on cognitive resources, can be stopped voluntarily, and operates within conscious awareness. The processes coinciding with "miserly" processing were presumed to be relatively more automatic and less controlled than the processes coinciding with "scientific" processing.

Though of great heuristic use, the mapping of DPM processes onto the automatic–controlled distinction introduces a number of measurement problems. Most basically, this mapping confounds the critical distinction between operating principles and operating conditions (Gawronski & Bodenhausen, 2009; Gawronski, Sherman, & Trope, Chapter 1, this volume; Sherman, 2006). Operating *principles* refer to the qualitative nature of the cognitive processes that translate inputs into outputs. That is, they describe what the process does (e.g., activation of associations, information integration, inhibition, propositional reasoning). In contrast, *operating conditions* refer to the conditions under which a given process operates (e.g., when motivation and processing capacity are high; Moors & De Houwer, 2006).

Importantly, demonstrating the conditions under which a process operates does not necessarily reveal anything about the qualitative nature of the process. For example, because inhibition processes may proceed in a relatively automatic or controlled fashion (Calanchini & Sherman, 2013; Moskowitz, Chapter 27, this volume), identifying a process of interest as operating automatically (an operating condition) does not necessarily reveal anything about whether the process is inhibitory in nature (an operating principle). Rather, positive identification of the inhibitory nature of the process requires research that directly examines indications of inhibition. Likewise, demonstrating the operating principles of a process does not necessarily reveal anything about the operating conditions of that process. Thus, knowing that a process is inhibitory in nature does not necessarily reveal anything about whether the process operates in a relatively automatic or controlled fashion. Rather, positive identification of the operating conditions of the process requires research that directly examines indications of the features of automaticity (intentionality, efficiency, awareness, susceptibility to inhibition).

Nevertheless, research on DPMs has frequently identified operating principles from operating conditions and vice versa, rather than by directly measuring each. In terms of the former, operating principles have been inferred from markers of automaticity and control, including use of different types of judgment content (e.g., category cues vs. individuating information) that are presumed to be used more or less automatically and different types of measures (e.g., implicit versus explicit) that are presumed to reflect more or less automatic processing. The identification of a process as relatively automatic or controlled (its operating conditions) is then used to infer its operating principles (e.g., activation of associations, information integration, inhibition, propositional reasoning), not because the operating principles have been directly measured, but because evidence of automaticity or control is consistent with the assumed operating conditions of the process in question. For example, the fact that behavioral responses on implicit measures seem to reflect features of automatic processing has been taken as evidence that those responses must be driven by a process that is assumed to operate automatically, such as the activation of associations. In a similar fashion, DPMs often attempt to identify operating conditions via indications of the operating principles of the process in question, rather than by directly testing the operating conditions. For example, evidence that a process involves recourse to propositional beliefs is typically used to infer that the process cannot be automatic in nature, an inference that may be misplaced (e.g., De Houwer, Chapter 35, this volume).

DPMs are fundamentally concerned with identifying the operating principles of the cognitive processes that transform inputs into outputs. Most DPMs also are interested in identifying the operating conditions of those processes, so that they may be distinguished as reflecting "scientific" versus "miserly" modes of processing. However, operating principles and operating conditions should not be used to infer one another. Rather, both principles and conditions must be independently established.

Behavioral Effects as Proxies for Operating Principles

Additional measurement problems for DPMs derive from the use of behavioral proxy measures to identify both operating principles and operating conditions. As far as operating principles are concerned, one fundamental challenge for DPMs (and, indeed, for all of cognitive and social cognitive psychology) is that many of the mental processes described in the models are not directly observable. Rather, the operation of these processes must be inferred from people's responses on behavioral measures. Two different methods have been widely used to accomplish such inferences.

Content Proxies

Many DPMs have attempted to measure distinct processes, their operating principles, and the extent of their use by examining the influence of different types of information in various judgment tasks. In this method, the use of different types of information is assumed to reflect the operation of distinct cognitive processes. For example, prominent DPMs of persuasion (Chaiken, 1980; Petty & Cacioppo, 1986), impression formation (Brewer, 1988; Fiske & Neuberg, 1990), and dispositional attribution (Gilbert, Pelham, & Krull, 1988) are based on this approach. In these models, the use of one kind of information (e.g., peripheral cues, category-based information, dispositional cues) is thought to reflect one dual process (e.g., peripheral processing, categorization, trait inference) and the use of another kind of information (e.g., argument strength, individuating information, situational cues) is thought to reflect the other dual process (e.g., central route processing, individuation, situational correction).

A problem with this approach is that it infers the operation of specific processes from the relationships among inputs (e.g., categorical and individuating information) and outputs (e.g., judgment stereotypicality) without directly measuring the processes of interest (e.g., categorization; individuation). To the extent that the input–output relationship is influenced by alternative or additional processes, the measurement outcome will be a poor proxy for the unmeasured processes of interest (e.g., De Houwer, 2011; De Houwer, Gawronski, & Barnes-Holmes, in press). For example, stereotype application and inhibition processes also influence trait judgments. This problem is exacerbated when multiple processes are inferred from a single behavioral outcome (e.g., judgment stereotypicality), as it may be impossible to assess the extent to which that outcome is due to more of one process (categorization), less of the other process (individuation), or a combination of both.

Task Proxies

A second strategy for inferring the operating principles of cognitive processes in DPMs has been to use separate measures as proxies for the two processes. For example, research on stereotyping sometimes uses implicit measures to assess the activation of associations in memory and explicit measures to assess the inhibition of stereotypic responses (e.g., Devine, 1989). As another example, research on attitudinal processes may use implicit measures to assess associative processing and explicit measures to assess propositional processing (e.g., Strack & Deutsch, 2004).

However, in relying on different tasks to infer different processes, there is always the risk that observed differences are due not to the hypothesized differences in the nature of the underlying processes but, instead, to other processes that may contribute to performance on the tasks. To the extent that task performance is influenced by alternative or additional processes, task performance will be a poor proxy for the unmeasured processes of interest (e.g., De Houwer, 2011; De Houwer et al., in press). For example, responses on many implicit measures are determined not only by activated associations but also by processes that determine the correct task response, processes that override the activated associations, and so forth (e.g., Sherman et al., 2008). Responses on explicit measures are influenced by a wide range of different processes, including associative processes. The nature of this problem is well illustrated by the example of research on implicit and explicit memory systems, in which task dissociations supporting the implicit–explicit distinction were reinterpreted as reflecting the operation of perceptual versus conceptual processing (e.g., Roediger, 1990). In the same way, observed differences on implicit and explicit measures of evaluation may reflect features of the tasks that are not directly related to the distinction of interest (e.g., between associative and propositional processing; Payne, Burkley, & Stokes, 2008; Sherman et al., 2008).

Behavioral Effects as Proxies for Operating Conditions

DPMs also have used behavioral outcomes as proxies for operating conditions, with similar complications. Both content and task dissociations have been used to infer the operating conditions of the processes in question.

Content Proxies

Many DPMs have attempted to assess operating conditions by examining the influence of different types of information in various judgment tasks. In this method, the use of different types of information is assumed to reflect relatively automatic versus controlled processes. For example, the aforementioned DPMs of persuasion (Chaiken, 1980; Petty & Cacioppo, 1986), impression formation (Brewer, 1988; Fiske & Neuberg, 1990), and dispositional attribution (Gilbert et al., 1988) assume that the use of one kind of information (e.g., peripheral cues, categories, dispositional cues) reflects relatively automatic (unintentional, efficient, unaware, or lack of susceptibility to inhibition) processes, whereas the use of another kind of information (e.g., argument strength, individuating information, situational cues) reflects relatively controlled processes.

A major problem for this approach is that although some kinds of information (e.g., category identity) may often be accessed and applied more easily than other kinds of information (e.g., individuating information), it also is possible to reverse the situation (e.g., Erb et al., 2003; Krull & Dill, 1996; Kunda & Thagard, 1996; Trope & Gaunt, 2000). Which kind of information is more easily accessed and applied often depends on the design of the task, the specific configuration of the information, the context, or perceivers' goals. Thus, it is inherently problematic to equate different types of content with the distinction between automatic and controlled operating conditions. Content is not a strong proxy for operating conditions.

In order to solve this problem, more recent versions of these models typically dissociate content and operating conditions (Brewer & Feinstein, 1999; Fiske, Lin, & Neuberg, 1999; Petty & Wegener, 1999), proposing that all kinds of information (peripheral cues, categories, argument strength, individuating information) may be processed in either an automatic or a controlled manner. However, though this resolves the theoretical problem, a measurement problem remains. In these types of models, in any given experiment, the use of different content remains the only way to indicate the operation of two different processes that vary in features of automaticity–control. As such, proxy assumptions about content and operating conditions remain necessary.

It is possible to manipulate directly which kind of information (e.g., categorical vs. individuating information; disposition vs. situational information; source cues vs. message strength) is relatively accessible and easy to use. However, manipulating one type of information to be easier to use, then showing that it is, in fact, easier to use does not reflect on the operating conditions of the underlying processes of interest (categorization vs. individuation; trait inference vs. situational correction; peripheral vs. central route processing). Rather, because specific content is used to instantiate the underlying processes, this does not tell us about those processes per se, only about those processes when they are instantiated in a way that makes one or the other relatively easy to accomplish.

Task Proxies

A second strategy for inferring the operating conditions of cognitive processes in DPMs has been to use separate measures as proxies for automatic and controlled processing. For example, researchers often assume that responses on implicit measures reflect processes that operate automatically, whereas responses on explicit measures reflect processes that operate in a controlled fashion (e.g., Devine, 1989; Fazio, Jackson, Dunton, & Williams, 1995; Greenwald, McGhee, & Schwartz, 1998). However, although implicit measures are certainly less susceptible to control than are explicit measures, responses on both types of measures reflect the influence of both relatively automatic and controlled processes (Calanchini & Sherman, 2013; Sherman et al., 2008). In fact, observed differences on implicit and explicit measures may not reflect differences in the extent of automatic versus controlled processing at all, as is almost unanimously assumed. Rather, such differences may reflect the influence of automatic processes, controlled processes, or both (Calanchini & Sherman, 2013; Sherman et al., 2008).

Summary

Attempts to test DPMs have been fraught with a variety of measurement problems. When operating principles and operating conditions are confounded and each is used to infer the other, neither may be measured with precision. The use of content and task dissociation proxies to measure operating principles and operating conditions also is problematic. To the extent that the content–tasks reflect operating principles and conditions beyond those of interest, then the content–tasks will be poor proxies for the operating principles and conditions they are meant to represent. Thus, when the processes in process models are not measured directly, significant problems with testing the models may arise.

CONCEPTUALIZING AND QUANTIFYING INTERACTIONS AMONG PROCESSES

Another challenge for DPMs is how to characterize and measure the joint and interactive influences of multiple processes. There are many ways to conceptualize the manner in which the dual processes in a DPM interact to produce behavior (e.g., Gilbert, 1999; Klauer & Voss, 2008). The most basic type of model is one in which the two processes are represented as distinct alternatives that do not co-occur. A number of early content proxy dissociation models took this form (e.g., Brewer, 1988; Chaiken, 1980; Petty & Cacioppo, 1986). In these models, which of the two processes guides behavior is determined by moderators having to do with the actor's motivation and ability to think carefully about the issue at hand. Obviously, these kinds of models are not well suited for considering the simultaneous, independent, and interactive contributions of the processes.

Other models propose that behavior is driven by a combination of the two processes. One variant of this approach suggests that dual processes represent two ends of a continuum (e.g., Fiske et al., 1999; Fiske & Neuberg, 1990). This sort of model imposes a hydraulic relationship between the two processes: As one increases, the other must decrease. As a result, the two processes are not independent, and it is difficult to determine the contribution of each. Movement along the continuum may reflect increased or decreased use of one process, the other process, or both. This type of model is particularly problematic when considering the distinction between automatic and controlled processes, as it requires that automatic processes are enhanced when controlled processes are diminished, and vice versa. However, it is clear that automatic and controlled processing are frequently independent of one another (e.g., Jacoby, Toth, & Yonelinas, 1993) or even positively correlated (e.g., increases in automatic processing are accompanied by increases in controlled processing; Jacoby, Begg, & Toth, 1997).

Other variants of combinatorial models permit simultaneous and distinct contributions of each process to behavior. For example, the newer versions of content proxy models that theoretically dissociate content and operating conditions also have incorporated the idea that dual processes may simultaneously influence behavior (e.g., Brewer & Feinstein, 1999; Petty & Wegener, 1999). The two processes (e.g., heuristic and systematic processes) may contribute in an additive or interactive fashion (e.g., Chen & Chaiken, 1999). Interactive processes may take a variety of forms. One process (e.g., heuristic processing) may bias the manner in which the other process (e.g., systematic processing) operates. Alternatively, one process may constrain the influence of the other one. The most common variant of this type of model is one in which the more controlled process constrains the more automatic one when the actor possesses sufficient motivation and ability (e.g., Devine, 1989; Gilbert et al., 1988).

Conceptually, in contrast to either–or models or continuum models, joint influence models permit the independent assessment of each of the dual processes. However, in practice, the previously described measurement problems complicate these efforts. In the content proxy measurement strategy, inferences about the interactions between the two processes still depend on assumptions about which type of content reflects which type of process. Likewise, inferences about how these interactions are moderated by operating conditions may be based on proxy assumptions about the relative ease of using different pieces of information. Absent an independent means of establishing the operating conditions of the two processes, researchers run the risk of circular reasoning (e.g., whichever content is more influential under cognitive load is assumed to represent the more automatic process, thereby supporting a constraint model). Moreover, the extent of the influence of each of the processes often is inferred from a single behavioral outcome (e.g., judgment stereotypicality, extent of persuasion), rather than from distinct measures of the contributions of the two processes to the outcome. As is the case with continuum models, this restricts the ability to infer whether the single outcome is due to more of one process (e.g., category use, association activation), less of the other process (e.g., individuation, overcoming biased associations), or both (Sherman et al., 2008).

Finally, in the task proxy measurement strategy, there simply is no means to assess the simultaneous contributions of the dual processes, because they are each measured with a different dependent variable. This severely limits the ability to articulate the nature of the dual processes and the ways in which they interact to produce behavior.

FORMAL PROCESS MODELS

One increasingly common solution to these problems is the use of formalized mathematical process models of behavior (for an overview, see Sherman, Klauer, & Allen, 2010). These models seek to identify and quantify the processes that account for outcomes on measures of behavior (e.g., judgments, error rates, reaction times) via a set of variables (or parameters) and a set of equations that establish relationships among the variables. The variables in the equations represent the hypothesized component processes (operating principles; e.g., activation of associations, information integration, inhibition) that result in distinct responses on the measure of interest. The equations define the manner in which the processes interact to produce those responses. Solving the equations yields estimates of the extents of the processes.

Of most importance to the concerns raised in this chapter, an inherent feature of formal models is that the outcomes of measures are not assumed to act as proxies for the cognitive operations that produced those outcomes. Instead, the proposed underlying processes are directly linked to observed input–output relations via mathematical formulations that estimate the extents of the different processes. In this way, formal models provide a method for identifying and estimating operating principles without recourse to either content-based or task-based measurement proxies. Moreover, formal models demand a specification of the manner in which underlying processes interact to produce behavior, and provide a proxy-free means of testing those specifications. Before delving into these issues, we feel that it would be helpful to provide a concrete example of a formal model that may be used to illustrate these points.

A Brief Example

A wide variety of process models have been proposed to account for performance on a number of social cognitive measurement tasks in recent years (e.g., Klauer, Voss, Schmitz, & Teige-Mocigemba, 2007; Krieglmeyer & Sherman, 2012; Meissner & Rothermund, 2013; Mierke & Klauer, 2003; Nadarevic & Erdfelder, 2011; Payne, 2001; Payne, Hall, Cameron, & Bishara, 2010; Rothermund, Wentura, & De Houwer, 2005; Stahl & Degner, 2007). Here, we briefly introduce the Quad model (Conrey, Sherman, Gawronski, Hugenberg, & Groom, 2005; Sherman et al., 2008) to illustrate the application of a formal model. The Quad model proposes that four qualitatively distinct processes contribute to performance on implicit measures of evaluation and knowledge: (1) activation of biased associations (AC), (2) detection of correct responses (D), (3) overcoming biased associations when they conflict with correct responses (OB), and (4) guessing (G) when there is no other basis for responding. The model is depicted as a processing tree in Figure 9.1. Each path represents a likelihood, and processing parameters with lines leading to them are conditional upon all preceding parameters. For instance, OB is conditional upon both AC and D. Similarly, G is conditional upon the lack of AC (1 – AC) and the lack of D (1 – D). Note that these conditional relationships do not imply a serial or temporal order in the onset and conclusion of the different processes. Rather, these relationships are mathematical descriptions of the manner in which the parameters interact and constrain one another to produce behavior. Thus, AC, D, and OB may occur simultaneously. However, in determining a response, the status of OB determines whether AC or D drives responses when they are in conflict.

The conditional relationships described by the model form a system of equations that predicts the number of correct and incorrect responses in the compatible (e.g., pairing black faces and negative words on an Implicit Association Test [IAT]) and incompatible trials (e.g., pairing black faces and positive words on an IAT) of an implicit measure. The model's predictions are then compared with the actual data to determine

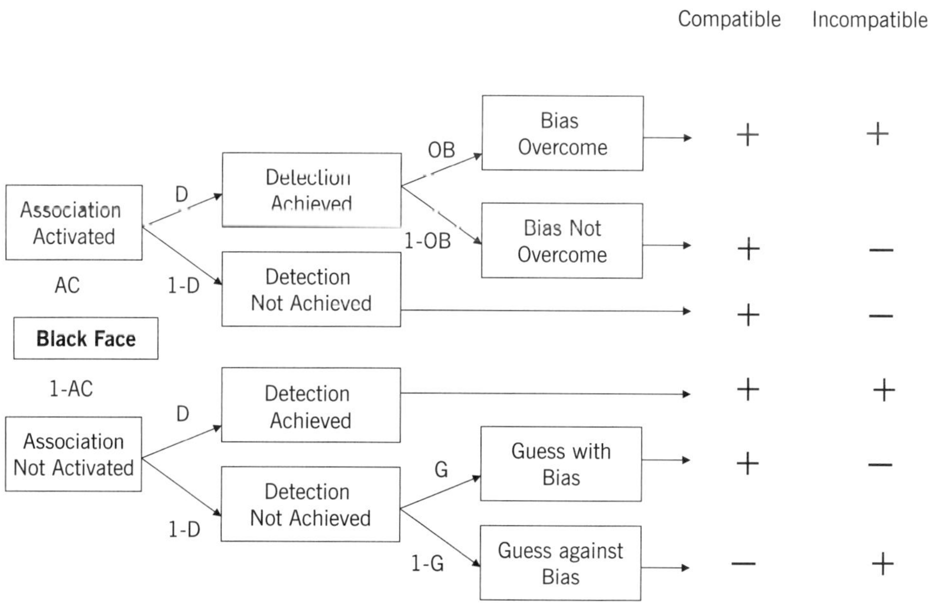

FIGURE 9.1. The Quadruple Process model. Each path represents a likelihood. Parameters with lines leading to them are conditional upon all preceding parameters. The columns on the right side of the figure depict correct (+) and incorrect (–) responses as a function of process pattern.

the model's ability to account for the data. A chi-square estimate is computed for the difference between the predicted and observed errors. To best approximate the model to the data, the four parameter values are changed through maximum likelihood estimation until they produce a minimum possible value of the chi-square. The final parameter values that result from this process are interpreted as relative levels of the four processes. We describe applications of the Quad model in more detail below.

Advantages of Formal Models

Formal modeling offers a number of important advantages over traditional DPM approaches. First, conceptually, formal models presume that the behavioral outcomes of measures are not isomorphic with the processes that are hypothesized to produce those outcomes. Thus, although behavioral outcomes provide the raw material from which process estimates are derived, the distinction between output and process is clear. Pragmatically, the extents of the processes are not inferred based on raw outcomes alone, but rather are estimated via mathematical formulations that directly tie the processes to input–output relations in the measurement task.

Second, by estimating the extents of different processes that contribute to performance on a single task that presents the same content in all conditions, formal models avoid the problem of relying on content or task proxies that may be poor indicators of the processes.

Third, formal models permit the independent and simultaneous measure of multiple distinct processes. Because the role of each process in producing an outcome is mathematically specified, the processes can be assessed independently of one another. This contrasts with process inferences made from judgment tasks, in which it is often impossible to know whether the outcome was based on more of one process (categorization), less of another process (individuation), or a combination of both.

Fourth, the act of formalizing a theory into a mathematical model demands a level of theoretical specificity that typically is not observed in verbally formulated models. In particular, the interactive and determinative relationships among the processes must be defined explicitly and transformed into a set of mathematical propositions that are hypothesized to lead to specific outcomes. The theory must commit itself to a mathematical instantiation that can be directly tested against the data.

A fifth and related point is that the extent to which the assumptions of a formal model can account for behavior can be directly evaluated via model-fitting procedures. DPMs are notorious for their ability to assimilate a wide variety of findings, sometimes including data that would seem to violate the predictions of the models. This has led to concerns that DPMs may be unfalsifiable (e.g., Gawronski, 2013; Gawronski et al., Chapter 1, this volume; Keren & Schul, 2009). By contrast, model-fitting procedures (e.g., goodness-of-fit indices) provide a way in which to demonstrate clearly that formal models may be unable to account for relevant data. Moreover, competing formal models may be directly compared in their ability to account for a set of findings, yielding the possibility of incrementally improving process theories.

Finally, formalized theories permit more precise measures of processes than do traditional DPMs. This is because formal models link the proposed processes to mathematical equations that are solved to yield specific numerical estimates of the extent of each process. This approach may be contrasted with the standard measurement approach for verbally formulated theories, in which content or task outcome proxies are used to infer the relative extents (more vs. less) to which different processes occurred but cannot provide point estimates of the extents of those processes.

Operating Principles Must Be Independently Validated

It is important to note that applying and/or fitting a model provides estimates of the process parameters but, in itself, cannot validate the psychological meanings of those parameters. That is, whether the parameters reflect their intended processes must be established independently via construct validation studies that build a nomological network linking theoretical propositions about the processes, known operationalizations of the proposed construct, and empirical data (Cronbach & Meehl, 1955). For example, if a parameter is meant to represent the extent of activation of associations (AC), then that parameter should be responsive to the extent to which a novel target has been associated with specific attributes during learning (e.g., Sherman et al., 2008). This parameter also should vary with stimulus manipulations designed to increase the likelihood of associations being activated (e.g., the category prototypicality of different targets; Krieglmeyer & Sherman, 2012). If a parameter is meant to reflect a stimulus detection process (D), then that parameter should respond to manipulations of the perceptual clarity of stimuli (Krieglmeyer & Sherman, 2012). If a parameter is meant to represent an inhibition process (e.g., OB), then this might be supported by showing that general inhibition training or instructions that encourage inhibition increase the extent of the process (e.g., Krieglmeyer & Sherman, 2012), by correlating the parameter with known group differences (e.g., alcohol and aging are known to interfere with inhibition; Gonsalkorale, Sherman, & Klauer, 2009; Gonsalkorale, Sherman, & Klauer, in press; Sherman et al., 2008), by showing that the parameter correlates with other known measures of inhibition, or by showing that it predicts inhibition-relevant behavior (e.g., Gonsalkorale, von Hippel, Sherman, & Klauer, 2009). As with all psychological constructs, careful work is required to establish convergent validity, divergent validity, predictive validity, and so forth.

Operating Conditions Must Be Independently Validated

Likewise, the conditions under which the different processes operate cannot be assumed from the design of a formal model, and must be established through independent research. In terms of DPMs, this issue is most relevant in considering the extent to which a given process operates automatically or requires control, because this is the operating process distinction around which DPMs have been built. As such, the extent to which a given process meets the various criteria of automaticity–control (intentionality, efficiency, awareness, susceptibility to inhibition) must be demonstrated with independent empirical evidence. For example, if a parameter is meant to reflect an efficient process, this might be demonstrated by showing that the parameter is unaffected by a cognitive load or a short response deadline.

THE RELATIONSHIP BETWEEN THE QUAD MODEL AND DUAL-PROCESS THEORIES

In the remainder of this chapter, we describe in some detail the ways in which the Quad model has been used to elucidate empirical and theoretical issues in the dual-processes literature. Beyond describing the specific contributions of the Quad model, this discussion is meant to illustrate more broadly the manner in which formal models may be strategically applied to advance our understanding of the processes that contribute to cognition and behavior (see also Klauer, Chapter 10, and Payne & Cameron, Chapter 8, this volume). Before doing this, it is useful to consider in general terms the relationship between the Quad model and DPMs.

Quad Model Processes Correspond to Prevalent DPM Processes

The Quad model was not developed for the purpose of addressing DPMs. Rather, the model was developed with the more pragmatic goal of identifying the processes that contribute to performance on the IAT (Greenwald et al., 1998). It was only during the early stages of validating the model that we recognized that the processes specified in the Quad model corresponded closely to the operating principles of the processes that are very commonly included in DPMs. Specifically, AC corresponds closely to the conception of simple associations or habitual responses that are triggered by stimuli in most DPMs of attitudes (e.g., Fazio, 1990; Wilson, Lindsey, & Schooler, 2000), persuasion (e.g., Chaiken, 1980; Petty & Cacioppo, 1986), stereotyping (e.g., Brewer, 1988; Devine, 1989; Fiske & Neuberg, 1990), prejudice (e.g., Fazio et al., 1995; Greenwald et al., 1998), and judgment (e.g., Epstein, 1994; Sloman, 1996). D corresponds closely to stimulus detection processes that serve to provide an accurate representation of the environment in DPMs of persuasion (e.g., Chaiken, 1980; Petty & Cacioppo, 1986), person perception (e.g., Brewer, 1988; Fiske & Neuberg, 1990), and memory (e.g., Jacoby, 1991). Finally, OB corresponds to self-regulatory processes that attempt to inhibit unwanted or inappropriate responses in DPMs, such as Devine's (1989) model of stereotyping or Wegner's (1994) model of thought suppression.[1]

A Mea Culpa *about Operating Conditions*

Recognition of the similarities between the Quad model parameters and DPM processes influenced the manner in which we described the model and its purposes, and not always in a positive way. Though we are now vigilant in distinguishing between operating principles and operating conditions, this has not always been the case. On some occasions, we made the distinction clear (Sherman, 2006). However, in adopting the DPM framework for describing the Quad model parameters, we also frequently adopted the confound between operating principles and operating conditions often found in the DPM literature. As such, our descriptions of the processes measured by the Quad model were frequently presented as a contrast between automatic (activation of associations) and controlled (detection; overcoming bias) processes. Our empirical work with the model was frequently described as examining the contributions of automatic and controlled processing to the measure of interest.

Nevertheless, rather than assume that the Quad model parameters corresponded to automatic and controlled processes, in a number of studies we attempted to verify independently the operating conditions of the parameters. For instance, time pressure was shown to decrease detection and overcoming bias, but not activation of associations (Conrey et al., 2005), suggesting that AC is a more efficient process than D or OB. Neuroimaging also linked detection with activation in both the dorsal anterior cingulate cortex and the dorsolateral prefrontal cortex, areas of the brain associated with implementing control (Beer et al., 2008). Other research showed that overcoming bias is impaired by alcohol consumption (Sherman et al., 2008) and decreases with age (Gonsalkorale, Sherman, et al., 2009; Gonsalkorale et al., in press), attesting to its status as a controlled, inhibitory process. Though these data support some of our initial assumptions about the extent to which the Quad model processes possess features of automaticity and control, we no longer frame our research in terms of operating conditions, focusing instead on the more central question of operating principles. The extent to which cognitive processes can be described as definitively automatic or controlled, including those measured by the Quad model, is a complicated matter, to which we return later.

How Many Processes Should a Process Model Have?

The Quad model has often been portrayed as a competitor to DPMs because it proposes four rather than two processes. However, in our view, the number of processes described by the model is a rather insignificant factor in comparing our approach with those of DPMs (Sherman, 2006). Instead, it is the means by which the proposed processes are measured and the specification of how those processes interactively influence behavior that most significantly differentiate the Quad model from most DPMs. Thus, despite the different numbers of processes described by the two models, the Process Dissociation (PD) model (Payne, 2001) and the Quad model share much in common, whereas the PD model is quite different from other DPMs despite the fact that they all propose two processes.

The fundamental problem with a debate about the appropriate number of processes to consider is that there are a practically limitless number of candidate processes one might identify. Broadly described processes, such as *encoding*, may be divided into many subprocesses (e.g., selection, attention, construal, attribution, representation), which may be further divided (e.g., attention capture, attention maintenance, attention switching), and so on. Any process can be described at many different levels of breadth. Thus, it is futile to argue about the "real" number of processes that contribute to any behavior. Rather, researchers should identify the processes of interest based on theoretical considerations (i.e., which processes are most relevant to the goals of the research). Much more important than the number of processes to be considered is that those processes and their operation be adequately described and measured.

A Brief Survey of Quad Model Applications of Relevance to DPMs

The most natural application of the Quad model has been to address the problem of task confounds and the multicomponent nature of responses on implicit measures of evaluation. Implicit measures were devised to overcome the "willing" and "able" problems associated with self-report (or explicit) measures—that respondents may conceal their true evaluations due to self-presentational concerns or be unable to report accurately evaluations that are inaccessible to introspection. Implicit measures minimize these problems by assessing evaluations without directly requesting that respondents report them, for example, by structuring the task in a manner that conceals what is being measured (e.g., evaluative priming; Fazio et al., 1995) or by making responses difficult to control (e.g., IAT; Greenwald et al., 1998). These features of implicit measures have led to the widely held belief that responses on the measures reflect only the respondent's automatically activated mental associations (e.g., Fazio & Towles-Schwen, 1999; Greenwald et al., 1998). In turn, this has led to the development of a whole family of DPMs based on the distinction between implicit and explicit processes, representations, or systems that correspond to the distinction between automatic and controlled operating conditions (e.g., Fazio et al., 1995; Greenwald et al., 1998; Lieberman, Gaunt, Gilbert, & Trope, 2002; Rydell & McConnell, 2006; Strack & Deutsch, 2004; Wilson et al., 2000). However, as we argued earlier, there are a number of problems with interpreting dissociations between implicit and explicit task performance as reflecting only the distinction between automatic and controlled processes. First, this approach promotes a confound between operating principles (e.g., associative vs. propositional processes) and their supposed operating conditions (automaticity vs. control). Second, there is the problem that observed differences on implicit and explicit measures may be due not to the hypothesized differences in operating principles or operating conditions but, instead, to some other feature that differs between the tasks. This is because measures are not process-pure indicators of single operating principles (e.g., activation of associations) or operating conditions (e.g., automaticity). As such, the different measures may be poor proxies for operating principles and conditions. Finally, because each process must be measured with a separate implicit or explicit task, it is impossible to assess the independent and joint contributions of the dual processes to a single response. Thus, for example, it is impossible to distinguish between a person who has strongly activated, biased associations but can overcome them and a person who has weakly activated associations but cannot overcome them. Application of the Quad model and other formal models avoids all of these problems.

Multiple Processes Contribute to Implicit Task Performance

The first and most basic question we asked in our research on the Quad model is whether it provides a good account of implicit task performance. At this point, we have fitted the model to scores of datasets and have consistently found that it accounts well for performance on both the IAT and various priming tasks (Sherman et al., 2008). Because it is necessary to show that the model's parameters are measuring the processes we claim they are measuring, we aimed other early research at establishing the construct validity of the parameters. For example, the facts that OB is negatively correlated with reaction time bias on implicit measures and is diminished among older adults and the inebriated is consistent with our claim that the parameter measures a self-regulatory process that inhibits the influence of biased associations. As described earlier, we also sought to investigate empirically the operating conditions of the model parameters, showing that AC is less dependent on processing resources than D or OB, for example. A more extensive summary of this work, which is beyond the scope of this chapter, may be found elsewhere (e.g., Sherman et al., 2008, 2010).

Having validated the model in a number of ways, most of our subsequent research has turned to elucidating the processes that account for important implicit evaluation effects. We have been particularly interested in identifying the processes that account for the malleability of implicit evaluations, variability in implicit evaluations among different respondents, and the ability of implicit evaluations to predict behavior. As described earlier, responses on implicit measures of evaluation are commonly thought to reflect only the associations that are automatically activated in performing the task, and implicit measure outcomes are most often described as reflecting solely the extent of biased associations. This understanding of implicit measures constrains interpretations of implicit evaluation malleability, variability, and behavioral prediction. If the measures only reflect underlying associations, then any change, variability, or predictiveness of the measures must, by definition, be due only to associations in memory (e.g., the same stimuli activate different associations, the same associations are activated to a different extent, or the associations themselves are altered; Blair, 2002; Gawronski & Sritharan, 2010). In contrast, the Quad model provides a means of directly assessing the influence of four distinct processes on these outcomes. We have now accumulated a substantial body of evidence indicating that these important effects are not due solely to associations that are activated in performing the tasks. What follows is a very brief description of some of this work. Expanded treatments may be found in Sherman et al. (2008; 2010).

Implicit Evaluation Malleability

One important class of implicit evaluation effects is the demonstration that implicit evaluations can be altered by a variety of interventions (e.g., Blair, 2002). Consistent with the common view, we have shown that some of these effects, such as increases in implicit bias following ego threat (Allen & Sherman, 2011) and decreases in bias upon exposure to favorable outgroup exemplars (Gonsalkorale, Allen, Sherman, & Klauer, 2010), or racially diverse contexts (Soderberg & Sherman, 2013), are related only to changes in the AC parameter. However, other interventions that reduce bias, such as counterprejudicial training, are associated with both reductions in AC and enhanced D (Calanchini, Gonsalkorale, Sherman, & Klauer, 2013). In still other cases, malleability effects do not appear to be related at all to activated associations. For example, the finding that placing outgroup members in positive social contexts reduces implicit bias was shown to be related only to enhanced OB instigated by the context (Allen, Sherman, & Klauer, 2010).

Implicit Evaluation Variability

Another important class of implicit evaluation effects is the observation of individual differences in implicit evaluations among different groups of respondents. Here, too, we observed that some group differences, such as those between black and white participants, are related only to differences in the AC parameter. However, other group differences, such as those between people who are internally but not externally motivated to control prejudice (high Internal Motivation to Respond without Prejudice Scale [IMS]–low External Motivation to Respond without Prejudice Scale [EMS]) and other people, are related to differences in both AC and D (in this case, lower AC and higher D among high IMS–low EMS respondents; Gonsalkorale, Sherman, Allen, Klauer, & Amodio, 2011). In still other cases, associations appear to have nothing to do with group differences in implicit evaluations. We have found that the tendency for older people to demonstrate higher levels of implicit prejudice than younger people is related only to reduced OB among older respondents (Gonsalkorale, Sherman, et al., 2009; Gonsalkorale et al., in press).

Implicit Evaluations Predicting Behavior

In other research, implicit evaluations are used to predict a variety of important behaviors. Here, too, we find evidence for the influence of multiple processes. For example, Gonsalkorale, von Hippel, et al. (2009) found that the quality of interactions between white non-Muslims and a Muslim confederate was predicted by an interaction between AC and OB. Specifically, when participants had low AC estimates of negative associations with Muslims, their level of OB was unrelated to how much they were liked by the confederate. In contrast, participants with high AC estimates of negative associations with Muslims were liked to the extent that they had high OB estimates. Thus, the ability to overcome negative associations predicted the quality of the interaction only when those associations were strong.

THEORETICAL IMPLICATIONS FOR THE DUAL-PROCESS APPROACH

This research on the Quad model has a number of important implications for the theoretical status of operating principles and operating conditions within the dual-process approach, particularly DPMs based on the distinction between implicit and explicit processes (e.g., Fazio et al., 1995; Greenwald et al., 1998; Lieberman et al., 2002; Rydell & McConnell, 2006; Strack & Deutsch, 2004; Wilson et al., 2000). The following discussion focuses primarily on task dissociation DPMs.

Operating Principles

A fundamental underpinning of many of these DPMs is that implicit and explicit measures reflect the operation of qualitatively distinct processes that reflect distinct operations. Though a wide variety of processes are recognized to contribute to responses on explicit measures across these models, they all share the assumption that implicit measures primarily (or only) reflect the activation of associations in memory. Implicit measures are used as proxies for measuring underlying associations, and responses on implicit measures are considered to be isomorphic with the associations that give rise to those responses.

Research on the Quad model raises serious objections to this assumption. The AC parameter of the model measures the extent to which the activation of evaluative associations influences responses on implicit measures. However, D represents an accuracy-oriented process that cannot be achieved solely through the passive activation of associations in memory. OB represents a self-regulatory process that overcomes the activated associations when necessary. As such, D and OB (and sometimes G) appear to be nonassociative processes (Calanchini & Sherman, 2013). Nevertheless, our research has clearly demonstrated the critical role played by these processes in implicit evaluation effects. In some cases, implicit evaluation malleability, variability, and behavior prediction are related to both associative and nonassociative processes. In other cases, associative processes appear to have nothing to do with these outcomes, and are based entirely on nonassociative components of task performance.

One of the primary goals of DPMs is to describe the operating principles by which stimulus inputs are translated into behavioral outputs. Based on research with the Quad model and other formal models of implicit task performance that include nonassociative processes (Klauer et al., 2007; Krieglmeyer & Sherman, 2012; Meissner & Rothermund, 2013; Mierke & Klauer, 2003; Nadarevic & Erdfelder, 2011; Payne, 2001; Payne et al., 2010; Rothermund et al., 2005; Stahl & Degner, 2007), it is now abundantly clear that the practice of using implicit measures as proxies for associative processing obstructs the accurate identification of operating principles. To specify and test more effectively the operating principle components of DPMs, we strongly advocate that they be uncoupled from the use of specific types of proxy content and proxy measures. The use of formal models, which allow researchers to quantify the contributions of multiple distinct processes to a given behavioral outcome, is one useful way to measure processes without relying on such proxies.

Operating Conditions

Just as DPMs based on the distinction between implicit and explicit processes assume that implicit measures reflect associative processes, so, too, do they assume that these measures reflect automatic processes. Because implicit measures either conceal what is being measured or hinder respondents' ability to control outcomes on the measures intentionally, many researchers assume that responses reflect only automatic processes that are initiated unintentionally, operate efficiently, cannot be inhibited, and operate outside of conscious awareness. We certainly do not question that implicit measures permit less control than explicit measures. Nevertheless, work with the Quad model clearly shows that the D and OB components of implicit task performance possess some features of controlled processing. For example, the fact that both of these processes are curtailed by a response deadline, that D is linked to activation in both the dorsal anterior cingulate cortex and the dorsolateral prefrontal cortex, and that OB is impaired by old age and alcohol consumption all reveal signatures of controlled processing. Yet, at the same time, these processes are sufficiently efficient to influence behavior within the constraints of measures that are very difficult to control (for a review, see Calanchini & Sherman, 2013). These results fit comfortably within a growing body of research indicating that, like any other cognitive process, processes that work to achieve control over automatically activated associations, habits, or impulses may themselves become automatized in certain ways (e.g., Glaser & Knowles, 2008; Monteith, Lybarger, & Woodcock, 2009; Moskowitz, Chapter 27, this volume).

Following the lead of Jacoby (1991) and others, we have argued since the advent of our work on the Quad model that performance on any task must reflect both automatic and controlled processes. At this point, it also is apparent that many specific processes possess features of both automaticity and control, even those that occur within the course of completing an implicit measure. In general terms, this is not a particularly novel insight. Bargh (1994) urged researchers to think about the four "horsemen" of automaticity as dissociable, and noted that few processes would be likely to possess all four of the features of automaticity (unintentional; efficient; unaware; cannot be inhibited). Unfortunately, few researchers (ourselves included) have consistently taken this advice to heart. However, this complication raises particularly difficult challenges for DPMs that are based on the distinction between automatic and controlled processing (Gawronski et al., Chapter 1, and Moors, Chapter 2, this volume). If particular processes cannot be clearly identified as automatic or controlled, then how can they be placed into categories of processes, mental representations, or systems that are defined in terms of the distinction between automaticity (or implicit) and control (or explicit)? This problem threatens the ontological status of the distinction that these DPMs wish to make.

SUMMARY

In this chapter, we have argued that the absence of sound measurement methods has hindered the development and utility of DPMs. At the core of many of the problems is the commonplace confounding of operating principles and operating conditions. We believe it is time for the dual-process approach to be divorced from the distinction between automatic and controlled processes, representations, or systems. Questions pertaining to automaticity and control should be viewed as empirical in nature but not as definitional features of the processes of interest or as the primary basis for categorizing qualitatively distinct processes together in DPMs (Moors & De Houwer, 2006). It is increasingly apparent that the operating principles of qualitatively distinct processes are not tightly associated with the automatic–controlled distinction. Many processes can operate in more or less automatic fashion, and all processes possess features of both automaticity and control. Progress in developing and testing DPMs also has been hindered by the use of content and task proxies for inferring operating principles and conditions. We advocate formal modeling as a proxy-free means to identify the nature of and estimate the extent of underlying cognitive processes by mathematically linking those processes to relations between stimulus inputs and behavioral outputs, specifying not only the qualitative nature of the processes but also the manner in which those processes interact to produce behavior.

ACKNOWLEDGMENTS

Preparation of this chapter was partially supported by Grant No. KR 3742/1-1 from the German Science Foundation to Regina Krieglmeyer.

NOTE

1. In many previous descriptions of the Quad model, we also drew links between the G

parameter and response biases that influence behavior only when D fails (e.g., Jacoby, 1991). However, this effort was misguided. Whether a bias influences responses independently of D or only when D fails is not logically tied to the qualitative nature (operating principles) of the process. For example, in Payne's (2001) work, the *A* parameter represents the activation of biased associations (much like AC in the Quad model). However, these associations influence behavior only when Detection (the C parameter in Payne's work) fails. In contrast, associations may influence behavior independently of Detection in the Quad model. Thus, although the conditions of influence of association activation differ in the models in terms of independence from detection, the operating principles that define the nature of the processes are highly similar in the two models.

REFERENCES

Allen, T. J., & Sherman, J. W. (2011). Ego threat and intergroup bias: A test of motivated-activation versus self-regulatory accounts. *Psychological Science, 22,* 331–333.

Allen, T. J., Sherman, J. W., & Klauer, K. C. (2010). Social context and the self-regulation of implicit bias. *Group Processes and Intergroup Relations, 13,* 137–149.

Bargh, J. A. (1994). The four horsemen of automaticity: Awareness, intention, efficiency, and control in social cognition. In R. S. Wyer, Jr., & T. K. Srull (Eds.), *Handbook of social cognition* (2nd ed., pp. 1–40). Hillsdale, NJ: Erlbaum.

Beer, J. S., Stallen, M., Lombardo, M. V., Gonsalkorale, K., Cunningham, W. A., & Sherman, J. W. (2008). The Quadruple Process model approach to examining the neural underpinnings of prejudice. *NeuroImage, 43,* 775–783.

Blair, I. V. (2002). The malleability of automatic stereotypes and prejudice. *Personality and Social Psychology Review, 6,* 242–261.

Brewer, M. B. (1988). A dual process model of impression formation. In T. K. Srull & R. S. Wyer (Eds.), *Advances in social cognition* (Vol. 1, pp. 1–36). Hillsdale, NJ: Erlbaum.

Brewer, M. B., & Feinstein, A. S. H. (1999). Dual processes in the cognitive representations of persons and social categories. In S. Chaiken & Y. Trope (Eds.), *Dual-process theories in social psychology* (pp. 255–270). New York: Guilford

Calanchini, J., Gonsalkorale, K., Sherman, J. W., & Klauer, K. C. (2013). Counter-prejudicial training reduces activation of biased associations and enhances response monitoring. *European Journal of Social Psychology, 43,* 321–325.

Calanchini, J., & Sherman, J. W. (2013). Implicit attitudes reflect associative, non-associative, and non-attitudinal processes. *Social and Personality Psychology Compass, 7*(9), 654–667.

Chaiken, S. (1980). Heuristic versus systematic processing and the use of source versus message cues in persuasion. *Journal of Personality and Social Psychology, 39,* 752–766.

Chen, S., & Chaiken, S. (1999). The Heuristic–Systematic Model in its broader context. In S. Chaiken & Y. Trope (Eds.), *Dual-process theories in social psychology* (pp. 73–96). New York: Guilford Press.

Conrey, F. R., Sherman, J. W., Gawronski, B., Hugenberg, K., & Groom, C. J. (2005). Separating multiple processes in implicit social cognition: The quad model of implicit task performance. *Journal of Personality and Social Psychology, 89,* 469–487.

Cronbach, L. J., & Meehl, P. E. (1955). Construct validity in psychological tests. *Psychological Bulletin, 52,* 281–302.

De Houwer, J. (2011). Why the cognitive approach in psychology would profit from a functional approach and vice versa. *Perspectives on Psychological Science, 6,* 202–209.

De Houwer, J., Gawronski, B., & Barnes-Holmes, D. (in press). A functional-cognitive framework for attitude research. *European Review of Social Psychology.*

Devine, P. G. (1989). Stereotypes and prejudice: Their automatic and controlled components. *Journal of Personality and Social Psychology, 56,* 5–18.

Epstein, S. (1994). Integration of the cognitive and psychodynamic unconscious. *American Psychologist, 49,* 709–724.

Erb, H., Kruglanski, A. W., Chun, W. Y., Pierro, A., Mannetti, L., & Spiegel, S. (2003). Searching for commonalities in human judgement: The parametric unimodel and its dual mode alternatives. *European Review of Social Psychology, 14,* 1–47.

Fazio, R. H. (1990). Multiple processes by which attitudes guide behavior: The MODE model as an integrative framework. *Advances in Experimental Social Psychology, 23,* 75–109.

Fazio, R. H., Jackson, J. R., Dunton, B. C., & Williams, C. J. (1995). Variability in automatic activation as an unobtrusive measure of racial attitudes: A bona fide pipeline? *Journal of Personality and Social Psychology, 69*, 1013–1027.

Fazio, R. H., & Towles-Schwen, T. (1999). The MODE model of attitude-behavior processes. In S. Chaiken & Y. Trope (Eds.), *Dual-process theories in social psychology* (pp. 97–116). New York: Guilford Press.

Fiske, S. T., Lin, M., & Neuberg, S. L. (1999). The continuum model: Ten years later. In S. Chaiken & Y. Trope (Eds.), *Dual-process theories in social psychology* (pp. 231–254). New York: Guilford Press.

Fiske, S. T., & Neuberg, S. L. (1990). A continuum model of impression formation: From category-based to individuation processes as a function of information, motivation, and attention. In M. P. Zanna (Ed.), *Advances in experimental social psychology* (Vol. 23, pp. 1–74). San Diego: Academic Press.

Fiske, S. T., & Taylor, S. E. (1984). *Social cognition.* Reading, MA: Addison-Wesley.

Gawronski, B. (2013). What should we expect from a dual-process theory of preference construction in choice? *Journal of Consumer Psychology, 23*, 556–560.

Gawronski, B., & Bodenhausen, G. V. (2009). Operating principles versus operating conditions in the distinction between associative and propositional processes. *Behavioral and Brain Sciences, 32*, 207–208.

Gawronski, B., & Sritharan, R. (2010). Formation, change, and contextualization of mental associations: Determinants and principles of variations in implicit measures. In B. Gawronski, & B. K. Payne (Eds.), *Handbook of implicit social cognition: Measurement, theory, and applications* (pp. 216–240). New York: Guilford Press.

Gilbert, D. T. (1999). What the mind's not. In S. Chaiken & Y. Trope (Eds.), *Dual process theories in social psychology* (pp. 3–11). New York: Guilford Press.

Gilbert, D. T., Pelham, B. W., & Krull, D. S. (1988). On cognitive busyness: When person perceivers meet persons perceived. *Journal of Personality and Social Psychology, 54*, 733–740.

Glaser, J., & Knowles, E. D. (2008). Implicit motivation to control prejudice. *Journal of Experimental Social Psychology, 44*, 164–172.

Gonsalkorale, K., Allen, T. J., Sherman, J. W., & Klauer, K. C. (2010). Mechanisms of group membership and exemplar exposure effects on implicit attitudes. *Social Psychology, 41*, 158–168.

Gonsalkorale, K., Sherman, J. W., Allen, T. J., Klauer, K. C., & Amodio, D. M. (2011). Accounting for successful control of implicit racial bias: The roles of association activation, response monitoring, and overcoming bias. *Personality and Social Psychology Bulletin, 37*, 1534–1545.

Gonsalkorale, K., Sherman, J. W., & Klauer, K. C. (2009). Aging and prejudice: Diminished regulation of automatic race bias among older adults. *Journal of Experimental Social Psychology, 45*, 410–414.

Gonsalkorale, K., Sherman, J. W., & Klauer, K. C. (in press). Measures of implicit attitudes may conceal differences in implicit associations: The case of anti-aging bias. *Social and Personality Psychology Science.*

Gonsalkorale, K., von Hippel, W., Sherman, J. W., & Klauer, K. C. (2009). Bias and regulation of bias in intergroup interactions: Implicit attitudes toward Muslims and interaction quality. *Journal of Experimental Social Psychology, 45*, 161–166.

Greenwald, A. G., McGhee, D. E., & Schwartz, J. L. K. (1998). Measuring individual differences in implicit cognition: The Implicit Association Test. *Journal of Personality and Social Psychology, 74*, 1464–1480.

Heider, F. (1958). *The psychology of interpersonal relations.* New York: Wiley.

Jacoby, L. L. (1991). A process dissociation framework: Separating automatic from intentional uses of memory. *Journal of Memory and Language, 30*, 513–541.

Jacoby, L. L., Begg, I. M., & Toth, J. P. (1997). In defense of functional independence: Violations of assumptions underlying the process-dissociation procedure. *Journal of Experimental Psychology: Learning, Memory, and Cognition, 23*, 484–495.

Jacoby, L. L., Toth, J. P., & Yonelinas, A. P. (1993). Separating conscious and unconscious influences of memory: Measuring recollection. *Journal of Experimental Psychology: General, 122*, 139–154.

Kelley, H. H. (1967). Attribution theory in social psychology. In D. Levine (Ed.), *Nebraska Symposium on Motivation* (Vol. 15, pp. 192–240). Lincoln: University of Nebraska Press.

Keren, G., & Schul, Y. (2009). Two is not always better than one: A critical evaluation of two-systems theories. *Perspectives on Psychological Science, 4*, 533–550.

Klauer, K. C., & Voss, A. (2008). Effects of race on responses and response latencies in the weapon identification task: A test of six models. *Personality and Social Psychology Bulletin, 34*, 1124–1140.

Klauer, K. C., Voss, A., Schmitz, F., & Teige-Mocigemba, S. (2007). Process components of the Implicit Association Test: A diffusion-model analysis. *Journal of Personality and Social Psychology, 93*, 353–368.

Krieglmeyer, R., & Sherman, J. W. (2012). Disentangling stereotype activation and stereotype application in the Stereotype Misperception Task. *Journal of Personality and Social Psychology, 103*, 205–224.

Krull, D. S., & Dill, J. C. (1996). On thinking first and responding fast: Flexibility in social inference processes. *Personality and Social Psychology Bulletin, 22*, 949–959.

Kunda, Z., & Thagard, P. (1996). Forming impressions from stereotypes, traits, and behaviors: A parallel-constraint-satisfaction theory. *Psychological Review, 103*, 284–308.

Lieberman, M. D., Gaunt, R., Gilbert, D. T., & Trope, Y. (2002). Reflection and reflexion: A social cognitive neuroscience approach to attributional inference. *Advances in Experimental Social Psychology, 34*, 199–249.

March, J. G., & Simon, H. A. (1958). *Organizations*. Oxford, UK: Wiley.

Meissner, F., & Rothermund, K. (2013). Estimating the contributions of associations and recoding in the Implicit Association Test: The ReAL model for the IAT. *Journal of Personality and Social Psychology, 104*, 45–69.

Mierke, J., & Klauer, K. C. (2003). Method-specific variance in the Implicit Association Test. *Journal of Personality and Social Psychology, 85*, 1180–1192.

Monteith, M. J., Lybarger, J. E., & Woodcock, A. (2009). Schooling the cognitive monster: The role of motivation in the regulation and control of prejudice. *Social and Personality Psychology Compass, 3*, 211–226.

Moors, A., & De Houwer, J. (2006). Problems with dividing the realm of processes. *Psychological Inquiry, 17*, 199–204.

Nadarevic, L., & Erdfelder, E. (2011). Cognitive processes in implicit attitude tasks: An experimental validation of the Trip Model. *European Journal of Social Psychology, 41*, 254–268.

Payne, B. K. (2001). Prejudice and perception: The role of automatic and controlled processes in misperceiving a weapon. *Journal of Personality and Social Psychology, 81*, 181–192.

Payne, B. K., Burkley, M., & Stokes, M. B. (2008). Why do implicit and explicit attitude tests diverge?: The role of structural fit. *Journal of Personality and Social Psychology, 94*, 16–31.

Payne, B. K., Hall, D. L., Cameron, C. D., & Bishara, A. J. (2010). A process model of affect misattribution. *Personality and Social Psychology Bulletin, 36*, 1397–1408.

Petty, R. E., & Cacioppo, J. T. (1986). The elaboration likelihood model of persuasion. *Advances in Experimental Social Psychology, 19*, 123–205.

Petty, R. E., & Wegener, D. T. (1999). The Elaboration Likelihood Model: Current status and controversies. In S. Chaiken & Y. Trope (Eds.), *Dual process theories in social psychology* (pp. 41–72). New York: Guilford Press.

Roediger, H. L. (1990). Implicit memory: Retention without remembering. *American Psychologist, 9*, 1043–1056.

Rothermund, K., Wentura, D., & De Houwer, J. (2005). Validity of the salience asymmetry account of the Implicit Association Test: Reply to Greenwald, Nosek, Banaji, and Klauer (2005). *Journal of Experimental Psychology: General, 134*, 426–430.

Rydell, R. J., & McConnell, A. R. (2006). Understanding implicit and explicit attitude change: A systems of reasoning analysis. *Journal of Personality and Social Psychology, 91*, 995–1008.

Schneider, W., & Shiffrin, R. M. (1977). Controlled and automatic human information processing: I. Detection, search, and attention. *Psychological Review, 84*, 1–66.

Sherman, J. W. (2006). On building a better process model: It's not only how many, but which ones and by which means. *Psychological Inquiry, 17*, 173–184.

Sherman, J. W., Gawronski, B., Gonsalkorale, K., Hugenberg, K., Allen, T. J., & Groom, C. J. (2008). The self-regulation of automatic associations and behavioral impulses. *Psychological Review, 115*, 314–335.

Sherman, J. W., Klauer, K. C., & Allen, T. J. (2010). Mathematical modeling of implicit social cognition: The machine in the ghost.

In B. Gawronski & B. K. Payne (Eds.), *Handbook of implicit social cognition: Measurement, theory, and applications* (pp. 156–175). New York: Guilford Press.

Shiffrin, R. M., & Schneider, W. (1977). Controlled and automatic human information processing: II. Perceptual learning, automatic attending and a general theory. *Psychological Review*, *84*, 127–190.

Sloman, S. A. (1996). The empirical case for two systems of reasoning. *Psychological Bulletin*, *119*, 3–22.

Soderberg, C. K., & Sherman, J. W. (2013). No face is an island: How implicit bias operates in social scenes. *Journal of Experimental Social Psychology*, *49*, 307–313.

Stahl, C., & Degner, J. (2007). Assessing automatic activation of valence: A multinomial model of EAST performance. *Experimental Psychology*, *54*, 99–112.

Strack, F., & Deutsch, R. (2004). Reflective and impulsive determinants of social behavior. *Personality and Social Psychology Review*, *8*, 220–247.

Trope, Y., & Gaunt, R. (2000). Processing alternative explanations of behavior: Correction or integration? *Journal of Personality and Social Psychology*, *79*, 344–354.

Tversky, A., & Kahneman, D. (1974). Judgment under uncertainty: Heuristics and biases. *Science*, *185*, 1124–1131.

Wegner, D. M. (1994). Ironic processes of mental control. *Psychological Review*, *101*, 34–52.

Wilson, T. D., Lindsey, S., & Schooler, T. Y. (2000). A model of dual attitudes. *Psychological Review*, *107*, 101–126.

CHAPTER 10

Random-Walk and Diffusion Models

Karl Christoph Klauer

Random-walk and diffusion models are models of the processes by which speeded decisions on stimuli are made. The central idea in this kind of model is that a decision is based on the accumulation of information relevant to the decision. When there is no imperative stimulus, then the accumulation is slow and random; when there is such a stimulus, the accumulation is rapid. At some point in time, the decision maker feels that enough information has accrued for a decision to be made, at which point a decision is made and a response is initiated. These models address both response accuracy and response times.

Consider as a running example the "shooter" paradigm. Here, participants are required to make speeded responses in discriminating between target persons who are holding a weapon and unarmed target persons who are holding a harmless object. Participants are to respond "Shoot" if the target holds a weapon and "Don't shoot" if the target holds a harmless object (Correll, Park, Judd, & Wittenbrink, 2002). Targets can be white or black persons. In this example, random-walk and diffusion models model response accuracy and response times for shoot–don't shoot decisions.

The models considered in this chapter build on a sequential view of processing stages, with early encoding processes followed by a stage of perceptual analysis, evidence interpretation and accumulation to a decision, and a final stage of response execution. As we will see, the model parameters are linked to important psychological constructs characterizing the decision process. For example, they capture speed–accuracy tradeoffs, response biases, and the efficiency with which decision-relevant evidence is accumulated.

Many dual-process and dual-system frameworks in social psychology (e.g., Smith & DeCoster, 2000; Strack & Deutsch, 2004; Gawronski & Bodenhausen, 2006) distinguish between two types of processes, one of which autonomously and quickly suggests a default judgment, decision, or behavioral response, termed, for example, *impulsive* or *associative*. The default response can be modified, overwritten, or amplified by a second type of process that operates more slowly, effortfully, and in a controlled, rule-based fashion. It comes into play to the extent to which processing resources and motivation create favorable circumstances for the effortful process to operate. For example, in the shooter paradigm, a black target might associatively trigger an impulse to respond "Shoot" based on the automatic activation of stereotypical associations linking black people with the presence of weapons and threat in general. In one dual-process model, such impulses would capture the response unless controlled processes of the second type intervene and replace the impulsive response with a response that is based on a more controlled and complete analysis of the scene (Payne, 2001). In dual-process and dual-system models, the two types of processes are seen as qualitatively different, with one relying on the activation of associations, and the other on, for example, the rule-based manipulation of propositions, and they derive response proposals relatively independently, leading to the possibility of a conflict that then needs to be resolved.

This architecture is not easily mapped on the information-accumulation framework of random-walk and diffusion models. The process of evidence accumulation is unitary, and there is no provision for alternative processes by which an independent response tendency or impulse could be derived. Nor is there an apparatus for conflict resolution. Automatic influences are instead mediated by preattentive processes subserving the accumulation process itself, as I explain in more detail later. Such processes codetermine aspects to which the stimulus attention is directed, which evidence is spontaneously perceived to be relevant, how speed–accuracy tradeoffs are set, and so forth. For example, in the shooter paradigm, preattentive processes might bias perceptual analyses to focus on human faces early on, and meaning-extraction interpretative subprocesses might then associate black people's faces with threat, thereby biasing the interpretation of ambiguous pieces of evidence in the ongoing evidence accumulation. For example, a longish metal tube might with greater likelihood be disambiguated as the barrel of a gun than as a large pen in early stages of information accumulation when the target person is black. In other words, the information-accumulation framework favors the view that automatic or associative influences insinuate themselves into the process of evidence accumulation by shaping its parameters and settings rather than by driving independent alternative processes. Therefore, one lesson that can be learned from random-walk and diffusion models is that a dual-system model of the kind sketched earlier is not the only explanation of data from a given decision paradigm if and when a random-walk or diffusion model fits the data well.

Within the information-accumulation framework, several modeling choices have to be made, and how this is done leads to the major models discussed in the literature (Luce, 1986). One aspect is what it means to accumulate information and how information accrual is modeled. A second question concerns the *stopping rule:* What is the criterion for terminating the information accrual? A third question regards the *decision rule:* Once information accrual has terminated, what is the basis for making a decision?[1] Finally, one of the goals is to model the variability in responses and response latencies, necessitating a plausible mechanism whereby variability is introduced in the process.

Let us walk through these choices one by one. What does it mean to accumulate information? Bits of information are invariably modeled numerically. That is, what is accumulated is numbers, with their size and sign encoding the decision-relevant bits of information in the stimulus. One major distinction is whether the bits of information accrue continuously or in discrete portions. Do we, in other words, think of the decision process as analogous to reading a meter that changes continuously in time or do we treat it as unfolding in discrete time quanta analogously to taking fast snapshots the way a movie camera does? This distinction leads to the distinction between continuous stochastic processes such as the diffusion model and discrete-time stochastic processes, as implemented in classical random-walk models. An orthogonal distinction concerns the number of meters or counters that are monitored. Is evidence accumulated separately for each decision option, so that there is a separate counter or meter for each decision option, leading to so-called *accumulator models*, or is the evidence summarized in one counter or meter, with positive increments encoding bits of information favoring one decision and negative increments favoring the other decision, as in *random-walk* and *diffusion* models? In the latter case, the accumulated evidence is a relative value, gauging the evidence for one option relative to the other option. Random-walk and diffusion models are therefore most readily implemented for binary decisions with just two options.

What is the criterion for terminating the information accrual? The most frequent choice is to postulate the existence of criterion values or thresholds that, when crossed, both terminate the information accrual process and determine the decision. In models with just one counter or meter, two thresholds are placed on the counter scale. The accumulation process is assumed to start from a point between the two thresholds, and as soon as one of them is crossed, the accumulation process is terminated and a decision is made. If the lower threshold is passed, then the decision is made in favor of the decision option that is associated with negative increments, whereas crossing the upper threshold is tantamount to a decision for the option associated with positive increments. In accumulator models, on the other hand, the absolute evidence for each decision option is accrued separately. Typically, a threshold is postulated for each counter, and a decision is made as soon as one of the counters exceeds one of the thresholds. Again, this fixes the decision; it is the one associated with the counter whose value exceeds its associated threshold. But other possibilities for stopping rules and decision-making rules have been investigated (e.g., Audley, 1960; Audley & Pike, 1965).

How can variability be introduced into the process? There are many possibilities, not all of which have been systematically explored. First, variability might reside in the stimuli. For example, in social psychology, a frequently used task is that of speeded evaluative decisions in which stimuli have to be sorted into the categories "good" or "bad" as rapidly as possible. Stimuli typically differ in how well they represent these categories, leading to variability in the speed and accuracy with which evaluative decisions are made across stimuli. Variability can also reside in the observer; one possibility is noise in the nervous system leading to variability within each individual evidence-accumulation process; another possibility is that of variability at a larger time scale due to fluctuations in attention and/or resource allocation to the task at hand. Variability can also be introduced into the threshold values governing the termination of the accumulation process and the decision made. Finally, variability may exist in the starting values of accumulators or evidence counters due to (1) residual activation stemming from previous trials or (2) extraneous sources or (3) too early, anticipatory, starts of the accumulation process, prior to signal onset (Laming, 1968).

Within the space spanned by these modeling options, several models have been formulated and explored. Let us consider a brief history of these models, beginning with the most simple models and some of the challenges these encounter. Most work has focused on binary decisions.

A SIMPLE ACCUMULATOR

LaBerge (1962) proposed a simple accumulator model, which he referred to as *recruitement theory*. Here, bits of information are binary and favor either decision option A or option B (LaBerge also admitted the possibility of nondiagnostic bits of information favoring neither option). Once a stimulus is presented, bits of information come in at discrete points in time and augment a count in favor of option A, with probability p, or a count in favor of decision B, with probability $q = 1 - p$. For example, in the shooter paradigm, perceiving a crouching person holding an object with both hands pointed away from the body might add to a count in favor of a weapon decision; perceiving that the object held appears to have a brownish, soft surface texture at first sight might add to a count in favor of a harmless object such as a wallet. The parameter p depends on the stimulus; if it requires decision A, $p_A > q_A$ is usually assumed to hold; if it requires decision B, $p_B < q_B$ is assumed. The accumulation is terminated as soon as the counter for option A exceeds a given threshold k_A or the counter for option B exceeds a given threshold k_B, whichever occurs earlier, and the decision (A or B) is determined by which threshold was crossed.

These few assumptions are sufficient to generate a probability distribution for the joint probabilities of the decision outcome (A vs. B) and the number of bits of information that have to be sampled to reach a decision. Because sampling occurs in discrete time quanta, this latter number is thought to be proportional to the decision latency itself. The proportionality constant needs to be estimated from the data and thereby introduces a new parameter delta. The accumulator model, like the other models considered in this chapter, is a model of the decision and the decision latency; observed response latencies also contain components related to the initial encoding of stimuli and the execution of responses. For example, in the shooter paradigm, an initial analysis of the scene is likely to determine regions of interest in which to look for a weapon or a harmless object. Once a decision is reached, an overt response is initiated, which is typically a keypress in the shooter paradigm. These nondecision stages are usually lumped together in an additive time constant *r* to be added to the decision latency to yield the predictions for the observable response latencies. This modeling choice implies that these nondecision stages can only delay the expression of a decision as an observable response, but they do not by themselves have the capability to change the decision. The new parameter *r* can, however, be made to depend on the type of stimulus, whether it requires decision *A* or *B*, and on the type of response, whether the response indicating decision *A* or that indicating decision *B* is made (Voss, Voss, & Klauer, 2010).

A SIMPLE RANDOM-WALK MODEL

Let us contrast the simple accumulator with a simple random-walk model. Here there is only one counter, but the bits of information to be accrued are again binary. They take on values –1 and 1 depending upon whether a given bit favors decision option *B* or option *A*, respectively. The probability *p* with which incoming bits of information favor decision option *A* rather than *B* is again assumed to depend on the nature of the stimulus; stimuli that require decision option *A* according to the participant's task are assumed to yield values of *p* larger than ½; stimuli requiring decision *B* are assumed to be associated with values of *p* smaller than ½. Negative and positive thresholds, k_B and k_A, are placed on the counter scale. Accumulation begins with a counter value of zero and is terminated as soon as one of the thresholds is crossed, in which case the decision is determined by which boundary was crossed. Again, a proportionality constant delta and a residual constant *r* are needed to complete the model.

Both models are obviously very similar, the major difference being whether information is accumulated in separate counters, one for each decision option, or in just one counter for the relative evidence for option *A* relative to option *B*. Many variants of these models have been studied. For example, in the accumulator model, as in the random-walk model, the bits of information can be modeled as normally distributed instead of as binary (Heath, 1981; Vickers, 1970; see also Link, 1975; Link & Heath, 1975). By making time quanta for sampling information arbitrarily small, continuous versions of the discrete accumulator and random-walk models can be approximated. The continuous version of a random-walk model is called a diffusion process. In the classical diffusion model, the counter variable is incremented by a normally distributed random variable, and the average rate of increments is called the drift rate v, where the sign (and size) of the drift rate depends on the stimulus: Stimuli requiring decision *A* are assumed to be associated with positive v; those requiring decision *B*, with negative v. In what follows, before turning to differences between the two classes of models, I focus on some common problems of the simple accumulator and random-walk–diffusion models, and on modifications aimed at addressing these shortcomings.

TIME TO DECISION AND ACCURACY

One empirical problem concerns the relationship between the time to decision and the accuracy of the decision as decision time increases. In a standard reaction time task, it is assumed that participants do not respond until a threshold is crossed. A simpler situation is given if the amount of time allowed for decision making is controlled, usually by providing a signal that indicates when to respond. Following Usher and McClelland (2001), let us call this paradigm *time-controlled*. A time-controlled decision is simpler to model inasmuch as the stopping rule and the threshold parameters associated with it can be left out of the model. The decision made is now assumed to depend upon the difference in counter states in accumulator models and on the state of the counter in the random-walk models at the time of the response signal. In accumulator models, decision *A* is made if the counter for *A* exceeds the counter for *B*, and decision *B* is made otherwise. In random-walk models, decision *A* is made if the counter state at the time of the response signal is positive; otherwise decision *B* is made.

One simple prediction obtained for both classes of models is that as processing time is increased, decision accuracy should approach perfect accuracy. This is an adequate approximation in many cases, but for difficult perceptual discriminations there are cases in which accuracy remains below perfect performance even with unlimited processing time (Swensson, 1972). For example, in the shooter paradigm, pictures are usually presented with high resolution and contrast, so that, given unlimited time, a correct decision is usually reached. On the other hand, watching similar but dimly lit scenes may make for a difficult perceptual discrimination, with considerable uncertainty remaining even if inspection time is unlimited. This is one motivation for modifications of random-walk–diffusion models and accumulator models. In the context of diffusion models, one option is to introduce trial-by-trial variability into the drift rate (Ratcliff & Rouder, 1998). In the context of accumulator models, one option is to introduce spontaneous decay into the counter variables (Usher & McClelland, 2001). Both devices lead to an asymptotic upper bound on the level of accuracy that can be obtained given unlimited processing time. As pointed out by Ratcliff and Smith (2004), accumulator models with decay can, however, still predict arbitrarily high accuracy levels if response thresholds are set sufficiently far apart.

DISCRIMINABILITY AND CORRECT AND FALSE RESPONSE LATENCY

Turning to standard reaction time paradigms, differential predictions from the random-walk–diffusion models and the accumulator models have prompted some investigation of the relationship of response latencies for correct and wrong responses. All models predict response latencies to decrease for correct responses as the stimuli pertaining to decision option *A* and those associated with *B* are made easier to discriminate. Simple random-walk–diffusion models make a counterintuitive prediction for error latencies: These should also decrease as the decision task becomes easier. In contrast, simple accumulator models predict that error latencies should increase as the decision task becomes easier. Figure 10.1 shows a latency-discriminability function that plots the ease of discriminating between the stimuli requiring decision *A* and those associated with *B* on the horizontal axis against mean response latency on the vertical axis. The horizontal axis is divided into a left part for error latencies and a right part for correct response latencies. Discriminability is lowest at the center of the horizontal scale and increases going outward from the center to the left (errors) and right (correct responses).

Simple random-walk–diffusion models predict symmetrical U-shaped functions relating discriminability and latency when plotted in the format of Figure 10.1. Latencies should be largest in the least discriminable conditions and decrease for both correct and false responses as discriminability increases. In contrast, the simple accumulator models predict this decrease only for correct responses, whereas latencies for false responses should increase as discriminability increases.

Empirically, the limited data that have been collected suggest that the fastest participants are characterized by the symmetrical U-shaped function relating discriminability and latency predicted by simple random-walk–diffusion models. The slowest participants, on the other hand, exhibit the pattern predicted by the simple accumulator models. In between, U shaped relationships are observed so that latencies for false responses first increase as discriminability increases up to a point, but then decrease as discriminability is further increased (see Figure 10.1 for a typical example; for summaries of the relevant research, see Ratcliff & Smith, 2004; Usher & McClelland, 2001). None of the simple models is capable of accounting for the full range of observed relationships.

This has motivated further modifications. In diffusion models, adding the possibility of variability in the starting point of the information accumulation in addition to trial-by-trial drift-rate variance yields

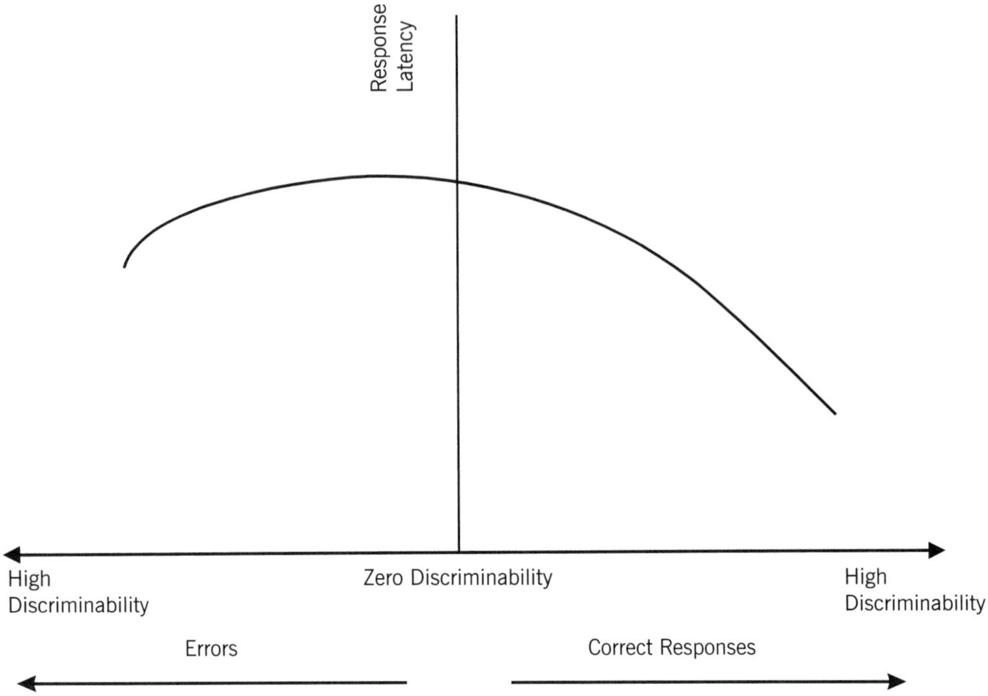

FIGURE 10.1. A latency–discriminability function. Discriminability on the horizontal axis increases, going outward from a condition of lowest discriminability at the center of the scale in both directions. The vertical axis plots mean response latency. In the left half of the plot, latencies of false responses are shown; in the right half, correct response latencies are shown.

the desired flexibility. Specifically, trial-by-trial drift-rate variance introduces the possibility of error latencies larger than correct response latencies (Ratcliff & Rouder, 1998); introducing starting-point variability, on the other hand, makes it possible for the model to accommodate faster errors than correct responses (Laming, 1968; Ratcliff & Rouder, 1998). Taken together, these choices define the Ratcliff diffusion model (Ratcliff, 1978) that has frequently been used to model data from binary decision tasks in various domains of psychological inquiry, as briefly reviewed below.

In accumulator models, adding lateral inhibition between the two accumulators in addition to spontaneous decay yields the desired flexibility. Lateral inhibition introduces a competition or negative correlation between the two counters that make the accumulator model more similar to random-walk models, which can be seen as implementing a perfectly negative correlation between the two counters. Having a parameter regulating the extent of counter competition therefore allows the model to extrapolate between the asymmetrical discriminability-latency functions predicted by the simple accumulator model and the peaked, symmetrical discriminability-latency functions predicted by the simple random-walk–diffusion model. These choices define Usher and McClelland's (2001) leaky, competing accumulator model.

Both of these models appear to account for typical datasets reasonably well (Ratcliff & Smith, 2004; Usher & McClelland, 2001). The leaky, competing accumulator model has the advantage that it generalizes more naturally to tasks with more than two decision options than does the Ratcliff diffusion model.

The Ratcliff diffusion model has, however, been applied much more frequently; therefore, I focus on that model in the remainder of the chapter. An important reason for the greater popularity of the Ratcliff diffusion model is probably the fact that it is easier to estimate and fit the diffusion model than the leaky, competing accumulator model. In fact, several programs have been developed for the purpose such as Fast-dm (Voss & Voss, 2007), Diffusion Model Analysis Toolbox (DMAT; Vandekerckhove & Tuerlinckx, 2007, 2008), and EZ-diffusion (Wagenmakers, van der Maas, & Grasman, 2007; Wagenmakers, van der Maas, Dolan, & Grasman, 2008). Another reason for the popularity of the Ratcliff diffusion model may reside in the fact that some of its model parameters have natural affinities with a number of important psychological processes and settings assumed to underlie decisions. Although I focus on the diffusion model in what follows, it is important to be aware that there are alternative possibilities such as the leaky, competing accumulator model. In fact, there is an excess of modeling possibilities in this area, and only a few possibilities have been systematically explored so far (see Ratcliff & Smith, 2004, for a systematic exploration of four models from the information-accumulation framework).

THE RATCLIFF DIFFUSION MODEL

Figure 10.2 shows a summary of the model. Relative evidence for decision option *A* or *B* is plotted along the vertical axis. Accumulation begins at a starting point on that axis. In the Ratcliff diffusion model, the starting point is a random variable with a uniform distribution ranging within an interval from z_l to z_u with $z_l > 0$ and mean value z. There are two decision thresholds. The lower threshold for decision *B* is arbitrarily fixed to zero; the position of the upper threshold is a free parameter a with $a > z_u$. Evidence accumulates with mean drift rate ν. The drift-rate parameter quantifies the direction (toward upper or lower threshold) and speed with which evidence accumulates. The accumulation process is, however, inherently stochastical, as symbolized by the random trajectory shown in Figure 10.2. Thus, drift rate quantifies the average or expected speed and direction of evidence accumulation, whereas the stochastic component introduces variability in the responses (sometimes the "wrong" threshold is crossed due to noise) and in response latencies. As already mentioned, the drift rate is itself assumed to be a random variable in the model introducing trial-by-trial variability; it is modeled as a normally distributed variable with variance η^2. Finally, nondecision components of response latencies due to encoding of the stimuli and response execution are summarized in one residual term that is assumed to follow a uniform distribution over an interval ranging from t_l to t_u with mean value t_0.

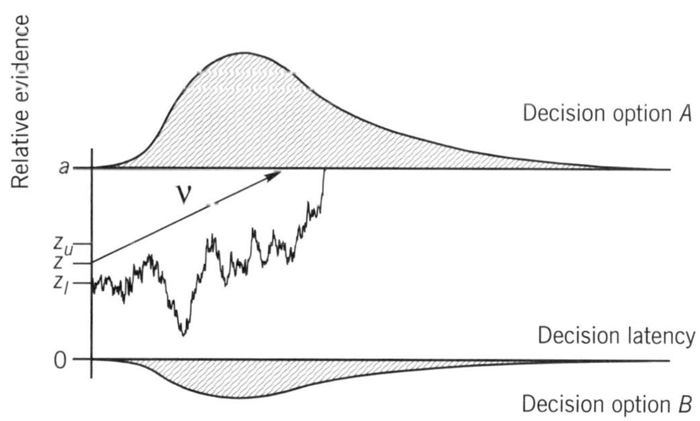

FIGURE 10.2. Graphical depiction of the Ratcliff diffusion model. Evidence is accumulated on the vertical scale as relative evidence toward decision option *A* relative to option *B*. The horizontal axis is the decision-latency axis. Evidence accumulation begins at a random starting point between z_l and z_u. It is a noisy process with a trend captured by mean drift rate ν. A decision is reached when one of the response thresholds is crossed. The upper threshold is the one for decision option *A*, the lower threshold the one for decision option *B*. The thresholds are separated by an amount that is given by parameter *a*.

Some of these parameters affect response accuracy and latency in transparent and readily interpretable ways, suggesting an association of these parameters with psychological constructs such as speed–accuracy tradeoffs, efficiency of discrimination, or response bias. Specifically, the larger the absolute value of mean drift rate, the faster and the more consistently the decision option in the direction in which drift rate points is reached. In other words, increases in the absolute drift rate cause the decision performance to increase in both speed and accuracy. This suggests that mean drift rate is a function of both the discriminability of the stimuli and the decision maker's overall level of discriminatory ability as determined by his or her amount of processing capacity, attention to the task, and practice in the task, among others. For example, in the shooter task, drift rate is limited by the resolution of the picture, by how high its contrast is, and by the size of the critical object (i.e., the weapon or the harmless object). It is also limited by the amount of processing resources the perceiver is willing to invest, for example, in terms of directing attention to the critical object and keeping it focused on that object until a decision can be made.

Threshold separation parameter *a*, on the other hand, is tied to speed–accuracy tradeoffs. If the two thresholds are far apart (*a* is large), much information must accumulate before a decision is made, leading to accurate, but slow decisions. Conversely, for small *a*, one of the two thresholds will be crossed relatively quickly, but relatively small random fluctuations will suffice to cross the "wrong" threshold, leading to fast, but relatively less accurate responses. In other words, parameter *a* seems well suited to capture speed–accuracy tradeoffs, that is, the settings governing the compromise between the requirement to reach a decision fast and the requirement to reach a correct decision; this is a compromise that participants have to find for any speeded choice task.

Shifting the mean starting point of evidence accumulation, *z*, away from one of the thresholds and toward the other threshold, leads to more frequent and faster responses associated with the closer threshold. This predisposes the parameter to capture a decision or response bias in favor of the decision associated with the nearer threshold. For example, in the shooter paradigm, preattentive processes may direct attention to human faces before attention can be directed to the critical object that is held by the target person. Stereotypical associations linking black people with threat more strongly than white targets may then lead to a starting point for the subsequent evidence accumulation that is closer to the threshold for weapons in the case of black targets than in the case of white targets. This would lead to faster correct "shoot" decisions along with more erroneous "shoot" decisions for black than for white targets.

Finally, the nondecision component adds a random amount of time to the response latencies. It thereby models all those factors that delay responses without the capability of changing responses. Early perceptual and late motor processes are usually attributed to this component. The influences of the variability parameters on responses and response latency are less transparent and more difficult to characterize. In consequence, possible psychological interpretations of the variability parameters for trial-by-trial variability in the drift rate η, in starting point, $z_u - z_l$, and in nondecision component, $t_u - t_l$, are less frequently offered, although I noted some possibilities earlier.

From this brief summary, it is clear that the model conceives of the processes that intervene between stimulus presentation and response as being organized in separable stages. After a stage of initial encoding, a stage of evidence accumulation is entered, which is followed by a stage of response execution once a decision has been reached. Based on how the parameters influence the predicted responses and their predicted latencies, the threshold separation parameter *a* can furthermore be tentatively aligned with speed–accuracy tradeoffs, mean starting point *z*, with response or decision bias, and mean drift rate ν, with overall performance level or efficiency of discrimination, with these other processes partialed out.

Model Parameters and Psychological Constructs

The link between model parameters on the one hand and psychological constructs, such as decision bias, speed–accuracy setting, and efficiency of discrimination, on the other suggests that the model parameters should be differentially sensitive to experimental manipulations and differences in variables assumed to covary with these processes. For example, if mean drift rate indexes the discriminatory performance in a way that partials out differences in speed–accuracy tradeoffs and decision biases, in perceptual speed and response-execution speed, then it should be sensitive both to stimulus-related variables determining the discriminability of the stimuli associated with the two response options and to participant-related variables determining the momentary discriminatory ability, establishing convergent validity. In contrast, it should not respond, for example, to manipulations of speed–accuracy tradeoffs, response bias, or response-execution difficulty, if it is to exhibit divergent or disciminant validity. Analogously, threshold separation parameter a should respond to manipulations of the speed–accuracy tradeoff, such as rewarding participants for accurate responses versus rewarding them for fast responses (convergent validity), but it should not respond to the manipulations targeting the drift rate as just described or manipulations targeting decision bias, response-execution speed, and so forth (discriminant validity). Mean starting point z should respond to manipulations of decision bias, such as rewarding participants more for correct A responses than for correct B responses (convergent validity) and, again, it should show discriminant or divergent validity inasmuch as it should not be sensitive to the kinds of manipulations that are believed to affect the efficiency of discrimination, speed–accuracy tradeoffs, decision biases, and so forth.

Research using the model has to some extent borne out these expectations. For example, using a color discrimination task, Voss, Rothermund, and Voss (2004) found that threshold separation parameter a was increased when accuracy motivation was induced, mean drift rates were lowered when stimuli were made harder to discriminate, and the nondecision component was increased when a more difficult form of response was required. The nondecision component was, however, also increased in the condition with increased accuracy motivation, suggesting that speed–accuracy tradeoffs also affect the speed of response execution, not just the decision process.

Furthermore, in a condition with response handicap, response execution was made more difficult: Participants were told to use the same finger for both keypress responses; in the control condition, they used different fingers. This had the expected effect on the nondecision component: t_0 was increased in the condition with handicap relative to the control condition, but it also led to an increase in (absolute) drift rates, as well as to an effect on mean starting point z. This may mean that the manipulation of response handicap also affected the psychological processes tentatively aligned with drift rate and mean starting point (i.e., the efficiency of discrimination and decision bias, respectively). Another possibility is that the model parameters do not succeed in dissociating psychological processes in the assumed manner as cleanly as hoped for; that is, the findings might reflect a lack of discriminant validity of drift-rate parameter as a measure of the efficiency of discrimination, and of the mean starting point parameter as a measure of decision bias. In a second experiment, Voss et al. (2004) found that mean starting points tracked a manipulation of response bias via differential payoff for the different decision options.

Taken together, Voss et al.'s (2004) results demonstrate convergent validity for the investigated parameters, but they also suggest potential problems in regard to discriminant validity. That is, the parameters were responsive to manipulations of the psychological processes with which they were tentatively linked (convergent validity), but drift rate, mean starting point, and nondecision component were also affected by manipulations of psychological processes tentatively linked to other parameters, suggesting a lack of discriminant validity.

The diffusion model is silent on the issue of the controlled or automatic nature of the processes captured by its parameters beyond the tentative interpretations in terms of psychological constructs just described. These constructs, on the other hand, are not easily mapped on the distinction between controlled and automatic processes. Each of them probably represents a complex mixture of controlled and automatic components. For example, response bias can be adjusted strategically in order to maximize one's payoff or chances of being correct (Luce, 1986; Macmillan & Creelman, 2005). On the other hand, it is plausible that task-irrelevant stimuli presented, for example, as prime stimuli in priming paradigms (e.g., Fazio, Sanbonmatsu, Powell, & Kardes, 1986; Payne, 2001) might exert subtle influences via response biases, as already explained for the shooter paradigm.

Similarly, speed–accuracy settings can to some extent be influenced by the participant's strategies, but they probably also comprise a less consciously controlled, bottom-up component responsible for adjusting speed–accuracy settings (1) in response to the perceived task difficulty or experienced fluency of task execution, (2) to maintain an acceptable error rate, or (3) in response to other subtle markers of performance (Botvinick, Braver, Barch, Carter, & Cohen, 2001).

Efficiency of discrimination, finally, refers to a controlled process in the sense that the discrimination unfolds conditional on the attempt to follow task instructions; it is also controlled in the sense that it depends on the processing resources strategically invested in the task. For example, it is likely to depend on the amount of effort invested and on the extent to which one intentionally focuses attention on the task rather than on other external and internal events and processes. But, of course, it is also dependent on the overall amount of available processing capacity and on the quality of perceptual analysis of stimuli, and on stimulus-related aspects that are not under the participant's control, such as the resolution and contrast of the presented scenes and the sizes of the critical objects in the shooter paradigm. Moreover, unless the sources of incoming bits of information are carefully monitored, evidence accumulation is likely to be involuntarily contaminated to some extent by irrelevant stimuli or distracters in the perceptual field that bear decision-relevant features, accounting for misattribution phenomena. For example, in the shooter paradigm, the race of the target person may not only bias the setting of the starting point of evidence accumulation and thereby response bias, but it may also be a cue used in disambiguating ambiguous pieces of evidence during evidence accumulation, as already explained, and thereby affect the efficiency of evidence accumulation. Or, perceiving a black target may directly add to the counter for evidence in favor of the presence of a weapon due to stereotypical associations with threat.

THE RATCLIFF DIFFUSION MODEL AS A CAUSAL MODEL

The linkages between the model parameters and psychological constructs that were discussed in the previous two sections motivate the use of the diffusion model in investigating the causal mediation of observed effects. For example, in research on motivated perception and cognition, it has been demonstrated that interpreting ambiguous situations is not a purely data-driven process; it can be biased toward positive interpretations by top-down influences. In one paradigm, Voss, Rothermund, and Brandtstätter (2008) used a color discrimination task similar to the one used by Voss et al. (2004). One of the two colors to be discriminated signaled a financial gain or loss, irrespective of the participants' responses in the discrimination task, whereas the other color was not associated with any consequence. This led to a response bias in favor of the color with the more positive financial consequences; that is, there was a tendency to decide in favor of the more positive color more frequently and faster than in favor of the less positive color—an optimistic bias that was especially pronounced for the most ambiguous stimuli.

The purpose of Voss et al.'s (2008) diffusion model analyses was to evaluate two causal hypotheses regarding the psychological mediation of this bias: Does it reflect a (possibly strategic) decision or response bias, or does it reflect a top-down effect on evidence accumulation, so that the sensitivity for bits of evidence in favor of the more positive color is increased? Based on the previously discussed linkages, the former possibility should map optimistic bias in the data on the mean starting point parameter z; the latter possibility should map it on an effect on drift rates. Both predictions received support, and Voss et al. (2008) concluded that the optimistic bias reflects the combined effect of a positivity bias in decision bias and an increased efficiency in processing the more positive kind of information.

Another example is Brendl, Markman, and Messner's (2001) analysis of the Implicit Association Test (IAT; Greenwald, McGhee, & Schwartz, 1998) in terms of a random-walk model. This analysis decomposes the IAT effect into a compatibility effect in the efficiency of evidence accumulation, and a compatibility effect on speed–accuracy settings. However, no attempt was made to fit an actual random-walk or diffusion model to IAT data.

Applying the Ratcliff diffusion model to investigate causal hypotheses is an ambitious and informative endeavor with considerable potential for gaining insights into meditational processes that would be difficult to obtain otherwise. Reaping these gains rests on the validity of the linkages between psychological constructs and model parameters, and ideally these linkages should be validated in studies modeled after the one by Voss et al. (2004), sketched earlier, for each new area of application of the model. A more cautious use of the model is as a measurement tool.

THE RATCLIFF DIFFUSION MODEL AS A MEASUREMENT MODEL

Another potentially useful manner of applying the Ratcliff diffusion model is as a tool to provide useful indices of targeted aspects of participants' performance in a theoretically motivated and principled manner. For example, scoring in the IAT is an issue that has received considerable attention (Greenwald, Nosek, & Banaji, 2003). Greenwald et al. have made it clear that there are many ways in which the IAT effect can be quantified, and they investigated a number of ad hoc indices vis-à-vis a number of desirable outcomes and psychometric criteria that are expected to be optimized by a reasonable index (e.g., being highly reliable).

One motivation for studying different scoring methods stems from the fact that performance on the IAT and differences between participants' performance is affected by many factors, such as differences between participants in overall speed, in cognitive skills, in speed–accuracy settings, and so forth (Blanton et al., 2009; Greenwald & Sriram, 2010; Klauer, Schmitz, Teige-Mocigemba, & Voss, 2010). Studying the different scoring methods is motivated in part by the desire to correct for such differences, with the goal to isolate the variance due to the differences between participants that are of interest in applying the IAT, that is, the individual differences in implicit attitudes (in attitude IATs). Simply quantifying IAT effects in terms of only the observed latencies, as was originally done, or in terms of only the accuracies, as is done in the Quad model (Conrey, Sherman, Gawronski, Hugenberg, & Groom, 2005) is probably not sufficient to factor out these undesired sources of variance, such as differences between participants in speed–accuracy settings. In fact, the most successful scoring methods, known as the *D* scores, amalgamate both latency and accuracy data in a way that is likely to factor out differences between participants in speed–accuracy tradeoffs to some extent.

Applying the diffusion model provides a more principled way of mapping latency data and accuracy data on a common metric (Spaniol, Madden, & Voss, 2006) that may approximate this goal. Klauer, Voss, Schmitz, and Teige-Mocigemba (2007) applied the Ratcliff diffusion model to IAT data by analyzing the compatible and the incompatible blocks of the IAT separately. This allowed them to compute an IAT effect separately for drift rates, threshold separation parameters, and nondecision component. Based on the relationship of these parameters to response frequencies and latencies, it seemed likely that the IAT effect in terms of drift rates would partial out differences in speed–accuracy tradeoffs (threshold separation parameters), and differences in response–execution speed and perceptual speed (nondecision component) to some extent. In other words, the diffusion model analyses provide a set of IAT-derived indices that may be useful in separating the different variance components that contribute to IAT data and to the IAT effect.

In fact, the IAT effect in terms of drift rate was found to capture the attitude-related variance of interest (it correlated with an external attitude criterion), whereas systematic method variance in the IAT was mapped on the IAT effect in terms of threshold separation parameters (systematic method variance was operationalized by the variance shared by IATs with unrelated contents; Klauer et al., 2007). These results suggest that the Ratcliff diffusion model may be useful as a measurement model of the IAT by providing separate and principled quantifications of method-related variance components and attitude-related variance components in the IAT. Based on these initial results, a more systematic exploration of the model-derived indices and their comparison with the *D* scores is desirable.

Unlike its use as a causal model, the Ratcliff diffusion model here functions basically as a scoring method suggesting a number of scores with the potential to partial out variance due to the psychological constructs tentatively linked to the different parameters. However, these tentative links are taken as motivation for the model-derived scores rather than as valid assumptions of the analysis, and the usefulness of the indices thus derived in terms of psychometric properties such as consistency, reliability, and validity must be corroborated empirically.

SUMMARY

Evidence accumulation is a natural framework within which to study choice and decision tasks. An important distinction in this framework is the one between accumulator models and random-walk–diffusion models. In modern versions, both of these classes of models are sufficiently flexible to describe the shapes of response frequency and latency data that are typically observed. Accumulator models are more easily generalized to situations with more than two decision options, whereas the Ratcliff diffusion model is more easily fitted to real data, and its parameters are more readily aligned with important psychological constructs of interest, such as efficiency of discrimination, speed–accuracy tradeoffs, and decision bias. Both classes of models suggest a rough separation of processing stages into (1) early encoding processes; (2) a stage of perceptual analysis, evidence interpretation, and accumulation to a decision; and (3) a stage of response execution; but the different model parameters and the psychological constructs to which they are linked are not easily mapped on the distinction between automatic and controlled processes. Moreover, the cognitive architecture implied by information-accumulation models is not compatible with the architecture underlying current social cognitive dual-process and dual-system models. Nevertheless, these models can be useful both as causal models, testing hypotheses about causal mediating paths that would otherwise be difficult to test, and as measurement tools, providing theoretically motivated indices of decision data that have the potential to partial out unwanted sources of variance in a principled manner.

NOTE

1. The second and third questions are often intertwined, that is, stopping and decision rules form a natural compound; but they can be dissociated as in paradigms in which information accrual is to be stopped as soon as an external signal indicates that a response deadline has been reached and a response is to be executed.

REFERENCES

Audley, R. J. (1960). A stochastic model for individual choice behavior. *Psychological Review, 67*, 1–15.

Audley, R. J., & Pike, A. R. (1965). Some stochastic models of choice. *British Journal of Mathematical and Statistical Psychology, 18*, 207–225.

Blanton, H., Jaccard, J., Klick, J., Mellers, B., Mitchell, G., & Tetlock, P. E. (2009). Strong claims and weak evidence: Reassessing the predictive validity of the IAT. *Journal of Applied Psychology, 94*, 567–582.

Botvinick, M., Braver, T., Barch, D., Carter, C., & Cohen, J. (2001). Conflict monitoring and cognitive control. *Psychological Review, 108*, 624–652.

Brendl, C. M., Markman, A. B., & Messner, C. (2001). How do indirect measures of evaluation work? Evaluating the inference of prejudice in the Implicit Association Test. *Journal of Personality and Social Psychology, 81*, 760–773.

Conrey, F. R., Sherman, J. W., Gawronski, B., Hugenberg, K., & Groom, C. (2005). Separating multiple processes in implicit social cognition: The quad model of implicit task performance. *Journal of Personality and Social Psychology, 89*, 469–487.

Corell, J., Park, B., Judd, C. M., & Wittenbrink, B. (2002). The police officer's dilemma: Using ethnicity to disambiguate potentially threatening individuals. *Journal of Personality and Social Psychology, 83*, 1314–1329.

Fazio, R. H., Sanbonmatsu, D. M., Powell, M. C., & Kardes, F. R. (1986). On the automatic activation of attitudes. *Journal of Personality and Social Psychology, 50*, 229–238.

Gawronski, B., & Bodenhausen, G. V. (2006). Associative and propositional processes in evaluation: An integrative review of implicit and explicit attitude change. *Psychological Bulletin, 132*, 692–731.

Greenwald, A. G., McGhee, D. E., & Schwartz, J. L. K. (1998). Measuring individual differences in implicit cognition: The Implicit Association Test. *Journal of Personality and Social Psychology, 74*, 1464–1480.

Greenwald, A. G., Nosek, B. A., & Banaji, M. R. (2003). Understanding and using the Implicit Association Test: I. An improved scoring algorithm. *Journal of Personality and Social Psychology, 85*, 197–216.

Greenwald, A. G., & Sriram, N. (2010). No measure is perfect, but some measures can be quite useful. *Experimental Psychology, 57*, 238–242.

Heath, R. A. (1981). A tandem random walk model for psychological discrimination. *British Journal of Mathematical and Statistical Psychology, 34*, 76–92.

Klauer, K. C., Schmitz, F., Teige-Mocigemba, S., & Voss, A. (2010). Understanding the role of executive control in the implicit association test: Why flexible people have small IAT effects. *Quarterly Journal of Experimental Psychology, 63*, 595–619.

Klauer, K. C., Voss, A., Schmitz, F., & Teige-Mocigemba, S. (2007). Process components of the Implicit Association Test: A diffusion-model analysis. *Journal of Personality and Social Psychology, 93*, 353–368.

LaBerge, D. A. (1962). A recruitment theory of simple behavior. *Psychometrika, 27*, 375–396.

Laming, D. R. J. (1968). *Information theory of choice-reaction times*. London: Academic Press.

Link, S. W. (1975). The relative judgment theory of two-choice response time. *Journal of Mathematical Psychology, 12*, 114–135.

Link, S. W., & Heath, R. A. (1975). A sequential theory of psychological discrimination. *Psychometrika, 40*, 77–105.

Luce, R. D. (1986). *Response times: Their role in inferring elementary mental organization*. New York: Oxford University Press.

Macmillan, N. A., & Creelman, C. D. (2005). *Detection theory: A user's guide* (2nd ed.). Mahwah, NJ: Erlbaum.

Payne, B. K. (2001). Prejudice and perception: The role of automatic and controlled processes in misperceiving a weapon. *Journal of Personality and Social Psychology, 81*, 181–192.

Ratcliff, R. (1978). A theory of memory retrieval. *Psychological Review, 85*, 59–108.

Ratcliff, R., & Rouder, J. N. (1998). Modeling response times for two-choice decisions. *Psychological Science, 9*, 347–356.

Ratcliff, R., & Smith, P. L. (2004). A comparison of sequential sampling models for two-choice reaction time. *Psychological Review, 111*, 333–367.

Smith, E. R., & DeCoster, J. (2000). Dual-process models in social and cognitive psychology: Conceptual integration and links to underlying memory systems. *Personality and Social Psychology Review, 4*, 108–131.

Spaniol, J., Madden, D. J., & Voss, A. (2006). A diffusion model analysis of adult age differences in episodic and semantic long-term memory retrieval. *Journal of Experimental Psychology: Learning, Memory, and Cognition, 32*, 101–117.

Strack, F., & Deutsch, R. (2004). Reflective and impulsive determinants of social behavior. *Personality and Social Psychology Review, 8*, 220–247.

Swensson, R. G. (1972). The elusive trade-off: Speed versus accuracy in visual discrimination tasks. *Perception and Psychophysics, 12*, 16–32.

Usher, M., & McClelland, J. L. (2001). The time course of perceptual choice: The leaky, competing accumulator model. *Psychological Review, 108*, 550–592.

Vandekerckhove, J., & Tuerlinckx, F. (2007). Fitting the Ratcliff diffusion model to experimental data. *Psychonomic Bulletin and Review, 14*, 1011–1026.

Vandekerckhove, J., & Tuerlinckx, F. (2008). Diffusion model analysis with MATLAB: A DMAT primer. *Behavior Research Methods, 40*, 61–72.

Vickers, D. (1970). Evidence for an accumulator of psychophysical discrimination. *Ergonomics, 13*, 37–58.

Voss, A., Rothermund, K., & Brandtstätter, J. (2008). Interpreting ambiguous stimuli: Separating perceptual and judgmental biases. *Journal of Experimental Social Psychology, 44*, 1048–1056.

Voss, A., Rothermund, K., & Voss, J. (2004). Interpreting the parameters of the diffusion model: An empirical validation. *Memory and Cognition, 32*, 1206–1220.

Voss, A., & Voss, J. (2007). Fast-dm: A free program for efficient diffusion model analysis. *Behavior Research Methods, 39*, 767–775.

Voss, A., Voss, J., & Klauer, K. C. (2010). Separating response-execution bias from decision bias: Arguments for an additional parameter in Ratcliff's diffusion model. *British Journal of Mathematical and Statistical Psychology, 63*, 539–555.

Wagenmakers, E.-J., van der Maas, H. L. J., Dolan, C. V., & Grasman, R. P. P. P. (2008). EZ does it!: Extensions of the EZ-diffusion model. *Psychonomic Bulletin and Review, 15*, 1229–1235.

Wagenmakers, E.-J., van der Maas, H. L. J., & Grasman, R. P. P. P. (2007). An EZ-diffusion model for response time and accuracy. *Psychonomic Bulletin and Review, 14*, 3–22.

PART IV

ATTITUDES AND EVALUATION

CHAPTER 11

The MODE Model

Attitude–Behavior Processes as a Function of Motivation and Opportunity

Russell H. Fazio and Michael A. Olson

First proposed in 1990, the MODE model aims to describe the multiple processes by which attitudes can affect judgments and behavior (Fazio, 1990). The model focuses on a basic distinction between two general classes of attitude-to-behavior processes—spontaneous versus deliberative—and considers *M*otivation and *O*pportunity to serve as the major *DE*terminants of which process is likely to operate.

The spontaneous process highlights a mechanism by which attitudes can guide behavior without the involvement of any conscious reflection on the part of the individual. Instead, by virtue of its automatic[1] activation from memory when the individual's encounters the attitude object, the attitude influences how the object is construed in the immediate situation—either directly, such as when the activated evaluation forms the immediate appraisal (e.g., an immediate "yuk" reaction), or indirectly, such as when it biases perceptions of the qualities of the object. In effect, the automatically activated attitude serves as a filter through which the object is viewed, just as suggested by the field's long-standing emphasis on the constructive nature of perception (e.g., Asch, 1940; Bruner, 1957; Hastorf & Cantril, 1954). Once activated, attitudes color perceptions of the object, and ensuing judgments or behaviors are a spontaneous reaction to these immediate perceptions. Thus, without any conscious consideration of one's attitude, and without any necessary awareness of its influence, one's behavioral response to an object can be guided by the attitude through a process initiated by its automatic activation. In other words, behavior emerges as a downstream consequence of the automatically activated attitude.

In striking contrast are situations in which individuals deliberate about the costs and benefits of pursuing a particular action and, in so doing, consider their attitudes toward the behavioral alternatives and decide upon a behavioral plan (e.g., Ajzen, 1991; Ajzen & Fishbein, 1980). Of course, any such deliberation requires some expenditure of effort. Hence, the individual must not only be motivated to engage in the effortful analysis but also have the opportunity (i.e., the time and the resources) to do so.

The MODE model also notes that the influence of attitudes on behavior sometimes may involve "mixed" processes that involve a combination of automatic and controlled components. Any controlled component within a mixed sequence requires, once again, that the individual be both motivated to engage in the necessary cognitive effort and have the opportunity to do so. Thus, one might be motivated to gauge the appropriateness, or even counter the influence, of an automatically activated attitude. That motivation might stem from an enhanced desire for accuracy (e.g., Schuette & Fazio, 1995), a sense of accountability (e.g., Sanbonmatsu & Fazio, 1990), a concern with social desirability (e.g., Fazio, Jackson, Dunton, & Williams, 1995), or, as in much of the research that has been conducted concerning racial attitudes and prejudice, motivations to control prejudiced reactions (e.g., Dunton & Fazio, 1997). Opportunity, from the perspective of the MODE model, is essentially a gating mechanism. One must have the resources and the time for the motivated processing. Provided the opportunity exists, an individual can counter or even correct for the influence of the automatically activated attitude. However, if the individual is fatigued or cognitively depleted, or if the situation demands an immediate response, then there will be little opportunity to engage in motivated deliberation. In that case, judgment or behavior is likely to be influenced by the automatically activated attitude, regardless of any relevant motivational concerns.

EARLY TESTS OF THE MODE MODEL

Measuring and Manipulating Attitude Accessibility

Early research testing the MODE model focused on the model's reasoning regarding attitudinally biased perceptions and, in particular, the role of attitude accessibility. The model argues that any such influence on how the object is construed is initiated by the automatic activation of the attitude from memory. Thus, initial tests of the model were based on research demonstrating that the likelihood of automatic attitude activation varied as a function of the associative strength between the attitude object and the individual's evaluation of the object. This work was rooted in a view of attitudes as object–evaluation associations in memory and in research demonstrating that the strength of such associations could both be measured by latency of response to an attitudinal query and enhanced by repeated attitudinal expression (e.g., Fazio, Chen, McDonel, & Sherman, 1982; Fazio, Powell, & Herr, 1983). Faster responses to a direct query regarding one's attitude were indicative of a stronger object–evaluation association and greater attitude accessibility. Importantly, the latency with which individuals responded to an attitudinal query predicted the likelihood of automatic attitude activation upon mere presentation of the attitude object as a prime in an evaluative priming procedure (Fazio, Sanbonmatsu, Powell, & Kardes, 1986. This procedure examined the extent to which identifying the connotation of a target adjective (e.g., *disgusting*) was facilitated by prior presentation of an attitude object (e.g., *anchovies*). Such facilitation was observed for trials in which the participant's attitude toward the prime was congruent with the valence of the target adjective. However, this priming effect varied as a function of the latency with which the participant could express his or her attitude toward the object when asked to do so directly. Objects characterized by faster response latencies produced stronger priming effects, and therefore more evidence of automatic attitude activation upon mere presentation of the object as a prime, than did objects to which the participant had responded relatively slowly when asked to express attitudes. This finding meant that latency of response to an attitudinal query could serve adequately as a proxy for the likelihood of automatic attitude activation, thus permitting tests of the MODE model's postulate that attitudinally biased perceptions should vary as a function of the accessibility of the attitude from memory.

In addition, rehearsal of one's attitude as a result of the need to respond to multiple attitudinal queries led both to faster latencies of response to a final query (e.g., Powell & Fazio, 1984) and to stronger effects when that attitude object was employed as a prime in the evaluative priming procedure (Fazio et al., 1986). Thus, attitude rehearsal enhanced the likelihood of automatic attitude activation. This finding also served as a basis for much of the early research testing the MODE model. Repeated attitudinal expression was employed as an experimental manipulation that was predicted to enhance the relation between attitudes and perceptions, judgments, or behavior. In many cases, both the measurement and the experimental approaches were pursued in the interest of providing converging evidence for the moderating role of attitude accessibility.

Before moving on to research concerning the consequences of attitude accessibility, we wish to emphasize that the underlying view of attitudes as object–evaluation *associations* of varying strength is not intended to imply that attitudes develop only via an associative learning mechanism. From the very outset (Fazio et al., 1982), the framework emphasized that attitudes can be based on reasoning relative to the value of the attributes of the attitude object, behavioral experience with the outcomes yielded by interaction with the object, inferences from observation of one's own behavior, the emotions that the object evokes, evaluative conditioning processes, and so forth. Many routes exist to the development of an attitudinal representation sufficiently strong to activate the evaluation when the object is encountered (see Fazio, 2007, for a more detailed presentation of the conceptualization of attitudes).

Accessible Attitudes Shape Construals

The importance of attitude accessibility as a moderating variable was documented in studies concerning the appraisal of information related to the attitude object. For example, in a study of the 1984 presidential election, Fazio and Williams (1986) found that respondents' attitudes toward the candidates predicted impressions of their performance during the televised debates. However, this relation grew stronger as attitude accessibility increased. A similar moderating role was evident in judgments of purported empirical evidence regarding the deterrent efficacy of capital punishment (Lord, Ross, & Lepper, 1979). Participants viewed research that reached a conclusion supportive of their attitudes as better conducted than research reaching the opposing conclusion. In two studies, one involving measurement of attitude accessibility via latency of response to a direct query and the other involving experimental manipulation of attitude accessibility via repeated attitudinal expression, Houston and Fazio (1989) found this effect to vary as a function of the accessibility of attitudes toward the death penalty. Biased processing was more evident for individuals with more accessible attitudes. Thus, new information about an attitude object appears to be colored by attitudes, especially more accessible attitudes.

Accessible attitudes also play an important role in the construal of multiply categorizable objects. Many objects, people, or events often can be construed in multiple ways. Yogurt can be construed as a health food or as a dairy product, a flu shot as an injection or as an immunization. In experiments involving the rehearsal of attitudes toward one of two potential categorizations, Smith, Fazio, and Cejka (1996) demonstrated that the more attitude-evoking possibility is more likely to dominate the categorization process. In other words, the object is likely to be construed in terms of the potential categorization toward which the individual has the more accessible attitude (for related evidence, see Fazio & Dunton, 1997; Young & Fazio, 2013).

The Roles of Motivation and Opportunity

According to the MODE model, the impact of attitudes will be reduced when individuals have both the motivation and the opportunity to deliberate about the available information and, in so doing, overcome the influence of any preexisting attitude. Research indicates that, under appropriate conditions, individuals faced with the need to make a decision will expend the effort to consider the available details instead of relying on earlier-formed attitudes. Sanbonmatsu and Fazio (1990) constructed a set of statements regarding two department stores in a way that the decision to buy a camera from one of the stores provided an indication of the process by which the decision was reached. The statements describing the various departments of one store were generally more positive than the statements regarding the other, with the exception of the camera department; the generally inferior store had the better camera department. After exposure to the stimulus information under instructions to form an overall evaluation of each store, participants were asked to imagine that they needed a new camera and to indicate the store at which they would shop. An attitude-based decision process would promote shopping at the generally superior store, despite its inferior camera department. In contrast, a decision to shop at the generally inferior store would suggest that an individual engaged in the effort of retrieving the original attribute details from memory and recognized the superiority of its camera department. Especially given that participants had been encouraged to form overall impressions of the two stores (not differentiated impressions of each department within each store), the attribute-based decision process was clearly the more effortful.

Participants were more likely to choose the store indicative of attribute-based processing only when they were both motivated to deliberate and had the opportunity to do so. Motivation was enhanced for some participants by leading them to believe that their store selections would be compared to those of other participants in the session and that they would have to explain their decisions publicly. Opportunity was manipulated by placing half the participants under time pressure. When either motivation was low or individuals needed to make their decisions quickly, they were relatively more likely to choose the store indicative of an attitude-based process (i.e., the generally superior store) despite its weaker camera department. When both motivation and opportunity were high, participants were more likely to choose the store with the better camera department. These findings have important implications for the reasoned-action process upon which Ajzen and Fishbein (1980) focused—deliberation that involves the "computation" of attitudes toward the act in question by integration of one's evaluation of relevant beliefs regarding the behavioral alternative. Such effortful reflection is likely to occur only when people are both properly motivated and have sufficient opportunity to deliberate.

Further evidence regarding the importance of an accuracy motivation is provided by research that has examined the relation between accessible attitudes and judgments of new information related to the attitude object. Using the capital punishment paradigm mentioned earlier, Schuette and Fazio (1995) replicated the earlier finding concerning the moderating role of attitude accessibility on the relation between attitudes toward the death penalty and judgments of empirical research. Participants for whom attitude accessibility had been enhanced by their being induced to express their attitudes repeatedly in an ostensibly separate experiment showed more evidence of attitudinally biased processing than did individuals who had expressed their attitudes only once. However, this effect was further moderated by a manipulation intended to motivate some participants to deliberate more extensively about the details of the capital punishment studies. They were told that the same research had been evaluated by a panel of experts, and that the very purpose of the study in which they were participating was to examine whether educated laypersons could analyze study reports carefully enough to reach judgments that matched expert opinion. Moreover, the judgments of the participants in any given session were to be shared openly and serve as the basis for a discussion concerning why each did or did not match the panel's views. This information led to less attitudinally biased judgments of the quality of the two capital punishment studies, even among those who had rehearsed their attitudes toward the death penalty. Thus, correspondence between attitudes and judgments was strong only in the cell of the experimental design involving higher attitude accessibility and lower accuracy motivation. Apparently, when individuals are properly motivated, they attend to information in a more objective and thorough fashion, constructing a judgment that is more likely to avert the influence of even a relatively accessible attitude.

More Recent Tests of the MODE Model

As noted earlier, initial tests of the MODE model relied on consideration of the moderating role of attitude accessibility. The more spontaneous attitude-to-behavior process was more evident for individuals with more accessible attitudes, presumably because their attitudes were relatively more likely to be automatically activated upon their encountering the attitude object. The development of the evaluative priming paradigm, from a procedure designed to test hypotheses regarding automatic attitude activation as a function of the strength of object–evaluation associations (Fazio et al., 1986) to a measurement tool that provided an estimate of the attitude automatically activated by the presentation of the attitude object (Fazio et al., 1995), offered a new approach to testing the model. The use of this tool, as well other implicit measures of attitude that followed (e.g., Greenwald, McGhee, & Schwartz, 1998; Payne, Cheng, Govorun, & Stewart, 2005), allowed for examination of the relation between an estimate of the attitude activated when the attitude object was encountered and related judgments or behavior. Moreover, the extent to which this relation varied as a function of motivation and opportunity could be examined. As a result, it became possible to test the model's predictions in new ways (for reviews, see Fazio & Towles-Schwen, 1999; Olson & Fazio, 2009). The resulting wave of research also led to the examination of forces beyond accuracy motivation or accountability that might evoke deliberative processing. In particular, research concerning racial prejudice began to examine how the relation between estimates of automatically activated racial attitudes and race-related judgments or behaviors was moderated by motivation to control prejudiced reactions (Fazio et al., 1995; Dunton & Fazio, 1997).

MODE MODEL INSIGHTS REGARDING PREJUDICE

The interaction of more spontaneous and more deliberative processes is a well-documented dynamic in the domain of prejudice, with various theoretical views arguing for important roles for each (e.g., Devine, 1989; Dovidio & Gaertner, 2004). Our belief is that the MODE model provides an overarching framework to explain a variety of the fascinating phenomena documented in prejudice research, and offers clarity for a number of ambiguities in the literature.

Automatically Activated Racial Attitudes

Since the interplay of automatic and controlled processes was first introduced to the study of prejudice (Devine, 1989; Gaertner & Dovidio, 1986), implicit social cognition research has blossomed, as has the use of its chief tools, implicit measures of attitudes (for reviews, see Fazio & Olson, 2003; De Houwer, 2009; Wittenbrink & Schwarz, 2007). Our priming technique for assessing automatically activated racial attitudes (Fazio et al., 1995) involves the brief presentation of faces of given races as a prime, followed by clearly valenced target adjectives that participants are to identify as positive or negative as quickly and accurately as possible. If one's attitude toward black people is negative and sufficiently strong, perception of a black face should spontaneously evoke a negative response. If the target word that immediately follows this face is negative, one will be relatively quick to identify its valence (and relatively slow to identify its valence if it is positive). The procedure includes a cover story to obscure our interest in race, and in addition to the multiple black and white primes of primary interest, additional white and other-race fillers are included to minimize participant awareness further. Indeed, participants remain oblivious to our interest in prejudice throughout the procedure.

It is also important to note that participants are under instructions to study the briefly presented face primes, so that they can pick them out later in a recognition task, ostensibly for the purpose of testing whether judging word meaning is such an automatic skill that they can perform the task well even they are assigned something else to do at the same time. Other than this, they are not instructed to process the face primes in any particularly way (e.g., by categorizing them as black or white as in the Implicit Association Test (IAT); for research concerning such categorization, see Fazio & Dunton, 1997; Jones & Fazio, 2010; Olson & Fazio, 2003). Thus, the priming technique provides a window into respondents' spontaneous, unfettered evaluative reactions to black and white individuals, categorized by race only to the extent that participants naturally do so. The view turns out to vary: while some white respondents evidence anti-black bias, some do not, and others exhibit a pro-black bias. Thus, instead of assuming relatively homogenous automatic prejudice across individuals (e.g., Devine, 1989), the MODE model recognizes meaningful variability in individuals' attitudes, variability that, as we describe next, has proven predictive of many race-related judgments and behaviors.

An exhaustive review of the predictive validity of priming measures is unnecessary for our present purposes (for a more complete review, see Cameron, Brown-Iannuzzi, & Payne, 2012). Furthermore, the MODE model does not make simple, main effect predictions per se regarding relations between automatically activated racial attitudes and behavior; such attitudes are argued to influence behavior only in the absence of motivation or opportunity. Nevertheless, we highlight a few studies in which such main effects—likely owing to a dearth of moderating factors—have been observed.

In an initial investigation, white respondents interacted with a black female researcher after completing the priming measure (Fazio et al., 1995). Although unaware of participants' responses during the priming procedure, she found that participants characterized by more negative automatically activated attitudes were less friendly and less interested in their interaction. In a similar study involving an interaction between white participants and a black experimenter (Dovidio, Kawakami, Johnson, Johnson, & Howard, 1997), automatic bias assessed by a priming measure related to less eye contact and other negative, nonverbal behaviors while interacting the black experimenter. More negative attitudes toward blacks on the measure also correlate with reports of more negative recent interactions with black people (Towles-Schwen & Fazio, 2001).

The priming measure has proven predictive of more complex race-related judgments as well. In one such study, participants were recruited purportedly to evaluate the quality of student essays (Jackson, 1997). Each essay included a biographical sketch and race-revealing photo. Again, the attitude estimate derived from the priming measure proved predictive: Participants with more negative attitudes toward blacks evaluated an essay written by a black individual more harshly. In a similar study, participants evaluated a number of purported applications for a position in the Peace Corps (Olson & Fazio, 2007). These materials were rich in information, containing resumes, personal essays, and questionnaire responses, and included materials from black and white candidates previously matched on their credentials. Again, participants' automatically activated attitudes predicted their evaluations of the black relative to the matched white candidate.

Motivated Processes Relevant to Racial Prejudice

Several motives relevant to racial contexts have been addressed in the literature, including motivations to avoid racial conflict, to abide by societal norms, or to be nonprejudiced in one's own and others' eyes (e.g., Dunton & Fazio, 1997; Plant & Devine, 1998), as well as more general goals like self-enhancement and comprehension (Kunda & Spencer, 2003) and those discussed earlier (e.g., accuracy). Here we will address the most relevant motives, i.e., those to avoid racial conflict and to be non-prejudiced.

The Motivation to Control Prejudiced Reactions (MCPR) scale (Dunton & Fazio, 1997), a 17-item questionnaire with two factors, was designed for this purpose. It assesses two distinct motives relevant to interracial contexts. The first, dubbed "Concern for Acting Prejudiced" (or, "Concern") gauges one's desire to appear unprejudiced to oneself and to others, and includes items such as "I feel guilty when I have a negative thought or feeling about a black person." The second factor, "Restraint to Avoid Dispute" (or, "Restraint") addresses one's desire to avoid race-related conflict, whether with or about blacks, and includes items such as "If I were participating in a class discussion and a black student expressed an opinion with which I disagreed, I would be hesitant to express my own viewpoint."

Much has been learned about the nature of the two motivations. The Concern factor, for example, correlates highly with measures of humanitarianism–egalitarianism, but the Restraint factor does not (Fazio & Hilden, 2001). In a study of childhood experiences (Towles-Schwen & Fazio, 2001), Concern was associated with reports of more positive interactions with blacks throughout childhood and relatively unprejudiced parents, whereas Restraint was associated with fewer and less positive interactions with blacks and reports of greater parental prejudice. Thus, Concern appears to be more approach-oriented and Restraint, more avoidance-oriented (see also Plant, Devine, & Peruche, 2010).

A recent study supports the notion that individuals with high Restraint are more avoidant (Olson & Fazio, 2007). Here, participants were required to report verbally to an audience their evaluations of candidates they had evaluated for the Peace Corps (as described earlier). According to judges' ratings, participants' public remarks corresponded to their private ratings, as one would expect. However, this relation was attenuated for individuals with high Restraint, suggesting they obfuscated their discussion of the black candidate, causing the judges to struggle to grasp their recommendations.

In a study that demonstrates the Concern factor's orientation toward personal standards, participants who completed the MCPR in an earlier session partook in a study on "reactions to commercials," in which they viewed several commercials, including a clever one designed to lead viewers inadvertently to exhibit a prejudiced response (Fazio & Hilden, 2001). It showed a black man while describing a series of violent crimes. Viewers assume that the pictured man is the criminal in question, but they later learn that he is the police officer who apprehended him. In response to this trickery, most participants reported feeling agitated, particularly if they scored high on either of the motivation factors. High-Concern individuals, however, also reported feeling guilty, suggesting that they experienced a violation of an internal standard of conduct (e.g., Higgins, 1987).

Mixed Processes

The MODE model pays particular attention to *mixed processes,* that is, interactions between automatic and controlled processes. As discussed earlier, opportunity acts as a "gate" through which motivated processes can influence judgments and behavior. When the gate is open, as it usually is in the studies we summarize below, motivated processes are predicted to interact with racial attitudes to influence outcomes. We first discuss research documenting moderating effects of Concern, followed by those involving Restraint.

One of the first tests of interactive effects involved a study in which participants also completed the Modern Racism Scale (MRS; McConahay, 1986), an often-used explicit measure of prejudice (Fazio et al., 1995; Olson, 2009). Its items require respondents to indicate their agreement with various statements, such as "Blacks should not push themselves where they are not wanted." This scale's original purpose was to provide a more subtle means of assessing prejudice toward blacks. However, as a verbal "behavior," responses to it—or to any measure that directly queries people about their attitudes—occur further downstream and are therefore susceptible to the influence of motivated processes. Consistent with the model, correspondence between automatically activated racial attitudes, as assessed by the priming measure and the MRS, was observed for people with low Concern; their attitudes appeared to guide their responses spontaneously. For more motivated individuals, there was little correspondence (see also Degner & Wentura, 2008; Payne, 2001; Payne et al., 2005). In fact, to the extent that the priming measure revealed automatic prejudice, highly motivated individuals appeared to overcorrect for their attitudes, to the point that they appeared less prejudiced than individuals characterized by positive scores on the priming measure. Thus, the MRS appears to conflate prejudice and motivation to avoid it, a problem that, we suspect, has the potential to beset any explicit measure of prejudice (Olson, 2009).

A major hurdle to more harmonious intergroup relations is avoidance of social situations in which encounters with outgroup members are likely. Research conducted by Towles-Schwen and Fazio (2003) demonstrates the MODE model's ability to predict such (un)willingness to enter situations. In this research, participants indicated their willingness to pursue situations (sit down at a crowded public table with the individual, go on a date, etc.) with a variety of potential interaction partners (a person in a wheelchair, an obese person, an Asian, a black individual, etc.). Compared to a condition in which the interaction partner was unspecified, participants indicated a willingness to enter situations with a black partner that corresponded to their automatically activated attitudes toward blacks—so long as they were not motivated to indicate otherwise. More motivated individuals, however, corrected for their prejudice and reported a greater willingness to enter these interactions. Hence, attitudes appeared to guide peoples' willingness to enter into interactions with blacks spontaneously among the less motivated, but correction for prejudice was observed among more Concern-motivated individuals.

The Restraint factor has evidenced consistent patterns of corrections for automatic prejudice in accordance with the MODE model in other studies. These studies generally involve forming an impression of a black individual, a point to which we return later. For example, Dunton and Fazio (1997) asked participants to describe their impressions of the "typical black male undergraduate," and then rate the valence of their thoughts. As expected, automatically activated racial attitudes predicted thought ratings for those low in Restraint motivation, suggesting a spontaneous application of prejudice to impression formation. More motivated respondents corrected for their prejudice; their impressions were similar in valence to those with racial attitudes opposite their own (i.e., motivated individuals with negative prejudice reported impressions similar to less motivated pro-black individuals, and motivated individuals with positive prejudice reported impressions similar to less motivated pro-white individuals).

We reported similar findings in a more recent study on first impressions of individuals in various social and occupational contexts (Olson & Fazio, 2004). Here, after collecting motivation and attitude estimate data, we asked participants to provide their impressions of a variety of black, white, and other-race individuals who were depicted in different occupations. Critical pairs of black and white targets were matched in terms of gender and the status and independence of their occupations (e.g., a white male professor, a black male minister). Participants rated targets on various traits, and from these we created an index of their preference for black relative to white targets within the pairs. As in Dunton and Fazio's (1997) research discussed earlier, automatically activated racial attitudes predicted the black–white trait index for those with relatively low Restraint. Higher-Restraint individuals evidenced correction for prejudice; those with more negative automatic attitudes toward blacks corrected their impressions in a pro-black direction, and those with more positive attitudes corrected in a pro-white direction.

The Roles of Correctional Goals and Social Context

The studies we have just reviewed provide consistent evidence in support of the MODE model's tenets, particularly the notion that automatically activated racial attitudes should predict race-related judgments and behavior in the absence of motivation or opportunity. Correction for prejudice has been consistently observed among motivated individuals. A broader look at this research, however, reveals two themes that speak to the nature of the motives that moderate the relation between attitudes and behavior in this domain. The first has implications for the correctional goal implied by the different motives. In studies showing moderating effects of the Concern motive, correction is seen most among prejudiced individuals (e.g., Fazio et al., 1995). Specifically, prejudiced, Concern-motivated individuals correct for prejudice in a way that makes them appear more positive toward blacks, but Concern-motivated individuals who already have pro-black automatic responses show less correction. Hence, it appears that Concern motivation has a unidirectional, "pro-black" manifestation, which is consistent with research suggesting its ties to egalitarianism. On the other hand, moderating effects of Restraint show a more bidirectional correction pattern (e.g., Olson & Fazio, 2004; Towles-Schwen & Fazio, 2006), suggesting that Restraint-motivated individuals are correcting for both prejudice *against* blacks and prejudice *in favor of* blacks. While it might seem counterintuitive that a class of motivated individuals would correct for a pro-black bias when the general thrust of such motives would seem to draw them in the opposite direction, recall that high Restraint serves the goal of avoiding race-related conflict. Such conflict might obviously stem from accusations of prejudice against blacks, but it is likely that it might also stem from a fear of appearing overly favorable toward blacks (i.e., "reverse discrimination").

A second theme to emerge from the studies we reviewed is that the Concern motive appears to operate in judgments of groups, whereas the Restraint motive appears to operate in individual contexts. We have speculated (Olson & Fazio, 2009) that Concern motivation may stem from an interest in redressing historical inequalities regarding blacks as a social group. Restraint, in being more conflict-avoidance-oriented, is likely to be more individual in its focus, because the sort of conflict feared by those characterized by this motive is largely interpersonal. Indeed, a meaningful way in which the various motives relevant to racial prejudice might be distinguished has to do with whether they are group- or individual-oriented. Individual-level motives, in addition to Restraint, might include comprehension and self-enhancement (e.g., Kunda & Spencer, 2003), and more specific motives regarding liking or disliking a target (e.g., Sinclair & Kunda, 1999). Group-level motives, in addition to Concern, might include *social dominance orientation* (the desire for clear hierarchical distinctions between groups; Pratto, Sidanius, Stallworth, & Malle, 1994), as well as recently discussed ideologies such as multiculturalism and color blindness (e.g., Plaut, 2010). If such a distinction truly cleaves nature at its joints, then the intriguing possibility arises that one's individual-level and group-level motives might be dissociated. For instance, one might be motivated to avoid prejudice toward groups but not toward individuals, or vice versa.

Zabel and Olson (2013) recently tested these ideas in an extension of Olson and Fazio's (2004) research described earlier. As before, the MCPR and priming measure were administered to participants who later provided their impressions of people in various occupational roles. Prior to the impression task (and premised on the notion that social targets can be flexibly construed, e.g., Fazio & Dunton, 1997), participants were primed to construe social targets at either the group level or the individual level. Those in the former condition were shown pictures of 20 individuals, analogous to those used in the impression task, and for each were asked to speculate in open-ended fashion, "What makes this person a member of a group?" In the latter condition, participants responded to the same photos by listing "What makes this person an individual?" As expected, those primed to construe the targets at the individual level showed a moderating effect of the Restraint motive on the attitude estimate's relation to their impressions of black versus white targets, replicating Olson and Fazio (2004). However, the data were surprising for those primed to construe the targets as group members, for whom Concern was expected to be the operative moderating motive. Here, those higher in Concern reported more positive evaluations of *all* targets, both black and white. Perhaps such a strategy is an effective means of appearing nonprejudiced to the self and others in contexts where it can be applied.

In a follow-up study, the "like everyone" option was revoked and participants were forced to provide pairwise preference judgments of the matched black–white targets (given the interest in the Concern motive here, all participants were primed to construe the targets at the group level). The anticipated Attitude Estimate × Concern interaction was found: Less motivated individuals' impressions appeared to be guided by their automatically activated attitudes, and motivated individuals showed a pattern of correction for negative racial bias. Hence, it does appear that Restraint is a motive that operates in individual contexts, and Concern is a motive that operates in group contexts.

The Role of Opportunity

We confess to having pursued empirical evidence for the role of the MODE model's opportunity variable with less vigor than we have pursued motivational variables. Thankfully, others' recent work includes findings that support the moderating role of opportunity in the prejudice domain. Perhaps the most obvious operationalization of the opportunity variable is time. Given time constraints, the model predicts that motivated processes are less able to influence verbal and behavioral responses, allowing greater influence of automatic ones. This is just what Ranganath, Smith, and Nosek (2008) found: Explicit measures of prejudice (as well as attitudes toward a variety of other objects) loaded on a common factor with implicit measures that tap more automatic responses only when participants reported their attitudes under strict time constraints (for parallel findings in the self-esteem domain, see also Koole, Dijksterhuis, & van Knippenberg, 2001). Analogous findings from studies asking respondents to report their "immediate" or "gut" reactions (vs. more deliberative responses) have been reported across a variety of domains (e.g., Gawronski & LeBel, 2008; Jordan, Whitfield, & Zeigler-Hill, 2007; Kendrick & Olson, 2012).

The opportunity variable also can be viewed in terms of the current level of resources an individual has available to exercise control in the service of some goal. Research documents that a depleted state leaves the individual more prone to the influence of the automatically activated attitude. For example, Govorun and Payne (2006) demonstrated that a resource-depleting Stroop color-naming task diminished the controlled component of a process dissociation procedure in a weapons identification task, leaving a greater role for automatic processes to guide judgments.

Alcohol consumption is yet another interesting way of considering the opportunity factor, as it has deleterious effects on working memory and response inhibition (e.g., Finn, Justus, Mazas, & Steinmetz, 1999). It is an ability to inhibit one's potentially automatic responses and instead choose a more deliberate route that the opportunity factor affords, and alcohol likely compromises this ability (Houben, Wiers, & Jansen, 2011). Bartholow, Dickter, and Sestir (2006) examined the effects of alcohol consumption on self-regulatory processes in stereotyping. They found that moderate alcohol consumption did not affect the automatic activation of prejudiced associations, suggesting, as the MODE model argues, that relatively automatic processes are unaffected by variables that compromise more deliberate ones. However, alcohol did impair peoples' ability to inhibit prejudiced responses on a "go–stop" task, which is precisely what manipulations of the opportunity factor are predicted to do (for analogous findings beyond the prejudice domain, see Hofmann & Friese, 2008). In another study, participants completed both implicit and explicit measures of prejudice after consuming alcohol or not (Loersch, Bartholow, Manning, Calanchini, & Sherman, 2012). Consistent with the model and the research already described indicating implicit–explicit correspondence when either motivation or opportunity is low, these two measurement types aligned for those under the effects of alcohol, but not for those who were not.

Research on cognition and aging parallels the work on alcohol. Put brusquely, being old is like being drunk, in that both decrease inhibitory processing capacity (Hasher, Zacks, & May, 1999). Consistent with this reasoning, earlier work by Von Hippel, Silver, and Lynch (2000) showed that older adults have difficulty stemming prejudiced thoughts. More recently, and in support of the MODE model, Stewart, Von Hippel, and Radvansky (2009) clarified through a process dissociation procedure that older adults do not show any more activation of automatic prejudice than do younger adults, but their prejudice is more likely to be expressed because of their reduced ability to inhibit prejudices, in other words, because of a reduction in opportunity (see also Gonsalkorale, Sherman, & Klauer, 2009).

Finally, certain behaviors are less susceptible to control by their very nature, thus providing a naturally occurring means of assessing the role of opportunity. These include both nonverbal behavior (DePaulo, 1992) and chonic, long-term behavior that cannot possibly be monitored at all times. Less controllable behaviors should be less susceptible to the influence of motivated processes. Consistent with this reasoning, automatic race-related bias has been found to "leak" into the nonverbal channels despite any motivation participants might have to conceal it (e.g., Dovidio, Kawakami, & Gaertner, 2002; Dovidio et al., 1997; McConnell & Leibold, 2001). Furthermore, it is likely that long-term, repeated interactions will allow perceivers a glimpse into their automatically activated racial attitudes, because no behavior can be constantly monitored at all times. Such is the case for college roommates, and in a recent study (Towles-Schwen & Fazio, 2006), white students randomly assigned to share a dormitory room with a black student were more likely to have their roommate relationships dissolve to the extent that the priming measure revealed automatic racial bias.

BEYOND PREJUDICE

We have focused our attention primarily on research concerning prejudice largely because it is a domain in which automatically-activated attitudes and relevant motivations are readily observed to compete for dominance. However, considerable research beyond the domain of prejudice also supports the MODE model. For example, much like in the interracial roommate research described above, automatically-activated attitudes toward one's romantic relationship partner can affect relationship outcomes in the long-term, despite any motivation to do otherwise. A recent 4-year longitudinal study of newlyweds found that one's automatically-activated attitude toward one's spouse (as measured by an evaluative priming procedure) is a better predictor of long-term changes in marital satisfaction than are self-reports (McNulty, Olson, Meltzer, & Shaffer, 2013). This prospective relation across the four years was mediated by partners' perceptions of problems in the relationship, suggesting that strong automatic attitudes toward one's partner influence basic perceptions of the relationship (see also Fazio, Ledbetter, & Towles-Schwen, 2000). Romantic relationships are also more likely to dissolve, in the long term, to the extent that one's partner evokes less positive automatic responses (Lee, Rogge, & Reis, 2010). We would suggest that motivated bolstering of one's appraisal of a romantic relationship grows increasingly difficult over the long term and, hence, the influence of automatically-activated attitudes becomes all the more evident.

At least in the moment of assessment, however, reports of relationship satisfaction do provide opportunity for the influence of motivated processes. Research on close relationships has found that the relation between automatically-activated attitudes toward a romantic partner and self-reports of satisfaction with the relationship varies as a function of individuals' motivation to believe that the relationship is thriving. Scinta and Gable (2007) assessed such motivation in a sample of dating couples by inquiring about the extent to which individuals' experienced "barriers to exit" the relationship. Believing that one had invested considerably in the relationship and had few relationship alternatives enhanced the motive to view the relationship favorably. Among those for whom this motivation was relatively low, the relation between automatic attitudes toward the partner and reports of satisfaction assumed exactly the form one would expect: more positive attitudes were associated with greater satisfaction. However, as "barriers to exit" increased, this relation attenuated and eventually reversed. Among those with a strong motivation to believe in the relationship, individuals with less positive automatically-activated attitudes toward their partner actually reported greater satisfaction than those with more positive attitudes. Other research regarding romantic relationships is relevant to the opportunity postulate of the MODE model. Operationalizing opportunity as an individual difference variable concerning resource capacity, Murray et al. (2011) found working memory capacity to moderate the relation between attitudes toward the partner and various outcome measures. The relation was attenuated among individuals with the stronger capacity to deliberate about the partner and the state of the relationship (see also Murray, Gomillion, Holmes, Harris, & Lamarche, 2013; Murray, Lupien, & Seery, 2012).

Motivation and opportunity also have proven critical in the domain of self-control. Just as the MODE model predicts, impulsive behavior has been found to vary as a function of motivation to behave otherwise and the extent to which the individual has the resources to counter those impulses. For example, in research by Hofmann, Rauch, and Gawronski (2007), the amount of candy that participants consumed depended on their automatically activated attitudes toward candy, their motivation to monitor and control their diet, and whether they had recently undergone a resource-depleting emotional suppression task. Among the resource-depleted participants, candy consumption was predicted primarily by attitudes, whereas those with fuller resources acted more in accord with their dietary motivation. Parallel findings were obtained by Hofmann and Friese (2008) when resource capacity was manipulated via alcohol consumption. Whereas dietary restraint was the more important predictor of candy consumption among the sober participants, alcohol intake enhanced the relation between attitudes toward candy and candy consumption.

Similarly, because a happy mood state signals that all is well, whereas sadness motivates more deliberative processing, mood states have been shown to moderate the relation between attitudes and behavior (Holland, de Vries, Hermsen, & van Knippenberg, 2012). Preference for candy bars versus apples (as assessed by a personalized IAT) predicted choice behavior when participants had been made to feel happy, but less so when they were made to feel sad. In the latter condition, participants' beliefs about the attributes of candy bars versus apples proved more influential.

Individual differences in working memory capacity also play a critical role in self-regulation (Hofmann, Gschwendner, Friese, Wiers, & Schmitt, 2008). Essentially, automatic attitudes toward a given temptation more strongly influenced behavior for individuals with lower working memory capacity, whereas self-regulatory goals relevant to the temptation were more effective in guiding behavior among those higher in capacity. More recent experimental evidence takes this a step further. Extensive training designed to enhance the working memory capacity of problem drinkers increased their ability to control automatic impulses to drink and led to reductions in alcohol use (Houben et al., 2011). Thus, greater resource capacity lessened the influence of the problem drinkers' automatically activated positivity toward alcohol.

IMPLICATIONS FOR IMPLICIT AND EXPLICIT MEASURES OF ATTITUDES

By now we hope it is clear that the MODE model speaks directly to the current debate about the role of implicit and explicit measures of attitudes in terms of both their interrelations and their relations to judgments and behavior. Although no measure is process-pure (e.g., Conrey, Sherman, Gawronski, Hugenberg, & Groom, 2005) and effective means of partitioning automatic and controlled inputs exist (e.g., Jacoby, 1991), a well-supported premise to most research employing both implicit and explicit measures is that the former taps relatively automatic processes and the latter taps relatively controlled, propositional processes (e.g., Fazio & Olson, 2003; Gawronski & Bodenhausen, 2011; Rydell & McConnell, 2006). As we have discussed, the model predicts that automatically activated attitudes will guide behavior in the absence of either motivation or opportunity to do otherwise. Its straightforward prediction is that implicit measures should generally correlate with explicit measures (which are in essence verbal behaviors and are therefore further downstream in the attitude–behavior process) in the absence of one of these moderating variables.

Numerous studies have revealed precisely the moderating pattern predicted by the model: Implicit measures relate reliably to explicit measures when motivation is low (e.g., low motivation to control prejudice: Fazio et al., 1995; Dasgupta & Rivera, 2006; low need for cognition: Conner, Perugini, O'Gorman, Ayres, & Prestwich, 2007; Florack, Scarabis, & Bless, 2001), or opportunity is lacking (e.g., time pressure: Koole et al., 2001; Ranganath et al., 2008). Important differences between implicit measurement varieties notwithstanding (see Hofmann, Gawronski, Gschwendner, Le, & Schmitt, 2005), it is telling that this basic pattern has been observed across a wide array of implicit measurement types in addition to priming (e.g., IAT: Dasgupta & Rivera, 2006; affect misattribution procedure [AMP]: Payne et al., 2005; Extrinsic Affective Simon Task [EAST]: Degner & Wentura, 2008), and across a wide range of attitudinal domains beyond prejudice (e.g., the self: Olson, Fazio, & Hermann, 2007; relationships: Scinta & Gable, 2007).

More important than questions about correlations between measures is when each measurement type best predicts behavior. A loose consensus has emerged within the field that implicit measures are better predictors of less controllable behavior, and explicit measures are better predictors of more controllable behavior. However, the MODE model's emphasis on mixed processes—interactions instead of main effects—argues otherwise. Its spontaneous attitude-to-behavior route predicts that automatically activated attitudes can influence any attitude-related behavior, regardless of its controllability, in the absence of motivation or opportunity to do otherwise. Consistent with this reasoning, a simple mapping of implicit measures to less controllable behavior and of explicit measures to more controllable behavior is not what the literature reveals. Instead, implicit measures have proved predictive of all sorts of behavior on the controllability continuum, including quite controllable behaviors, such as verbal evaluations of social targets (e.g., Jackson, 1997), real hiring decisions by employers (e.g., Agerström & Rooth, 2011), career decisions (e.g., Von Hippel, Brener, & Von Hippel, 2008), voting (e.g., Payne et al., 2010), and sexual assault (Widman & Olson, 2013).

Finally, we observe that not long ago, implicit and explicit measures were not so far apart. Indeed, early forays into implicit measurement revealed remarkable correspondence with explicit reports (Fazio & Olson, 2003). Likely this was because the measures assessed attitudes about which there was little motivation to interfere with accurate explicit reporting (e.g., flowers vs. insects: Greenwald et al., 1998; cockroaches vs. puppies: Fazio et al., 1986). Here, clear implicit–explicit correspondence was the rule. The original impetus for the priming measure was to assess an attitudinal strength variable (i.e., attitude accessibility), not to uncover some different attitudinal representation altogether (e.g., Wilson, Lindsey, & Schooler, 2000). Researchers have been tempted to identify separate automatic/unconscious and controlled/conscious attitudes in domains where reliable implicit–explicit dissociations have been observed (e.g., self-esteem; Spalding & Hardin, 1999), but here, too, the two measurement types correlate under conditions specified by the model (e.g., Olson et al., 2007; see also Lebel, 2010). Thus, we contend that it is more appropriate to explain measurement dissociations in terms of conceptually different attitude-to-behavior processes than in terms of independent attitudinal systems.

CONCLUSION

Over the past 20 or so years, the MODE model has served as a theoretical framework for understanding attitude–behavior relations in a variety of domains, including impression formation, impulsive behavior, prejudice, and close relationships, to name a few. It also provides insight into relations between implicit and explicit measures in these and other domains. It is the interaction between automatic and controlled components under conditions specified by the model—motivation and opportunity—that is central to its ability to provide such broad explanatory power.

NOTE

1. In accord with Shiffrin and Dumais's (1981) characterization of automaticity, we use the term *automatic* to refer to the inescapable initiation of a response to a given stimulus. Encountering the attitude object activates the associated evaluation without the individual's intent, even if he or she is attempting to engage in some other task. Any such activation need not reach the level of awareness, but the activation does increase the likelihood that the evaluation will influence subsequent information procssing (Bruner, 1957; Higgins, 1996). See Fazio (2007) for a more elaborate discussion of "automatic" attitude activation.

REFERENCES

Agerström, J., & Rooth, D. O. (2011). The role of automatic obesity stereotypes in real hiring discrimination. *Journal of Applied Psychology, 96*(4), 790–805.

Ajzen, I. (1991). The theory of planned behavior. *Organizational Behavior and Human Decision Processes, 50*, 179–211.

Ajzen, I., & Fishbein, M. (1980). *Understanding attitudes and predicting social behavior.* Englewood Cliffs, NJ: Prentice Hall.

Asch, S. E. (1940). Studies in the principles of judgments and attitudes: II. Determination of judgments by group and by ego standards. *Journal of Social Psychology, 12*, 433–465.

Bartholow, B. D., Dickter, C. L., & Sestir, M. A. (2006). Stereotype activation and control of race bias: Cognitive control of inhibition and its impairment by alcohol. *Journal of Personality and Social Psychology, 90*(2), 272–287.

Bruner, J. S. (1957). On perceptual readiness. *Psychological Review, 64*, 123–152.

Cameron, C. D., Brown-Iannuzzi, J. L., & Payne, B. K. (2012). Sequential priming measures of implicit social cognition: A meta-analysis of associations with behavior and explicit attitudes. *Personality and Social Psychology Review, 16*, 330–350.

Conner, M. T., Perugini, M., O'Gorman, R., Ayres, K., & Prestwich, A. (2007). Relations between implicit and explicit measures of attitudes and measures of behavior: Evidence of moderation by individual difference variables. *Personality and Social Psychology Bulletin, 33*(12), 1727–1740.

Conrey, F. R., Sherman, J. W., Gawronski, B., Hugenberg, K., & Groom, C. (2005). Separating multiple processes in implicit social cognition: The quad model of implicit task performance. *Journal of Personality and Social Psychology, 89*, 469–487.

Dasgupta, N., & Rivera, L. M. (2006). From automatic antigay prejudice to behavior: The moderating role of conscious beliefs about gender and behavioral control. *Journal of Personality and Social Psychology, 91*(2), 268–280.

Degner, J., & Wentura, D. (2008). The Extrinsic Affective Simon Task as an instrument for indirect assessment of prejudice. *European Journal of Social Psychology, 38*(6), 1033–1043.

De Houwer, J. (2009). Comparing measures of attitudes at the functional and procedural level: Analysis and implications. In R. E. Petty, R. H. Fazio, & P. Briñol (Eds.), *Attitudes: Insights from the new implicit measures* (pp. 361–390). Mahwah, NJ: Erlbaum.

DePaulo, B. M. (1992). Nonverbal behavior and self-presentation. *Psychological Bulletin, 111*, 203–243.

Devine, P. G. (1989). Stereotypes and prejudice: Their automatic and controlled components. *Journal of Personality and Social Psychology, 56*(1), 5–18.

Dovidio, J. F., & Gaertner, S. L. (2004). Aversive racism. In M. P. Zanna (Ed.), *Advances in experimental social psychology* (Vol. 36, pp. 1–51). San Diego: Academic Press.

Dovidio, J. F., Kawakami, K., & Gaertner, S. L. (2002). Implicit and explicit prejudice and interracial interaction. *Journal of Personality and Social Psychology, 82*(1), 62–68.

Dovidio, J. F., Kawakami, K., Johnson, C., Johnson, B., & Howard, A. (1997). On the nature of prejudice: Automatic and controlled processes. *Journal of Experimental Social Psychology, 33*(5), 510–540.

Dunton, B. C., & Fazio, R. H. (1997). An individual difference measure of motivation to control prejudiced reactions. *Personality and Social Psychology Bulletin, 23*(3), 316–326.

Fazio, R. H. (1990). Multiple processes by which attitudes guide behavior: The MODE model as an integrative framework. In M. P. Zanna (Ed.), *Advances in experimental social psychology* (Vol. 23, pp. 75–109). New York: Academic Press.

Fazio, R. H. (2007). Attitudes as object-evaluation associations of varying strength. *Social Cognition, 25*, 664–703.

Fazio, R. H., Chen, J., McDonel, E. C., & Sherman, S. J. (1982). Attitude accessibility, attitude–behavior consistency, and the strength of the object–evaluation association. *Journal of Experimental Social Psychology, 18*, 339–357.

Fazio, R. H., & Dunton, B. C. (1997). Categorization by race: The impact of automatic and controlled components of racial prejudice. *Journal of Experimental Social Psychology, 33*, 451–470.

Fazio, R. H., & Hilden, L. E. (2001). Emotional reactions to a seemingly prejudiced response: The role of automatically activated racial attitudes and motivation to control prejudiced reactions. *Personality and Social Psychology Bulletin, 27*(5), 538–549.

Fazio, R. H., Jackson, J. R., Dunton, B. C., & Williams, C. J. (1995). Variability in automatic activation as an unobstrusive measure of racial attitudes: A bona fide pipeline? *Journal of Personality and Social Psychology, 69*(6), 1013–1027.

Fazio, R. H., Ledbetter, J. E., & Towles-Schwen, T. (2000). On the costs of accessible attitudes: Detecting that the attitude object has changed. *Journal of Personality and Social Psychology, 78*, 197–210.

Fazio, R. H., & Olson, M. A. (2003). Implicit measures in social cognition research: Their meaning and use. *Annual Review of Psychology, 54*(1), 297–327.

Fazio, R. H., Powell, M. C., & Herr, P. M. (1983). Toward a process model of the attitude–behavior relation: Accessing one's attitude upon mere observation of the attitude object. *Journal of Personality and Social Psychology, 44*, 723–735.

Fazio, R. H., Sanbonmatsu, D. M., Powell, M. C., & Kardes, F. R. (1986). On the automatic activation of attitudes. *Journal of Personality and Social Psychology, 50*, 229–238.

Fazio, R. H., & Towles-Schwen, T. (1999). The MODE model of attitude–behavior processes. In S. Chaiken & Y. Trope (Eds.), *Dual process theories in social psychology* (pp. 97–116). New York: Guilford Press.

Fazio, R. H., & Williams, C. J. (1986). Attitude accessibility as a moderator of the attitude–perception and attitude–behavior relations: An investigation of the 1984 presidential election. *Journal of Personality and Social Psychology, 51*, 505–514.

Finn, P. R., Justus, A., Mazas, C., & Steinmetz, J. E. (1999). Working memory, executive processes and the effects of alcohol on Go/No-Go learning: Testing a model of behavioral regulation and impulsivity. *Psychopharmacology, 146*, 465–472.

Florack, A., Scarabis, M., & Bless, H. (2001). When do associations matter?: The use of automatic associations toward ethnic groups in person judgments. *Journal of Experimental Social Psychology, 37*(6), 518–524.

Gaertner, S. L., & Dovidio, J. F. (1986). The aversive form of racism. In J. F. Dovidio & S. L. Gaertner (Eds.), *Prejudice, discrimination, and racism* (pp. 61–89). Orlando, FL: Academic Press.

Gawronski, B., & Bodenhausen, G. V. (2011). The associative–propositional evaluation model: Theory, evidence, and open questions. *Advances in Experimental Social Psychology, 44*, 59–127.

Gawronski, B., & LeBel, E. P. (2008). Understanding patterns of attitude change: When implicit measures show change, but explicit measures do not. *Journal of Experimental Social Psychology, 44*(5), 1355–1361.

Gonsalkorale, K., Sherman, J. W., & Klauer, K. C. (2009). Aging and prejudice: Diminished regulation of automatic race bias among older adults. *Journal of Experimental Social Psychology, 45*, 410–414.

Govorun, O., & Payne, B. K. (2006). Ego depletion and prejudice: Separating automatic and controlled components. *Social Cognition, 24*, 111–136.

Greenwald, A. G., McGhee, D. E., & Schwartz, J. L. (1998). Measuring individual differences in implicit cognition: The Implicit Association Test. *Journal of Personality and Social Psychology, 74*(6), 1464–1480.

Hasher, L., Zacks, R. T., & May, C. P. (1999). Inhibitory control, circadian arousal, and age. In D. Gopher & A. Koriat (Eds.), *Attention and performance XVII: Cognitive regulation of performance: Interaction of theory and application* (pp. 653–675). Cambridge, MA: MIT Press.

Hastorf, A. H., & Cantril, H. (1954). They saw a game: A case study. *Journal of Abnormal and Social Psychology*, 49, 129–134.

Higgins, E. T. (1987). Self-discrepancy: A theory relating self and affect. *Psychological Review, 94*(3), 319–340.

Higgins, E. T. (1996). Knowledge activation: Accessibility, applicability, and salience. In E. T. Higgins & A. W. Kruglanski (Eds.), *Social psychology: Handbook of basic principles* (pp. 133–168). New York: Guilford Press.

Hofmann, W., & Friese, M. (2008). Impulses got the better of me: Alcohol moderates the influence of implicit attitudes toward food cues on eating behavior. *Journal of Abnormal Psychology, 117*(2), 420–427.

Hofmann, W., Gawronski, B., Gschwendner, T., Le, H., & Schmitt, M. (2005). A meta-analysis on the correlation between the Implicit Association Test and explicit self-report measures. *Personality and Social Psychology Bulletin, 31*(10), 1369–1385.

Hofmann, W., Gschwendner, T., Friese, M., Wiers, R., & Schmitt, M. (2008). Working memory capacity and self-regulatory behavior: Towards an individual differences perspective on behavior determination by automatic versus controlled processes. *Journal of Personality and Social Psychology, 95*, 962–977.

Hofmann, W., Rauch, W., & Gawronski, B. (2007). And deplete us not into temptation: Automatic attitudes, dietary restraint, and self-regulatory resources as determinants of eating behavior. *Journal of Experimental Social Psychology*, 43, 497–504.

Holland, R. W., de Vries, M., Hermsen, B., & van Knippenberg, A. (2012). Mood and the attitude–behavior link: The happy act on impulse, the sad think twice. *Social Psychological and Personality Science, 3*, 356–364.

Houben, K., Wiers, R. W., & Jansen, A. (2011). Getting a grip on drinking behavior: Training working memory to reduce alcohol abuse. *Psychological Science, 22*(7), 968–975.

Houston, D. A., & Fazio, R. H. (1989). Biased processing as a function of attitude accessibility: Making objective judgments subjectively. *Social Cognition, 7*, 51–66.

Jackson, J. R. (1997). *Automatically activated racial attitudes*. Unpublished doctoral dissertation, Indiana University, Bloomington, IN.

Jacoby, L. L. (1991). A process dissociation framework: Separating automatic from intentional uses of memory. *Journal of Memory and Language, 30*(5), 513–541.

Jones, C. R., & Fazio, R. H. (2010). Person categorization and automatic racial stereotyping effects on weapon identification. *Personality and Social Psychology Bulletin, 36*, 1073–1085.

Jordan, C. H., Whitfield, M., & Zeigler-Hill, V. (2007). Intuition and the correspondence between implicit and explicit self-esteem. *Journal of Personality and Social Psychology, 93*(6), 1067–1079.

Kendrick, R. V., & Olson, M. A. (2012). When feeling right leads to being right in the reporting of implicitly-formed attitudes, or how I learned to stop worrying and trust my gut. *Journal of Experimental Social Psychology, 48*(6), 1316–1321.

Koole, S. L., Dijksterhuis, A., & van Knippenberg, A. (2001). What's in a name: Implicit self-esteem and the automatic self. *Journal of*

Personality and Social Psychology, 80, 669–685.

Kunda, Z., & Spencer, S. J. (2003). When do stereotypes come to mind and when do they color judgment?: A goal-based theoretical framework for stereotype activation and application. *Psychological Bulletin, 129*, 522–544.

Lebel, E. P. (2010). Attitude accessibility as a moderator of implicit and explicit self-esteem correspondence. *Self and Identity, 9*, 195–208.

Lee, S., Rogge, R. D., & Reis, H. T. (2010). Assessing the seeds of relationship decay: Using implicit evaluations to detect the early stages of disillusionment. *Psychological Science, 21*(6), 857–864.

Loersch, C., Bartholow, B. D., Manning, M., Calanchini, J., & Sherman, J. W. (2012). *Intoxicated prejudice: The influence of alcohol consumption on implicit and explicit measures of racial attitudes.* Unpublished manuscript, University of Colorado. Boulder.

Lord, C. G., Ross, L., & Lepper, M. R. (1979). Biased assimilation and attitude polarization: The effects of prior theories on subsequently considered evidence. *Journal of Personality and Social Psychology, 37*, 2098–2109.

McConahay, J. B. (1986). Modern racism, ambivalence, and the modern racism scale. In J. F. Dovidio & S. L. Gaertner (Eds.), *Prejudice, discrimination, and racism* (pp. 91–125). Orlando, FL: Academic Press.

McConnell, A. R., & Leibold, J. M. (2001). Relations among the Implicit Association Test, discriminatory behavior, and explicit measures of racial attitudes. *Journal of Experimental Social Psychology, 37*, 435–442.

McNulty, J. K., Olson, M. A., Meltzer, A. L., & Shaffer, M. J. (2013). Though they may be unaware, newlyweds implicitly know whether their marriage will fail. *Science, 342*, 119–120.

Murray, S. L., Gomillion, S., Holmes, J. G., Harris, B., & Lamarche, V. (2013). The dynamics of relationship promotion: Controlling the automatic inclination to trust. *Journal of Personality and Social Psychology, 104*, 305–334.

Murray, S. L., Lupien, S. P., & Seery, M. D. (2012). Resilience in the face of romantic rejection: The automatic impulse to trust. *Journal of Experimental Social Psychology, 48*, 845–854.

Murray, S. L., Pinkus, R., Holmes, J. G., Harris, B., Gomillion, S., Aloni, M., et al. (2011). Signaling when (and when not) to be cautious and self-protective: Impulsive and reflective trust in close relationships. *Journal of Personality and Social Psychology, 101*, 485–502.

Olson, M. A. (2009). Measures of prejudice. In T. Nelson (Ed.), *Handbook of prejudice* (pp. 367–381). New York: Psychology Press.

Olson, M. A., & Fazio, R. H. (2003). Relations between implicit measures of prejudice: What are we measuring? *Psychological Science, 14*, 636–639.

Olson, M. A., & Fazio, R. H. (2004). Trait inferences as a function of automatically activated racial attitudes and motivation to control prejudiced reactions. *Basic and Applied Social Psychology, 26*, 1–11.

Olson, M. A., & Fazio, R. H. (2007). Discordant evaluations of blacks affect nonverbal behavior. *Personality and Social Psychology Bulletin, 33*, 1214–1224.

Olson, M. A., & Fazio, R. H. (2009). Implicit and explicit measures of attitudes: The perspective of the MODE model. In R. E. Petty, R. H. Fazio, & P. Briñol (Eds.), *Attitudes: Insights from the new implicit measures* (pp. 19–64). Mahwah, NJ: Erlbaum.

Olson, M. A., Fazio, R. H., & Hermann, A. D. (2007). Reporting tendencies underlie discrepancies between implicit and explicit measures of self-esteem. *Psychological Science, 18*, 287–291.

Payne, B. K. (2001). Prejudice and perception: the role of automatic and controlled processes in misperceiving a weapon. *Journal of Personality and Social Psychology, 81*, 181–192.

Payne, B. K., Cheng, C. M., Govorun, O., & Stewart, B. D. (2005). An inkblot for attitudes: Affect misattribution as implicit measurement. *Journal of Personality and Social Psychology, 89*, 277–293.

Payne, B. K., Krosnick, J. A., Pasek, J., Lelkes, Y., Akhtar, O., & Tompson, T. (2010). Implicit and explicit prejudice in the 2008 American presidential election. *Journal of Experimental Social Psychology, 46*, 367–374.

Plant, E. A., & Devine, P. G. (1998). Internal and external motivation to respond without prejudice. *Journal of Personality and Social Psychology, 75*, 811–832.

Plant, E. A., Devine, P. G., & Peruche, M. B. (2010). Routes to positive interracial interactions: Approaching egalitarianism or avoiding prejudice. *Personality and Social Psychology Bulletin, 36*, 1135–1147.

Plaut, V. C. (2010). Diversity science: Who needs it? *Psychological Inquiry*, *21*(2), 168–174.

Powell, M. C., & Fazio, R. H. (1984). Attitude accessibility as a function of repeated attitudinal expression. *Personality and Social Psychology Bulletin*, *10*, 139–148.

Pratto, F., Sidanius, J., Stallworth, L. M., & Malle, B. F. (1994). Social dominance orientation: A personality variable predicting social and political attitudes. *Journal of Personality and Social Psychology*, *67*, 741–763.

Ranganath, K. A., Smith, C. T., & Nosek, B. A. (2008). Distinguishing automatic and controlled components of attitudes from direct and indirect measurement methods. *Journal of Experimental Social Psychology*, *44*, 386–396.

Rydell, R. J., & McConnell, A. R. (2006). Understanding implicit and explicit attitude change: A systems of reasoning analysis. *Journal of Personality and Social Psychology*, *91*, 995–1008.

Sanbonmatsu, D. M., & Fazio, R. H. (1990). The role of attitudes in memory-based decision making. *Journal of Personality and Social Psychology*, *59*, 614–622.

Schuette, R. A., & Fazio, R. H. (1995). Attitude accessibility and motivation as determinants of biased processing: A test of the MODE model. *Personality and Social Psychology Bulletin*, *21*, 704–710.

Scinta, A., & Gable, S. L. (2007). Automatic and self-reported attitudes in romantic relationships. *Personality and Social Psychology Bulletin*, *33*, 1008–1022.

Shiffrin, R. M., & Dumais, S. T. (1981). The development of automatism. In J. R. Anderson (Ed.), *Cognitive skills and their acquisition* (pp. 111–140). Hillsdale, NJ: Erlbaum.

Sinclair, L., & Kunda, Z. (1999). Reactions to a black professional: Motivated inhibition and activation of conflicting stereotypes. *Journal of Personality and Social Psychology*, *77*, 885–904.

Smith, E. R., Fazio, R. H., & Cejka, M. A. (1996). Accessible attitudes influence categorization of multiply categorizable objects. *Journal of Personality and Social Psychology*, *71*, 888–898.

Spalding, L. R., & Hardin, C. D. (1999). Unconscious unease and self-handicapping: Behavioral consequences of individual differences in implicit and explicit self-esteem. *Psychological Science*, *10*, 535–539.

Stewart, B. D., Von Hippel, W., & Radvansky, G. A. (2009). Age, race, and implicit prejudice using process dissociation to separate the underlying components. *Psychological Science*, *20*, 164–168.

Towles-Schwen, T., & Fazio, R. H. (2001). On the origins of racial attitudes: Correlates of childhood experiences. *Personality and Social Psychology Bulletin*, *27*, 162–175.

Towles-Schwen, T., & Fazio, R. H. (2003). Choosing social situations: The relation between automatically activated racial attitudes and anticipated comfort interacting with African Americans. *Personality and Social Psychology Bulletin*, *29*, 170–182.

Towles-Schwen, T., & Fazio, R. H. (2006). Automatically activated racial attitudes as predictors of the success of interracial roommate relationships. *Journal of Experimental Social Psychology*, *42*, 698–705.

Von Hippel, W., Brener, L., & Von Hippel, C. (2008). Implicit prejudice toward injecting drug users predicts intentions to change jobs among drug and alcohol nurses. *Psychological Science*, *19*, 7–11.

Von Hippel, W., Silver, L. A., & Lynch, M. E. (2000). Stereotyping against your will: The role of inhibitory ability in stereotyping and prejudice among the elderly. *Personality and Social Psychology Bulletin*, *26*, 523–532.

Widman, L., & Olson, M. (2013). On the relationship between automatic attitudes and self-reported sexual assault in men. *Archives of Sexual Behavior*, *42*(5), 813–823.

Wilson, T. D., Lindsey, S., & Schooler, T. Y. (2000). A model of dual attitudes. *Psychological Review*, *107*, 101–126.

Wittenbrink, B., & Schwarz, N. (Eds.). (2007). *Implicit measures of attitudes*. New York: Guilford Press.

Young, A. I., & Fazio, R. H. (2013). Attitude accessibility as a determinant of object construal and evaluation. *Journal of Experimental Social Psychology*, *49*, 404–418.

Zabel, K., & Olson, M. A. (2013). *Construal level moderates correction of automatic racial bias in impression formations*. Unpublished manuscript, University of Tennessee, Knoxville, TN.

CHAPTER 12

The Elaboration Likelihood and Metacognitive Models of Attitudes

Implications for Prejudice, the Self, and Beyond

Richard E. Petty and Pablo Briñol

In this chapter we describe two models that are useful for understanding how attitudes are structured and how they change or resist change over time. We begin with a discussion of the elaboration likelihood model (ELM), a dual-route (but multiprocess) approach to persuasion, then describe the metacognitive model (MCM), which posits two fundamental processes involved in the underlying structure of attitudes. After briefly describing each approach, we discuss their interrelationship and conclude with applications of these approaches to understanding prejudice and self-evaluations.

THE ELM

The ELM (Petty & Cacioppo, 1981, 1986) is one of the earliest social psychological theories that distinguished thoughtful from nonthoughtful determinants of judgment (Chaiken & Trope, 1999; see Petty & Briñol, 2012, for a recent review). The ELM proposes that attitudes, as well as nonevaluative judgments, can be modified by processes that involve relatively high or low amounts of issue, or object-relevant, thinking, but the processes producing the judgment and the consequences that occur differ depending on the amount of thought involved. The ELM holds that there are numerous specific processes of attitude change that operate along the elaboration continuum (e.g., classical conditioning and use of decision heuristics require relatively little thought and operate at the low end of the continuum, but expectancy–value and cognitive response processes require higher degrees of thought and operate along the upper end of the continuum). The assortment of specific processes that occur along the low end of the continuum are collectively referred to as *peripheral route* mechanisms of persuasion, whereas the assortment of processes operating along the high end of the continuum are collectively referred to as *central route* mechanisms of persuasion.

Whether attitude change occurs as the result of relatively high or low amounts of thought matters for determining not only what judgment is formed but also how consequential that judgment is. Specifically, the more a judgment is based on thinking, the more it tends to persist over time, resist attempts at change, and have consequences for other judgments and behavior (see Petty, Haugtvedt, & Smith, 1995). Thus, even if two different processes result in the same judgment or the same extent of influence, the strength of these judgments can differ. For example, when variables such as emotion or a highly credible source produce persuasion through low thinking processes (e.g., serving as input to a simple heuristic), the attitudes formed are less persistent, resistant to change, and predictive of behavior than when the same amount of change is produced by these variables via high thinking processes (e.g., biasing the thoughts generated; see Petty & Krosnick, 1995, for a review of attitude strength research).

There are at least two important caveats to the ELM attitude strength predictions. First, the predictions are about deliberative attitudes—those that individuals report on explicit self-reports. Second, even on explicit measures of attitudes, not all of the strength consequences need to covary. For example, an attitude classically conditioned to be positive over many trials (low elaboration process) might be as stable over time as one that was made more positive because people carefully processed strong arguments about the advocacy (high elaboration process). However, the classically conditioned attitude would be weaker in the sense that it is less likely to resist an explicit attempt at counterpersuasion than an attitude based on reasoned argument. This is because when attitudes are conditioned, people have less ability to defend those attitudes from attack compared to when they have a substantive basis (Petty & Cacioppo, 1986). However, as we see shortly in addressing the MCM, on a measure of automatic attitude activation (implicit measure), the conditioned attitude can still be quite resistant to change (Petty, Tormala, Briñol, & Jarvis, 2006).

In addition to establishing the importance of the elaboration continuum for attitude change and strength, the ELM articulates the key mechanisms by which variables (e.g., source credibility, emotion) produce changes in attitudes along this continuum (see Figure 12.1). According to the ELM, when either motivation or ability to think is low, variables tend to serve as simple cues to influence. As cues, variables produce an outcome that is consistent with their valence (i.e., variables evaluated positively lead to more persuasion). When motivation and ability to think are high, variables serve in other roles, such as biasing thoughts or serving as arguments (pieces of evidence). When thinking is not constrained to be high or low by other factors, then variables determine how much thinking is done. There is much research supporting the notion that these different mechanisms operate under the conditions expected by the ELM (e.g., see Petty & Wegener, 1998, 1999). That is, any given feature of the persuasive setting (whether part of the source, message, recipient, or context), can serve as a simple cue, an issue-relevant argument, bias the thoughts that come to mind, or affect the motivation or ability to think about the message.

More recently, the ELM has incorporated another psychological process called *self-validation* (Petty, Briñol, & Tormala, 2002). Unlike previous mechanisms of attitude change that focus on primary or first-order cognition (i.e., amount and direction of thoughts), this new process emphasizes secondary or metacognition (Briñol & DeMarree, 2012; Jost, Kruglanski, & Nelson, 1998; Petty, Briñol, Tormala, & Wegener, 2007). The key notion of self-validation is that generating thoughts is not sufficient for them to have an impact on judgment. Rather, one must also have sufficient confidence in one's thoughts (*cognitive validation*) or feel good about them (*affective validation*). Thoughts that are not perceived as valid or that are disliked are mentally discarded. Thus, one of the core self-validation notions is that a host of familiar variables (happiness, source credibility, power, self-affirmation, etc.) that have already proven useful in other roles can also affect judgments by influencing whether or not people rely on their own thoughts (see Briñol & Petty, 2009a, for a review).

In summary, the ELM is a comprehensive theory of attitude formation and change (and other social judgments) that specifies the processes by which the numerous source, message, recipient, and context factors known to influence attitudes operate (see Briñol & Petty, 2012, for a review of the ELM in historical context). According to the ELM, the specific processes by which these variables operate under different elaboration conditions are seen as distinct mechanisms of influence, though the processes requiring higher thinking share the feature of producing attitudes that are more durable and impactful than the processes requiring lower thinking (for discussions regarding *lumping* vs. *splitting* of psychological processes, see Petty & Briñol, 2006a; Petty, Wheeler, & Bizer, 1999).

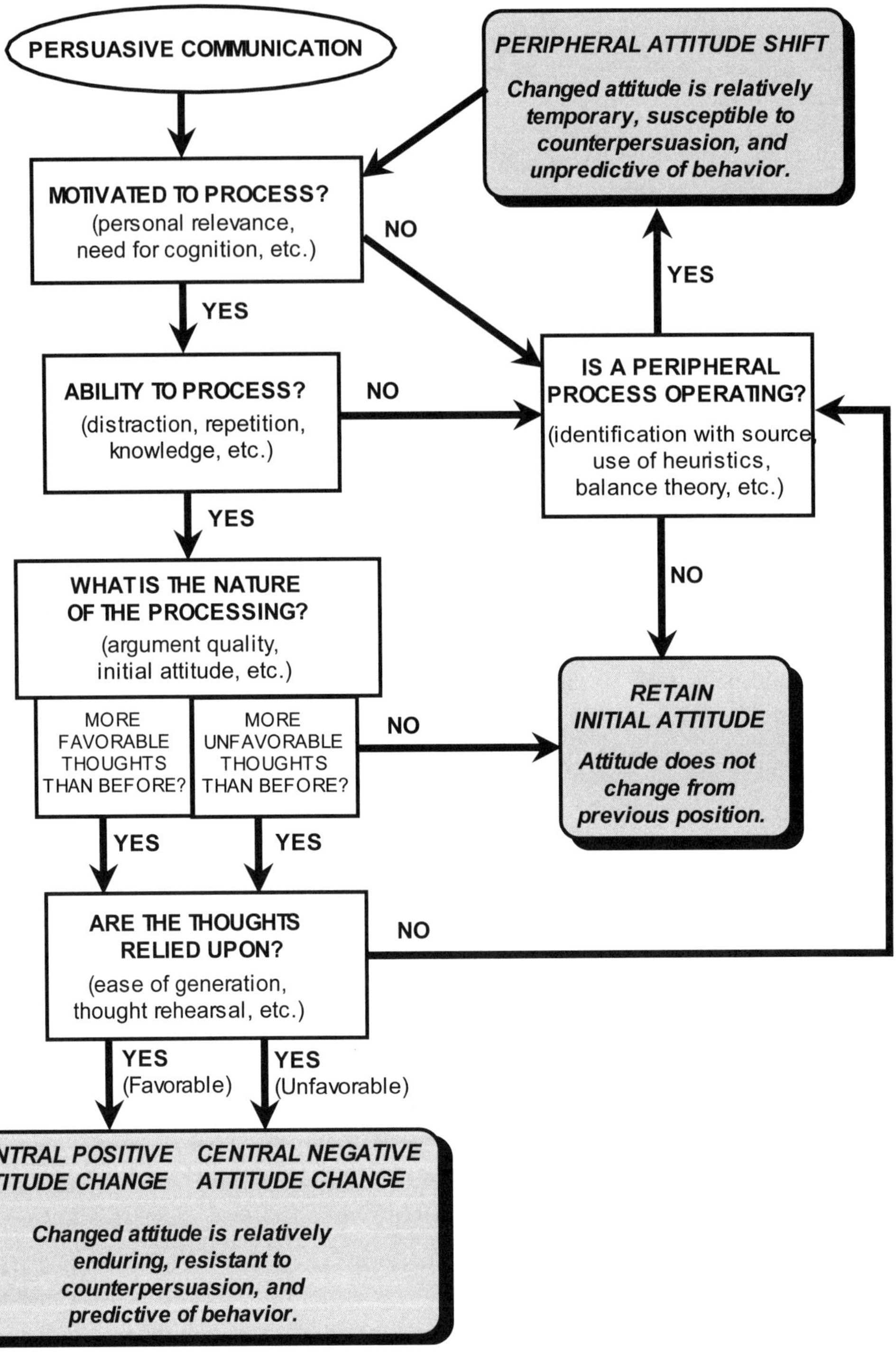

FIGURE 12.1. Schematic depiction of the ELM.

ILLUSTRATION: THE ELM APPLIED TO EMOTION

As an illustration of the utility of the multiple roles or processes along the elaboration continuum notion of the ELM, consider how a person's incidental emotions can impact evaluative judgments (Petty, Fabrigar, & Wegener, 2003). First and most simply, when thinking is constrained to be low (e.g., due to many distractions), an experienced emotion tends to serve as a simple associative cue or input to an affect heuristic and produce an evaluation consistent with its valence (e.g., Petty, Schumann, Richman, & Strathman, 1993). Thus, if one is feeling positive (e.g., happy) when evaluating a message, the message will be evaluated more favorably and induce more persuasion than if one is feeling negative (e.g., sad, angry). When thinking is high, however, one's emotions serve in other roles. First, emotions can be evaluated as evidence. Thus, whereas feeling fear would induce negative evaluations of virtually any object when used as a simple cue under low thinking conditions, when evaluated as evidence under high thinking conditions, feeling fear in response to a new automobile would cause it to be evaluated negatively, but feeling fear in response to a new horror film would cause it to be evaluated positively, since that is the desired emotion in that situation (see also, Martin, 2000; Pierro, Mannetti, Kruglanski, & Sleeth-Keppler, 2004).

In addition, when thinking is high, emotions can bias the ongoing thoughts. For example, positive consequences are more likely to come to mind and be seen as more likely to occur when people are in a happy rather than sad state (e.g., DeSteno, Petty, Wegener, & Rucker, 2000; Petty et al., 2003). And, as noted earlier, there is one more process by which recipient variables such as emotions can operate when thinking is high—affecting the use of one's thoughts. For example, Briñol, Petty, and Barden (2007) showed that if people are generating favorable thoughts about themselves or a new proposal, then they will be more persuaded if they are feeling happy following thought generation, because happiness instills confidence in the positive thoughts people just generated and/or makes them feel good about their thoughts, leading them to use their thoughts more than when they are feeling sad. However, if people are generating unfavorable thoughts (e.g., because message arguments are weak), then these same feelings of happiness lead to *less* persuasion, because people are more likely to rely on their negative thoughts and use these in forming their judgments.

Finally, when the likelihood of thinking is not constrained to be high or low by other variables, then emotions can affect the extent of thinking. For example, people might think about messages more when in a sad than in a happy state because sadness either signals a problem to be solved (Schwarz, Bless, & Bohner, 1991) or conveys a sense of uncertainty that might be addressed with additional thought (Tiedens, & Linton, 2001; see also Wegener, Petty, & Smith, 1995; Ziegler, 2013). If people process a message more when in a sad than in a happy state, then this means that they would be more persuaded by cogent arguments when sad than when happy but less persuaded by specious arguments.

Various theories of emotion and social judgment have incorporated one or more of the processes highlighted by the ELM (e.g., see Forgas, 2001; Schwarz et al., 1991). Notably, the ELM organizes these processes together into one overarching framework, and holds that these same processes can be used to understand not only the impact of incidental emotions but also a plethora of other, very different variables. For example, depending on the message recipient's extent of thinking, factors such as source credibility, attractiveness, and majority–minority status have been found to influence persuasion by the very same mechanisms by which emotions influence attitudes—serving as simple cues, biasing the thoughts of message recipients, serving as pieces of evidence relevant to the central merits of the issue, affecting thought use, and determining the amount of information processing that occurs (see Briñol & Petty, 2009b, for a review of multiple roles for source factors).

THE MCM OF ATTITUDE STRUCTURE

As just articulated, the ELM deals with the multiple processes by which variables can influence attitudes along the elaboration continuum and points to different consequences of these processes. Another model that is useful for understanding attitudes focuses on their underlying structure. According to our MCM (Petty, 2006; Petty & Briñol, 2006b; Petty, Briñol, & DeMarree, 2007), attitudes consist of evaluative associations (positive and negative) along with validity tags that can be represented in various ways, such as confidence–doubt. The MCM also explains how different attitude structures and attitude change techniques can lead to different results on implicit (automatic) and explicit (deliberative self-report) measures of attitudes. Briefly described, the MCM holds that automatic evaluative associations only determine explicit attitude measures to the extent that people endorse these associations. However, evaluative associations—whether endorsed or not—can affect implicit attitude measures (also see Gawronski & Bodenhausen, 2006). That is, the perceived validity tags tend not to influence implicit measures, at least not until these tags become so well learned that they are automatically activated (Maddux, Barden, Brewer, & Petty, 2005).

On the one hand, the MCM agrees with the commonly held view that for many attitude objects, one evaluation (relatively positive or negative) is dominant and represents the integration of knowledge about the object (see Fazio, 1995, for a review). For example, the top panel of Figure 12.2 shows a person with an explicitly positive attitude toward smoking. In such situations, this evaluation would come to mind upon encountering the attitude object, though the speed at which this occurs can vary (e.g., see Bargh, Chaiken, Raymond, & Hymes, 1996; Fazio et al., 1986).

On the other hand, according to the MCM, people can develop an attitude structure in which attitude objects are linked to both positivity and negativity separately (see also Cacioppo, Gardner, & Berntson, 1997), and tag these evaluations with varying degrees of confidence. These validating (or invalidating) metacognitions can vary in the strength of their association to the linked evaluation, and the strength of these links determines the likelihood that the perceived validity of the evaluation will be retrieved along with the evaluation itself. Most notably, perhaps, the MCM goes beyond the idea that attitude validation is solely an online

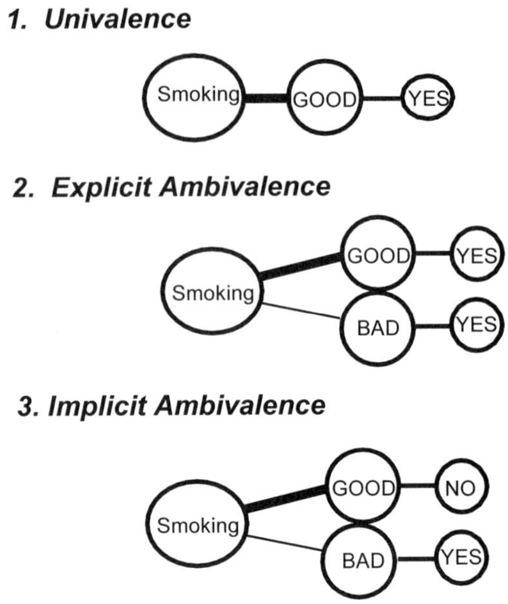

FIGURE 12.2. The MCM of attitude structure depiction of univalence (Panel 1), explicit ambivalence (Panel 2), and implicit ambivalence (Panel 3). Based on Petty (2006) and Petty and Briñol (2009).

process (e.g., Gawronski & Bodenhausen, 2006) and contends that perceived validities, like the evaluations themselves, can be stored for later retrieval. That is, the MCM assumes that just as it is adaptive to store evaluations to guide decision making and action (Fazio, 1995), so too is it adaptive to know whether any activated evaluation is a reliable guide without having to determine this on the spot. To the extent that the retrieval of validity tags becomes automatic, it even becomes possible for people to correct quickly for undesired evaluations that might come to mind. Furthermore, just as evaluative associations can be context-specific (Gawronski, Rydell, Vervliet, & De Houwer, 2010), so too can people learn to associate invalidity tags with evaluations more in some contexts than in others (e.g., see Maddux et al., 2005). Although the storage of validity tags might not be applied to every single context (e.g., it might not be likely for very new attitudes; Boucher & Rydell, 2012), some preliminary evidence is consistent with the possibility of storage of validity tags. For example, certainty has been found to predict certainty-related outcomes even when the certainty is measured at a separate occasion from the predicted outcome (e.g., Bassili, 1996; Wells, Olson, & Charman, 2003).

Importantly, the MCM argues that although people might not rely upon evaluative links that are associated with doubt (i.e., that are invalidated) when deliberatively responding to explicit measures, those automatic associations can still influence more automatic measures, and can therefore produce what we have called *implicit ambivalence*—a form of evaluative conflict that results from explicit–implicit attitude discrepancies (see Petty & Briñol, 2009, for a review). In fact, an important contribution of the MCM is the distinction between explicit and implicit forms of ambivalence. Sometimes a person holds both positive and negative evaluations to be valid, and this person's attitude is best described as being *explicitly ambivalent,* because both positive and negative associations come to mind and are endorsed (e.g., de Liver, van der Pligt, & Wigboldus, 2007; see Panel 2 of Figure 12.2). At other times, however, people might have two opposite accessible evaluations come to mind, but one is seen as valid whereas the other is rejected (see Panel 3 of Figure 12.2). A denied evaluation can be a past attitude (e.g., "I used to like smoking, but now it is disgusting"; Petty et al., 2006) or an association that was never endorsed but nonetheless automatically comes to mind for other reasons (e.g., from continuous stereotypical depictions in the media; Olson & Fazio, 2009). In such cases, the MCM refers to the attitude structure as one of implicit ambivalence. Even though people do not endorse opposite evaluations of the same attitude object (i.e., they are not explicitly ambivalent) they can nevertheless feel uncomfortable about such attitude objects without knowing the specific source of the conflict (see Rydell, McConnell, & Mackie, 2008; Petty, Briñol, & Johnson, 2012). This discomfort is consequential in that it leads people to process more carefully information associated with the object of their ambivalence (Petty et al., 2006; Briñol, Petty, & Wheeler, 2006).

LINKS BETWEEN THE ELM AND THE MCM

Although the MCM and the ELM were developed independently, they are linked in several ways. First, the ELM is related to the MCM through the concept of *elaboration* and the subsequent notion of *attitude strength.* As noted earlier, the degree of thinking (elaboration) is important in the ELM at least for two reasons. First, the extent of elaboration (how motivated and able people are to think about an issue) determines the role that variables will play in affecting attitudes (serve as a simple associative or inferential cue, bias processing, etc.). Second, greater amounts of elaboration are postulated to produce attitudes that are stronger (more durable and impactful). Thus, the ELM postulates changes in attitude structure that are fleshed out by the MCM.

According to the ELM, increased elaboration enhances attitude strength in at least two ways. First, elaboration strengthens the object–evaluation association (i.e., makes some evaluations more accessible than others). Thus, a small number of evaluative thoughts to a proposal likely produce a weak evaluative association, whereas a large number of evaluatively congruent thoughts produces a stronger evaluative association (cf. Bizer & Krosnick, 2001). The stronger the evaluative association (i.e., the more easily the attitude comes to mind), the more likely the evaluation is to persist over time and have an impact on judgment and behavior (see Fazio, 1995, for a review).

More uniquely, the MCM highlights another consequence of elaboration in the structure of attitudes. That is, the accessibility of an evaluation is separate from its perceived validity. For example, a large number of subliminal classical conditioning trials could produce a new evaluation that was highly accessible, but would do little for the perceived validity of the evaluation. However, extensive processing of issue-relevant arguments could produce an evaluation that was just as accessible as one produced with many conditioning trials, but the former attitude would likely be seen as higher in validity than the latter. Indeed, research shows that enhanced elaboration is associated with attitude certainty (Barden & Petty, 2008), and increased attitude certainty increases the strength consequences of attitudes (Gross, Holtz, & Miller, 1995; Petty, Briñol, Tormala, et al., 2007).

Related to the previous point, another link between the ELM and the MCM comes from the concept of *metacognitive validation*. Similar to the work on self-validation mentioned earlier, which suggests that thoughts (positive or negative) determine judgments more as trust in them increases (Petty et al., 2002), the MCM assumes that evaluative associations have a greater impact on deliberative judgments when validity tags indicate confidence. Thus, the MCM is similar to the self-validation process of the ELM in highlighting the importance of considering the validity associated with mental constructs, but it differs in the particular constructs of interest. Whereas the ELM research examines online assessment of certainty in one's salient thoughts (e.g., in response to persuasive proposals), the MCM research examines certainty in automatic associations that are stored in memory and assumes that these validity judgments can be stored and retrieved at a later point in time. Similar to research on self-validation, which shows that metacognitive confidence increases the use of primary cognition, the MCM holds that the more confidence people have in the validity of their automatic evaluations, the more these associations will be reflected in deliberative (explicit) measures of attitudes.

IMPLICATIONS FOR THE STUDY OF PREJUDICE

Now that we have described the ELM and the MCM, we explain how the basic principles of these models can be applied to the formation, change, and structure of particular attitudes. As a first example, consider the accumulated work on prejudice, which has suggested that attitudes toward minority groups can be influenced by a variety of low-deliberation processes, such as mere exposure (Pettigrew & Tropp, 2006) and classical conditioning (Dovidio, Gaertner, & Kawakami, 2003). Indeed, many contemporary theories of prejudice presumably focused on these subtle processes of influence because modern prejudice itself was thought to be subtle and covert (e.g., Dovidio, 2001). However, low-effort processes are not the only means of attitude change. As noted earlier, attitude formation and change can also be produced by highly deliberative processes. For example, Pettigrew (1998) proposed that "learning about others" is a critical step in how intergroup contact improves intergroup relations (Allport, 1954). In accord with this notion, there are numerous examples of how prejudice can be reduced by attendance at diversity seminars, and by learning new information about other social groups (Fisher, 1968; Rudman, Ashmore, & Gary, 2001).

As noted earlier, the ELM predicts that the process by which prejudice is created or transformed is consequential for the *strength* of the resulting attitudes. One relevant set of studies providing evidence for the importance of the amount of thinking in the domain of prejudice was conducted by Cárdaba, Briñol, Horcajo, and Petty (2013). These authors presented to participants either a persuasive message that contained compelling arguments in favor of a minority group or a control message on an irrelevant topic, and varied the amount of thinking by manipulating the targets' ability or motivation to think about the message. The results showed that even when the obtained reduction in prejudice was equivalent under low and high thinking conditions, there were important benefits of high-elaboration prejudice reduction. That is, although both high and low thinking processes were associated with a reduction in the extremity of prejudiced attitudes, the reductions in prejudice produced by high thinking processes were more persistent and resistant to subsequent attacks than equivalent changes produced by less thoughtful mechanisms (also see Wegener, Clark, & Petty, 2006).

Furthermore, by processing persuasive messages in favor of increasing tolerance toward minority groups, not only are deliberative measures of attitudes modified but so too are automatic responses assessed with implicit measures (Briñol, Petty, & McCaslin, 2009; Maio, Haddock, Watt, & Hewstone, 2009). As was the case for explicit measures, the greater the elaboration, the more consequential the subsequent changes that are observed for implicit measures. In one set of studies, for example, high-elaboration implicit attitude change for one attitude object was more likely to spread automatically and produce change in a semantically related attitude object (see Horcajo, Briñol, & Petty, 2010).

The studies described so far illustrate the importance of considering the concept of extent of *elaboration* in order to account for the consequences of both explicit and implicit attitude change. As noted, *validation* is the other concept that is critical for both the ELM and the MCM. Specifically, the ELM postulates that variables such as stereotypes can influence judgments by affecting not only the amount and direction of processing (primary cognition) but also the use of thoughts (secondary cognition) via changes in the perceived validity of those thoughts. The accumulated research suggests that the *timing* of the variable (i.e., whether it comes before or after thought generation) is one critical moderator of whether any given variable works by affecting primary or secondary cognitive processes (Briñol & Petty, 2009).

In most of the research on stereotyping and prejudice, group category membership (e.g., the race of the target) is presented *before* acquisition of individuating information. When such information precedes information processing, research has shown that stereotypes can influence attitudes and perceptions in the various ways articulated earlier, which include serving as a judgmental heuristic (for a review, see Bodenhausen, Macrae, & Sherman, 1999) or by biasing one's thoughts about a target person or his or her message (e.g., Wegener et al., 2006). Importantly, it seems plausible that learning of someone's group membership "after the fact" might allow stereotypes to influence perceptions in a completely different way—by affecting confidence in one's already generated thoughts. In two experiments testing this possibility, Clark, Wegener, Briñol, and Petty (2009) gave participants information about a target person, followed by a description designed to activate stereotypes. When processing capacity was high, greater thought confidence was generated when the group stereotype information was consistent rather than inconsistent with thoughts about the initial information that was processed. Thus, if judging a poorly performing student and generating unfavorable thoughts about that student, confidence in those thoughts was higher when it was subsequently revealed that the poorly performing student was of low rather than high socioeconomic status (SES). The opposite was true when judging a student who performed well. As a result, when SES stereotypes matched the performance, raters were more likely to recommend remedial classes for the low-performing student and gifted classes for the high-performing student. When processing capacity was low, however, stereotypes served their familiar heuristic role in judgment, and thought confidence played no role in judgment-related recommendations.

The Clark et al. (2009) study demonstrated the important role that stereotypes can play in the validation of accessible thoughts and the subsequent impact of those thoughts on deliberative judgments. As noted, the concept of validation is also important with respect to the potential impact of automatic associations on explicit and implicit measures of attitudes. That is, although people might not use automatically activated evaluations when deliberatively responding to explicit measures if those evaluations are associated with explicit doubt, those automatic associations can still influence more automatic measures of prejudice. And, as noted earlier, when discrepancies exist between explicit and implicit measures of attitudes, implicit ambivalence results. This ambivalence (as indexed by discrepancies between explicit and implicit racial attitudes) can motivate people to process race-relevant information and might account for earlier studies showing that low-prejudice white individuals are especially likely to scrutinize information from (Petty, Fleming, & White, 1999) or about (Fleming, Petty, & White, 2005 black individuals. The notion of implicit ambivalence suggests that not *all* low-prejudice individuals scrutinize information from or about blacks, but mostly those who also tend to be high in automatic prejudice (i.e., possess an implicit–explicit discrepancy).

In a series of studies examining the implicit ambivalence notion in the racial domain, Johnson, Petty, Briñol, and See (2013) found that as the discrepancy in students' implicit and explicit attitudes increased (i.e., more negative automatic attitudes than explicit attitudes or more positive automatic attitudes than explicit ones), they engaged in more processing of a message on a topic relevant to black individuals (e.g., advocating a program to hire more black faculty members at their university), or on a racially irrelevant topic if the source of the message was black rather than white. Because the direction of the discrepancy did not further qualify the results, this means that among participants who were low in explicit prejudice, primarily those who were high in implicit prejudice engaged in greater scrutiny of the race-relevant message, but among participants who were high in explicit prejudice, those who were low in implicit prejudice engaged in the greatest scrutiny. Overall, then, the results are compatible with the predictions derived from the implicit ambivalence notion of the MCM (see Petty et al., 2012, for a review on ambivalence in racial attitudes).

IMPLICATIONS FOR THE STUDY OF THE SELF

As a second illustration of the utility of the ELM and the MCM, consider the numerous parallels that exist between the literatures on attitudes and the self. To start, DeMarree, Petty, and Briñol (2007a, 2007b) argue that attitudes can be conceptualized as part of the self and the self can be viewed as an attitude object much like any other. Thus, the concepts of elaboration–strength and validation can be applied to the study of the self.

Based on the attitudes literature, one can make the straightforward prediction that evaluations of the self that are the result of more deliberative thinking are more likely to be impactful and durable than self-evaluations based on less thought. Some indirect evidence for this possibility comes from work on ambivalence and perceived knowledge. For example, the self-evaluation of individuals who have consistent (vs. inconsistent) self-related thoughts tends to be less malleable (Riketta & Ziegler, 2007), and more predictive of subsequent search information (Woike & Baumgardner, 1993). Also, self-perceptions for which participants' are perceived to have high (vs. low) knowledge have been found to be more predictive of behavior. In addition, when self-evaluations are highly accessible (as would be the case when they are based on high thought), these evaluations are more resistant to change and have a greater impact on information processing (DeMarree, Petty, & Strunk, 2010). Although these examples focus on the consistency, accessibility, and perceived amount of knowledge of self-relevant thoughts or attitudes, the results can be seen as conceptually consistent with the idea that increased thinking leads to enhanced judgmental strength of self-attitudes.

In a more direct test of this notion, Gascó, Briñol, and Horcajo (2010) changed participants' self-attitudes through either a persuasive procedure involving high elaboration (self-persuasion) or a less engaging procedure involving a reduced amount of thinking (passive exposure). Participants in the high thinking condition were requested to actively generate reasons why they liked their bodies. Previous research has shown that self-evaluations can be increased after thinking about one's strengths (e.g., Tice, 1992), and this particular procedure based on self-persuasion has been used successfully in previous studies of attitude change (e.g., Briñol, McCaslin, & Petty, 2012; Briñol, Gascó, Petty, & Horcajo, 2013). In contrast, participants in the low thinking condition were merely exposed to positive self-affirmations about their bodies, selected from a pretested intervention program in the treatment of attitudes toward the body and found to increase the favorability of body attitudes. As expected, participants in both the high and low thought groups showed more favorable attitudes toward their bodies than those in the control group. In addition, although the treatments were equally effective in changing attitudes, the strength associated with those attitudes was significantly different depending on the amount of thinking involved in the process of change. Specifically, attitudes were stronger in the high rather than low thinking treatment. Participants in the high thinking conditions perceived their attitudes to be more valid and more resistant to change than did those in the low thinking conditions.

The other critical concept besides elaboration in both the ELM and the MCM is validation. People can validate any accessible mental contents, including self-related cognitions (see Briñol, DeMarree, & Petty, 2010, for a review on validation of self-relevant cognitions). First, similar to the literature on attitude strength, showing that attitude certainty is associated with more impactful attitudes (see Petty et al., 1995), self-beliefs that are held with greater confidence are also more predictive of behavior (Setterlund & Niedenthal, 1993), more stable (Pelham, 1991; Pelham & Swann, 1994) and resistant to change (Swann & Ely, 1984; Swann, Pelham, & Chidester, 1988) than those held with doubt (see DeMarree et al., 2007a, 2007b, for reviews).

Second, in addition to being applied to attitudes, self-esteem, and other self-views, the concept of validation through certainty has also been found to moderate the impact of self-relevant thoughts on subsequent self-related attitudes or judgments. In one illustration, Briñol and Petty (2003, Experiment 4) examined whether confidence in self-relevant thoughts could be impacted in a manner similar to the way thoughts about other objects and issues are impacted. In this research, participants were required to think about and write down their best or worst qualities (thought-direction manipulation) using their dominant or nondominant hand. Then, participants rated their confidence in their thoughts and reported their self-esteem. Because writing with the nondominant hand occurs very infrequently and is difficult, and whatever is written with the nondominant may appear "shaky," the authors found, as expected, that using the nondominant hand decreased people's confidence in the thoughts they had just listed. As a consequence of the differential thought confidence, the effect of the direction of thoughts (positive–negative) on current self-esteem was significantly greater when participants wrote their thoughts with the dominant rather than the nondominant hand. Similar findings were obtained in follow-up research in which Briñol, Petty, and Wagner (2009) asked participants to write down their best or worst qualities while sitting with their backs erect, pushing their chests out (i.e., confident posture) or slouched forward with their backs curved (i.e., doubtful posture). Importantly, in these studies thought confidence mediated the influence of self-relevant thoughts on self-evaluation.

Finally, as was the case in the domain of racial attitudes, it seems reasonable that explicit–implicit self-evaluation discrepancies might be associated with implicit ambivalence and therefore be consequential. In one study testing the notion that explicit–implicit self-discrepancies could lead to enhanced information processing of self-relevant information (Briñol et al., 2006, Experiment 4), undergraduates' self-evaluations were assessed with both automatic (Implicit Association Test [IAT]; Greenwald & Farnham, 2000) and deliberative (Rosenberg, 1965) self-esteem measures. Then the absolute value of the difference between the two standardized measures was calculated as the index of discrepancy. Next, participants were exposed to either a strong or weak message about eating vegetables that was framed as self-relevant or not.

As predicted, the results of this study revealed that when the message was framed as self-relevant, the extent of explicit–implicit discrepancy interacted with argument quality to affect attitudes. The greater the discrepancy, the more participants differentiated strong from weak arguments, indicating greater information processing. However, when the same strong and weak messages were framed as irrelevant to the self (i.e., the message was said to be about the properties of vegetables rather than one's health), discrepancy did not interact with argument quality to predict attitudes. This suggests that explicit–implicit discrepancies do not lead to motivation to process all information—only those that are relevant to the object for which the discrepancy exists. Furthermore, as was the case with racial attitude discrepancies, the direction of the discrepancy (i.e., was implicit self-esteem greater or less than explicit self-esteem?), did not further moderate the results.

In summary, the previous two sections of this chapter have provided brief illustrations of two of the areas of application of the ELM and the MCM: prejudice and the self. Although we chose these specific domains because of their traditional importance within social psychology, the two theoretical models that are the subject of this chapter have proven useful in many other domains relevant to social psychology (ranging from numerical anchoring effects [Blankenship, Wegener, Petty, Detweiler-Bedell, & Macy, 2008] to health communication [Briñol & Petty, 2006]) and also have provided a valuable framework to other related disciplines (e.g., marketing and advertising; educational communication; and legal, organizational, and environmental psychology, to name just a few; see Haugtvedt & Kasmer, 2008; Petty, Barden, & Wheeler, 2009; Rucker & Petty, 2006; Rucker, Petty, & Priester, 2007).

LINKS TO AUTOMATIC VERSUS CONTROLLED PROCESSING

As highlighted in this chapter, two of the key concepts of the ELM and the MCM are *elaboration* (e.g., the elaboration continuum anchored by the central and peripheral routes to persuasion) and *validation*. These two concepts can be related to the classic distinction between automatic and controlled information processing (Schneider & Shiffrin, 1977). Beginning with elaboration, the ELM distinguishes between judgment processes that require relatively high versus low degrees of effortful thinking. Thus, one might wonder how this thinking continuum maps onto the features of automatic versus controlled information processing identified by Bargh (1994). In general, we view the information-processing features he identified (i.e., awareness, intention, efficiency, and control) as largely orthogonal to the ELM mechanisms that occur along the elaboration continuum (cf. Petty, Cacioppo, Strathman, & Priester, 1994). For example, although people tend to be more aware of high than of low thinking processes and often engage in them deliberately (i.e., intentionally), and low thinking processes typically unfold with greater efficiency and may be less likely to be controlled, this is not invariably the case. One can intentionally choose to use, and to be aware of using, a heuristic when not thinking very much but not be aware of being influenced by that same heuristic under high thinking conditions (Petty, 1994, 2001). Similarly, one's thoughts can be biased by one's mood under high thinking conditions without awareness or intention. Indeed, if people became aware of the biasing impact of mood, they would likely intend to correct for it (Wegener & Petty, 1997). And, just as people can attempt to correct for (control) biasing factors of which they have become aware under high thinking conditions, they likewise control for biases that are perceived to operate under low thinking conditions (Petty, Wegener, & White, 1998).[1]

Within the MCM, extensive elaboration can enhance the accessibility of object–evaluation links, as well as the perceived validity of those evaluations. The enhanced accessibility of evaluations due to elaboration means that such attitudes are more likely to come to mind spontaneously (i.e., unintentionally, efficiently) and inevitably (i.e., uncontrollably), though people may be aware of these gut reactions (Loersch, McCaslin, & Petty, 2011). However, attitudes also can be made highly accessible via nonelaboration-based processes, such as exposing one to many trials of subliminal evaluative conditioning or merely rehearsing one's attitude (see Fazio & Olson, 2003). Thus, there is no necessary connection between elaboration and automatically activated evaluations in the MCM.

With respect to validation processes, we have explained how this metacognitive process can influence (1) the use of thoughts in forming attitudes (in the ELM), (2) which evaluations are expressed on both implicit and explicit measures (in the MCM), and (3) which attitudes guide behavior. As was the case with elaboration, we view validation processes as able to occur in a relatively automatic or controlled fashion. For example, people can become more confident in a thought or an evaluation because they are feeling happy, but be unaware of this influence and therefore unlikely to control it. On the other hand, people can intentionally decide to rely on a thought or evaluation because it stems from a highly credible source and choose not to control this outcome (though they could if they wished). And, accessing validity tags to evaluations can become automatic if highly practiced.

CONCLUSION

The ELM is a theory about the core processes responsible for attitude change and the strength of the attitudes that result from those processes. One of the key attributes of the ELM is that it provided the field with a useful framework from which to understand the moderation (e.g., by amount of thinking) and mediation (by automatic, deliberative, or metacognitive processes) of social judgment. The MCM, a theory about the structure of attitudes, holds that objects can be linked to both positive and negative evaluations, each of which is associated with some degree of perceived validity. The theory can account for discrepancies in automatic versus deliberative attitudes, as well as postulate unique states, such as implicit ambivalence.

In summary, in this chapter we have noted that the two concepts of elaboration and validation serve as links between the ELM and the MCM. Increased elaboration enhances the durability and impact of attitudes by increasing not only the strength (accessibility) of object–evaluation associations but also the perceived validity of those evaluations. Given the integrative potential of these ideas, the two conceptual models reviewed here have shed light on a variety of phenomena that are relevant not only to attitude change but also numerous other judgments, ranging from the study of prejudice to the study of the self.

NOTE

1. Furthermore, we do not see the fundamental mechanisms by which variables have their impact on judgment as invariably linked to any particular mental system (affective/cognitive, impulsive/reflective, approach/avoidance, perceptual/knowledge). For example, low and high thinking processes can operate both within the cognitive and the affective system (see Petty & Briñol, 2006a, for further discussion). Thus, the different core processes of influence that we outlined can operate within and across systems.

REFERENCES

Allport, G. W. (1954). *The nature of prejudice.* Reading, MA: Addison-Wesley.

Barden, J., & Petty, R. E. (2008). The mere perception of elaboration creates attitude certainty: Exploring the thoughtfulness heuristic. *Journal of Personality and Social Psychology, 95,* 489–509.

Bargh, J. A. (1994). The four horsemen of automaticity: Awareness, efficiency, intention, and control in social cognition. In R. S. Wyer, Jr. & T. K. Srull (Eds.), *Handbook of social cognition* (2nd ed., pp. 1–40). Hillsdale, NJ: Erlbaum.

Bargh, J. A., Chaiken, S., Raymond, P., & Hymes, C. (1996). The automatic evaluation effect: Unconditional automatic attitude activation with a pronunciation task. *Journal of Experimental Social Psychology, 32,* 104–128

Bassili, J. N. (1996). Meta-judgmental versus operative indices of psychological properties: The case of measures of attitude strength. *Journal of Personality and Social Psychology, 71,* 637–653.

Bizer, G. Y., & Krosnick, J. A. (2001). Exploring the structure of strength-related attitude features: The relation between attitude importance and attitude accessibility. *Journal of Personality and Social Psychology, 81,* 566–586.

Blankenship, K. L., Wegener, D. T., Petty, R. E., Detweiler-Bedell, B., & Macy, C. L. (2008). Elaboration and consequences of anchored estimates: An attitudinal perspective on numerical anchoring. *Journal of Experimental Social Psychology, 44,* 1465–1476.

Bodenhausen, G. V., Macrae, C. N., & Sherman, J. W (1999). On the dialectics of discrimination: Dual processes in social stereotyping. In S. Chaiken & Y. Trope (Eds.), *Dual-process theories in social psychology* (pp. 271–290). New York: Guilford Press.

Boucher, K. L., & Rydell, R. J. (2012). Impact of negation salience and cognitive resources on negation during attitude formation *Personality and Social Psychology Bulletin, 38,* 1329–1342.

Briñol, P., & DeMarree, K. G. (Eds.). (2012). *Social metacognition.* New York: Psychology Press.

Briñol, P., DeMarree, K. G., & Petty, R. E. (2010). Processes by which confidence (vs. doubt) influences the self. In R. Arkin, K. Oleson, & P. Carroll (Eds.), *Handbook of the uncertain self* (pp. 13–35). New York: Psychology Press.

Briñol, P., Gascó, M., Petty, R. E., & Horcajo, J. (2013). Treating thoughts as material objects can increase or decrease their impact on evaluation. *Psychological Science, 24,* 41–47.

Briñol, P., McCaslin, M. J., & Petty, R. E. (2012). Self-generated persuasion: Effects of the target and direction of arguments. *Journal of Personality and Social Psychology, 102,* 925–940.

Briñol, P. & Petty, R. E (2003). Overt head movements and persuasion: A self-validation analysis. *Journal of Personality and Social Psychology, 84*, 1123–1139.

Briñol, P., & Petty, R. E. (2006). Fundamental processes leading to attitude change: Implications for cancer prevention communications. *Journal of Communication, 56*, 81–104.

Briñol, P., & Petty, R. E. (2009a). Persuasion: Insights from the self-validation hypothesis. In M. P. Zanna (Ed.), *Advances in experimental social psychology* (Vol. 41, pp. 69–118). New York: Elsevier.

Briñol, P., & Petty, R. E. (2009b). Source factors in persuasion: A self-validation approach. *European Review of Social Psychology, 20*, 49–96.

Briñol, P., & Petty, R. E. (2012). The history of attitudes and persuasion research. In A. Kruglanski & W. Stroebe (Eds.), *Handbook of the history of social psychology* (pp. 285–320). New York: Psychology Press.

Briñol, P., Petty, R. E., & Barden, J. (2007). Happiness versus sadness as determinants of thought confidence in persuasion: A self-validation analysis. *Journal of Personality and Social Psychology, 93*, 711–727.

Briñol, P., Petty, R. E., & McCaslin, M. J. (2009). Changing attitudes on implicit versus explicit measures: What is the difference? In R. E. Petty, R. H. Fazio, & P. Briñol (Eds.), *Attitudes: Insights from the new implicit measures* (pp. 285–326). New York: Psychology Press.

Briñol, P., Petty, R. E., Wagner, B. (2009). Body postures effects on self-evaluation: A self-validation approach. *European Journal of Social Psychology, 39*, 1053–1064.

Briñol, P., Petty, R. E., & Wheeler, S. C. (2006). Discrepancies between explicit and implicit self-concepts: Consequences for information processing. *Journal of Personality and Social Psychology, 91*, 154–170.

Cacioppo, J. T., Gardner, W. L., & Berntson, G. G. (1997). Beyond bipolar conceptualizations and measures: The case of attitudes and evaluative space. *Personality and Social Psychology Review, 1*, 3–25.

Cárdaba, M. M. A., Briñol, P., Horcajo, J., & Petty, R. E. (2013). The effect of need for cognition on the stability of prejudiced attitudes toward South American immigrants. *Psicothema, 25*, 73–78.

Chaiken, S., & Trope, Y. (Eds.). (1999). *Dual process theories in social psychology.* New York: Guilford Press.

Clark, J. K., Wegener, D. T., Briñol, P., & Petty, R. E. (2009). Discovering that the shoe fits: The self-validating role of stereotypes. *Psychological Science, 20*, 846–852.

De Liver, Y., van der Pligt, J., & Wigboldus, D. (2007). Positive and negative associations underlying ambivalent attitudes. *Journal of Experimental Social Psychology, 43*, 319–326.

DeMarree, K. G., Petty, R. E., & Briñol, P. (2007a). Self and attitude strength parallels: Focus on accessibility. *Social and Personality Psychology Compass, 1*, 441–468.

DeMarree, K. G., Petty, R. E., & Briñol, P. (2007b). Self-certainty: Parallels to attitude certainty. *International Journal of Psychology and Psychological Therapy, 7*, 141–170.

DeMarree, K. G., Petty, R. E., & Strunk, D. R. (2010). Self-esteem accessibility as attitude strength: On the durability and impactfulness of accessible self-esteem. *Personality and Social Psychology Bulletin, 36*, 628–641.

DeSteno, D., Petty, R. E., Wegener, D. T., & Rucker, D. D. (2000). Beyond valence in the perception of likelihood: The role of emotion specificity. *Journal of Personality and Social Psychology, 78*, 397–416.

Dovidio, J. F. (2001). On the nature of contemporary prejudice: The third wave. *Journal of Social Issues, 57*, 829–849.

Dovidio, J. F., Gaertner, S. L., & Kawakami, K. (2003). The Contact Hypothesis: The past, present, and the future. *Group Processes and Intergroup Relations, 6*, 5–21.

Fazio, R. H. (1995). Attitudes as object–evaluation associations: Determinants, consequences, and correlates of attitude accessibility. In R. E. Petty & J. A. Krosnick (Eds.), *Attitude strength: Antecedents and consequences* (pp. 247–283). Hillsdale, NJ: Erlbaum.

Fazio, R. H., & Olson, M. A. (2003). Implicit measures in social cognition research: Their meaning and use. *Annual Review of Psychology, 54*, 297–327.

Fazio, R. H., Sanbonmatsu, D. M., Powell, M. C., & Kardes, F. R. (1986). On the automatic activation of attitudes. *Journal of Personality and Social Psychology, 50*, 229–238.

Fisher, F. L. (1968). Influences of reading and discussion on the attitudes of fifth graders toward American Indians. *Journal of Educational Research, 62*, 130–134.

Fleming, M. A., Petty, R. E., & White, P. H. (2005). Stigmatized targets and evaluation: Prejudice as a determinant of attribute scrutiny and polarization. *Personality and Social Psychology Bulletin, 31*, 496–507.

Forgas, J. P. (2001). *The handbook of affect and social cognition*. Mahwah, NJ: Erlbaum.

Gascó, M., Briñol, P., & Horcajo, J. (2010). Cambio de actitudes hacia la imagen corporal: El efecto de la elaboración sobre la fuerza de las actitudes [Attitude change toward body image: The role of elaboration on attitude strength]. *Psicothema, 22*, 77–82.

Gawronski, B., & Bodenhausen, G. V. (2006). Associative and prepositional processes in evaluation: An integrative review of implicit and explicit attitude change. *Psychological Bulletin, 132*, 692–731.

Gawronski, B., Rydell, R. J., Vervliet, B., & De Houwer, J. (2010). Generalization versus contextualization in automatic evaluation. *Journal of Experimental Psychology: General, 139*, 683–701.

Greenwald, A. G., & Farnham, S. D. (2000). Using the Implicit Association Test to measure self-esteem and self-concept. *Journal of Personality and Social Psychology, 79*, 1022–1038.

Gross, S. R., Holtz, R., & Miller, N. (1995). Attitude certainty. In R. E. Petty & J. A. Krosnick (Eds.), *Attitude strength: Antecedents and consequences* (pp. 215–245). Hillsdale, NJ: Erlbaum.

Haugtvedt, C. P., & Kasmer, J. A. (2008). Attitude change and persuasion. In C. P. Haugtvedt, P. M. Herr, & F. R. Kardes (Eds.), *Handbook of consumer psychology* (pp. 419–436). New York: Erlbaum.

Horcajo, J., Briñol, P., & Petty, R. E. (2010). Consumer persuasion: Indirect change and implicit balance. *Psychology and Marketing, 27*, 938–963.

Johnson, I., Petty, R. E., Briñol, P., & See, M. (2014). *Watchdog: A new look from the implicit ambivalence perspective*. Unpublished manuscript, Ohio State University, Columbus.

Jost, J. T., Kruglanski, A. W., & Nelson, T. O. (1998). Social meta-cognition: An expansionist review. *Personality and Social Psychology Review, 2*, 137–154.

Loersch, C., McCaslin, M. J., & Petty, R. E. (2011). Exploring the impact of social judgeability concerns on the interplay of associative and deliberative attitude processes. *Journal of Experimental Social Psychology, 47*, 1029–1032.

Maddux, W. W., Barden, J., Brewer, M. B., & Petty, R. E. (2005). Saying no to negativity: The effects of context and motivation to control prejudice on automatic evaluative responses. *Journal of Experimental Social Psychology, 41*, 19–35

Maio, G. R., Haddock, G., Watt, S. E., & Hewstone, M. (2009). Implicit measures in applied contexts: An illustrative examination of antiracism advertising. In R. E. Petty, R. H. Fazio, & P. Briñol (Eds.), *Attitudes: Insights from the new implicit measures* (pp. 327–357). New York: Psychology Press.

Martin, L. L. (2000). Moods do not convey information: Moods in context do. In J. P. Forgas (Ed.), *Feeling and thinking: The role of affect in social cognition* (pp. 153–177). Cambridge, UK: Cambridge University Press.

Olson, M. A., & Fazio, R. H. (2009). Implicit and explicit measures of attitudes: The perspective of the MODE model. In R. E. Petty, R. H. Fazio, & P. Briñol (Eds.), *Attitudes: Insights from the new implicit measures* (pp. 19–64). New York: Psychology Press.

Pelham, B. W. (1991). On confidence and consequence: The certainty and importance of self-knowledge. *Journal of Personality and Social Psychology, 60*, 518–530.

Pelham, B. W., & Swann, W. B., Jr. (1994). The juncture of intrapersonal and interpersonal knowledge: Self-certainty and interpersonal congruence. *Personality and Social Psychology Bulletin, 20*, 349–357.

Pettigrew, T. F. (1998). Intergroup contact theory. *Annual Review of Psychology, 49*, 65–85.

Pettigrew, T. F., & Tropp, L. (2006). A meta-analytic test of intergroup contact theory. *Journal of Personality and Social Psychology, 90*, 751–783.

Petty, R. E. (1994). Two routes to persuasion: State of the art. In G. d'Ydewalle, P. Eelen, & P. Bertelson (Eds.), *International perspectives on psychological science* (Vol. 2, pp. 229–247). Hillsdale, NJ: Erlbaum.

Petty, R. E. (2001). Subtle influences on judgments and behaviors: Who is most susceptible? In J. Forgas & K. D. Williams (Eds.), *Social influence: Direct and indirect processes* (pp. 129–146). Philadelphia, PA: Psychology Press.

Petty, R. E. (2006). A metacognitive model of attitudes. *Journal of Consumer Research, 33*(1), 22–24.

Petty, R. E., Barden, J., & Wheeler, S. C. (2009). The elaboration likelihood model of persuasion: Developing health promotions to produce sustained behavior change. In R. J. DiClemente, R. A. Crosby, & M. Kegler (Eds.), *Emerging theories in health promotion practice and research* (2nd ed., pp. 185–214). San Francisco: Jossey-Bass.

Petty, R. E., & Briñol, P. (2006a). Understanding social judgment: Multiple systems and processes. *Psychological Inquiry, 17,* 217–223.

Petty, R. E., & Briñol, P. (2006b). A metacognitive approach to "implicit" and "explicit" evaluations: Comment on Gawronski and Bodenhausen (2006). *Psychological Bulletin, 132,* 740–744.

Petty, R. E., & Briñol, P. (2009). Implicit ambivalence: A meta-cognitive approach. In R. E. Petty, R. H. Fazio, & P. Briñol (Eds.), *Attitudes: Insights from the new implicit measures* (pp. 119–161). New York: Psychology Press.

Petty, R. E. & Briñol, P. (2012). The Elaboration Likelihood Model: Three decades of research. In P. A. M. Van Lange, A. Kruglanski, & E. T. Higgins (Eds.), *Handbook of theories of social psychology* (pp. 224–245). London: Sage.

Petty, R. E., Briñol, P., & DeMarree, K. G. (2007). The meta-cognitive model (MCM) of attitudes: Implications for attitude measurement, change, and strength. *Social Cognition, 25,* 609–642.

Petty, R. E., Briñol, P., & Johnson, I. (2012). Implicit ambivalence. In B. Gawronski & F. Strack (Eds.), *Cognitive consistency: A unifying concept in social psychology* (pp. 178–201). New York: Guilford Press.

Petty, R. E., Briñol, P., & Tormala, Z. L. (2002). Thought confidence as a determinant of persuasion: The self-validation hypothesis. *Journal of Personality and Social Psychology, 82,* 722–741.

Petty, R. E., Briñol, P., Tormala, Z. L., & Wegener, D. T. (2007). The role of metacognition in social judgment. In A. W. Kruglanski & E. T. Higgins (Eds.), *Social psychology: Handbook of basic principles* (2nd ed., pp. 254–284). New York: Guilford Press.

Petty, R. E., & Cacioppo, J. T. (1981). *Attitudes and persuasion: Classic and contemporary approaches.* Dubuque, IA: Brown.

Petty, R. E., & Cacioppo, J. T. (1986). The Elaboration Likelihood Model of persuasion. *Advances in Experimental Social Psychology, 19,* 123–205.

Petty, R. E., Cacioppo, J. T., & Strathman, A., & Priester, J. R. (1994). To think or not to think?: Exploring two routes to persuasion. In S. Shavitt & T. C. Brock (Eds.), *Persuasion: Psychological insights and perspectives* (pp. 113–147). Needham Heights, MA: Allyn & Bacon.

Petty, R. E., Fabrigar, L. R., & Wegener, D. T., (2003). Emotional factors in attitudes and persuasion. In R. J. Davidson, K. R. Scherer, & H. H. Goldsmith (Eds.), *Handbook of affective sciences* (pp. 752–772). Oxford, UK: Oxford University Press.

Petty, R. E., Fazio, R. H., & Briñol, P. (2009a). The new implicit measures: An overview. In R. E. Petty, R. H. Fazio, & P. Briñol (Eds.), *Attitudes: Insights from the new implicit measures* (pp. 3–18). New York: Psychology Press.

Petty, R. E., Fazio, R. H., & Briñol, P. (Eds.). (2009b). *Attitudes: Insights from the new implicit measures.* New York: Psychology Press.

Petty, R. E., Fleming, M. A., & White, P. (1999). Stigmatized sources and persuasion: Prejudice as a determinant of argument scrutiny. *Journal of Personality and Social Psychology, 76,* 19–34.

Petty, R. E., Haugtvedt, C., & Smith, S. M. (1995). Elaboration as a determinant of attitude strength: Creating attitudes that are persistent, resistant, and predictive of behavior. In R. E. Petty & J. A. Krosnick (Eds.), *Attitude strength: Antecedents and consequences* (pp. 93–130). Mahwah, NJ: Erlbaum.

Petty, R. E., & Krosnick, J. A. (Eds.). (1995). *Attitude strength: Antecedents and consequences.* Mahwah, NJ: Erlbaum.

Petty, R. E., Schumann, D. W., Richman, S. A., & Strathman, A. J. (1993). Positive mood and persuasion: Different roles for affect under high and low elaboration conditions. *Journal of Personality and Social Psychology, 64,* 5–20.

Petty, R. E., Tormala, Z. L., Briñol, P., & Jarvis, W. B. G. (2006). Implicit ambivalence from attitude change: An exploration of the PAST Model. *Journal of Personality and Social Psychology, 90,* 21–41.

Petty, R. E., & Wegener, D. T. (1998). Attitude change: Multiple roles for persuasion variables. In D. Gilbert, S. Fiske, & G. Lindzey (Eds.), *The handbook of social psychology* (4th ed., Vol. 1, pp. 323–390). New York: McGraw-Hill.

Petty, R. E., & Wegener, D. T. (1999). The Elaboration Likelihood Model: Current status and controversies. In S. Chaiken & Y. Trope (Eds.), *Dual process theories in social psychology* (pp. 41–72). New York: Guilford Press.

Petty, R. E., Wegener, D. T., & White, P. (1998). Flexible correction processes in social judgment: Implications for persuasion. *Social Cognition, 16*, 93–113.

Petty, R. E., Wheeler, S. C., & Bizer, G. Y. (1999). Is there one persuasion process or more?: Lumping versus splitting in attitude change theories. *Psychological Inquiry, 10*, 156–163.

Pierro, A., Mannetti, L., Kruglanski, A. W., & Sleeth-Keppler, D. (2004). Relevance override: On the reduced impact of cues under high motivation conditions of persuasion studies. *Journal of Personality and Social Psychology, 86*, 252–264.

Riketta, M., & Ziegler, R. (2007). Self-ambivalence and reactions to success versus failure. *European Journal of Social Psychology, 37*, 547–560.

Rosenberg, M. (1965). *Society and the adolescent self-image*. Princeton, NJ: Princeton University Press.

Rucker, D. D., & Petty, R. E. (2006). Increasing the effectiveness of communications to consumers: Recommendations based on the elaboration likelihood and attitude certainty perspectives. *Journal of Public Policy and Marketing, 25*, 39–52.

Rucker, D. D., Petty, R. E., & Priester, J. R. (2007). Understanding advertising effectiveness from a psychological perspective: The importance of attitudes and attitude strength. In G. J. Tellis & T. Ambler (Eds.), *The handbook of advertising* (pp. 73–88). Thousand Oaks, CA: Sage.

Rudman, L. A., Ashmore, R. D., & Gary, M. L. (2001). "Unlearning" automatic biases: The malleability of implicit prejudice and stereotypes. *Journal of Personality and Social Psychology, 81*, 856–868.

Rydell, R. J., McConnell, A. R., & Mackie, D. M. (2008). Consequences of discrepant explicit and implicit attitudes: Cognitive dissonance and increased information processing. *Journal of Experimental Social Psychology, 44*, 1526–1532.

Schneider, W., & Shiffrin, R. M. (1977). Controlled and automatic human information processing: I. Detection, search, and attention. *Psychological Review, 84*, 1–66.

Schwarz, N., Bless, H., & Bohner, G. (1991). Mood and persuasion: Affective status influence the processing of persuasive communications. In M. Zanna (Ed.), *Advances in experimental social psychology* (Vol. 24, pp. 161–197). San Diego: Academic Press.

Setterlund, M. B., & Niedenthal, P. M. (1993). "Who am I? Why am I here?": Self-esteem, self-clarity, and prototype matching. *Journal of Personality and Social Psychology, 65*, 769–780.

Swann, W. B., & Ely, R. J. (1984). A battle of wills: Self-verification versus behavioral confirmation. *Journal of Personality and Social Psychology, 46*, 1287–1302.

Swann, W. B., Pelham, B. W., & Chidester, T. R. (1988). Change through paradox: Using self-verification to alter beliefs. *Journal of Personality and Social Psychology, 54*, 268–273.

Tice, D. M. (1992). Self-concept change and self-presentation: The looking glass self is also a magnifying glass. *Journal of Personality and Social Psychology, 63*, 435–451.

Tiedens, L. Z., & Linton, S. (2001). Judgment under emotional certainty and uncertainty: The effects of specific emotions on information processing. *Journal of Personality and Social Psychology, 81*, 973–988.

Wegener, D. T., Clark, J. K., & Petty, R. E. (2006). Not all stereotyping is created equal: Differential consequences of thoughtful versus non-thoughtful stereotyping. *Journal of Personality and Social Psychology, 90*, 42–59.

Wegener, D. T., & Petty, R. E. (1997). The flexible correction model: The role of naive theories of bias in bias correction. In M. P. Zanna (Ed.), *Advances in experimental social psychology* (Vol., 29, pp. 141–208). San Diego: Academic Press.

Wegener, D. T., Petty, R. E., & Smith, S. M. (1995). Positive mood can increase or decrease message scrutiny: The hedonic contingency view of mood and message processing. *Journal of Personality and Social Psychology, 69*, 5–15.

Wells, G. L., Olson, E. A., & Charman, S. D. (2003). Distorted retrospective eyewitness reports as functions of feedback and delay. *Journal of Experimental Psychology: Applied, 9*, 42–52.

Woike, B. A., & Baumgardner, A. H. (1993). Global-specific incongruencies in self-worth and the search for self-knowledge. *Personality and Social Psychology Bulletin, 19*, 290–295.

Ziegler, R. (2013). Mood and processing of proattitudinal and counterattitudinal messages. *Personality and Social Psychology Bulletin, 39*, 482–495.

CHAPTER 13

The Associative–Propositional Evaluation Model

Operating Principles and Operating Conditions of Evaluation

Bertram Gawronski and Galen V. Bodenhausen

Conflicting evaluative responses to the same object, individual, or social group can be vexingly commonplace in everyday life (Conner & Armitage, 2008). For example, we may experience spontaneous apprehension and discomfort when encountering members of stigmatized groups even though we intellectually abhor prejudice and wish to express solidarity with minorities. Analogously, people can feel a strong romantic attraction toward another person despite firmly believing that this person is not a good match. Although these two examples are quite distinct, both are characterized by a conflict between spontaneous evaluative responses and deliberate evaluative judgments. One valuable approach to studying such evaluative conflicts is to compare people's responses on traditional self-report measures (e.g., attitude scales, likability ratings) to their responses on performance-based paradigms (e.g., Implicit Association Test, sequential priming). Conceptually, deliberate evaluative judgments on the former type of measures can be described as *explicit evaluations* in the sense that their evaluative meaning is explicit in the observed response (e.g., participants explicitly report their agreement or disagreement with an evaluative statement about an attitude object). Conversely, spontaneous evaluative responses on the latter type of measures can be described as *implicit evaluations* in the sense that their evaluative meaning is implicit in the observed response (e.g., evaluative responses are inferred from participants' latencies in responding to positive and negative words that are preceded by brief presentations of an attitude object). Over the past years, a substantial body of research has documented the possibility of dissociations between implicit and explicit evaluations, including different antecedents, different consequences, and discrepant evaluations of the same object.

The main goal of the current chapter is to review the core assumptions of our associative–propositional evaluation (APE) model, which explains dissociations between implicit and explicit evaluations in terms of their underlying mental processes (Gawronski & Bodenhausen, 2006a, 2006b, 2007, 2011). Whereas implicit evaluations are assumed to be the behavioral outcome of *associative processes*, explicit evaluations are conceptualized as the behavioral outcome of *propositional processes*. By making specific assumptions about mutual interactions between associative and propositional processes, the APE model implies a wide range of predictions about the conditions under which implicit and explicit evaluations show either converging or diverging patterns of responses. These predictions and relevant empirical evidence are extensively reviewed elsewhere (Gawronski & Bodenhausen, 2011), and we therefore refrain from providing elaborate discussions of these aspects in this chapter. Instead, we focus on how the distinction between associative and propositional processes relates to the distinction between automatic and controlled processes that has shaped dual-process theorizing for the last three decades (see Gawronski & Creighton, 2013). Our central argument is that the associative–propositional distinction refers to the principles that define *what* a particular process is doing. In contrast, the automatic–controlled distinction refers to empirical claims about *when* that process is operating. Although the two dichotomies are sometimes assumed to overlap, the APE model draws a sharp line between operating principles and operating conditions (Gawronski & Bodenhausen, 2007, 2009). In this spirit, we first explain the defining features of associative and propositional processes and then outline the manner in which the two processes are assumed to operate in an automatic versus controlled fashion. To resolve some common misconceptions about the APE model, we also address the difference between our dual-process distinction in terms of associative and propositional processes and cognate conceptualizations in terms of dual systems and dual representations.

OPERATING PRINCIPLES

As we noted earlier, the associative–propositional distinction refers to the operating principles that define what a given process is doing. In the APE model, we specify *associative processes* as the activation of mental associations on the basis of feature similarity and spatiotemporal contiguity; *propositional processes* are defined as the validation of momentarily activated information on the basis of logical consistency. These general definitions can be further specified on the basis of whether they refer to the expression or the formation of evaluative representations.

Expression of Evaluative Representations

A central assumption in research on attitudes is that encountering a stimulus can elicit a positive or negative response by activating stored evaluative representations in memory. In the APE model, we assume that principles of similarity matching determine the activation of mental concepts that represent the encountered stimulus (e.g., Afrocentric features of a face activating the concept *African American*), which can spread to other concepts that are associatively linked with the stimulus (e.g., activation of the concept *African American* spreading to the associated stereotypical attribute *hostile*). To the extent that the associated concepts have a positive or negative connotation, their activation is assumed to produce a spontaneous gut response that is in line with the valence of these concepts (*implicit evaluation*).

An important aspect of the similarity matching principle is that stimuli do not have to be perceptually identical across time and contexts to elicit the same evaluative response. Instead, configurations of input stimuli that pass a critical threshold of similarity are sufficient to activate the same mental representation (Smith, 1996). For example, relatively Afrocentric facial features can activate black stereotypes even when they are present in the faces of individuals who are categorized as white (Blair, Judd, & Fallman, 2004). In addition, the principle of similarity matching implies that even unknown stimuli can elicit spontaneous evaluative responses to the extent that they resemble a previously encountered stimulus with a stored evaluative representation. For example, unknown individuals may elicit a spontaneous positive or negative response by virtue of their resemblance to people we know (Gawronski & Quinn, 2013).

Another important aspect of the similarity matching principle is that associative activation is not an all-or-none process, such that encountering a given object would activate each and every concept that is associated with that object in memory. Instead, objects tend to activate only a limited subset of associated concepts. Which subset of associated concepts is activated in response to a given object is assumed to depend on the overall configuration of input stimuli, including both the target object and the context in which it is encountered. For example, encountering a black person in a jazz bar may activate the stereotypical attribute *musical*, whereas the same black person may activate the stereotypical attribute *criminal* if that person is encountered in a dark alley (for a review, see Gawronski & Sritharan, 2010). Hence, an attitude object may elicit distinctly different implicit evaluations depending on the particular context in which it is encountered. However, the activation of associated concepts is not entirely context-driven, because it is constrained by the preexisting structure of mental links in memory. After all, different contexts can modulate the activation of concepts in response to a given object only if these concepts are part of the mental representation of that object.

A central feature of associative activation is that it is independent of subjective truth or falsity. Specifically, we assume that the principles of similarity matching determine the activation of associated concepts regardless of whether the activated link is considered valid or invalid. For example, encountering a Muslim-looking man may activate the concept *terrorism* even if a person rejects the implied connection between Muslims and terrorism (Devine, 1989). According to the APE model, the validity of activated links is determined by a process of propositional validation. Specifically, we assume that activated information is regarded as valid unless the default process of affirming the validity of activated information produces an inconsistent set of beliefs. The central idea underlying these assumptions is that although consistency does not guarantee accuracy, inconsistency is an unambiguous indicator of an erroneous component in one's system of beliefs (Gawronski, 2012). In such cases, the momentarily considered set of information needs to be updated, which involves a reassessment of the validity of each component.

With regard to evaluative responses, we assume that the affective gut reactions resulting from associatively activated concepts are translated into the format of a propositional statement (e.g., a negative affective reaction toward object *X* is transformed into propositional statements such as "I dislike *X*" or "*X* is bad"). To the extent that the propositional evaluation implied by an affective gut response is consistent with other momentarily considered propositions, it may be endorsed in a verbal evaluative judgment (*explicit evaluation*). If, however, the overall set of momentarily considered propositions is inconsistent, the inconsistency has to be resolved to avoid aversive feelings of dissonance (Festinger, 1957). In general, propositional evaluations of a given object may be assessed for their consistency with (1) nonevaluative propositions about states of affairs and (2) propositional evaluations of other attitude objects (Jones & Gerard, 1967). To the extent that a set of momentarily considered propositions is inconsistent, consistency may be restored either by rejecting one of the involved propositions (i.e., reversing the subjective truth value of that proposition) or by searching for an additional proposition that resolves the inconsistency (Gawronski & Strack, 2004). For example, the propositional implication of a negative affective reaction to minority members (e.g., "I dislike African Americans") may be inconsistent with the propositional evaluation of another attitude object (e.g., "Negative evaluations of disadvantaged groups are wrong") and nonevaluative propositions about states of affairs (e.g., "African Americans are a disadvantaged group"). Thus, the inconsistency between the three propositions may lead to a rejection of the negative affective reaction as a valid basis for an evaluative judgment (e.g., "I like African Americans"). However, consistency may also be restored by rejecting either the nonevaluative proposition about states of affairs (e.g., "African Americans are not a disadvantaged group") or the propositional evaluation of another relevant attitude object (e.g., "Negative evaluations of disadvantaged groups are okay."). Whereas the former case should result in a dissociation between implicit and explicit evaluations, the two kinds of evaluations should show converging negative responses in the latter cases (Gawronski, Peters, Brochu, & Strack, 2008).

In addition to such "bottom-up" effects of associative on propositional processes, the APE model also includes specific assumptions about "top-down" effects of propositional thinking on associative processes. Specifically, we assume that processes of propositional reasoning can influence associative processes by activating new information in the course of validating activated information. For example, if people are motivated to believe in the validity of a particular proposition, they may engage in a selective search for information that supports the validity of that proposition (Kunda, 1990). In such cases, biased retrieval of information from memory can activate associated concepts of a particular valence, which produces correspondence between implicit and explicit evaluations in a top-down fashion (Peters & Gawronski, 2011a).

An important factor in such top-down effects is whether propositional reasoning involves an affirmation or negation of the relevant information. Specifically, we argue that merely negating a particular proposition (i.e., reversing its truth value) is insufficient to deactivate the associative link underlying this proposition. In fact, negations often lead to ironic effects, such that the activation level of the underlying association is enhanced rather than reduced (e.g., Gawronski, Deutsch, Mbirkou, Seibt, & Strack, 2008). For example, negating the proposition "old people are bad drivers" may enhance the associative link between the concepts *old people* and *bad drivers*, thereby leading to a dissociation between implicit and explicit evaluations (Deutsch, Gawronski, & Strack, 2006). This situation is different if processes of propositional reasoning involve an affirmation of new information. For example, affirming the proposition "old people are good drivers" may strengthen the association between the concepts *old people* and *good drivers*, thereby increasing the correspondence between implicit and explicit evaluations. Thus, if a person is motivated to hold a positive (negative) impression of an attitude object, but experiences a negative (positive) affective reaction toward that object, the individual may engage in a directed memory search to retrieve positive (negative) information about the object, which should promote a positive (negative) evaluation for both explicit and implicit evaluations. If, however, the positive (negative) impression is maintained by merely negating the negative (positive) evaluation implied by the affective gut response (i.e., without retrieving supportive positive or negative information), explicit and implicit evaluations should show a dissociation, such that explicit evaluations reflect the desired positive (negative) evaluation, whereas implicit evaluations should reflect the original negative (positive) response.

Formation of Evaluative Representations

Before an evaluative representation can be activated, it has to be formed on the basis of some kind of learning experience. In the APE model, we distinguish between two conceptually distinct processes of forming evaluative representations depending on whether they are based on associative or propositional principles. Drawing on our general definition of associative processes, *associative learning* can be specified as the formation of associative links between mental concepts on the basis of observed spatiotemporal contiguities. The central assumption underlying this definition is that observed co-occurrences between objects and events result in a coactivation of their corresponding mental concepts, which in turn creates an associative link between the two. Repeatedly observing the same co-occurrences strengthens this link, which facilitates the spread of activation from one concept to the other upon encountering one of the two associated stimuli. An illustrative example of associative learning is *evaluative conditioning* (EC; see De Houwer, Thomas, & Baeyens, 2001), in which repeated pairings of a conditioned stimulus (CS) with a positive or negative unconditioned stimulus (US) can produce a mental association between the CS and the US in memory. As a result, subsequent presentations of the CS spread to the representation of the US, which produces an evaluative response to the CS that is in line with the valence of the US (e.g., Walther, Gawronski, Blank, & Langer, 2009).

In contrast to the associative principle of mere coactivation, *propositional learning* is defined as the formation of evaluative representations on the basis of propositional information that is regarded as valid. This definition is based on our conceptualization of propositional processes as being concerned with the validity of momentarily activated information. Propositional learning may be based on new information that is presented in the format of propositional statements (e.g., persuasive arguments asserting the quality of a consumer product). Alternatively, propositional learning can be based on propositional inferences about observed stimulus events in the environment (e.g., co-occurrences between stimulus events can trigger propositional inferences about their causal relation). Whereas the former case involves the acquisition of externally provided propositional information, the latter case involves the acquisition of self-generated propositional information. Yet, in both cases, the new information has to pass a process of propositional validation. This validity assessment is equivalent to the one involved in the expression of evaluative representations, such that new propositional information may be regarded as either true or false depending on its consistency with other momentarily considered propositions.

Although associative and propositional learning represent distinct mechanisms of forming evaluative representations, their outcomes are assumed to interact in a manner that is similar to the mutual interactions in the expression of evaluative representations. First, associatively formed representations may provide the input for propositional inferences, implying a bottom-up effect of associative on propositional processes. Thus, whether or not the evaluation implied by an associatively formed representation is regarded as valid depends on the consistency of this evaluation with other momentarily considered propositions (e.g., Gawronski & LeBel, 2008). Second, propositional processes may influence associative processes in a "top-down" fashion when externally provided or self-generated propositions create new mental links in memory (e.g., Whitfield & Jordan, 2009). As we outlined earlier, an important determinant of such top-down effects is whether the involved inferences entail an affirmation or negation of the relevant information. Whereas the affirmation of a given proposition should create an evaluative representation that is in line with the meaning of that proposition, negating a given proposition is claimed to have ironic effects.[1]

An important aspect of the distinction between associative and propositional learning is that the same stimulus event may influence evaluative representations through two simultaneously operating processes (Gawronski & Bodenhausen, 2006a). For example, repeated co-occurrences of a CS and a valenced US may create a mental link between the two stimuli through processes of associative learning. At the same time, the observed co-occurrences may provide the basis for self-generated propositions about their evaluative meaning (e.g., propositional inferences about the CS being a cause of the positive or negative event represented by the US), which may influence the evaluative representation through processes of propositional learning. This distinction is important, because it qualifies the conceptual equation of *evaluative conditioning* and *associative learning* that we endorsed in the initial presentation of the APE model (for a more detailed discussion, see Gawronski & Bodenhausen, 2011). To the extent that EC can be defined as the change in the evaluation of a CS due to its pairing with a valenced US (De Houwer, 2007), EC effects may be the result of either associative or propositional learning (e.g., Gawronski, Balas, & Creighton, in press). Yet a theoretical challenge is to identify the conditions under which the effect of observed co-occurrences on evaluative responses is mediated by associative or propositional learning (or both). This question pertains to the operating conditions of associative and propositional processes, which we discuss in the following section (cf. Gawronski & Bodenhausen, 2007, 2011).

OPERATING CONDITIONS

Whereas the associative–propositional distinction refers to the operating principles that define *what* a particular process is doing, the automatic–controlled distinction refers to empirical claims about *when* that process is operating (e.g., when there is no conscious awareness; when there is no intention to start the process; when cognitive resources are reduced; when there is a goal to alter or stop the process; see Bargh, 1994). According to the APE model, there is no one-to-one mapping between operating principles and operating conditions, such that associative processes would operate automatically, whereas propositional processes operate in a controlled fashion (Gawronski & Bodenhausen, 2009). Instead, both associative and propositional processes have automatic and controlled aspects. Moreover, each type of process involves different components, which require separate consideration in a thorough analysis of operating conditions. Because different features of automatic processing need not co-occur, we also deem it important to distinguish between the unique roles of awareness, intentionality, efficiency, and controllability (see Table 13.1). Impor-

TABLE 13.1. Overview of Associative and Propositional Process Components in the Formation versus Expression of Evaluative Representations and the APE Model's Assumptions about Their Operating Conditions (i.e., Awareness, Intentionality, Efficiency, Controllability).

		Awareness	Intentionality	Efficiency	Controllability
			Formation		
Associative learning	Formation of mental representations on the basis of observed spatiotemporal contiguities	Independent of conscious awareness	Unintentional, although antecedents may involve intentional exposure to particular contiguities	Efficient, although attentional distraction may undermine encoding of contiguities	Uncontrollable, although effects of associative learning can be concealed by processing goals
Propositional learning	Formation of mental representations on the basis of propositional information that is regarded as valid	Dependent on conscious awareness	Unintentional storage possible in the absence of memorization goal	Mere consideration of proposition efficient, although comprehension may require more resources when information is complex	Controllable through invalidation, although limited to propositional level
			Expression		
Associative activation	Activation of mental concepts through similarity matching and spread of activation	Experiential awareness of affective gut responses; processes and mental concepts that give rise to affective gut responses can be unconscious	No intention required, although intentional activation possible	Efficient, although effortful activation possible	Controllability depends on adopted control strategy (i.e., affirmation vs. negation)
Propositional validation	Default affirmation of the validity of activated information	No awareness required, although conscious reassessment of validity possible	No intention required, although intentional reassessment of validity possible	Efficient, although effortful reassessment of validity possible	Controllable through negation of validity
	Monitoring (in)consistency between activated information	No awareness required, although conscious monitoring possible; inconsistency raises conscious awareness	No intention required, although intentional monitoring possible	Required resources depend on amount of information and complexity of inferences	Uncontrollable
	Resolution of inconsistency between activated information	Reassessment of activated information involves conscious awareness of processing steps (e.g., reversal of truth value, search for information that resolves inconsistency)	Intentional	Required resources depend on amount of information and complexity of inferences	Controllable through change in preferred strategy to resolve inconsistency
	Report of outcome of validation process	Conscious	Intentional	Efficient	Controllable

tantly, whereas the distinction between associative and propositional processes is purely conceptual, any claims about their operating conditions are empirical and therefore have to be assessed on the basis of relevant evidence.

Awareness

Expression

Conscious awareness is commonly defined in terms of introspective access to mental processes or mental contents. Empirically, lack of introspective access can be established through participants' inability to verbally report a mental process or mental content. In the APE model, we argue that people usually have *experiential access* to their affective gut reactions resulting from associatively activated concepts, and that they often rely upon these reactions in making propositional evaluative judgments. Still, people also sometimes reject their affective gut reactions as a basis for an evaluative judgment when these reactions are inconsistent with other momentarily considered propositions. However, such dissociations between affective gut reactions and evaluative judgments do not imply that the affective gut reactions are introspectively inaccessible.

Note, however, that although people may be experientially aware of the affective gut reactions resulting from activated associations, they may sometimes be unaware of the processes that gave rise to these reactions (Gawronski, Hofmann, & Wilbur, 2006). For example, people may show a positive or negative gut response toward an unfamiliar individual on the basis of that person's similarity to a known individual. However, they may not be able to identify the similarity between the two individuals as the cause of their affective gut response (e.g., Günyadin, Zayas, Selcuk, & Hazan, 2012). In terms of the APE model, such effects can be explained by the principle of similarity matching that characterizes the process of associative activation. In this example, the resemblance between the two individuals may activate evaluative concepts that are associated with the known individual, thereby eliciting an affective gut response that is in line with the valence of these concepts. Yet the particular content of these associations may remain unconscious even when people are experientially aware of the affective gut reaction resulting from these associations. In other words, people may be experientially aware of their affective gut reactions to a person or object, but they may sometimes be unaware of the particular associations that are responsible for these reactions.

As for propositional processes, we assume that conscious awareness is not required for the default process of affirming the validity of activated information, although people may sometimes engage a conscious reassessment of the validity of that information. Similar considerations apply to the process of monitoring the consistency of momentarily activated information. In many cases, this monitoring process may operate outside of conscious awareness, even though people can certainly monitor their belief systems consciously to identify potential inconsistencies. However, inconsistency between activated information is assumed to raise conscious awareness, which in turn supports the resolution of inconsistency (Morsella, Zarolia, & Gazzaley, 2012). In such cases, the necessary reassessment of the activated information involves conscious awareness of the involved processing steps, such as the negation (i.e., reversal of the truth value) of a particular proposition or the search for information that resolves the inconsistency. The behavioral process of reporting an evaluative judgment generally occurs under conscious awareness.

Formation

Associative learning is commonly assumed to be independent of people's awareness of the relevant contiguities that are responsible for the formation of new associative links. The APE model generally agrees with this contention. Yet several studies found that EC effects were smaller (e.g., Hofmann, De Houwer, Perugini, Baeyens, & Crombez, 2010) or fully attenuated (e.g., Pleyers, Corneille, Luminet, & Yzerbyt, 2007) when participants failed to remember the relevant CS–US pairings. These findings have led some researchers to reject the hypothesis that observed CS–US contiguities can influence evaluative representations through an unconscious process of associative learning (e.g., Mitchell, De Houwer, & Lovibond, 2009). However, there are a number of methodological issues that have to be taken into account when interpreting the relation between memory performance and evaluation. First, it is important to note that current approaches to measure memory for CS–US pairings confound effects of contingency memory and conditioned attitudes, thereby biasing results in favor of the conclusion that contingency memory is a necessary precondition for EC effects. If the confounded influences are disentangled by means of process dissociation (Jacoby, 1991), EC effects tend to emerge even in absence of contingency memory (Hütter, Sweldens, Stahl, Unkelbach, & Klauer, 2012). Second, although memory measures are certainly suitable to investigate the contribution of propositional knowledge of CS–US relations to EC effects at the time of expressing an evaluative response, they remain ambiguous about the role of conscious awareness during the formation of an evaluative representation (Gawronski & Walther, 2012). This ambiguity is due to the fact that (1) memory measures are unable to distinguish between encoding-related and retrieval-related effects, and (2) the relation between memory performance and evaluation is merely correlational, which limits conclusions about causal relations between memory performance and EC effects. As a result, any possible data pattern can be interpreted in at least two different ways, which undermines the suitability of memory measures to investigate whether evaluative learning can occur outside of conscious awareness. As outlined in detail by Gawronski and Walther (2012), a stringent test of this hypothesis requires experimental approaches in which awareness of CS–US pairings is manipulated during encoding.[2] To be sure, memory measures can be very useful to study the contribution of propositional knowledge to EC effects at the time of expressing an evaluative response (e.g., Balas & Gawronski, 2012). However, such influences should not be confused with unconscious influences of CS–US pairings at the time of forming an evaluative representation.

Whereas associative learning is assumed to be independent of conscious awareness, propositional learning generally requires conscious awareness. This hypothesis is based on evidence that externally provided propositional statements cannot be encoded outside of awareness (Baars, 2002; Greenwald, 1992). What is usually extracted from a propositional statement under suboptimal processing conditions is the presence of individual stimuli and their co-occurrence, but not the propositional meaning of the statement. Similarly, conscious awareness is assumed to be required for the self-generation of propositions in response to stimulus events. Of course, to the extent that people are consciously aware of the contiguity of two stimuli, associative and propositional learning may jointly influence the evaluative representation of these stimuli (e.g., Gawronski et al., in press). Yet lack of conscious awareness should eliminate the effects propositional learning, leaving associative learning as the only mechanism that can produce representational changes.

Intentionality

Expression

In general terms, a process can be described as *unintentional* if it is instigated in the absence of a person's intention to start that process (Bargh, 1994). Applied to evaluative responses, it has been argued that the activation of evaluative associations—and therefore the affective gut reactions resulting from these associations—occurs regardless of the intention to evaluate an object (e.g., Bargh, Chaiken, Raymond, & Hymes, 1996). In line with this contention, the APE model assumes that the activation of evaluative associations in memory can indeed occur unintentionally, thereby meeting the second criterion of automaticity. However, it is important to note that evaluative associations can also be activated intentionally. For example, an individual may intentionally search for particular information in memory, and the evaluative associations that are activated through this search may influence this person's affective responses to the relevant target object (e.g., Peters & Gawronski, 2011a). Thus, even though the activation of evaluative associations—and therefore the affective gut reactions resulting from these associations—does not require intention, evaluative associations can also be activated intentionally.

As for propositional processes, we argue that intention is not required for the default process of affirming the validity of activated information, even though individuals may sometimes engage in an intentional reassessment of the validity of that information. Similar to our assumptions about awareness, we assume that such intentional reassessments will occur when the overall set of activated information is inconsistent. In such cases, people will intentionally restore consistency by either negating (i.e., reversing the truth value of) a particular proposition or by searching for information that resolves the inconsistency. In addition, we argue that the monitoring of (in)consistency occurs unintentionally (Morsella et al., 2012), even though people may sometimes engage in an intentional assessment of the consistency of their beliefs. The behavioral process of reporting an evaluative judgment is generally intentional.

Formation

Associative learning can be described as *unintentional* in the sense that the learning process itself does not require the goal to form a new association. However, associative learning can certainly have intentional antecedents, such that people may intentionally expose themselves to repeated co-occurrences to facilitate their acquisition (e.g., intentional exposure to pairs of words in the learning of a foreign language).

Similar considerations apply to propositional learning. Once an externally provided or self-generated proposition is considered, its content may be stored in memory even when people do not have the goal to memorize it. Of course, the goal to memorize the content of a given proposition may facilitate its storage, but such a goal is not a necessary precondition. In fact, a substantial body of evidence suggests that alternative processing goals (e.g., impression formation) can be more effective in producing a strong memory trace than memorization goals (e.g., Hamilton, Katz, & Leirer, 1980). The same is true for the process of self-generating a new proposition, which also does not require an intention to instigate this process. Although self-generated propositions can certainly be the result of intentional inferences about stimulus relations, they can be purely "stimulus-driven" in the sense that they spring from activated associations when people unintentionally notice a systematic relation between stimuli.

Efficiency

Expression

A process can be described as *efficient* if it operates even under conditions of reduced cognitive resources. Applied to evaluative responses, it is commonly assumed that evaluative associations are activated in response to a particular stimulus even when cognitive resources are scarce. The APE model generally agrees with the contention that associative processes are highly efficient. However, this efficiency does not imply that evaluative associations cannot be activated in an effortful manner. Even though evaluative associations—and therefore the affective gut reactions resulting from these associations—do not require cognitive effort to become activated, they can also be activated through the effortful retrieval of evaluative information from memory (e.g., Peters & Gawronski, 2011a).

As for propositional processes, we argue that the default process of affirming the validity of activated information is highly efficient in the sense that it occurs even under conditions of reduced cognitive resources. However, the situation is different for the monitoring and the resolution of inconsistency. In many situations, the monitoring of momentarily activated information may occur efficiently through the unconscious and unintentional operation of the brain's conflict monitoring system (Botvinic, Cohen, & Carter, 2004). However, when people engage in a conscious and intentional assessment of particular pieces of information, limits in working memory capacity will constrain (1) how much information they can hold simultaneously in memory and (2) the complexity of syllogistic inferences they can perform to assess the consistency of this information. To the extent that the amount of relevant information is rather small and the complexity of the required inferences is low, the identification and resolution of inconsistency will require few cognitive resources (e.g., Richter, Schroeder, & Wöhrmann, 2009). If, however, the amount of relevant information is large or the required inferences are relatively complex, the cognitive resources that are required for the identification and resolution of inconsistency will be more substantial (e.g., Martinie, Olive, & Milland, 2010). In other words, we do not assume that propositional processes are cognitively effortful per se. Rather, processes of propositional reasoning can be more or less effortful depending on the complexity of the inferences that are involved. For example, high levels of complexity are often involved when motivational concerns bias the direction of propositional reasoning, in that people engage in an elaborate search for information that validates a desired conclusion or invalidates an undesired conclusion (e.g., Moreno & Bodenhausen, 1999). The behavioral process of reporting the outcome of these validation processes usually requires few cognitive resources. What does require more cognitive resources is the mental process of reaching an evaluative conclusion, not the behavioral process of reporting that conclusion.

Formation

According to the APE model, the formation of mental links through associative learning is resource-independent, although attentional distraction may sometimes disrupt associative learning if it undermines the encoding of the relevant contiguities (e.g., Pleyers, Corneille, Yzerbyt, & Luminet, 2009). Thus, when investigating the proposed resource-independence of associative learning, we deem it important to distinguish between different aspects of working memory capacity (see Baddeley, 2010). Whereas capacity constraints on episodic memory (e.g., concurrent rehearsal of a complex digit-string) should leave associative learning unaffected, capacity constraints on perceptual processing (e.g., concurrent attention to numbers in a two-back task) may reduce the effects of associative learning to the extent that it undermines the perceptual encoding of the relevant stimulus contiguities (see also Custers & Aarts, 2011; Field & Moore, 2005).

As for propositional learning, we assume that the mere consideration of a given proposition does not require substantial amounts of cognitive resources, although greater elaboration can certainly strengthen the resulting mental links (Craik & Lockhart, 1972). Nevertheless, comprehension of externally provided propositional information may require more resources if this information is highly complex. The same is true for the self-generation of propositional information given that limited cognitive resources can constrain the complexity of self-generated information.

Controllability

Expression

Another important characteristic that has been used to describe associative processes is the notion of controllability. In technical terms, a process can be described as *uncontrollable* if it operates despite a person's intention to terminate that process. Thus, whereas the intentionality criterion refers to the goal of starting a process, the controllability criterion refers to the goal of altering or stopping a process (Bargh, 1994). Applied to the current question, one could argue that the activation of evaluative associations—and therefore of the affective gut reactions resulting from these association—is uncontrollable if this activation process cannot be altered or terminated. We argue that the activation of evaluative associations is controllable to some extent. However, the overall success in controlling the activation of evaluative associations is assumed to depend on the nature of the adopted control strategy. According to the APE model, the most critical factor in this regard is whether the adopted control strategy implies a negation of information that is already activated or an affirmation of new information. As outlined earlier, negating the validity of an affective gut reaction is assumed to reduce the influence of this reaction on evaluative judgments. However, it may not eliminate the affective gut reaction per se, as mere negations do not necessarily deactivate the associations that gave rise to this reaction. In contrast, affirming new evaluative information typically activates new associations in memory, which tend to influence the affective gut reactions resulting from activated associations in the intended direction.

As for propositional processes, we argue that the default process of affirming the validity of activated information is generally controllable, because activated information can always be negated. However, the process of monitoring the (in)consistency of activated information is most likely uncontrollable, in that it cannot be altered or stopped. The process of inconsistency resolution is generally controllable given that people may change the preferred strategy to resolve inconsistency. For example, instead of rejecting one of the involved propositions as false, a person may search for information that resolves the inconsistency (or vice versa). The behavioral process of reporting an evaluative judgment is generally controllable given that a person can always report a different judgment voluntarily.

Formation

In the APE model, we assume that associative learning is uncontrollable in the sense that observed contiguities can create mental links despite the goal of not forming an association between the relevant stimuli (e.g., Gawronski et al., in press). A more complex question is whether associative learning can be intentionally altered (rather than stopped). Several studies have shown that EC effects of repeated CS–US pairings can be reversed when the CSs were assumed to have a "negative" relation to the USs (e.g., the CS dislikes the US; the CS is an enemy of the US; see Fiedler & Unkelbach, 2011; Förderer & Unkelbach, 2012). Although these findings seem to suggest that associative learning can be altered by higher-order processing goals, there is evidence that reversed EC effects resulting from "negative" CS–US relations may conceal unqualified associative effects that can be uncovered under particular conditions. For example, Langer, Walther, Gawronski, and Blank (2009) presented participants with several CS–US pairs and additional information indicating that the two stimuli have either a positive relation (i.e., like each other) or a negative relation (i.e., dislike each other). Subsequently, the original valence of the USs was reversed, such that participants received negative information about positive USs and positive information about negative USs (see Walther et al., 2009). Participants in a control condition were presented with neutral information about the USs. Results in the control condition showed a standard EC effect when the CSs and the USs had a positive relation, but a reversed EC effect when the CSs and the USs had a negative relation (see also Fiedler & Unkelbach, 2011; Förderer & Unkelbach, 2012). More importantly, when the original valence of the USs was reversed, CS evaluations failed to produce the mirror image of the crossover interaction obtained in the control condition. Instead, there was only an unqualified main effect of US valence, such that CS evaluations directly reflected the new valence of the US that had been paired with a given CS regardless of whether the relation between the two stimuli was positive or negative. These results suggest that propositional inferences regarding "negative" CS–US relations can conceal associative effects to the extent that information about these relations is available during the encoding of CS–US pairings (for related findings, see Gawronski, Walther, & Blank, 2005). However, the same pairings simultaneously create an unqualified associative link between the CS and the US, which can be uncovered through subsequent revaluation of the USs.

As for the controllability of propositional learning, it is certainly possible to invalidate intentionally an externally provided or self-generated proposition. Such goal-dependent invalidation is conceptually equivalent to the effects of motivated reasoning, in which people may have a desire to confirm or disconfirm the validity of a given proposition. As with negation effects in motivated reasoning, however, the effectiveness of intentional invalidation is often limited to the propositional level, in that merely negating a particular proposition (i.e., reversing its truth value) is insufficient to deactivate the associative link underlying this proposition. The process of self-generating propositions can also be uncontrollable, in that such propositions may often be the "stimulus-driven" result of noticing a systematic relation between stimuli.

DUAL PROCESSES, DUAL SYSTEMS, OR DUAL REPRESENTATIONS?

The APE model is a dual-process theory in the sense that it distinguishes between two conceptually distinct processes on the basis of their operating principles. Whereas associative processes are defined as the *activation* of mental associations on the basis of feature similarity and spatiotemporal contiguity, propositional processes are defined as the *validation* of momentarily activated information on the basis of logical consistency. Deviating from this conceptualization, however, the APE model has sometimes been misinterpreted as a dual-system or dual-representation theory. Whereas dual-process theories limit their assumptions to the distinction between two kinds of mental processes (see Gawronski & Creighton, 2013), dual-system theories postulate systematic overlap between multiple distinct dualities (e.g., associative/automatic/experiential/holistic/slow-learning vs. propositional/controlled/rational/analytic/fast-learning) with the two categories of processes being supported by different mental or neural structures (e.g., Epstein, 1994; Kahneman, 2003; Lieberman, 2003; Sloman, 1996; Smith & DeCoster, 2000; Strack & Deutsch, 2004). A particular subset of dual-system theories is dual-representation theories, which propose the storage of two distinct memory representations of the same object (e.g., Rydell & McConnell, 2006; Wilson, Lindsey, & Schooler, 2000).

Although the APE model shares some assumptions with dual-system and dual-representation theories, it disagrees with both conceptualizations in fundamental ways (Gawronski & Bodenhausen, 2011). First, rejecting the notion of dual representations, the APE model does not assume a separate storage of associations and propositions in memory. Instead, all information is assumed to be stored in the form of associations, which may or may not pass a propositional assessment of validity. Second, the APE model does not assume systematic overlap between multiple distinct dualities, as proposed by dual-system theories. As we have outlined in detail in this chapter, we do not assume a one-to-one mapping between operating principles (associative vs. propositional) and operating conditions (automatic vs. controlled). We also do not assume systematic overlap of either distinction with other kinds of dualities (e.g., holistic vs. analytic, experiential vs. rational, slow-learning vs. fast-learning). Third, the APE model remains agnostic about whether associative and propositional processes are supported by distinct mental or neural structures. Although the notion of dual systems may provide useful links to basic concepts in neuroscience, we remain skeptical as to whether the brain can be meaningfully divided into two systems, considering that the brain includes multiple specialized regions that mutually interact with each other to produce a particular behavioral outcome. In fact, we doubt whether claiming that the two processes operate in two different systems provides any additional prediction over and above the ones that are already implied by the dual-process distinction.

An important issue in this context concerns the status of associations and propositions as mental entities. Although associative and propositional processes are conceptually distinct in the sense that they are characterized by nonoverlapping operating principles, a qualitative distinction between associations and propositions as conceptually distinct entities is more difficult to maintain (Gawronski & Bodenhausen, 2006b). According to the APE model, any association turns into a proposition if it is assigned a truth value. Conversely, any proposition depends on activated associations, because we do not propose an independent storage of propositions in memory. Thus, although the APE model distinguishes between associative and propositional processes as two conceptually distinct processes, the terms *association* and *proposition* should not be misinterpreted as implying two conceptually distinct mental entities.

Another important question in the context of memory representation concerns the storage of relational information. For example, the stimulus event *John is eating the sandwich* is inherently relational, in that it involves a clear structure between the actor (*John*), the described action (*eating*), and the object of the action (*sandwich*). Because associative memory has sometimes been described as being limited to unstructured, bidirectional links between concepts that do not include relational information (e.g., Lieberman, 2003), proponents of propositional models tend to reject the notion of associative memory on the grounds that memory representations are inherently relational (e.g., Mitchell et al., 2009). In response to this criticism, it is important to note that structural relations can certainly be accommodated in associative memory models that are based on distributed networks with multiple layers of excitatory and inhibitory links (Smith, 1996). Moreover, as we outlined earlier, the central distinction in the APE model is not between associative and propositional *representations*. Instead, we distinguish between associative and propositional *processes* on the basis of their nonoverlapping operating principles. Of course, any cognitive account has to accommodate the inherently relational structure of mental representation. However, this issue is fundamentally different from the dual-process distinction in the APE model, which defines associative and propositional processes in terms of their operating principles (i.e., activation vs. validation), not in terms of their underlying mental representations.

CONCLUSION

Our main goal in this chapter has been to explain how the distinction between associative and propositional processes relates to the distinction between automatic and controlled processes that has guided dual-process theorizing in the last three decades. We have argued that the associative–propositional distinction refers to what a given process is doing (*operating principles*), whereas the automatic–controlled distinction refers to empirical claims about when that process is operating (*operating conditions*). Although the two dichotomies are sometimes assumed to overlap, the APE model draws a sharp line between operating principles and operating conditions, in that both associative and propositional processes have automatic and controlled aspects. Although the APE model is primarily concerned with the role of associative and propositional processes in evaluation, its core assumptions are applicable to both evaluative and nonevaluative information, thereby providing the basis for a general theory of human thought.

ACKNOWLEDGMENTS

Preparation of this chapter was supported by grants from the Canada Research Chairs Program, the Social Sciences and Humanities Research Council of Canada, and the Ontario Ministry for Research and Innovation.

NOTES

1. Challenging the generality of such ironic effects, a recent study by Peters and Gawronski (2011b) found that negation can qualify the stored representations resulting from subjectively invalid propositions to the extent that the invalidation occurs within a sufficiently short interval after encoding. Nevertheless, there seem to be systematic limits in the processing of observed co-occurrences between stimuli that involve a contrastive relation (e.g., Moran & Bar-Anan, 2013).
2. In this context, it is important to distinguish between attention and awareness as two conceptually distinct aspects of encoding CS–US relations. Although attention to the relevant stimuli is likely required for both associative and propositional learning, associative learning may occur in the absence of conscious awareness to the extent that the relevant CS–US pairings are in the focus of attention (e.g., Custers & Aarts, 2011; Field & Moore, 2005).

REFERENCES

Baars, B. J. (2002). The conscious access hypothesis: Origins and recent evidence. *Trends in Cognitive Sciences, 6,* 47–52.

Baddeley, A. (2010). Working memory. *Current Biology, 20,* 136–140.

Balas, R., & Gawronski, B. (2012). On the intentional control of conditioned evaluative responses. *Learning and Motivation, 43,* 89–98.

Bargh, J. A. (1994). The four horsemen of automaticity: Awareness, intention, efficiency, and control in social cognition. In R. S. Wyer & T. K. Srull (Eds.), *Handbook of social cognition* (pp. 1–40). Hillsdale, NJ: Erlbaum.

Bargh, J. A., Chaiken, S., Raymond, P., & Hymes, C. (1996). The automatic evaluation effect: Unconditional automatic activation with a pronunciation task. *Journal of Experimental Social Psychology, 32,* 104–128.

Blair, I. V., Judd, C. M., & Fallman, J. L. (2004). The automaticity of race and Afrocentric facial features in social judgments. *Journal of Personality and Social Psychology, 87,* 763–778.

Botvinick, M. M., Cohen, J. D., & Carter, C. S. (2004). Conflict monitoring and anterior cingulate cortex: An update. *Trends in Cognitive Sciences, 8*, 539–546.

Conner, M., & Armitage, C. J. (2008). Attitudinal ambivalence. In W. D. Crano & R. Prislin (Eds.), *Attitudes and attitude change* (pp. 261–286). New York: Psychology Press.

Craik, F. I. M., & Lockhart, R. S. (1972). Levels of processing: A framework for memory research. *Journal of Verbal Learning and Verbal Behavior, 11*, 671–684.

Custers, R., & Aarts, H. (2011). Learning of predictive relations between events depends on attention, not on awareness. *Consciousness and Cognition, 20*, 368–378.

De Houwer, J. (2007). A conceptual and theoretical analysis of evaluative conditioning. *Spanish Journal of Psychology, 10*, 230–241.

De Houwer, J., Thomas, S., & Baeyens, F. (2001). Associative learning of likes and dislikes: A review of 25 years of research on human evaluative conditioning. *Psychological Bulletin, 127*, 853–869.

Deutsch, R., Gawronski, B., & Strack, F. (2006). At the boundaries of automaticity: Negation as reflective operation. *Journal of Personality and Social Psychology, 91*, 385–405.

Devine, P. G. (1989). Stereotypes and prejudice: Their automatic and controlled components. *Journal of Personality and Social Psychology, 56*, 5–18.

Epstein, S. (1994). Integration of the cognitive and psychodynamic unconscious. *American Psychologist, 49*, 709–724.

Festinger, L. (1957). *A theory of cognitive dissonance*. Evanston, IL: Row, Peterson.

Fiedler, K., & Unkelbach, C. (2011). Evaluative conditioning depends on higher order encoding processes. *Cognition and Emotion, 25*, 639–656.

Field, A. P., & Moore, A. C. (2005). Dissociating the effects of attention and contingency awareness on evaluative conditioning effects in the visual paradigm. *Cognition and Emotion, 19*, 217–243.

Förderer, S., & Unkelbach, C. (2012). Hating the cute kitten or loving the aggressive pit-bull: EC effects depend on CS–US relations. *Cognition and Emotion, 26*, 534–540.

Gawronski, B. (2012). Back to the future of dissonance theory: Cognitive consistency as a core motive. *Social Cognition, 30*, 652–668.

Gawronski, B., Balas, R., & Creighton, L. A. (in press). Can the formation of conditioned attitudes be intentionally controlled? *Personality and Social Psychology Bulletin*.

Gawronski, B., & Bodenhausen, G. V. (2006a). Associative and propositional processes in evaluation: An integrative review of implicit and explicit attitude change. *Psychological Bulletin, 132*, 692–731.

Gawronski, B., & Bodenhausen, G. V. (2006b). Associative and propositional processes in evaluation: Conceptual, empirical, and metatheoretical issues. Reply to Albarracín, Hart, and McCulloch (2006), Kruglanski and Dechesne (2006), and Petty and Briñol (2006). *Psychological Bulletin, 132*, 745–750.

Gawronski, B., & Bodenhausen, G. V. (2007). Unraveling the processes underlying evaluation: Attitudes from the perspective of the APE Model. *Social Cognition, 25*, 687–717.

Gawronski, B., & Bodenhausen, G. V. (2009). Operating principles versus operating conditions in the distinction between associative and propositional processes. *Behavioral and Brain Sciences, 32*, 207–208.

Gawronski, B., & Bodenhausen, G. V. (2011). The associative–propositional evaluation model: Theory, evidence, and open questions. *Advances in Experimental Social Psychology, 44*, 59–127.

Gawronski, B., & Creighton, L. A. (2013). Dual-process theories. In D. E. Carlston (Ed.), *The Oxford handbook of social cognition* (pp. 282–312). New York: Oxford University Press

Gawronski, B., Deutsch, R., Mbirkou, S., Seibt, B., & Strack, F. (2008). When "just say no" is not enough: Affirmation versus negation training and the reduction of automatic stereotype activation. *Journal of Experimental Social Psychology, 44*, 370–377.

Gawronski, B., Hofmann, W., & Wilbur, C. J. (2006). Are "implicit" attitudes unconscious? *Consciousness and Cognition, 15*, 485–499.

Gawronski, B., & LeBel, E. P. (2008). Understanding patterns of attitude change: When implicit measures show change, but explicit measures do not. *Journal of Experimental Social Psychology, 44*, 1355–1361.

Gawronski, B., Peters, K. R., Brochu, P. M., & Strack, F. (2008). Understanding the relations between different forms of racial prejudice: A cognitive consistency perspective. *Personality and Social Psychology Bulletin, 34*, 648–665.

Gawronski, B., & Quinn, K. A. (2013). Guilty by mere similarity: Assimilative effects of facial resemblance on automatic evaluation. *Jour-*

nal of Experimental Social Psychology, 49, 120–125.

Gawronski, B., & Sritharan, R. (2010). Formation, change, and contextualization of mental associations: Determinants and principles of variations in implicit measures. In B. Gawronski & B. K. Payne (Eds.), *Handbook of implicit social cognition: Measurement, theory, and applications* (pp. 216–240). New York: Guilford Press.

Gawronski, B., & Strack, F. (2004). On the propositional nature of cognitive consistency: Dissonance changes explicit, but not implicit attitudes. *Journal of Experimental Social Psychology, 40,* 535–542.

Gawronski, B., & Walther, E. (2012). What do memory data tell us about the role of contingency awareness in evaluative conditioning? *Journal of Experimental Social Psychology, 48,* 617–623.

Gawronski, B., Walther, E., & Blank, H. (2005). Cognitive consistency and the formation of interpersonal attitudes: Cognitive balance affects the encoding of social information. *Journal of Experimental Social Psychology, 41,* 618–626.

Greenwald, A. G. (1992). New Look 3: Reclaiming unconscious cognition. *American Psychologist, 47,* 766–779.

Günaydin, G., Zayas, V., Selcuk, E., & Hazan, C. (2012). I like you but I don't know why: Objective facial resemblance to significant others influences snap judgments. *Journal of Experimental Social Psychology, 48,* 350–353.

Hamilton, D. L., Katz, L. B., & Leirer, V. O. (1980). Cognitive representation of personality impression: Organizational processes in first impression formation. *Journal of Personality and Social Psychology, 39,* 1050–1063.

Hofmann, W., De Houwer, J., Perugini, M., Baeyens, F., & Crombez, G. (2010). Evaluative conditioning in humans: A meta-analysis. *Psychological Bulletin, 136,* 390–421.

Hütter, M., Sweldens, S., Stahl, C., Unkelbach, C., & Klauer, K. C. (2012). Dissociating contingency awareness and conditioned attitudes: Evidence of contingency-unaware evaluative conditioning. *Journal of Experimental Psychology: General, 141,* 539–557.

Jacoby, L. L. (1991). A process dissociation framework: Separating automatic from intentional uses of memory. *Journal of Memory and Language, 30,* 513–541.

Jones, E. E., & Gerard, H. B. (1967). *Foundations of social psychology.* New York: Wiley.

Kahneman, D. (2003). A perspective on judgment and choice: Mapping bounded rationality. *American Psychologist, 58,* 697–720.

Kunda, Z. (1990). The case for motivated reasoning. *Psychological Bulletin, 108,* 480–498.

Langer, T., Walther, E., Gawronski, B., & Blank, H. (2009). When linking is stronger than thinking: Associative transfer of valence disrupts the emergence of cognitive balance. *Journal of Experimental Social Psychology, 45,* 1232–1237.

Lieberman, M. D. (2003). Reflective and reflexive judgment processes: A social cognitive neuroscience approach. In J. P. Forgas, K. R. Williams, & W. von Hippel (Eds.), *Social judgments: Implicit and explicit processes* (pp. 44–67). New York: Cambridge University Press.

Martinie, M.-A., Olive, T., & Milland, L. (2010). Cognitive dissonance induced by writing a counterattitudinal essay facilitates performance on simple tasks but not on complex tasks that involve working memory. *Journal of Experimental Social Psychology, 46,* 587–594.

Mitchell, C. J., De Houwer, J., & Lovibond, P. F. (2009). The propositional nature of human associative learning. *Behavioral and Brain Sciences, 32,* 183–198.

Moran, T., & Bar-Anan, Y. (2013). The effect of object-valence relations on automatic evaluation. *Cognition and Emotion, 27,* 743–752.

Moreno, K. N., & Bodenhausen, G. V. (1999). Resisting stereotype change: The role of motivation and attentional capacity in defending social beliefs. *Group Processes and Intergroup Relations, 2,* 5–16.

Morsella, E., Zarolia, P., & Gazzaley, A. (2012). Cognitive conflict and consciousness. In B. Gawronski & F. Strack (Eds.), *Cognitive consistency: A fundamental principle in social cognition* (pp. 19–46). New York: Guilford Press.

Peters, K. R., & Gawronski, B. (2011a). Mutual influences between the implicit and explicit self-concepts: The role of memory activation and motivated reasoning. *Journal of Experimental Social Psychology, 47,* 436–442.

Peters, K. R., & Gawronski, B. (2011b). Are we puppets on a string?: Comparing the impact of contingency and validity on implicit and explicit evaluations. *Personality and Social Psychology Bulletin, 37,* 557–569.

Pleyers, G., Corneille, O., Luminet, O., & Yzerbyt, V. (2007). Aware and (dis)liking: Item-based analyses reveal that valence acquisition via evaluative conditioning emerges only when there is contingency awareness. *Journal of Experimental Psychology: Learning, Memory, Cognition, 33,* 130–144.

Pleyers, G., Corneille, O., Yzerbyt, V., & Luminet, O. (2009). Evaluative conditioning may incur attentional costs. *Journal of Experimental Psychology: Animal Behavior Processes, 35,* 279–285.

Richter, T., Schroeder, S., & Wöhrmann, B. (2009). You don't have to believe everything your read: Background knowledge permits fast and efficient validation of information. *Journal of Personality and Social Psychology, 96,* 538–558.

Rydell, R. J., & McConnell, A. R. (2006). Understanding implicit and explicit attitude change: A systems of reasoning analysis. *Journal of Personality and Social Psychology, 91,* 995–1008.

Sloman, S. A. (1996). The empirical case for two systems of reasoning. *Psychological Bulletin, 119,* 3–22.

Smith, E. R. (1996). What do connectionism and social psychology offer each other? *Journal of Personality and Social Psychology, 70,* 893–912.

Smith, E. R., & DeCoster, J. (2000). Dual-process models in social and cognitive psychology: Conceptual integration and links to underlying memory systems. *Personality and Social Psychology Review, 4,* 108–131.

Strack, F., & Deutsch, R. (2004). Reflective and impulsive determinants of social behavior. *Personality and Social Psychology Review, 8,* 220–247.

Walther, E., Gawronski, B., Blank, H., & Langer, T. (2009). Changing likes and dislikes through the backdoor: The US-revaluation effect. *Cognition and Emotion, 23,* 889–917.

Whitfield, M., & Jordan, C. H. (2009). Mutual influences of explicit and implicit attitudes. *Journal of Experimental Social Psychology, 45,* 748–759.

Wilson, T. D., Lindsey, S., & Schooler, T. Y. (2000). A model of dual attitudes. *Psychological Review, 107,* 101–126.

CHAPTER 14

The Systems of Evaluation Model

A Dual-Systems Approach to Attitudes

Allen R. McConnell and Robert J. Rydell

Consider the following everyday situations. New neighbors move in next door, and despite the fact that one's interactions with them are overtly quite pleasant, one experiences an uncomfortable feeling around them that defies explanation. Or consider the couple deciding between two vacation destinations, one in a cosmopolitan setting with great restaurants and museums, and the other offering pristine, sandy beaches. After much contemplation about which one would make them happier, they choose the city, yet they would have been happier had they gone to the ocean instead. Finally, there is the dieter's dilemma, in which one has to wrestle with passing up a tempting, calorie-laden dessert in order to pursue long-range goals associated with being healthier and happier with one's appearance in the mirror. Although cases involving impression formation, judgment and decision making, and self-regulation may seem disparate, we contend that, at a process level, there are important commonalities across these situations, and that approaching attitudes from a dual-systems perspective sheds light on their similarities.

When it comes to behavior, it seems reasonable that people should gravitate toward more attractive options. In the parlance of social psychology, people should pursue the most positive attitude objects before them and eschew the more negative ones. However, this supposition is not only contradicted by findings that attitudes often fail to predict behavior well (e.g., Fazio, 1986), but it also assumes that evaluative processes eventually converge on a singular evaluation for any object. In our chapter, we present an alternative to this latter assumption. Specifically, we outline our systems of evaluation model (SEM; McConnell, Rydell, Strain, & Mackie, 2008; Rydell & McConnell, 2006), which puts forward a dual-systems approach to attitude formation and change. The SEM posits that two dissociable systems of knowledge give rise to qualitatively different types of attitude object evaluations. In this chapter, we describe the basic tenets of the SEM, present research findings that support it, discuss the important consequences of holding discrepant implicit and explicit evaluations, and compare and contrast the SEM to other dual-systems and dual-process models of attitudes.

THE SEM

The SEM adopts as a starting point that people possess two partially independent mental systems with distinct properties and characteristics (e.g., Kahneman, 2003; Sloman, 1996; Strack & Deutsch, 2004;

Smith & DeCoster, 2000) that differ in the knowledge each uses and in how relevant information is processed. We assume that a *rule-based system* provides evaluations of attitude objects rendered by applying logic and deductive reasoning to symbolic forms of knowledge (e.g., language, mathematical formulas) relevant to the attitude object. For instance, one could reflect on the abstract qualities of beaches (e.g., soft sand, relaxing surf sounds) and, based on a formal analysis, report having a positive attitude toward beaches. Evaluations produced by the rule-based system, referred to as *explicit evaluations*, can typically be formed and modified relatively quickly, because logic and syllogisms are responsive to one's deliberate goals and deductive reasoning processes. Because explicit evaluations are grounded in logic and symbolic representations, their assessment is typically derived from measures that rely on similar processes to complete (common language-based attitude measures; e.g., a feeling thermometer).

On the other hand, we propose that there is an *associative system* in which evaluations of attitude objects are derived from many associations that are stored in memory and based on paired occurrences involving similarity and contiguity. Evaluations evoked by the associative system, referred to as *implicit evaluations*, typically are slower to form and change, because they are based on accumulated attitude object–evaluation pairings in memory. For example, many episodes of walking on a beach and being happy lead to a relatively strong association between "beach" and "positivity" in memory. Once established, the presentation of an attitude object should evoke a spontaneous evaluation relatively automatically, without intention or any effortful thoughtful production. Because implicit evaluations are produced from associations in memory, their assessment is typically rendered by measures that gauge associative strength in memory (e.g., Implicit Association Test, IAT; Greenwald, McGee, & Schwartz, 1998).

In the previous example, the rule-based system and the associative system led to the expression of positive attitudes toward beaches even though the underlying knowledge used by each system was quite different. And often, evaluations produced by the rule-based system and by the associative system are similar because one's repeated associations with an attitude object and one's abstract knowledge about it are relatively consonant. However, because the underlying knowledge and how that information is processed can differ between the rule-based and associative systems of evaluations, striking differences in the output of these systems may result. Sometimes these evaluative discrepancies are manufactured in the laboratory (e.g., using subliminal priming) to establish and evaluate the potential independence of these systems (e.g., Rydell, McConnell, & Mackie, 2008; Rydell, McConnell, Mackie, & Strain, 2006). However, there are many real-world circumstances in which meaningful asymmetries between implicit and explicit evaluations exist (e.g., Hofmann, Rauch, & Gawronski, 2007; Jellison, McConnell, & Gabriel, 2004). These discrepancies can be even more consequential, because research (e.g., Dovidio, Kawakami, & Gaertner, 2002; Rydell & McConnell, 2006) indicates that different behavioral outcomes are related to one's explicit evaluations (e.g., deliberate, strategic actions) and to one's implicit evaluations (e.g., spontaneous actions, nonverbal displays).

SUPPORT FOR THE SEM

Although one's implicit and explicit evaluations may often be of the same valence, laboratory experiments can produce dissociations between evaluations derived from the rule-based and associative systems to document the different processes underlying them. Because the associative system of evaluation is based on the accrual of many pairings between an attitude object and appraisals over time, the speed with which implicit evaluations form and change will typically be slower than the speed with which explicit evaluations form and change. Although some manipulations, such as imagining counterstereotypical exemplars or altering the context around the attitude object, may affect the expression of associative knowledge (see Blair, 2002), we contend that, all things being equal, evaluations produced by the associative system are slower to develop and change than attitudes generated by the rule-based system. This prediction has been borne out in a number of empirical studies.

For example, Rydell and McConnell (2006, Experiment 2) had participants form an impression about a novel target individual named Bob by reading 200 descriptions of his behavior. For the first 100 statements, the valence implied by the statements suggested that Bob either performed only desirable actions or performed only undesirable actions in order that participants form positive or negative initial impressions of Bob, respectively. Next, an additional 100 statements describing Bob were neutral in valence (i.e., did not imply positivity or negativity), mildly counterattitudinal (i.e., 20 of the opposite valence connoted by the first 100 statements followed by 80 neutral statements), or completely counterattitudinal (i.e., all 100 statements were of the opposite valence implied by the first 100 statements). After exposure to all 200 statements, participants offered explicit evaluations of Bob (liking scales, feeling thermometers, and semantic differentials) and implicit evaluations of Bob (using an IAT). Not surprisingly, both explicit and implicit evaluations of Bob reflected the valence of the initial 100 statements in the neutral condition. However, the signature of attitude change between explicit and implicit measures was quite different when the second 100 statements provided counterattitudinal information. Encountering just 20 counterattitudinal items in the mildly counterattitudinal condition resulted in a strong shift in explicit evaluations of Bob, away from the valence connoted in the initial 100 statements, but did not significantly alter implicit evaluations of Bob. Eventually, implicit evaluations did significantly shift toward the direction of the new information, but only when participants were exposed to 100 counterattitudinal statements (but the additional 80 counterattitudinal statements had very little impact on explicit evaluations of Bob). Overall, change in explicit evaluations revealed an asymptotic signature (i.e., fast change in response to initial counterattitudinal information but then very little change following extreme amounts of it), whereas change in implicit evaluations showed a linear signature (i.e., change was proportional to the amount of counterattitudinal information presented). As anticipated by the SEM, explicit evaluations changed quickly as participants integrated new information about Bob into their on-line impressions of him (see McConnell, Sherman, & Hamilton, 1994), whereas implicit evaluations required a considerable amount of counterattitudinal information to produce change, because the associative system more closely reflects the totality of information associated with the attitude object (see also Rydell, McConnell, Strain, Claypool, & Hugenberg, 2007).

If appraisals produced by the rule-based system reflect deliberation, then providing participants with explicit processing goals should affect perceivers' explicit evaluations more than their implicit evaluations, which should not be strongly influenced by processing goals. To test this prediction, Rydell and McConnell (2006, Experiment 3) had participants form impressions using "the Bob paradigm" previously described (e.g., 100 initial statements about Bob, followed by 100 additional items that were neutral, mildly counterattitudinal, or completely counterattitudinal) and complete the same measures of explicit and implicit evaluations of Bob. In addition, participants were given explicit processing goals either to rely on their first impressions of Bob (the default manner in which impressions of individuals are made; see McConnell et al., 1994) or not to rely on their first impressions. When participants were instructed to rely on their first impressions, the data for explicit and implicit evaluations of Bob replicated the previous study: Changes in explicit evaluations revealed the asymptotic signature, whereas changes in implicit evaluations revealed the linear signature described earlier. However, when participants were instructed not to rely on first impressions, their explicit evaluations of Bob showed a more linear rather than asymptotic trend (i.e., the additional 80 counterattitudinal items in the completely counterattitudinal condition slowly eroded participants' initial explicit evaluation of Bob), yet their implicit evaluations of Bob were not affected by the instructions to rely or not rely on their first impressions. Thus, providing participants with information-processing goals changed the nature of explicit evaluations but did not have any impact on implicit evaluations. From the SEM perspective, this is expected because explicit goals should affect the system of evaluation that is responsive to logic and reasoning (i.e., the rule-based system of evaluation) but should be less consequential for evaluations derived from paired associations in memory (i.e., the associative system of evaluation).

Although differential speed of change and differential responsiveness to deliberate processing goals between the two systems of evaluation are anticipated outcomes in the SEM, it is also assumed that each system of evaluation is sensitive to different forms of information. Each system could potentially draw upon all the information about the attitude object that is stored in memory to render an evaluation, but the SEM assumes that each system is sensitive to and therefore more likely to use different types of information, at least when multiple forms of information are available. For example, associative knowledge that is not available to conscious deliberation should affect implicit evaluations but not affect explicit evaluations as strongly. To test this prediction, Rydell et al. (2008) had participants form impressions in "the Bob paradigm." On each trial, a positive or negative word (e.g., *love, hate*) presented subliminally to participants was immediately replaced by an image of Bob's face on the computer monitor. Next, a sentence was presented that characterized one of Bob's behaviors. Thus, participants were exposed to information in a 2 (subliminal prime valence: positive vs. negative) × 2 (descriptive sentence valence: positive vs. negative) between-subjects design. Afterwards, participants provided their explicit and implicit evaluations of Bob. In short, implicit evaluations of Bob reflected the valence of the subliminal primes (i.e., more positive when the subliminal primes were positive, more negative when the subliminal primes were negative), whereas explicit evaluations of Bob reflected the valence implied by the statements (i.e., more positive following positive behavioral descriptions, more negative following negative behavioral descriptions). As predicted by the SEM, each system of evaluation was more influenced by information attuned to the form of knowledge underlying the rule-based (i.e., behavioral sentences) and associative (i.e., subliminal primes) systems of evaluation, reflecting the potential for these systems of evaluation to be completely dissociable (see Rydell et al., 2006, for additional evidence).

Admittedly, it may be unusual for an individual to receive forms of information that are completely at odds with each other (e.g., very positive behavioral descriptions and very negative subliminal cues). Although demonstrations such as these are important to test the hypothesized processes underlying explicit and implicit evaluations, one might conclude that such cases are extremely rare. However, we contend that there are probably a number of circumstances in which such evaluative dissociations naturally exist. Consider the conditions under which one is forming an impression of novel individuals such as new neighbors. Initial conversations with one's new neighbors might reveal a wealth of positive information about them (e.g., they tell positive stories about their families or hobbies). These verbal descriptions are probably important pieces of information for developing positive explicit evaluations of them. Yet what if other information about them was not verbal in nature, such as their being a member of a group associated with a pejorative stigma (e.g., they are obese). From the perspective of the SEM, one's explicit evaluations of these neighbors should be very positive (based on the positivity conveyed in their stories about themselves), but one's implicit evaluations of them might be very negative (based on the strength of association between obesity and negativity) when such a cue is irrelevant for one's deliberate information-processing goals.

This possibility was assessed in several studies by McConnell et al. (2008), who used a modified Bob paradigm that presented descriptions conveying that Bob performed positive or negative actions, along with an image of Bob's face. In some cases, Bob was a relatively thin, White man. In other cases (in different experiments), Bob was an obese man or an African American man. In cases where Bob was thin and white, implicit evaluations of him reflected the valence implied by his behaviors. However, when Bob was portrayed as obese or African American, implicit evaluations of him were negative even when his behaviors indicated that he performed nothing but positive actions. In short, the strong association between social group membership cues (e.g., weight, race) and negativity led to the formation of implicit evaluations of Bob that reflected group-based stigmas rather than his actions.

To explore this effect further, McConnell et al. (2008, Experiment 2) used the same paradigm but presented behaviors about a woman (Bobbie) who was presented as average in physical attractiveness, as physically unattractive, or as very physically attractive. When Bobbie was average in attractiveness, implicit evaluations of her reflected the valence of her actions. However, when she was portrayed as physically unattractive, implicit evaluations of her were negative even when she performed nothing but positive actions (replicating the effect observed with obesity and with African Americans). But most important, when Bobbie was very physically attractive, implicit evaluations of her were very positive even when her actions were exclusively negative in valence. Thus, when associated with a group membership cue strongly associated with valence (negative or positive), implicit evaluations were strongly influenced by this associative cue and not the actions described about the target individual. These results strongly support the dissociable systems outlined by the SEM.

If appraisals produced by the associative system reflect the accrual of evaluations over time, while assessments rendered from the rule-based system of evaluation are responsive to logic and deliberation, we might expect to see interesting asymmetries in how one's implicit and explicit evaluations predict one's *own* past behaviors. In one study that examined this possibility, Jellison et al. (2004) examined how gay men's implicit and explicit evaluations of sexual orientation predicted their past experiences. Specifically, they had men who identified as being primarily homosexual provide explicit reports of sexual orientation attitudes (using common paper-and-pencil measures of attitudes toward homosexuality) and implicit attitude measures toward sexual orientation (using a sexual orientation IAT). In addition, these men provided reports about their past personal experiences, including the frequency with which they had positive, gay-affirming experiences in their lives (e.g., attending gay-supportive religious services, subscribing to publications that cater to the gay community) and the extent to which they had disclosed their homosexuality to others (e.g., family members, coworkers). Jellison et al. anticipated that gay men's implicit sexual orientation evaluations would be a better predictor of their *frequency* of past positive gay experiences (presumably, many gay-affirming experiences would result in more positivity being associated with their sexual orientation in memory) but that gay men's explicit evaluations would be a better predictor of the extent to which they had disclosed their sexual orientation to others ("coming out" to others reflects a strategic, deliberate choice that results from a thoughtful analysis of the consequences of disclosing one's sexual orientation to others). Indeed, this is exactly what they found. The frequency of involvement in gay-affirming activities was uniquely predicted by gay men's implicit evaluations (i.e., having more positive past experiences was related to relatively more positive implicit evaluations of homosexuality), whereas disclosure of one's sexual orientation to others was uniquely predicted by gay men's explicit evaluations (i.e., more "coming out" was related to more positive explicit evaluations of homosexuality). Thus, Jellison et al. provided evidence that distinct forms of past experiences are related to one's implicit (e.g., frequency of past experiences) and explicit (e.g., strategic, deliberate actions) evaluations, which is in line with the expectations of the SEM (see Sinclair, Dunn, & Lowery, 2005, for similar findings regarding children's implicit racial prejudice and their parents' level of prejudice).

To summarize, a number of studies support important distinctions between rule-based and associative systems of evaluation. Measures of attitudes derived from these systems of evaluations can show striking differences and asymmetries. For example, explicit measures of attitudes that capture the rule-based system of evaluation can change very quickly to new information and are affected by explicit processing goals that guide one's impression formation objectives (Rydell & McConnell, 2006; Rydell et al., 2007). Implicit measures of attitudes that capture the associative system of evaluation, on the other hand, change more slowly and are unaffected by explicit processing goals

(Rydell & McConnell, 2006; Rydell et al., 2007), and are strongly influenced by cues involving group membership–valence associations (McConnell et al., 2008) and by cues that are subliminal in nature (Rydell et al., 2006). Finally, there is good evidence that the frequency of past experiences that can produce strong associations between attitude objects and evaluations in memory is uniquely related to one's implicit evaluations, whereas past actions involving the strategic performance of behaviors are uniquely predicted by one's explicit evaluations (Jellison et al., 2004). These strong dissociations seem best accounted for by a framework that views attitudes as the product of two discrete systems of evaluation.

CONSEQUENCES OF INCONSISTENT IMPLICIT AND EXPLICIT EVALUATIONS

The previous findings reveal that a number of conditions, either in the laboratory or in everyday life, can result in people holding different attitudes derived from the rule-based and associative systems of evaluation. When systems of evaluation are in conflict, what are the consequences? Below we outline a number of significant outcomes, including inconsistencies in behavior, felt ambivalence (negative arousal), affective forecasting errors, and difficulty in successful goal attainment. These effects can be quite far-reaching, and they underscore the value of considering how different attitudes can result from distinct systems of evaluation.

One of the most well documented outcomes of holding inconsistent implicit and explicit evaluations is observing divergent behaviors. In the domain of interracial interactions, there is considerable evidence that people's implicit racial prejudice (i.e., attitudes toward outgroup members, as indexed by association-based measures) uniquely predicts participants' nonverbal behaviors toward minority group members (e.g., McConnell & Leibold, 2001). Although explicit measures of attitudes can predict behavioral outcomes, implicit measures of attitudes, such as racial IATs, predict intergroup behaviors better than explicit measures of attitudes in contexts in which social sensitivity concerns are considerable (for a meta-analysis, see Greenwald, Poehlman, Uhlmann, & Banaji, 2009). Yet there is evidence that even with novel individual targets (instead of social group targets in which political correctness pressures may exist), implicit measures of attitudes can uniquely predict many subtle nonverbal behaviors that explicit measures cannot. For example, Rydell and McConnell (2006, Experiment 4) induced different explicit and implicit evaluations of a novel person using "the Bob paradigm." Afterwards, participants were told that they were going to interact with Bob in a different room in a "get acquainted" interaction. First, they reported on how much they would want to have social contact with Bob. Next, they moved to a different room to meet Bob, but upon arriving, only Bob's bookbag was there, and the experimenter suggested that Bob must have stepped out for a moment. Participants then grabbed a chair from against the wall and positioned it for the forthcoming interaction, which never took place. From these actions, two indices of behavior were computed: desire for future interaction (greater reported desire is an indicator of more positive behavior) and seating distance (less distance between Bob's bookbag and the chair positioned by the participant is an indicator of more positive behavior. Participants' greater desire for future interaction was uniquely predicted by participants' explicit evaluations being more positive toward Bob, and closer seating distance was uniquely predicted by participants' more positive implicit evaluations toward Bob. Thus, when interacting with a novel individual, participants' rule-based evaluations uniquely predicted a deliberate behavior (i.e., desire for future contact) and their associative evaluations uniquely predicted a spontaneous behavior (i.e., seating distance).

Because holding inconsistent beliefs can be aversive and arousing (e.g., Festinger, 1957), one might wonder whether holding inconsistent implicit and explicit evaluations might trigger felt ambivalence (or diffuse negative arousal caused by inconsistent evaluations of an attitude object but not attributed to that object, which is sometimes called *implicit ambivalence*). Indeed, there is suggestive evidence that this might be the case. Briñol, Petty, and Wheeler (2006) found that participants with greater discrepancies in explicit and implicit self-beliefs (e.g., one's own shyness) processed persuasive messages related to the domain of the discrepancy more extensively. Although Briñol et al. did not assess felt ambivalence in their study, greater attentional deployment in the service of making sense of one's discrepant feelings can result from experiencing felt ambivalence (Schwarz & Clore, 2007).

Accordingly, Rydell et al. (2008) examined how holding inconsistent explicit and implicit evaluations of Bob (using a modified Bob paradigm involving subliminal priming to induce implicit evaluations of Bob that diverged from written statements describing Bob's actions) might lead to experiencing the discomfort associated with discrepant implicit and explicit evaluations, which in turn might trigger greater information processing about a persuasive appeal authored by Bob. Explicit and implicit evaluations of Bob were then assessed. After assessing attitudes toward Bob, participants reported on how much they felt uncomfortable, uneasy, and bothered (a standard measure of negative arousal; Elliot & Devine, 1994). Later, they read an essay purportedly written by Bob advocating for the adoption of senior comprehensive exams that, based on a between-participants manipulation, featured either strong or weak arguments in support of that position, borrowing from a classic paradigm used in persuasion research (Petty & Cacioppo, 1986). Finally, participants reported their opinion about whether their university should institute senior comprehensive exams. Greater persuasion for strong than weak arguments would be evidence of more elaborative processing, consistent with greater scrutiny of Bob's arguments.

Overall, Rydell et al. (2008) found that the greatest evidence of elaborative processing was exhibited when participants' implicit and explicit evaluations were placed in opposition (e.g., negative subliminal primes coupled with positive behavioral sentences about Bob's actions). More important, the relation between implicit–explicit discrepancy and greater argument scrutiny was mediated by participants' report of negative arousal. That is, having greater implicit–explicit discrepancy appears to trigger discomfort, which in turn instigates greater attentional deployment (in this case, more scrutiny of Bob's arguments). A follow-up study by these authors introduced a self-affirmation manipulation, which eliminated these effects. Thus, it appears that when people hold inconsistent evaluations derived from the rule-based and associative systems of evaluation, greater information processing results (e.g., Briñol et al., 2006) and the negative arousal that is triggered induces this greater attentional deployment (Rydell et al., 2008). Returning to the example of the "new neighbors next door," it is possible that the *discomfort* one feels could result from having positive explicit evaluations of the neighbors (from the positive stories they share) but holding more negative implicit evaluations of them (from a pejorative group-association cue; McConnell et al., 2008).

In addition to felt ambivalence, it is possible that holding discrepant explicit and implicit evaluations might have broader judgment and decision-making implications. Our SEM account assumes that only evaluations from the rule-based system are available to individuals for full consideration and reflection. Thus, when people look into the future and attempt to anticipate what will make them happy, they can only draw on knowledge from the rule-based system, which ultimately may only represent a subset of the information that goes into their in-the-moment experiences (Gawronski & Bodenhausen, 2006). Indeed, the literature on affective forecasting shows that people routinely reveal systematic errors when predicting how they will feel (Wilson & Gilbert, 2003). Perhaps one source of affective forecasting errors is people's inability to take into account information from their associative system of evaluation when rendering forecasts about future events in which, ultimately, their in-the-moment enjoyment will be shaped by inputs from both systems of evaluation.

This premise was tested by McConnell, Dunn, Austin, and Rawn (2011), who had participants provide their explicit and implicit evaluations of chocolate and apples. Next, participants predicted how much they would enjoy eating each food item. Finally, they actually ate each food item and reported their actual enjoyment. When using their explicit and implicit evaluations as predictors, only their explicit evaluations uniquely predicted their forecasts (e.g., people who reported on a feeling thermometer that they especially liked chocolate more than apples anticipated that they would prefer chocolate to a greater degree). However, their actual in-the-moment enjoyment of the food items was predicted by both their explicit and implicit evaluations (greater positivity on both explicit and implicit measures predicted greater happiness while actually eating the food items). But most important, the magnitude of their misforecasts (i.e., being "off" in their predictions relative to their actual enjoyment) was uniquely predicted by their implicit evaluations. For example, when some *under*estimated how much they really would enjoy a piece of chocolate more than a piece of apple, the magnitude of their misforecast was predicted by their having an especially positive implicit evaluation of chocolate relative to apples. In other words, the information from their associative system (which may not be available for conscious reflection, according to the SEM) was unavailable at the time of the forecast, yet this knowledge contributed to their in-the-moment enjoyment. Thus, implicit evaluations can represent a blind spot in people's pursuit of happiness. When thinking about our couple that should have gone to the beach instead of the city for a vacation, perhaps there were many positive associations with beaches in memory that defied conscious access and articulation that, while walking on the beach, would have made the smell of fresh salt water and the feeling of warm sand between their toes especially delightful.

Finally, we would propose that implicit–explicit discrepancies might lead to unhappiness not only through affective forecasting errors but also self-regulatory failures. Many important goal-directed behaviors involve people's ability to focus on long-term goals (e.g., losing weight) and avoid short-term temptations (e.g., tasty desserts). When people lose the ability to engage in executive control, they often give in to temptation (e.g., Vohs & Heatherton, 2000). In a study that lends support to the tenets of the SEM, Hofmann et al. (2007) obtained measures of participants' explicit and implicit evaluations of a tempting food item (M&M's candies) and allowed participants to eat as many as they wanted as part of a purported product testing study. Half of their participants were first induced to have cognitive depletion, whereas control participants were not. For those who were not cognitively depleted, their explicit evaluations, but not their implicit evaluations of M&M's, predicted how much of the candy they ate. But in the cognitive depletion condition, implicit evaluations, not explicit evaluations, predicted M&M's consumption. Although Hoffmann et al. did not test the SEM explicitly in their study, we view their findings as quite supportive of it. When cognitive resources are diminished, behavior is less deliberate and action (in this case, eating M&M's) is therefore better predicted by implicit evaluations, because the associative system is not compromised by reductions in central executive resources. Thus, returning to the dieter's dilemma at the beginning of our chapter, the interplay of different systems of evaluation can help predict the individuals for whom reductions in cognitive resources will be especially problematic—those with greater implicit–explicit discrepancies.

SYSTEMS VERSUS PROCESSES: THE SEM IN RELATION TO OTHER ATTITUDE MODELS

The SEM was influenced by several dual-process models of attitudes, most notably the MODE model (motivation and opportunity as determinants; Fazio, 2007), the APE model (associative–propositional evaluation; Gawronski & Bodenhausen, 2006), and the MCM (metacognitive model; Petty, Briñol, & DeMarree, 2007). These models assume that attitudes are the product of two sometimes interrelated processes: an associative process that involves the activation of an association from memory, and a controlled process that, given motivation and cognitive capacity, can transform or invalidate the association accessed from memory. As such, they assume that a single evaluative response to an attitude object is refined over time both to provide the best fit with the context and past experience, and to remain consistent with other motivations and cognitions. The SEM departs from these models in two important ways by hypothesizing that (1) there are distinct systems (not distinct processes) that account for evaluations, and (2) these systems, while potentially interacting, can operate independently and concurrently.

Using the term *system* to describe and explain the joint effect of many different psychological processes that usually work in concert to produce a common output has been criticized (e.g., Keren & Schul, 2009). Two complaints often leveled against systems approaches are that theorizing in terms of systems leads to less specificity than theorizing in terms of processes, and that theorizing in terms of distinct systems does not engender the same level of integration or interaction between the systems as theorizing about distinct processes (e.g., Gawronski & Bodenhausen, 2006). However, we employ the term *system* in the SEM for two reasons. First, we believe more is gained by describing systems than by describing processes. Why might this be? In most dual-process models of attitudes, the associative process and the controlled process each can comprise several different processes; thus, each "process" in traditional dual-process models of attitudes may include many processes or underlying mechanisms. In terms of more associative processes, people must attend to relevant attitude objects, categorize them (either explicitly or implicitly), and integrate the immediate context with past experiences with the object. For more controlled processes, people can validate or invalidate certain evaluations, strive for consistency, embrace social norms, and engage in self-presentation or self-protection. These processes dynamically interact to determine the subsequent evaluation; moreover they are organized in such a way that they "work together." This approach does not reduce the value of understanding any one process within the system or of explicating how this process fits into the system as a whole; instead, it simply recognizes that these processes, when combined together, are part of a greater structure or system that renders evaluations.

Second, we believe that a systems approach more accurately explains the findings presented previously. Specifically, the data showing dissociations between implicit and explicit evaluations in response to presenting valence-inconsistent subliminal primes and behavioral statements about Bob (e.g., Rydell et al., 2006) are more in line with associative and rule-based systems that are sensitive to different types of information. Other attitude models would argue that both implicit and explicit evaluations should be, at least to some degree, affected by both behavioral statements and subliminal primes (cf. Whitfield & Jordan, 2009). That is, because they do not propose distinct evaluative systems that can use different forms of information, they have greater difficulty in explaining these dissociations. Perhaps other models could argue that certain correction processes eliminate the impact of subliminal primes or associative cues on explicit evaluations (e.g., Loersch, McCaslin, & Petty, 2012), but it is harder to understand why behavioral statements would not impact implicit evaluations when presented along with associative forms of information. For example, without putting forward different systems of evaluation, it is difficult to explain why implicit evaluations are more responsive to the valence of the behavioral statements when no associative cues are present but are relatively unaffected by these same behavioral statements when strong associative cues are also present (e.g., McConnell et al., 2008). In the next section of our chapter, we expand more on these findings and why they may occur.

Evidence of implicit–explicit dissociations is also integral to the second assumption of the SEM that is inconsistent with dual-process models of attitudes: The associative and rule-based systems can operate independently and concurrently. For example, it is hard to explain strong dissociations in response to valence-inconsistent subliminal primes and behavioral statements without assuming a relatively strong independence between systems that are operating in parallel. Although we acknowledge that it is difficult to provide unequivocal support for independent systems because implicit and explicit measures (like most psychological measures) are not process-pure (Sherman, 2006), these dissociations, especially because they occur with a diversity of associative cues (some of which may be unavailable to the individual and therefore less likely to be corrected for), provide initial evidence of independence (cf. Keren & Schul, 2009).

Another, related point involves work on explicit–implicit discrepancies, or *implicit ambivalence*. How would prominent dual-process models such as the MODE or the

APE explain implicit ambivalence findings (e.g., Petty et al., 2006)? If inconsistency is solely a function of propositional processes (Gawronski & Bodenhausen, 2006), why would explicit–implicit discrepancies have any impact on subsequent behavior when people are unaware of the discrepancy? Furthermore, any model that starts with a highly accessible attitude being activated from memory, then being altered by subsequent controlled processing, because of its sequential nature and the relative lack of influence of controlled processing on attitudes stored in memory, provides little or no opportunity for explicit–implicit discrepancies to lead to implicit ambivalence (Fazio, 2007). That is, because the MODE model predicts that attitudes are evaluative summaries stored in memory, where the process of forming this summary knowledge eliminates ambivalence, and proposes that more controlled processes have little impact or influence on this stored knowledge (Fazio, 2007), the MODE model seems to have difficulty in explaining implicit ambivalence findings. All of the "conflict resolution" in the MODE and the APE models takes place during controlled processing or by subsequent controlled behavior (e.g., biased information exposure). If there is no reason for controlled processing to occur because one cannot report any ambivalence (e.g., Petty et al., 2006), why would these effects occur?

However, we hasten to add two points. First, it should be noted that because each evaluative system is sensitive to specific types of information does not necessarily make it unresponsive to other forms of information. Rydell and McConnell (2006) showed that implicit evaluations can be influenced by the valence of the behavioral information presented in the absence of associative forms of information (e.g., subliminal primes, associative cues). Also, it has been shown in several lines of research that presenting subliminal primes can impact explicit evaluations (e.g., Murphy & Zajonc, 1993). Thus, it is clear that additional work is needed to understand better when and how associative and behavioral information presented in conjunction with one another selectively affects implicit and explicit evaluations, respectively. The SEM proposes that each system becomes more fully engaged with information to which it is most sensitive and neglects (at least in part) information to which it is less sensitive. Nonetheless, understanding the processes underlying this "engagement" and "neglect" will be important to explain better the attitudinal dissociations obtained in our work and how these systems of evaluation interact.

Finally, we would like to point out that the SEM is different from the dual attitude model (Wilson, Lindsey, & Schooler, 2000), which proposes that "older" attitudes are not replaced by "newer" attitudes when attitude change occurs; instead, these older attitudes are still present in memory and can impact behavior when cognitive resources are reduced. Although both models propose that relatively independent evaluations can exist, the SEM does not require that an attitude change manipulation is necessary to produce these distinct evaluations, nor does it assume that attitude change manipulations are ineffective insofar as "old" attitudes are not stored intact separately in memory from "new" attitudes. Instead, the SEM predicts when, how, and by which types of information evaluations based on each system are likely to form and change.

A MORE ELABORATED, BUT MORE SPECULATIVE, ACCOUNT OF THE SEM

In an effort to explicate the processes underlying somewhat amorphous concepts such as "engagement" and "neglect," as well as to provide a better explanation of how the associative and rule-based systems interact, we speculate on additional elements of the SEM. We start with two basic assumptions. First, systems provide a means to organize different types of mechanisms or processes that have similar features (e.g., Deutsch & Strack, 2006; Smith & DeCoster, 2000), which simply serve to transform inputs, in whatever form, to outputs. Second, all attitude-relevant information that is encoded could, in theory, serve as an input for any process.

Perceivers encode an array of potentially attitude-relevant information when they encounter, interact with, or learn about an attitude object. This information is not represented in a simple way (e.g., a coherent memory, a singular node or concept in an associative network) but is instead represented in a more distributed fashion, and some of these representations may be redundant with others. We use the term *codes* to describe these representations, which is similar to Anderson's (1978) view of mental representations within systems: "Well-designed systems tend to have special representations for the kinds of information they have to process frequently. These representations are designed to facilitate the kind of computations useful for this kind of information" (p. 273). Thus, many different codes that can be created during encoding in response to the same information (e.g., learning about an individual's behavior) are relevant to appraising an object and other object-specific information (e.g., context, goal relevance).

According to this extension of the SEM, specific types of codes should provide the most informative output of a process—with essentially the code that is most easily usable and has the greatest amount of informational value for the most accessible process. The accessibility of the code can also be based on recent or repeated use, with more commonly used codes for a process being the most accessible. A specific code also becomes more accessible if the context during retrieval is similar to the context during encoding, with the role of the context in code accessibility being due in large part to the extent to which the context garnered attention during encoding (Gawronski, Rydell, Verilet, & De Houwer, 2010; Rydell & Gawronski, 2009). In addition, codes that were encoded when certain goals were activated should be more accessible when those goals are also activated during retrieval. As with contexts, the extent to which goals were accessible during encoding should determine how accessible certain codes are to attitudinal processes when goals are activated.

The most important feature of codes for this elaboration of the SEM is the makeup of the code or the information contained within the code (e.g., Anderson, 1978; Wyer & Srull, 1989). Some types of codes should serve as "better" inputs (in terms of the ease with which they can lead to usable outputs) into associative processes. The *associative system* is defined in large part as an interrelated group of processes that utilize specific types of codes. Codes used by the associative system are not verbalizable, not easily used for attributions, not easily converted into propositions, and not easily used for syllogistic reasoning. People may be aware of the outputs of the processes based on these codes, but they should not, under most circumstances, be aware of the codes' existence, because they are unaware of the processes that transform these codes into output. On the other hand, other types of codes serve as "better" inputs into rule-based processes. These types of codes are verbalizeable, can be used when making attributions, can be part of propositions, and can be used in syllogistic reasoning. They also make up many aspects of our subjective experiences, especially if one assumes that the outputs of associative processes can be turned into propositions (e.g., Strack & Deutsch, 2004).

To a large extent, research on the SEM has been concerned with differentiating between the associative and rule-based systems in engineering situations where implicit and explicit attitude measures should presumably be most discrepant. As described earlier, Rydell et al. (2006) found that subliminal primes (100 primes of one valence presented before each behavior) influenced implicit evaluation measures, whereas behavioral information (50 positive and 50 negative descriptive behaviors about which participants received feedback to determine whether the target person performed good or bad actions) influenced explicit evaluation measures, creating a large discrepancy in valence between these measures. Findings such as these may be explained by subliminal primes and behavioral information creating qualitatively different types of codes that are accessible to and utilized by processes underlying the associative system and the rule-based system, respectively. Because codes generated by subliminal primes would likely be perceptual and not verbalizeable, these codes should impact mostly processes in the associative system and would be unlikely to impact processes in the rule-based system. Thus, these codes would lead participants to be "engaged" by these processes, and codes based on the behavioral information, at least in part, may be "neglected" by processes that comprise the associative system. In the most straightforward interpretation of Rydell et al.'s results, encoding behavioral information would provide codes that mostly serve as input for processes underlying the rule-based system. As a result, encoding behavioral information could lead to codes that almost exclusively serve as input for processes that are part of the rule-based system (i.e., codes that are "engaged" by the rule-based system and "neglected" by the associative system).

Such purity, however, seems somewhat unlikely. Instead, it seems more plausible that the behavioral information could lead to the generation of codes that could serve as input to processes in both the associative system and the rule-based system. For example, encoding behavioral information may lead to codes similar to those that underlie processes, such as spontaneous trait inferences (e.g., Winter & Uleman, 1984), which would likely be utilized by processes that are part of the associative system. In addition to these codes, other codes that serve as input for processes of the rule-based system would also be created. If so, the reason why Rydell et al. (2006) might find such large discrepancies between implicit and explicit attitude measures in this paradigm might be that the codes created by encoding behavioral information that influences processes in the associative system may be insensitive to negation (e.g., Deutsch, Gawronski, & Strack, 2006). That is, the valence of the behaviors, and not the feedback about the behaviors, influences these processes, whereas processes that are part of the rule-based system are sensitive to negation (i.e., they are influenced by both the valence of the behaviors and the feedback). Consistent with the idea that behavioral information has less influence on processes that are part of the associative system, Rydell et al. (2008) found that completely crossing the valence of the prime and the behavioral information showed that primes only influenced implicit attitude measures, and that behavioral information only influenced explicit measures. However, Whitfield and Jordan (2009), in a similar study, showed that both primes and behaviors influenced implicit and explicit attitude measures. This difference observed in the Rydell et al. (2008) findings may have been due to the way they presented behavioral information. Unlike Rydell et al., Whitfield and Jordan (2009) presented all positive or all negative behavioral information instead of using feedback to distinguish between positive and negative behavioral information. Given these differences, further research is needed to understand exactly how encoding behavioral information influences measures of implicit evaluation when inconsistent associative information is available.

Regardless, finding dissociations between implicit and explicit attitude measures does not mean, as noted earlier, that the associative and rule-based systems do not interact. For instance, in many cases, processes that are part of the associative system often support the processes involved in the rule-based system. Seeing a TV commercial for a politician may activate positive or negative affect via processes subsumed by the associative system. This affective reaction may be altered or corrected by considering other information about the candidate. Many processes that are part of the rule-based system (e.g., thinking about whether a friend's bad behavior when she was drunk should change one's liking for her) are likely supplemented and directed in large part by processes that are part of the associative system. For example, the propositional information used during this attributional process is likely guided by relatively automatic evaluations of drinking, the friend, and the self (see Strack & Deutsch, 2004, for a similar conceptualization of behavior). If so, how might these processes that are part of different systems interact?

These systems should interact at the level of codes in three main ways. First, they could interact as a result of the presence of codes that contain information that can be used by processes from both the associative and the rule-based system. This could occur because the codes have different features, or because distinct codes with different features are highly interrelated. Second, they could interact in a sequential manner, whereby the output from one type of process, for example, an associative process, provides information that can be used as a code for a process that is part of the rule-based system. Third, they could interact as a result of previous information processing involving both the associative and rule-based system, creating new codes that contain more complicated pieces of information that reduce the number of processes needed to render an evaluation.

Even when codes exist that lead to inconsistent evaluations by the associative and rule-based systems, the systems may interact for a different reason. When the output generated by the systems is highly discrepant in response to an attitude object, this may lead to sufficient arousal (Rydell et al., 2008) that, when attributed to the object (Rydell & Durso, 2012), would lead to increased utilization of processes underlying the rule-based system. Under certain conditions, there may be sufficient processing by the rule-based system, such that the output of this processing might "feed back" into the associative system (e.g., Gawronski & Bodenhausen, 2006). This may be why, for instance, presenting counterattitudinal information impacts implicit measures over time in accordance with the amount of counterattitudinal information presented (e.g., Rydell & McConnell, 2006). However, when there is a relatively large store of associative information (e.g., when the attitude object is a member of a stigmatized group), the impact of the interaction between the associative and rule-based systems would be negligible on implicit measures (e.g., McConnell et al., 2008).

A CAVEAT ABOUT METHODS

One limitation with empirical demonstrations of the SEM to date is that they rely on discrepancies between implicit and explicit evaluation measures to provide evidence for distinct systems. In addition to issues with the logic of "double-dissociation" experiments (e.g., Keren & Schul, 2009), we should reiterate that no measure is process-pure (e.g., Sherman, 2006). That is, there is not a one-to-one correspondence between a measure and a system. While modeling data may shed light on the interaction and how manipulations influence the associative system and the rule-based system, many still unaccounted for pieces of the puzzle are needed to provide evidence for a systems approach (or for that matter, a dual-process approach). Thus, there is a real need to develop measures, paradigms, and sophisticated modeling techniques to elucidate more fully the strengths and weaknesses of all current attitude models. Furthermore, there needs to be greater development of new methods. The most relevant criterion for these new measures, at least in our view, is that they should be designed to address important theoretical debates in the attitudes literature. Creating new measures is not enough. New measures must also address and possibly resolve current debates in the field.

CONCLUSION

In our chapter, we have outlined the SEM and reviewed empirical findings supporting many of its key predictions. The SEM stands apart from other attitude models by asserting that there are two distinct systems of evaluation, the associative system and the rule-based system, each of which can operate relatively independently of the other in terms of attitude formation and revision. Moreover, the SEM anticipates a number of important consequences that result from discrepancies between these two systems of evaluation, ranging from specific asymmetries in behavior to judgment and decision-making shortcomings. We contend that these outcomes are more difficult for existent dual-process models of attitudes to explain than they are for a dual-systems approach. As such, the SEM not only sheds light on a number of important theoretical issues in attitudes and persuasion research, but it also provides a process account that can help explain a variety of interesting phenomena revealed in impression formation (e.g., an odd but undeniably uncomfortable feeling one can have with new acquaintances), in judgment and decision making (e.g., why people might pick the wrong vacation destination), and in self-regulation (e.g., why dieters can have such a hard time putting down a tempting slice of cheesecake).

ACKNOWLEDGMENTS

This work was supported by the Lewis Endowed Professorship at Miami University.

REFERENCES

Anderson, J. R. (1978). Arguments concerning representations for mental imagery. *Psychological Review, 85*, 249–277.

Blair, I. V. (2002). The malleability of automatic stereotypes and prejudice. *Personality and Social Psychology Review, 6*, 242–261.

Briñol, P., Petty, R. E., & Wheeler, S. C. (2006). Discrepancies between explicit and implicit self-concepts: Consequences for information processing. *Journal of Personality and Social Psychology, 91,* 154–170.

Deutsch, R., Gawronski, B., & Strack, F., (2006). At the boundaries of automaticity: Negation as a reflective operation. *Journal of Personality and Social Psychology, 91,* 385–405.

Detsch, R., & Strack, F. (2006). Duality models in social psychology: From dual processes to interacting systems. *Psychological Inquiry, 17,* 166–172.

Dovidio, J. F., Kawakami, K., & Gaertner, S. L. (2002). Implicit and explicit prejudice and interracial interaction. *Journal of Personality and Social Psychology, 82,* 62–68.

Elliot, A. J., & Devine, P. G. (1994). On the motivational nature of cognitive dissonance: Dissonance as psychological discomfort. *Journal of Personality and Social Psychology, 67,* 382–394.

Fazio, R. H. (1986). How do attitudes guide behavior? In R. M. Sorrentino & E. T. Higgins (Eds.), *Handbook of motivation and cognition* (Vol. 1, pp. 204–243). New York: Guilford Press.

Fazio, R. H. (2007). Attitudes as object–evaluation associations of varying strength. *Social Cognition, 25,* 603–637.

Festinger, L. (1957). *A theory of cognitive dissonance.* Palo Alto, CA: Stanford University Press.

Gawronski, B., & Bodenhausen, G. V. (2006). Associative and propositional processes in evaluation: An integrative review of implicit and explicit attitude change. *Psychological Bulletin, 132,* 692–731.

Gawronski, B., Rydell, R. J., Vervliet, B., & De Houwer, J. (2010). Generalization versus contextualization in automatic evaluation. *Journal of Experimental Psychology: General, 139,* 682–701.

Greenwald, A. G., McGhee, D. E., & Schwartz, J. L. K. (1998). Measuring individual differences in implicit cognition: The Implicit Association Test. *Journal of Personality and Social Psychology, 74,* 1464–1480.

Greenwald, A. G., Poehlman, T. A., Uhlmann, E. L., & Banaji, M. R. (2009). Understanding and using the Implicit Association Test: III. Meta-analysis of predictive utility. *Journal of Personality and Social Psychology, 97,* 17–41.

Hofmann, W., Rauch, W., & Gawronski, B. (2007). And deplete us not into temptation: Automatic attitudes, dietary restraint, and self-regulatory resources as determinants of eating behavior. *Journal of Experimental Social Psychology, 43,* 497–504.

Jellison, W. A., McConnell, A. R., & Gabriel, S. (2004). Implicit and explicit measures of sexual orientation attitudes: Ingroup preferences and related behaviors and beliefs among gay and straight men. *Personality and Social Psychology Bulletin, 30,* 629–642.

Kahneman, D. (2003). A perspective on judgment and choice: Mapping bounded rationality. *American Psychologist, 58,* 697–720.

Keren, G., & Schul, Y. (2009). Two is not always better than one: A critical evaluation of two-system theories. *Perspectives on Psychological Science, 4,* 533–550.

Loersch, C., McCaslin, M. J., & Petty, R. E. (2011). Exploring the impact of social judgeability concerns on the interplay of associative and deliberative attitude processes. *Journal of Experimental Social Psychology, 47,* 1029–1032.

McConnell, A. R., Dunn, E. W., Austin, S. N., & Rawn, C. D. (2011). Blind spots in the search for happiness: Implicit attitudes and nonverbal leakage predict affective forecasting errors. *Journal of Experimental Social Psychology, 47,* 628–634.

McConnell, A. R., & Leibold, J. M. (2001). Relations among the Implicit Association Test, discriminatory behavior, and explicit measures of racial attitudes. *Journal of Experimental Social Psychology, 37,* 435–442.

McConnell, A. R., Rydell, R. J., Strain, L. M., & Mackie, D. M. (2008). Forming implicit and explicit attitudes toward individuals: Social group association cues. *Journal of Personality and Social Psychology, 94,* 792–807.

McConnell, A. R., Sherman, S. J., & Hamilton, D. L. (1994). On-line and memory based aspects of individual and group target judgments. *Journal of Personality and Social Psychology, 67,* 173–185.

Murphy, S. T., & Zajonc, R. B. (1993). Affect, cognition, and awareness: Affective priming with optimal and suboptimal stimulus exposures. *Journal of Personality and Social Psychology, 64,* 723–739.

Petty, R. E., Briñol, P., & DeMarree, K. G. (2007). The meta-cognitive model (MCM) of attitudes: Implications for attitude measurement, change, and strength. *Social Cognition, 25,* 657–686.

Petty, R. E., & Cacioppo, J. T. (1986). *Commu-*

nication and persuasion: Central and peripheral routes to attitude change. New York: Springer-Verlag.

Rydell, R. J., & Durso, G. R. O. (2012). Can I borrow a feeling?: Spillover of negative arousal from inconsistent information during attitude formation diminishes perceptions of well-being. *Journal of Experimental Social Psychology, 48*, 575–578.

Rydell, R. J., & Gawronski, B. (2009). I like you, I like you not: Understanding the formation of context dependent automatic evaluations. *Cognition and Emotion, 23*, 1118–1152.

Rydell, R. J., & McConnell, A. R. (2006). Understanding implicit and explicit attitude change: A systems of reasoning analysis. *Journal of Personality and Social Psychology, 91*, 995–1008.

Rydell, R. J., McConnell, A. R., & Mackie, D. M. (2008). Consequences of discrepant explicit and implicit attitudes: Cognitive dissonance and increased information processing. *Journal of Experimental Social Psychology, 44*, 1526–1532.

Rydell, R. J., McConnell, A. R., Mackie, D. M., Strain, L. M. (2006). Of two minds: Forming and changing valence inconsistent attitudes. *Psychological Science, 17*, 954–958.

Rydell, R. J., McConnell, A. R., Strain, L. M., Claypool, H. M., & Hugenberg, K. (2007). Implicit and explicit attitudes respond differently to increasing amounts of counterattitudinal information. *European Journal of Social Psychology, 37*, 867–878.

Schwarz, N., & Clore, G. L. (2007). Feelings and phenomenal experiences. In E. T. Higgins & A. W. Kruglanski (Eds.), *Social psychology: Handbook of basic principles* (2nd ed., pp. 385–407). New York: Guilford Press.

Sherman, J. W. (2006). On building a better process model: It's not only how many, but which ones and by which means? *Psychological Inquiry, 17*, 173–184.

Sinclair, S., Dunn, E. W., & Lowery, B. (2005). The influence of parental racial attitudes on children's automatic racial prejudice. *Journal of Experimental Social Psychology, 41*, 283–289.

Sloman, S. A. (1996). The empirical case for two systems of reasoning. *Psychological Bulletin, 119*, 3–22.

Smith, E. R., & DeCoster, J. (2000). Dual-process models in social and cognitive psychology: Conceptual integration and links to underlying memory systems. *Personality and Social Psychology Review, 4*, 108–131.

Strack, F., & Deutsch, R. (2004). Reflective and impulsive determinants of social behavior. *Personality and Social Psychology Review, 8*, 220–247.

Vohs, K. D., & Heatherton, T. F. (2000). Self-regulatory failure: A resource-depletion approach. *Psychological Science, 11*, 249–254.

Whitfield, M., & Jordan, C. J. (2009). Mutual influence of implicit and explicit attitudes. *Journal of Experimental Social Psychology, 45*, 748–759.

Wilson, T. D., & Gilbert, D. T. (2003). Affective forecasting. In M. P. Zanna (Ed.), *Advances in experimental social psychology* (Vol. 35, pp. 345–411). San Diego: Academic Press.

Wilson, T. D., Lindsey, S., & Schooler, T. Y. (2000). A model of dual attitudes. *Psychological Review, 107*, 101–126.

Winter, L., & Uleman, J. S. (1984). When are social judgments made?: Evidence for the spontaneousness of trait inferences. *Journal of Personality and Social Psychology, 47*, 237–251.

Wyer, R. S., & Srull, T. K. (1989). *Memory and cognition in its social context*. Hillside, NJ: Erlbaum.

PART V

SOCIAL PERCEPTION

CHAPTER 15

Controlled Processing and Automatic Processing in the Formation of Spontaneous Trait Inferences

Randy J. McCarthy and John J. Skowronski

Perceivers use the extracted trait implications of observed behaviors to make generalizations about the underlying dispositions of those performing the behaviors. For example, on hearing that Jeff published a scholarly article, perceivers may infer that Jeff is smart. The thought that Jeff is smart can feel as if it emerged effortlessly. It may even appear to the perceiver that smartness is an inherent property of Jeff or of Jeff's behaviors rather than a product of the perceiver's inferential processes.

Considerable evidence suggests that perceivers can make sense of incoming social information with minimal effort or awareness because of the rapid and unintentional application of knowledge structures to the interpretation of perceived behaviors. Indeed, such application often produces *spontaneous trait inferences* (STIs) in which the trait is seen as an inherent property of the actor. These spontaneous inferences can be made while encoding information about an actor and his or her behavior and are generated in the absence of an explicit goal to form trait inferences.

THIS CHAPTER'S THREE MAIN STI THEMES

In this chapter we discuss these STIs and conceptualize the relevant literature around three themes:

1. We explicitly couch STIs as phenomena that possess characteristics of both controlled processes and automatic processes.
2. We explicitly discuss the structure and characteristics of STIs that are stored in memory.
3. We introduce a distinction between *STI generation* (i.e., the actual inference of trait information, linking of the trait with an actor, and encoding the actor–trait dyad into memory) and *STI expression* (the effect that already-stored STIs have on subsequent processing and responding (for previous reviews of STIs, see Skowronski, Carlston, & Hartnett, 2008; Uleman, Newman, & Moskowitz, 1996; Uleman, Saribay, & Gonzales, 2008).

To provide a preview of the remainder of the chapter, we would like to briefly introduce each of these themes.

Theme 1: Automatic Processing and Controlled Processing in STIs

Our first theme addresses the extent to which STIs may exhibit characteristics of both automatic processing and controlled processing. Our view of automatic processing is taken from the taxonomy provided by Bargh (1994). Automatic processes (1) may be elicited without intent, (2) can proceed with few cognitive resources, (3) cannot be voluntarily stopped once started, and (4) can operate outside of awareness. Conversely, controlled processes are those not characterized by these features.

Throughout this chapter we relate STI research findings to the distinction between controlled processes and automatic processes. That STIs may sometimes appear to be automatic is straightforward: Because the defining characteristic of STIs (i.e., the spontaneity) is that they occur without intent, virtually by definition, STIs must possess some features of automaticity. However, STIs also possess characteristics that typify controlled processing. Thus, STIs are influenced by automatic processes in some ways but are controllable in other ways. Our discussion of STIs will reflect this duality.

Theme 2: STIs, Fast-Learning Memory, and Slow-Learning Memory

Our second theme reflects the cognitive structure of the trait information that is acquired about others. Theorists (e.g., Sloman, 1996; Smith & DeCoster, 2000) suggest that acquired trait knowledge can take two forms. One form is acquired by, and stored in, a "slow-learning" system that reflects knowledge about co-occurrences in the world. A second form is acquired by, and stored in, a "fast-learning" system in which knowledge is acquired via mechanisms such as language and inference-making.

We believe that exposure to trait-implying behaviors can cause information acquisition to occur in both systems. On the one hand, we suggest that exposure to trait-implying behaviors can cause the development and strengthening of associations between actors and traits in the slow-learning system. These associations should strengthen slowly as perceivers repeatedly encounter someone who performs a behavior relevant to a given trait. On the other hand, exposure to trait-implying behaviors can also imply acquisition of inferences about the actor. These should be acquired quickly and should reflect the fact that a trait is seen as a property of the actor (and is not just associated with the actor). In addition to elaborating on the idea of a dual-storage system in the context of STIs, in this chapter we outline some of the consequences of this idea.

Theme 3: STI Generation versus STI Expression

For our third theme we introduce a distinction between the formation of STIs and other cognitive processes associated with STIs. We apply the term *STI generation* when participants infer a trait concept and see that trait as a property of an actor. We use the term *STI expression* to refer to other cognitions that are relevant to STIs.

We make this *STI generation* versus *STI expression* distinction because it is not uncommon for these two concepts to be referred to synonymously in the academic literature. However, these concepts are not synonymous. To understand STIs and how they work, one needs to understand STI generation, the cognitive structures and processes that are involved in the storage of STIs, and the effects that STIs have on processing that occurs after trait inferences about the actors are produced and stored (i.e., STI expression). Moreover, we argue that STI generation and STI expression both exhibit characteristics of automatic processing and characteristics of controlled processing, and we describe research supporting this claim.

SETTING THE STAGE FOR STIs: KNOWLEDGE STRUCTURES LINKING BEHAVIORS AND TRAITS

STI generation assumes that perceivers possess knowledge structures indicating that behaviors are observable expressions of an actor's underlying disposition. These knowledge structures are accessed when encountering an actor's behaviors and are used to generate trait inferences about the actor. This is a seemingly straightforward idea. Making an inference that Donal is creative when seeing him construct an aesthetically pleasing artwork from scraps of wood necessarily implies the presence of stored knowledge linking the behavior (constructing pleasing artwork) to the trait (creative).

Evidence for this idea can be demonstrated by examining differences in the knowledge structures people possess and the subsequent STIs formed. If STIs are driven by these knowledge structures, then different knowledge structures should produce different STIs. Numerous examples of this idea can be found in research: (1) Parents at high risk for child physical abuse spontaneously form more negative, relative to positive, trait inferences from the observation of children's behaviors (Crouch et al., 2010); (2) aggressive individuals spontaneously encode ambiguously hostile behaviors in aggressive trait terms, whereas nonaggressive individuals encode these behaviors in nonaggressive trait terms (e.g., Zelli, Cervone, & Huesmann, 1996); and (3) individual differences in the trait of authoritarianism may guide subsequently formed STIs (e.g., Uleman, Winborne, Winter, & Shechter, 1986). Other studies have assessed differences in individual worldviews (often influenced by culture) and linked those differences to STI generation. For example, persons with individualistic (vs. collectivistic) worldviews are especially likely to believe that behaviors have an internal genesis and to possess knowledge structures prompting dispositional (vs. situational) interpretations of the behavior of others (e.g., Na & Kitayama, 2011; Zárate, Uleman, & Voils, 2001).

Other studies pointing to the importance of knowledge structures to the formation of inferences have explored the effect of knowledge structure accessibility on subsequent inferences. This is commonly done using the experimental technique known as *priming*, which is exemplified by a classic study exploring impression formation (Higgins, Rholes, & Jones, 1977). As part of a bogus "perceptual task" some participants were exposed to words associated with the construct of "reckless" and some were exposed to words associated with the construct of "adventurous." Later, in an ostensibly unrelated task, participants formed impressions of persons performing ambiguously reckless–ambiguous behaviors. Despite being exposed to the same behavior descriptions, participants exposed to the different primes made different judgments, and these judgments were consistent with the primed constructs.

In the Higgins et al. (1977) study the impressions formed were not spontaneous, but were elicited by experimental instructions. However, the logic of differential knowledge structure accessibility has been extended into STI research. For example, Newman and Uleman (1990) conducted two experiments in which different participants were subtly primed with different traits prior to reading a list of ambiguous behaviors. Their results showed that when priming occurred outside of awareness, participants spontaneously interpreted behaviors in terms of the primed trait. In other words, if "persistent" was activated by a prime, then a perceiver would see Mike's behavior "he would not take no as an answer" as persistent and judge Mike to be persistent. Thus, knowledge structure accessibility can influence interpretations of behaviors during their encoding and inferences made about actors based on those behaviors.

Knowledge structure accessibility research results show that repeated exposure to stimuli that temporarily heighten schema accessibility may ultimately produce chronic accessibility of the knowledge structures that guide impression formation (e.g., Higgins, King, & Mavin, 1982). Such results cause one to wonder whether individual differences, priming, and differences in chronic accessibility of schemas are at all related to one another; they seem to be. Bargh, Bond, Lombardi, and Tota (1986) conducted a study in which some participants were identified as having chronically accessible schemas of kindness (i.e., chronics) or not (i.e., nonchronics). The researchers also subliminally primed some participants with the trait "kind." Participants then completed a judgment task in which they interpreted a target's behaviors, then rated the target's kindness. The results were clear. The highest target trait ratings were provided by chronics who were also primed. The lowest trait ratings were provided by nonchronics who were not primed. Middling in their responses were nonprimed chronics and primed nonchronics.

Such results suggest that differences in knowledge structure accessibility can be caused by consistent pairing of stimuli and cognitions to the point that the stimuli can unintentionally elicit the application of knowledge structures. However, knowledge structure accessibility can also be temporarily heightened via priming. Thus, chronically accessible knowledge structures likely operate through the same cognitive mechanisms as temporarily accessible knowledge structures. To our knowledge, the additive effects of chronic and temporary schema accessibility have not been tested in the context of STIs. However, current theorizing about cognition and STIs suggests that such a study would produce results consistent with the data produced by Bargh et al. (1986).

STIs CAN OCCUR AT ENCODING AND DO NOT DEPEND ON MEMORY FOR BEHAVIORS

A battle that STI researchers continually fight is to demonstrate that measures of trait inferences are capturing STIs formed during behavior encoding and are not memory-based inferences. For example, if results suggest that perceivers believe Amanda to be smart, one might wonder whether this belief is based on a spontaneous inference formed during behavior encoding or derived from participants' ability to recall that Amanda published a paper in a scientific journal, with the inference formed using the recalled information only when the inference is requested.

This latter possibility indicates that it is especially tricky to measure STIs. Much like trying to see whether the light stays on when the refrigerator door is closed, the mere attempt at measuring STIs may prompt inference making. This measurement conundrum has been addressed in a few ways. First, researchers often use indirect measures to capture STIs. These methods attempt to measure the presence of STIs without asking participants to try and report any inferences about the actors. For example, the often-used false-recognition paradigm is ostensibly a recall accuracy task. Forming trait inferences based on recalled information is irrelevant to participants' goal to respond accurately. Thus, the systematic pattern of falsely recognizing traits that were never shown suggests the tacit influence of STIs.

However, though ambiguous as to the processes contributing to inference making, direct measures of inferences can be useful in the pursuit of STI evidence. For example, asking participants to provide trait ratings of an actor would seem to encourage recall and use of any information about an actor they have available. Thus, trait ratings may reflect both STIs and recalled information about the behaviors. However, it may be unclear from those trait ratings how much of each contributes to the observed ratings. So why would researchers ever use trait ratings to measure STIs? Because trait ratings provide information that some indirect measures do not. For example, STIs produce "halo effects" in trait ratings. This result suggests that STIs possess inferential properties (e.g., Carlston & Skowronski, 2005), something that is difficult to demonstrate using indirect measures.

Other ways in which the measurement conundrum has been addressed are (1) by comparing inferences that are thought to be made spontaneously to inferences that are thought to be made effortfully (e.g., Carlston & Skowronski, 1994; McCarthy & Skowronski, 2011a; Todorov & Uleman, 2002; Uleman & Moskowitz, 1994), and (2) by inhibiting participants' ability to use recalled information. For example, some researchers have statistically controlled for participants' ability to recall information on which the inferences were based (e.g., McCarthy & Skowronski, 2011b), omitted data from trials in which participants recognized behaviors (e.g., Carlston & Skowronski, 1994), or minimized behavior recall by including delays of up to a week between encoding and inference measurement (e.g., Carlston & Skowronski, 1994; Todorov & Uleman, 2004). In all cases participants' recall ability was independent of STI expression, indicating that the STIs, and not memory for the behaviors, were responsible for the observed results.

THE DUAL CHARACTERISTICS OF STI GENERATION: A LITTLE AUTOMATICITY, A LITTLE CONTROLLED PROCESSING

One issue that often emerged in this area is whether STIs are made automatically or whether they reflect controlled processing. A more nuanced view that is reflected in recent thinking is that outcomes can reflect some combination of automatic processing and controlled processing. We note that the data suggest that this conclusion applies to STIs.

STIs Can Exhibit Properties Reflecting Automaticity

STIs sometimes reflect at least three characteristics (e.g., Bargh, 1994) of automaticity. They can occur in the absence of conscious goals to make trait inferences (spontaneity). They can occur in the absence of awareness of the process of inference making (lack of awareness). They can occur in the face of diminished cognitive capacity (efficiency). Illustrative evidence on these points is presented in the paragraphs that follow.

STI Spontaneity

By definition, STIs are spontaneous. The characteristic of *spontaneity* refers to the fact that trait inferences can occur without external prompts or in the absence of conscious goals to generate inferences. Indeed, in typical STI studies, trait inferences are detectable even though participants are not instructed to infer traits. That is, evidence of inference making on later tasks indicates that even without instructing participants to form impressions about the actors, participants nonetheless do so (e.g., Carlston & Skowronski, 1994; Carlston, Skowronski, & Sparks, 1995; Todorov & Uleman, 2002).

Particularly strong evidence for spontaneity emerges when the inference-prompting information is thought by participants to be "irrelevant" to the central experimental task. For example, Winter, Uleman, and Cunniff (1985; see also Lupfer, Clark, & Hutcherson, 1990; Uleman, Moskowitz, Roman, & Rhee, 1993; Uleman, Newman, & Winter, 1992) presented trait-implicative behaviors as part of a "filler task" and still found evidence that participants generated inferences about the actors described in the filler task.

Lack of STI Awareness

STIs sometimes exhibit other characteristics of automaticity. For example, STIs can occur outside of the perceivers' awareness, a conclusion derived from research using a false-recognition paradigm (e.g., McCarthy & Skowronski, 2011a; Todorov & Uleman, 2002). This paradigm exposes participants to actors (identified via photographs) paired with behaviors. Some behavior descriptions both implied and contained a trait word (e.g., *He is generous and left a 45% tip*); other behavior descriptions implied but did not contain a trait word (e.g., *He left a 45% tip*). Presumably, in both types of trials, during encoding participants form actor–trait inferences. Later, participants saw the actors paired with a trait word (e.g., *generous*) and their task was to determine (*yes* or *no*) whether or not the trait word actually appeared in the behavior that was previously paired with the actor. In signal detection terms, participants could correctly identify traits that were actually shown (i.e., "hits") or erroneously identify traits that were implied but not shown (i.e., "false alarms"). In a third type of trial—a "control" trial—the to-be-recognized trait was neither shown nor implied by the behavior previously paired with the photograph. A reliable finding indicative of STI generation is that participants more often falsely identify traits as being in a sentence on false alarm trials than on control trials. Assuming that people are motivated to provide correct responses, these false identifications suggest that people are not aware that they are making these mistakes.

Additional evidence suggesting that STIs can be made without awareness was provided by Moskowitz and Roman (1992). In accordance with the well-established assimilation effect in priming research, they reasoned that tacit activation of a trait concept should cause perceivers to assimilate subsequently encountered information to the activated trait (e.g., Lombardi, Higgins, & Bargh, 1987). This is precisely what they found. Participants without an impression-formation goal who first read behaviors implying the traits *confident* and *persistent* rated the protagonist of a vignette they subsequently read as especially confident and persistent. Additionally, Moskowitz and Roman (1992) instructed other participants to form impressions of actors intentionally. They reasoned that these participants should have been especially aware of the constructs implied by the behaviors, and this awareness would induce them to be especially unlikely to assimilate subsequently encountered information to those constructs. Indeed, participants in this condition who read behaviors implying the traits *confident* and *persistent* subsequently rated the vignette protagonist as especially *un*confident and *non*persistent. In other words, in this study, intentionally inferred traits led to contrast effects in the processing of subsequently encountered information, but traits inferred spontaneously led to assimilation effects. This divergence in results between the encoding conditions strongly suggests that STIs in the tacit (no goal) condition were formed outside the awareness of the perceiver.

STI Efficiency

Data also suggest that STI production can be highly efficient. In experiments in which participants' cognitive resources are allocated to tasks such as rehearsing short groupings of digits, levels of STI production are sometimes comparable to those exhibited by participants' who devote all their cognitive resources to processing information about actor behaviors (e.g., Crawford, Skowronski, Stiff, & Sherer, 2007; Todorov & Uleman, 2003). Even in studies in which such cognitive load manipulations significantly diminished STI production, evidence for STI production was merely reduced, never eliminated (e.g., Wells, Skowronski, Crawford, Scherer, & Carlston, 2011).

STIs Can Exhibit Properties Reflecting Controlled Processing

It was evident early in STI research that there is a distinction to be made between *spontaneity* and *automaticity*. STIs are clearly unintentional, which is one characteristic of automatic processing. However, for an outcome to be fully automatic, the outcome must meet other criteria. Although it is true that STIs sometimes exhibit the automaticity-indicative properties of unintentionality, lack of awareness, and efficiency, it would be a mistake to conclude that STIs are fully automatic. Automatic processes should be resistant to manipulation or intervention, and that is definitely not a characteristic of STIs. Illustrative evidence is described in the sections that follow.

Cognitive Capacity Studies

One approach to showing that a process is not automatic is to demonstrate that it requires cognitive resources. This has been tried by a number of researchers, and evidence from STI studies that experimentally manipulated cognitive processing resources has been mixed.

Todorov and Uleman (2003) conducted a series of such studies using the false-recognition paradigm. In one study, the presentation time of actors paired with short behaviors was reduced to 2 seconds. This reduction in presentation time, although surely limiting participants' ability to engage in effortful processing, did not inhibit STI generation relative to a self-paced comparison group. In a second experiment, instructing participants to adopt a shallow processing goal (i.e., counting nouns) slightly reduced evidence of STI generation. Finally, participants completing a concurrent load task evinced STI generation comparable to that provided by participants who were not under cognitive load (see also Crawford et al., 2007; Lupfer et al., 1990; Winter et al., 1985).

In comparison, Uleman et al. (1992) found that concurrent load did affect STI generation. Results provided by Wells et al. (2011) similarly showed that as cognitive load increased and the cognitive resources available for actor–trait linking decreased, evidence for STI generation decreased. Wells et al. also found that similar results were evident in individuals with dispositionally varied working memory capacity. However, even here, persons with low working memory capacity experiencing high cognitive load yielded evidence of STI generation, albeit to a reduced degree. Nonetheless, a fair appraisal of results across all of these studies suggests that although STI generation is efficient, it does seem to require some degree of cognitive processing resources.

Processing Goal Studies

Other manipulations can similarly affect the extent to which trait inferences about actors are generated. These manipulations do not affect STIs by making finite cognitive resources scarce, but they demonstrate STIs' nonautomaticity by showing that STI generation and expression vary across conditions that alter cognitive processing. Such elasticity is inconsistent with the notion of automaticity. If a process is automatic, it should be immune to such manipulations.

Working from the belief that traits are elaborations of behaviors, some researchers have suggested that providing participants with goals that make elaborative thinking difficult should reduce the tendency to infer traits. One way to accomplish this is to provide participants with a goal to search for a series of letters while reading trait-implicative behaviors. In one experiment using this "grapheme search" manipulation (Uleman & Moskowitz, 1994) participants read trait-implicative behaviors and were given one of three sentence features to analyze: Some were told to search for graphemes; others were told to search for phonemes; and still others were told to determine the gender of the persons described. Evidence for STI generation was weakest in participants searching for graphemes, intermediate in those searching for phonemes, and strongest in participants determining actor gender (also see McCarthy & Skowronski, 2011a).

Documenting the effect of processing goals on STIs was also central to studies conducted by Crawford et al. (2007). Their results indicated that when participants were instructed to determine whether an informant was telling lies or telling the truth, STI generation was diminished. However, as effective as the lie detection instructions were at interfering with STI generation, more research is needed in to pinpoint the mechanism through which this manipulation operates. One interpretation is that determining whether an informant is being truthful requires working memory resources: Participants following these instructions may be introducing a self-imposed cognitive load while processing the stimuli. A second interpretation is that the lie detection instruction causes participants to make inferences about truthfulness instead of about the traits implied by the behaviors. Regardless of the exact explanation, the goal to detect whether the described behaviors were lies clearly interfered with STI generation.

Rim, Uleman, and Trope (2009) provided another example of conscious processing goals affecting STI generation. Construal-level theory (e.g., Trope & Liberman, 2010) suggests that psychologically distant objects are thought of more abstractly and schematically than are psychologically near objects. If traits are indeed abstractions made from behaviors, then the theory suggests that thinking about psychologically distant others should increase the likelihood that those persons' behaviors would be encoded in trait terms. As expected from the theory, Rim et al. (2009) found that those directly instructed to process information abstractly were especially likely to form STIs. Additional results showed that the behaviors of others who were spatially or temporally nearby prompted fewer STIs than the behaviors of spatially or temporally distant others.

AUTOMATIC PROCESSING AND CONTROLLED PROCESSING IN STI EXPRESSION

To this point we have focused on STI generation. in the next sections we discuss how already-formed STIs can affect subsequent cognition. We devote the first section to cognitive structures and cognitive processes that might be linked to STIs, and offer ideas about how acquired trait knowledge is stored. Specifically, we suggest that STIs may cause information to be stored simultaneously in one memory system that tracks associations and in another system responsible for the storage of conceptual knowledge.

In a second section that addresses STI expression, we argue that if STIs are indeed about actors' dispositions, and are not merely traits associated with actors, then one should be able to detect the unique signatures of these inferences. We also discuss the possible controllability of STI expression. Questions of interest are whether STIs become automatically accessible on seeing a person for whom an inference is held, and whether perceivers can inhibit the expression of STIs using controlled processing.

Acquiring and Storing Trait Knowledge via Dual-Processing Systems

One issue that has pushed STI research forward is the extent to which measurements of STIs merely reflect the formation of associations between actors and traits or whether they truly reflect inferences about the actors. Associations can merely index the fact that two events or concepts have been noted to co-occur. Inferences similarly track this co-occurrence, but with the addition of extra information. In the case of trait inferences, this extra information is that the trait is considered to be a property of the actor. Hence, one way to view inferences is in terms of "associations plus": Inferences not only reflect associative knowledge (Tom–kind) but also indicate the nature of the conceptual relation between the concepts that are involved in the association (Tom *is* kind).

Evidence of such duality might have been seen in a study described by Skowronski, Carlston, Mae, and Crawford (1998). In this study, some participants were told that actors, depicted by photos, were describing their own trait-implicative behaviors. It was expected that this belief should prompt participants to make inferences about the actors (i.e., STI condition). Participant responses in this condition suggested that they did so. However, other participants believed that actor–behavior pairs had nothing to do with each other and that pairs were created arbitrarily. It was expected that this condition should preclude making inferences about the people in the photos. Yet participants in this condition still responded as if the pairing had caused them to associate persons depicted in the photos with the traits implied by the behavior with which each photo was paired. This well-replicated effect has been dubbed spontaneous trait transference (STT).

The result fits with the notions that people can be associated with traits, that people can have trait inferences made about them, and that these two sources of stored trait knowledge are not the same. In pursuing these ideas, a number of experiments has explored whether responses in STI and STT conditions differ (they do), whether effects in STI and STT conditions are responsive to different manipulations (they are), and whether effects in STI and STT conditions seem to have different properties (they do). These results are reviewed in Skowronski et al. (2008), so there is no need to duplicate them here. However, it is useful to our purposes in this chapter to review some conclusions derived from that review (see also Goren & Todorov, 2009).

The first conclusion is that the intuition of Skowronski et al. (1998) seemed to be correct: There does seem to be a difference between trait knowledge acquired in STT conditions and trait knowledge acquired in STI conditions. For example, the trait knowledge acquired in STT and STI conditions accumulates at different rates (faster in STI than in STT). A second conclusion, one that is especially germane to our chapter, is the idea that the trait knowledge acquired in STI conditions seems to reflect "associations plus." One implication is that if one can cause inference-making mechanisms to be turned off or circumvented, the data in STI and STT conditions can be made to look the same. However, a second implication is that trait knowledge can be acquired about individuals via the formation and strengthening of actor–trait links, even when the mental mechanisms responsible for inference making about actors are shut down.

Such outcomes suggest the presence of, and simultaneous operation of, two mental mechanisms that foster information acquisition and retain different forms of information: One is associational in nature and the other is inferential in nature. One recent series of studies by McCarthy, Wells, Skowronski, and Carlston (2013) sought to collect data reflecting this distinction. Their studies compared how participants in STT conditions and STI conditions reacted to repeated pairings of informants with trait-implicative behaviors. In one study, informants describing either the self (STI) or another person (STT) were paired with one trait-implying behavior, five behaviors implying the same trait, or 10 behaviors implying the same trait. In a later task, participants tried to associate traits with informants such that they could recall the trait when cued with an informant photo. As in most studies, when a trait-implying behavior was presented only once, evidence of informant–trait linkage was greater in the STI condition than in the

STT condition. As the number of repetitions of informants and trait-implicative behaviors increased, data reflecting the strength of actor–trait associations also increased. However, the rate of increase was similar for STT and STI conditions. This similarity in acquisition rate occurred regardless of whether behaviors in the multiple-behavior condition were the same as the original behavior (no new information) or differed from the original behavior (converging implications condition).

The implication is that the difference in recall on the first trial reflected the differential impact of inference making (STI) and association (STT) on mental representations of the informants. In theory, on the first trial both STT and STI conditions produced informant–trait links, but in the STI condition additional information reflecting inferences about informants was extracted and stored. Thus, the view of McCarthy et al. (2013) was that repeated exposure to trait-implying behaviors did not affect the strength of informant–trait inferences but did affect the strength of informant–trait associations, even in the STI condition.

To understand this conclusion, contrast the results of this first study with results from a second study that used a trait ratings measure instead of a recall task. The researchers believed that in STI conditions the converging behaviors would add information that would be relevant to participants' judgments. Hence, judgments from behaviors with converging implications should be more extreme than judgments made from an equal number of identical trait-implicative behaviors. The data confirmed these expectations. However, in STT conditions, because informants were not describing themselves, no new information about informants should have been added with repeated behaviors, even when events were nonidentical but had converging implications. This implies that trait judgments in STT conditions ought to have been equally affected by repetition, regardless of whether the behaviors described were identical or nonidentical but had converging implications. These patterns were observed in the judgment data obtained in STT conditions.

The results of these two studies suggest three conclusions. First, in both STT and STI conditions, there is an association formed between informants and traits, and this can similarly be strengthened with repetition. Second, in STI conditions, the link that is formed can be viewed as "association-plus." That "plus" is an inference that labels the trait as a property of the actor. Third, while the association is not especially strengthened by presentation of behaviors with converging trait implications (compared to repetition of the same behavior), the inference is strengthened by the presentation of such converging behaviors. Such results are consistent with the view that spontaneous inferences cause changes both in the memory system that reflects informant–trait associative knowledge and in the memory system that reflects inferences that are made about informants based on the trait implications of the behaviors described.

Expressions of Acquired Trait Knowledge

Once formed and stored, the trait knowledge acquired after making STIs should affect responses on other tasks. The nature of such effects can point back to the inferential nature of acquired trait knowledge. For example, Kressel and Uleman (2010) demonstrated that participants identified actions preceded by traits (e.g., clumsy → stumble) faster than traits preceded by actions (e.g., stumble → clumsy). This paralleled the manner in which participants identified other causally related concepts (i.e., spark → fire vs. fire → spark), a result suggesting that mental representations of trait inferences contain causal relations to concepts such as behaviors. Furthermore, evidence from spontaneous causal inference research suggests that, in much the same manner as STIs, these causal implications have some elements of automaticity, in that they can emerge outside of awareness (e.g., Hassin, Bargh, & Uleman, 2002).

McCarthy and Skowronski (2011b) examined additional downstream consequences of the formation and storage of STIs. They reasoned that acquired trait knowledge could be used to make predictions about the future behaviors of persons about whom STIs were made. The behaviors about which the participants were making predictions were pretested, so that the trait implications of such behaviors were known. Thus, participants in the studies could predict whether actors would behave consistently with a spontaneously inferred disposition or not. The results were clear: They did. Participants predicted that actors would behave in a manner consistent with trait implications of the behaviors previously paired with the actors.

McCarthy and Skowronski (2011b) also wondered whether participants could refrain from using trait knowledge once it was spontaneously acquired. Exploring this, they told some participants that behaviors paired with actors were misleading so that attempts should be made *not* to use that information in behavior predictions. Although the extremity of the predictions was somewhat reduced by these instructions, participants' predictions about the actors remained consistent with the trait implications of the behaviors previously paired with the actors. Thus, participants were influenced by STIs, even when trying not to be. This suggests that some degree of automaticity exists when people apply their spontaneously acquired trait knowledge to other cognitions about actors. However, the reduction in ratings observed by McCarthy and Skowronski also suggests that controlled processing can contribute to the use of spontaneously derived trait knowledge.

These implications converge with results obtained by other researchers. For example, Uleman et al. (1996) used a recognition probe paradigm in which participants read trait-implicative behaviors. Immediately following the behavior descriptions, participants had to determine quickly and accurately whether a word appeared in the previously read behavior. When the to-be-recognized word was a trait implied by the previous behavior, participants exhibited more errors and longer decision latencies than when the to-be-recognized word was not implied. In Na and Kitayama's (2011) variation of this paradigm, behaviors were paired with actor photographs, thus allowing for STI–actor associations to develop. Later, seeing the actor facilitated participants' ability to recognize trait words implied by the behaviors previously paired with the actors.

These two findings may appear contradictory—in one instance, STIs facilitate responding on a later task; in the other, STIs prompt slow responses. However, in our view, these studies nicely highlight fact that the STI expression can cause effects on subsequent cognition via both controlled processing and automatic processing. In the Na and Kitayama (2011) studies, the spontaneously inferred traits were linked to actor photos. Thus, presentation of the photo should increase trait accessibility, which should facilitate recognition. Moreover, in this case, even if this accessibility-driven (and largely automatic) route to responding were unavailable (i.e., no inference was made), a correct response could still be produced by recalling the initial behavior–actor pairing. The important point is that on these trials, controlled processing does not conflict with automatic processing: both are working "in the same direction." However, in the Uleman et al. (1996) recognition probe paradigm—in which people immediately determine whether the trait appeared in a previously read behavior—they are not working "in the same direction." Instead, in the Uleman et al. study, the spontaneous activation of a trait caused by the presentation of trait-implicative behavior may conflict with accurate memory for the original behavior. In other words, in this paradigm, the two processes work against each other and cause slow and erroneous responding. Therefore, there is no contradiction in the results from these two paradigms. Whether responses are facilitated by prior exposure to a trait-implicative behavior or are impaired by a prior exposure depends entirely on the cognitive processes used to produce responses in that task.

Consider this point in the context of the different tasks used by Uleman et al. (1996) and Na and Kitayama (2011). Expression of a trait inference in these tasks can be due to two different processes. The first process is the retrieval of trait inferences formed during encoding. On seeing the person for whom an impression is held, trait information associated with that person may become accessible (e.g., Na & Kitayama, 2011). This increase in trait accessibility may influence subsequent responding outside of perceiver awareness. The second process is the effortful retrieval of information about the target of the inferences. That is, people can effortfully search their memories for information that is relevant to a trait judgment, and they can also have some discretion about how to use it.

Given this duality, on many measures, the exact mechanism responsible for the impact of exposure to trait-implicative behaviors can be unclear. That is, if one assesses the impact of such exposures on trait judgments, it is difficult to know whether an observed change in ratings is due to the influence of trait knowledge accessibility, effortful recall, or some unknown combination of the two.

Data from the false-recognition paradigm often used in STI research can be used to address this issue. The task is structured to create inner conflicts within participants as to whether a trait actually appeared in a behavior previously paired with an actor or not. The extent to which people accurately distinguish between traits internally generated during encoding and traits retrieved from episodic recall provides researchers with a sense of inference making during encoding.

However, correct responding on this task does *not* assess the extent to which the influence of STIs on trait recognition performance is attributable to automatic processes, and the extent to which performance is attributable to controlled processes. This is because on trials leading to hits (correct recognition of previously seen traits), actor–trait associations and effortful recall both favor the same response. A high hit rate can be due to strong actor–trait associations *or* to good behavior recall, *or* to a combination of the two. The situation differs for *false alarms* (incorrect decisions that a trait was previously seen when, in fact, it was implied): Actor–trait associations work *in opposition to* behavior recall. A low false-alarm rate can be due to weak actor–trait associations being expressed *or* to good behavior recall, *or* to a combination of the two.

The process dissociation procedure (PDP; Jacoby, 1991) specifies methods that can be applied to these data. Its methods and calculations allow separate examination of automatic influences and controlled influences on recognition responses.To do so, the PDP compares recognition performance on trials in which processes work in concert (i.e., trials on which people need to recognize trait words that were included in sentences correctly—*inclusion trials*) to trials in which processes work in opposition (i.e., trials on which people need to avoid false alarms—*exclusion trials*).

The logic of the PDP assumes that hits on inclusion trials are due to behavior recall or, when recall fails, to the influence of actor–trait associations. This is described mathematically as Hits = Recall + Associations/(1 – Recall). In this equation, the term *Recall* reflects accurate memory for behavioral information, and the term *Associations* is shorthand for the expression of actor–trait associations. Similarly, false alarms on exclusion trials are due to the actor–trait association becoming expressed and the failure of a correct recall inhibiting this expression. This is described mathematically as False Alarms = Associations/(1 – Recall). Thus, an index of recall is estimated by taking the difference between performance on inclusion trials and exclusion trials: Recall = Hits – False Alarms. This value is then used to estimate the influence of actor–trait associations: Associations = False Alarms/(1 – Recall).

To gain insight into the contributions that controlled and automatic processes made to the impact of STIs on responses to subsequent tasks, McCarthy and Skowronski (2011a) computed PDP-derived estimates of automatic processing and controlled processing from three studies that all used the false-recognition paradigm. In the first group, some participants were told to watch the computer screen during behavior encoding. Participants in a second group were told to form trait inferences during behavior encoding. Participants in a third group were told to search for the letters *ch* during encoding. It was hypothesized that the participants in this third group would be especially unlikely to form STIs. The results confirmed this prediction. Moreover, data from this third condition showed that relative to the other two conditions, the *ch* search manipulation significantly reduced the estimate of the influence of actor–trait associations during the trait recognition task. However, analyses of data from participants in all three conditions yielded similar recall estimates, suggesting that the influence of such processing was equal across the three conditions. These results might be interpreted to indicate that affecting the strength of trait inferences made during encoding uniquely affects the extent to which such knowledge automatically affects subsequent judgments, but does not affect the extent to which conscious recall of the behaviors or conscious recall of the traits implied by the behaviors affects subsequent judgments.

In a second study, McCarthy and Skowronski (2011a) again used the false-recognition paradigm and PDP methods to compute estimates of automatic processing and controlled processing. This study relied on the notion that different types of memory—semantic trait information and episodic behavioral information—have different decay rates. In the study, some participants experienced a relatively short interval between behavior encoding and the trait recognition task (~5 minutes); others experienced a longer interval (~20 minutes). Participants experiencing the brief time interval evinced significantly higher amounts of controlled processing relative to those in the long interval condition. Thus, as the time between encoding and trait recognition increased, participants were less able to inhibit the expression of the automatic processes. In comparison, as reflected the computed automatic processing estimates, the expression of automatic processes on the recognition task was unaffected by the time interval.

Finally, in a third study, participants reported their confidence level after making each decision in a trait recognition task. McCarthy and Skowronski (2011a) assumed that people had no insight into processes that were automatic, so the confidence estimates should be unrelated to the calculated estimates of automatic processing. In comparison, because confidence estimates rely on controlled processing, it was expected that such estimates should be related to the calculated estimates of controlled processing. Indeed, the data showed that self-reported decision confidence was associated with estimates of controlled processing but not with estimates of automatic processing.

These results suggest that even when motivated or instructed to avoid the influence of STIs, and even with the cognitive capacity to inhibit the influence of STIs, it seems that people's responses may still be influenced by STIs made at an earlier time. We contend that the reason for perceiviers' inability to inhibit STI expression is their lack of awareness of the extent to which STIs vary in accessibility and how such variations might affect their responses. Simply put, it is difficult for people to inhibit something for which they have no subjective feeling of influence. Therefore, it is not surprising that people do not perform very well the task of inhibition. Given this conclusion, it seems that the best way to avoid the potential biasing effects of STIs on later responses is to prevent STIs from being formed in the first place.

However, another important implication of these findings is that one needs to be cautious in one's claims about automatic influence. For example, results from the false-recognition paradigm often are cited as evidence for the automatic influence of STIs on subsequent responding. We believe that this conclusion is true only when one uses methods to decompose responding on the false-recognition task into separate components reflecting controlled processing and automatic processing. When this is done, it is clear that both automatic processes and controlled processes contribute to the effects that STIs have on subsequent responding. Moreover, the data suggest to us that the relative influence of STI-related automatic processing and controlled processing on any given task will depend on the exact characteristics of the task and the exact cognitive processes and structures that are needed to produce responses on that task.

SUMMARY: STIs AND THE DUAL-PROCESS VIEW

In our view, the accumulated results we describe in this chapter suggest that people often make STIs about actors when encountering trait-implicative actor behaviors. We also argue that the data suggest that (1) the STI results reported in the literature likely reflect elements of both automatic processing and controlled processing; (2) trait information extracted during STI generation can be stored in both the "fast-learning" conceptual knowledge system and in the "slow-learning" associative system; and (3) automatic processing and controlled processing exert their influence both during STI generation and STI expression. Finally, we also argue that the data point to the notion that processing is sometimes neither entirely automatic nor entirely controlled. Instead, task performance can simultaneously involve elements of both automatic and controlled processing. The relative importance of each will depend on the task and the circumstances in which the task is performed.

REFERENCES

Bargh, J. A. (1994). The four horsemen of automaticity: Intention, awareness, efficiency, and control as separate issues. In R. S. Wyer & T. K. Srull (Eds.), *Handbook of social cognition: Vol. 1. Basic processes* (2nd ed., pp. 1–40). Hillsdale, NJ: Erlbaum.

Bargh, J. A., Bond, R. N., Lombardi, W. J., & Tota, M. E. (1986). The additive nature of chronic and temporary sources of construct accessibility. *Journal of Personality and Social Psychology, 50,* 869–878.

Carlston, D. E., & Skowronski, J. J. (1994). Savings in the relearning of trait information as evidence for spontaneous inference generation. *Journal of Personality and Social Psychology, 66,* 840–856.

Carlston, D. E., & Skowronski, J. J. (2005). Linking versus thinking: Evidence for the different associative and attributional bases of spontaneous trait transference and spontaneous trait inference. *Journal of Personality and Social Psychology, 89,* 884–898.

Carlston, D. E., Skowronski, J. J., & Sparks, C. (1995). Savings in relearning: II. On the formation of behavior-based trait associations and inferences. *Journal of Personality and Social Psychology, 69,* 420–436.

Crawford, M. T., Skowronski, J. J., Stiff, C., & Sherer, C. R. (2007). Interfering with inferential, but not associative, processes underlying spontaneous trait inference. *Personality and Social Psychology Bulletin, 33,* 677–690.

Crouch, J. L., Milner, J. S., Skowronski, J. J., Farc, M. M., Irwin, L. M., & Neese, A. (2010). Automatic encoding of ambiguous child behavior in high and low risk for child physical abuse parents. *Journal of Family Violence, 25,* 73–80.

Goren, A., & Todorov, A. (2009). Two faces are better than one: Eliminating false trait associations with faces. *Social Cognition, 27,* 222–248.

Hassin, R. R., Bargh, J. A., & Uleman, J. S. (2002). Spontaneous causal inferences. *Journal of Experimental Social Psychology, 38,* 515–522.

Higgins, E. T., King, G. A., & Mavin, G. H. (1982). Individual construct accessibility and subjective impressions and recall. *Journal of Personality and Social Psychology, 43,* 35–47.

Higgins, E. T., Rholes, W. S., & Jones, C. R. (1977). Category accessibility and impression formation. *Journal of Experimental Social Psychology, 13,* 141–154.

Jacoby, L. L. (1991). A process dissociation framework: Separating automatic from intentional uses of memory. *Journal of Memory and Language, 30,* 513–541.

Kressel, L. M., & Uleman, J. S. (2010). Personality traits function as causal concepts. *Journal of Experimental Social Psychology, 46,* 213–216.

Lombardi, W. J., Higgins, E. T., & Bargh, J. A. (1987). The role of consciousness in priming effects on categorization. *Personality and Social Psychology Bulletin, 13,* 411–429.

Lupfer, M. B., Clark, L. F., & Hutcherson, H. W. (1990). Impact of context on spontaneous trait and situational attributions. *Journal of Personality and Social Psychology, 58,* 239–249.

McCarthy, R. J., & Skowronski, J. J. (2011a). The interplay of controlled and automatic processes in the expression of spontaneously inferred traits: A PDP analysis. *Journal of Personality and Social Psychology, 100,* 229–240.

McCarthy, R. J., & Skowronski, J. J. (2011b). What will Phil do next?: The influence of spontaneous trait inferences on behavior predictions. *Journal of Experimental Social Psychology, 47,* 321–332.

McCarthy, R. J., & Skowronski, J. J. (2012). *Disease avoidance goals interfere with the spontaneous inference of traits.*

McCarthy, R. J., Wells, B. M., Skowronski, J. J., & Carlston, D. (2013). *Behavior repetition differentially affects STT and STI: Evidence from a measure of association and a measure of trait judgment.*

Moskowitz, G. B., & Roman, R. J. (1992). Spontaneous trait inferences as self-generated primes: Implications for conscious social judgment. *Journal of Personality and Social Psychology, 62,* 728–738.

Na, J., & Kitayama, S. (2011). Spontaneous trait inference is culture-specific: Behavioral and neural evidence. *Psychological Science, 22,* 1025–1032.

Newman, L. S., & Uleman, J. S. (1990). Assimilation and contrast effects in spontaneous trait inference. *Personality and Social Psychology Bulletin, 16,* 224–240.

Rim, S., Uleman, J. S., & Trope, Y. (2009). Spontaneous trait inference and construal level theory: Psychological distance increases nonconscious trait thinking. *Journal of Experimental Social Psychology, 45*, 1088–1097.

Skowronski, J. J., Carlston, D. E., & Hartnett, J. L. (2008). Spontaneous impressions derived from observations of behavior: What a long, strange trip its been (and it's not over yet). In N. Ambady & J. J. Skowronski (Eds.), *First impressions* (pp. 313–333). New York: Guilford Press.

Skowronski, J. J., Carlston, D. E., Mae, L., & Crawford, M. T. (1998). Spontaneous trait transference: Communicators take on the qualities they describe in others. *Journal of Personality and Social Psychology, 74*, 837–848.

Sloman, S. A. (1996). The empirical case for two systems of reasoning. *Psychological Bulletin, 119*, 3–22.

Smith, E. R., & DeCoster, J. (2000). Dual-process models in social and cognitive psychology: Conceptual integration and links to underlying memory systems. *Personality and Social Psychology Review, 4*, 108–131.

Todorov, A., & Uleman, J. S. (2002). Spontaneous trait inferences are bound to actors' faces: Evidence from a false recognition paradigm. *Journal of Personality and Social Psychology, 39*, 549–562.

Todorov, A., & Uleman, J. S. (2003). The efficiency of binding spontaneous trait inferences to actors' faces. *Journal of Experimental Social Psychology, 39*, 549–562.

Todorov, A., & Uleman, J. S. (2004). The person reference process in spontaneous trait inferences. *Journal of Personality and Social Psychology, 87*, 482–493.

Trope, Y., & Liberman, N. (2010). Construal-level theory of psychological distance. *Psychological Review, 117*, 440–463.

Uleman, J. S., & Moskowitz, G. B. (1994). Unintended effects of goals on unintended inferences. *Journal of Personality and Social Psychology, 66*, 490–501.

Uleman, J. S., Moskowitz, G. B., Roman, R. J., & Rhee, E. (1993). Tacit, manifest, and intentional reference: How spontaneous trait inferences refer to persons. *Social Cognition, 11*, 321–351.

Uleman, J. S., Newman, L. S., & Moskowitz, G. B. (1996). People as flexible interpreters: Evidence and issues from spontaneous trait inference. In M. P. Zanna (Ed.), *Advances in experimental social psychology* (Vol. 28, pp. 211–279). San Diego: Academic Press.

Uleman, J. S., Newman, L., & Winter, L. (1992). Can traits be inferred automatically?: Spontaneous inferences require cognitive capacity at encoding. *Consciousness and Cognition, 1*, 77–90.

Uleman, J. S., Saribay, S. A., & Gonzalez, C. (2008). Spontaneous inferences, implicit impressions, and implicit theories. *Annual Review of Psychology, 59*, 329–360.

Uleman, J. S., Winborne, W. C., Winter, L., & Schecter, D. (1986). Personality differences in spontaneous trait inference at encoding. *Journal of Personality and Social Psychology, 51*, 396–403.

Wells, B. M., Skowronski, J. J., Crawford, M. T., Scherer, C. R., & Carlston, D. E. (2011). Inference making and linking both require thinking: Spontaneous trait inference and spontaneous trait transference both rely on working memory capacity. *Journal of Experimental Social Psychology, 47*, 1116–1126.

Winter, L., & Uleman, J. S. (1984). When are social judgments made?: Evidence for the spontaneousness of trait inferences. *Journal of Personality and Social Psychology, 47*, 237–252. [See correction in *Journal of Personality and Social Psychology, 50*, 355 (1986)]

Winter, L., Uleman, J. S., & Cunniff, C. (1985). How automatic are social judgments? *Journal of Personality and Social Psychology, 49*, 904–917. [See correction in *Journal of Personality and Social Psychology, 50*, 381 (1986)]

Zárate, M. A., Uleman, J. S., & Voils, C. I. (2001). Effects of culture and processing goals on the activation and binding of trait concepts. *Social Cognition, 19*, 295–323.

Zelli, A., Cervone, D., & Huesmann, L. R. (1996). Behavioral experience and social inferences: Individual differences in aggressive experience and spontaneous versus deliberate trait inference. *Social Cognition, 14*, 165–190.

CHAPTER 16

The Dynamic Interactive Model of Person Construal

Coordinating Sensory and Social Processes

Jonathan B. Freeman and Nalini Ambady

As you walk down a busy street, you happily glance around, momentarily glimpsing dozens if not hundreds of other people. As decades of research have shown, a mere glimpse of these individuals allows you to to place each of them quickly and efficiently into a number of relevant social categories. Most important, it seems, are sex, race, age, and emotion (Calder, Young, Perrett, Etcoff, & Rowland, 1996; Macrae & Bodenhausen, 2000), although it is becoming increasingly clear that other, more ambiguous categories may be automatically extracted as well, such as sexual orientation (Rule, Macrae, & Ambady, 2009). All this information may be availed to perceivers in just a fraction of a second. In the laboratory, for example, if a participant is asked explicitly to categorize a face by sex, response latencies generally hover around a half a second (e.g., Quinn & Macrae, 2005). Of course, reaction time tasks are accompanied by a large motor component (all the time required to convert cognitive representations into a hand movement), and event-related potential (ERP) findings suggest that such categorizations may be cognitively furnished within even shorter time periods (e.g., Freeman, Ambady, & Holcomb, 2010; Ito & Urland, 2003). Regardless, perceivers are able to extract categorical information rapidly from other people with impressive ease, so much so that the process appears to be mandatory.

It is only recently that social psychologists have become concerned with the perceptual processes culminating in social categorization. Traditionally, the focus has been on the consequences of categorization and the host of cognitive, affective, and behavioral effects that ensue. Consider, for example, two influential models of impression formation, Fiske and Neuberg's (1990) continuum model and Brewer's (1988) dual-process model. According to these models, from some array of available cues arises a dominant categorization (e.g., black), which then exerts a host of influences on impressions, memory, and behavior. It automatically activates related stereotypes (Devine, 1989), albeit conditionally (Gilbert & Hixon, 1991; Macrae & Bodenhausen, 2000), which then bias impressions in ways that are often stereotypically consistent. This category-based responding, however, may be tempered by a number of factors, such as attention or motivation. With the help of such intervening factors, these models posit that perceivers may move beyond categories and begin to rely more on individuating information, such as the observation that the target person pushed her friend.

In general, these models argue that perceivers by default resort to category-based responding, presumably because it maximizes cognitive efficiency and streamlines the demands of social interaction (also see

Allport, 1954). However, motivational states, such as the desire to be accurate, can move perceivers from category-based to more individuated impressions, involving a piecemeal integration of unique aspects of a target's behavior (Fiske & Neuberg, 1990). Inconsistencies between stereotypes and a target's behavior, or bad category fit, can also lead to more individuated impressions (Brewer, 1988). Moreover, attentional resources may limit perceivers' ability to move toward more individuated responding. As such, these person perception models aim to parse out the relative contributions of stereotypical and individuated information in forming impressions of others.

Although sharing a similar aim, Kunda and Thagard's (1996) parallel constraint satisfaction model takes a different approach, arguing that stereotypical and individuated information are given equal priority in person perception, and that both kinds of information are simultaneously integrated into a coherent impression through constraint satisfaction. This stands in contrast to Fiske and Neuberg's (1990) and Brewer's (1988) models, in that stereotypical information does not inherently receive more weight than individuating information. Instead, the Kunda and Thagard (1996) model assumes there are no fundamental differences in the representation of stereotypical and individuating information; all that matters is the strength of the information.

One important aspect common to all these models is that initial categorization provides the starting point, after which subsequent impressions, memory, or other social phenomena are predicted and explained. With a given categorization having taken place (e.g., black), the aim of these models is to understand the variety of factors that guide subsequent impressions and contribute to more category-based versus individuated responding. But what of initial categorization itself? Although these models have long acknowledged that perceivers tend to categorize spontaneously along a dominant dimension from brief exposure to another's face, the process underlying this remained relatively obscure.

Outside the social psychological literature, on the other hand, there has been an expansive body of work examining the mechanisms underlying face perception (e.g., Bruce & Young, 1986; Farah, Wilson, Drain, & Tanaka, 1998; Haxby, Hoffman, & Gobbini, 2000). By connecting insights from the social literature on social categorization to the cognitive and vision literatures on face perception, an emerging area of work has begun to forge the relationships between lower-level sensory processing and higher-order social cognition. This has often been referred to as *person construal* research. Traditional social psychological research focused on the aftermath of social categorization and its influences on downstream phenomena. Person construal research, on the other hand, aims to understand how perceptual cues and their bottom-up operations ultimately lead to particular social categorizations.

Thus, seminal models of person perception (Brewer, 1988; Fiske & Neuberg, 1990; Kunda & Thagard, 1996) have been enormously valuable for explaining high-level impressions and perceivers' differential reliance on categorical versus individuating information in judging others. However, they have not aimed to explain the initial categorization process itself. Instead, extant models have treated categorization as a rapid, straightforward process that triggers a number of consequential effects. This is consistent with a long tradition in social psychology, dating back to the seminal work of Allport (1954), who argued that categorizing others is a highly efficient and spontaneous, perhaps inevitable, phenomenon that the cognitive system uses to economize on mental resources. This quickly became a guiding principle in the field of person perception. Categorization, accordingly, allows us to avoid dealing with the complexities and inconsistencies inherent to other people, and instead to provide a convenient shortcut for social interaction.

Although this characterization is highly valuable and probably correct, one problem is that despite categorizations being highly rapid and efficient, each is also highly complex. And each is complex in ways that are not likely to be captured adequately by this "feed forward" approach, in which bottom-up cues feed activation forward onto a dominant category, which feeds activation forward onto related stereotypes, which then feed into a number of downstream effects (also see Johnson & Freeman, 2010). The main trouble is that there is potentially a great deal of feedback as well, in which stereotypes and higher-order social cognitive phenomena constrain lower levels of processing (e.g., category activation), thereby fundamentally altering basic perceptions. On encountering a middle-aged black man, for example, one dominant categorization has been argued often to arise (e.g., black), with the dominant category determined by a number of factors (Bodenhausen & Macrae, 1998). The stereotypes associated with this dominant category then figure into perceivers' impressions with some degree of priority (Brewer, 1988; Fiske & Neuberg, 1990; Kunda & Thagard, 1996) and become subject to a variety of downstream interpretative processes and, in some cases, inhibitory control (Bodenhausen & Macrae, 1998). What has not readily been considered, however, is that initial categorization—as automatic as it may be—could potentially be affected by the very stereotype activations and downstream processing that it triggers.

Recently, we proposed a dynamic interactive model of person construal, which provides a computational account of the real-time social categorization process and emphasizes its cyclical, ongoing, and interactive nature (Freeman & Ambady, 2011). The model posits an intimate interplay between bottom-up sensory cues and top-down social factors in driving the process of categorizing others. In this process, particular categorizations emerge from the ongoing interaction between lower-level sensory processing and higher-order social cognition. As such, ultimate categorizations (e.g., "He's a man!") are the stable end result of a dynamic process in which both bottom-up and top-down factors gradually constrain one another over time.

BOTTOM-UP, MEET TOP-DOWN

One of the most important considerations motivating the dynamic interactive model of person construal is how social category representations would be implemented in a human brain, and the dynamics involved in activating those representations. At the neural level, the representation of a social category would be reflected by a pattern of activity distributed across a large population of neurons. Thus, activating a social category representation would involve continuous changes in a pattern of neuronal activity (Smith & Ratcliff, 2004; Spivey & Dale, 2006; Usher & McClelland, 2001). Neuronal recordings in nonhuman primates have shown that, very soon after a face is presented, about half of a face's visual information rapidly accumulates in temporal cortex neurons, while the remaining half gradually accumulates over the following hundreds of milliseconds (Rolls & Tovee, 1995). This gradual evolution of a face's representation tends to involve a transition between initial coarse analysis of the face to a more fine-grained representation (Sugase, Yamane, Ueno, & Kawano, 1999). As such, during early moments of the categorization process, the transient interpretation of a face is partially consistent with multiple categories (e.g., both male or female), because the coarse "gist" available is partially suggestive of both categories. As more information accumulates and representations become more fine-grained, the pattern of neuronal activity dynamically sharpens into an increasingly confident representation (e.g., male), while other, competing representations (e.g., female) are naturally pushed out (Freeman, Ambady, Rule, & Johnson, 2008; Spivey & Dale, 2006; Usher & McClelland, 2001). One important function of this dynamic competition is the ability of the perceptual system to take the natural diversity that is inherent in others' sensory cues (e.g., slightly masculine features on a woman's face) and slot it into the rigid categories that are needed to so readily perceive other people.

Importantly, during those fuzzy hundreds of milliseconds it takes for the neuronal activity to achieve a stable pattern (~100% male or ~100% female), top-down factors—such as context, stereotypes, motivation, or attention—could also potentially exert an influence beyond bottom-up processing of facial cues, thereby partly determining the pattern toward which the system will gravitate (e.g., Bar, 2004; Grossberg, 1980; Spivey, 2007), thereby partly influencing social categorization. Accordingly, social categorization would incorporate not just another's facial cues (and vocal and bodily cues), but also top-down sources, rendering categorization always a compromise between the perceptual cues "actually" there and the baggage perceivers bring to the categorization process. Why would this be the case? Intuitively, we might expect that our basic perception of a visual stimulus, such as a face, would be immune to top-down factors and instead entail a veridical representation of the perceptual information before our eyes (see Marr, 1982). This was long presumed to be the case (e.g., Fodor, 1983; Pylyshyn, 1984; but see Bruner & Goodman, 1947). However, most researchers would now agree that human perception is a highly active and constructive process. To the extent that perception is for action and for guiding functionally adaptive interactions with the environment (Gibson, 1979), one might expect it to be able to be adjusted by top-down factors—such as expectations, motivations, or attention—so long as these factors may facilitate adaptive behavior.

The visual world, of course, is rife with ambiguous and conflicting information—ever more so in perceiving social targets—and it is the job of the perceptual system to construct coherent, meaningful percepts that the cognitive system can use to effect behavior. Consider, for example, the words in Figure 16.1A. A visual pass across the top of the figure and one effortlessly sees "CAT," and a visual pass across the bottom and one just as effortlessly sees "THE." If one were to cover up the first and last letters of each word, however, one would be quick to note that the middle letter "A" in CAT and middle letter "H" in THE are entirely identical. Yet when placed in the different contexts of surrounding letters, the identical letter stimulus is perceived one way ("A") or the other ("H") based on whichever helps the perceptual system construct the most coherent interpretation. More specifically, perceivers' expectations—in this case, based on stored lexical representations of "cat" and "the"—constrained the perceptual processing of the middle letler, biasing it in a way that agreed best with prior conceptual knowledge.

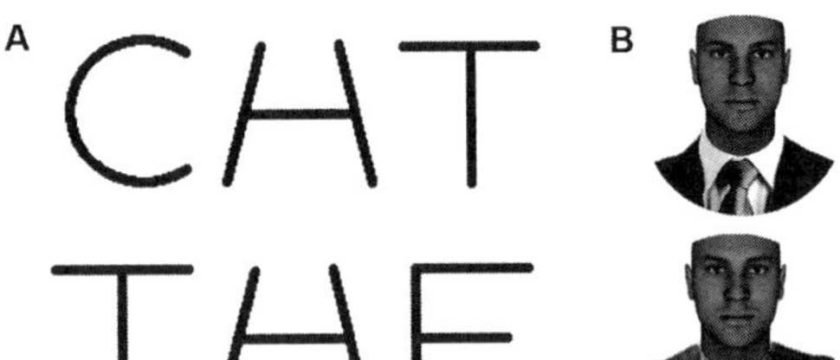

FIGURE 16.1. (A) The ambiguous middle letter is readily disambiguated by the surrounding letters based on prior conceptual knowledge. (B) A face's race may be similarly disambiguated by the surrounding context cues based on prior stereotype knowledge. From Freeman, Penner, Saperstein, Scheutz, and Ambady (2011). Copyright by the authors. Reprinted by permission.

Such influences of context are hardly limited to ambiguous stimuli. You may not have realized, for example, that the word *letter* in the last sentence of the previous paragraph in fact did not read *letter.* A *t* was switched for an *l,* but the processing of the other letters likely constrained processing of the *t,* biasing it toward an *l* to create a more coherent perception (i.e., forming *letter* rather than *letler*). The word recognition system was attracted to perceive *letter* as it had a preexisting conceptual representation for it, and the surrounding letters gave the system enough evidence to run with that interpretation. Reminiscent perhaps of the tendency for person perceivers to economize considerably on mental resources (Allport, 1954; Macrae & Bodenhausen, 2000), readers tend not to process every single letter of every word; in fact, they may skip whole words altogether (Sereno & Rayner, 2003). For a streamlined perceptual–cognitive pipeline, prior expectations and conceptual knowledge—and in some cases motivations as well (Balcetis & Dunning, 2006; Pauker et al., 2009)—are rapidly brought to bear on the basic processing of visual information, allowing context and expectations to fill in the patterns for which we are too lazy to seek fine-grained evidence.

What permits these influences of expectation on perception is the intimate exchange between bottom-up and top-down forces. Three decades ago, the pioneering work of McClelland and Rumelhart (1981) elegantly showed that such context effects naturally arise out of the dynamics of a simple network of interconnected artificial neurons—a connectionist network—in which representations of features, letters, and words recurrently feed activation back and forth with one another until settling on a best-fitting state. Returning to the CAT/THE example, bottom-up processing of the written text's features activates letter representations, which in turn activate conceptual representations of the words *cat* and *the,* which in turn exert top-down pressure back on the letter processing. Ultimately, this top-down feedback is able to bias the ambiguous middle letter toward an "A" interpretation in the context of CAT and toward an "H" interpretation in the context of THE. As such, it is the dynamic interaction between bottom-up and top-down information sources that yields such flexible and context-sensitive perception.

Our dynamic interactive model applies these seminal insights from the word recognition literature to person construal. A general diagram of the model appears in Figure 16.2. Technically, it is a recurrent connectionist network with stochastic interactive activation (McClelland, 1991). A number of pools are depicted; in specific instantiations of the model, each pool will contain a variety of nodes (e.g., *female, Asian, caring, male cues*). Specific details may be found in Freeman and Ambady (2011). The network provides an approximation of the kind of processing that might take place in a human brain (Rogers & McClelland, 2004; Rumel-

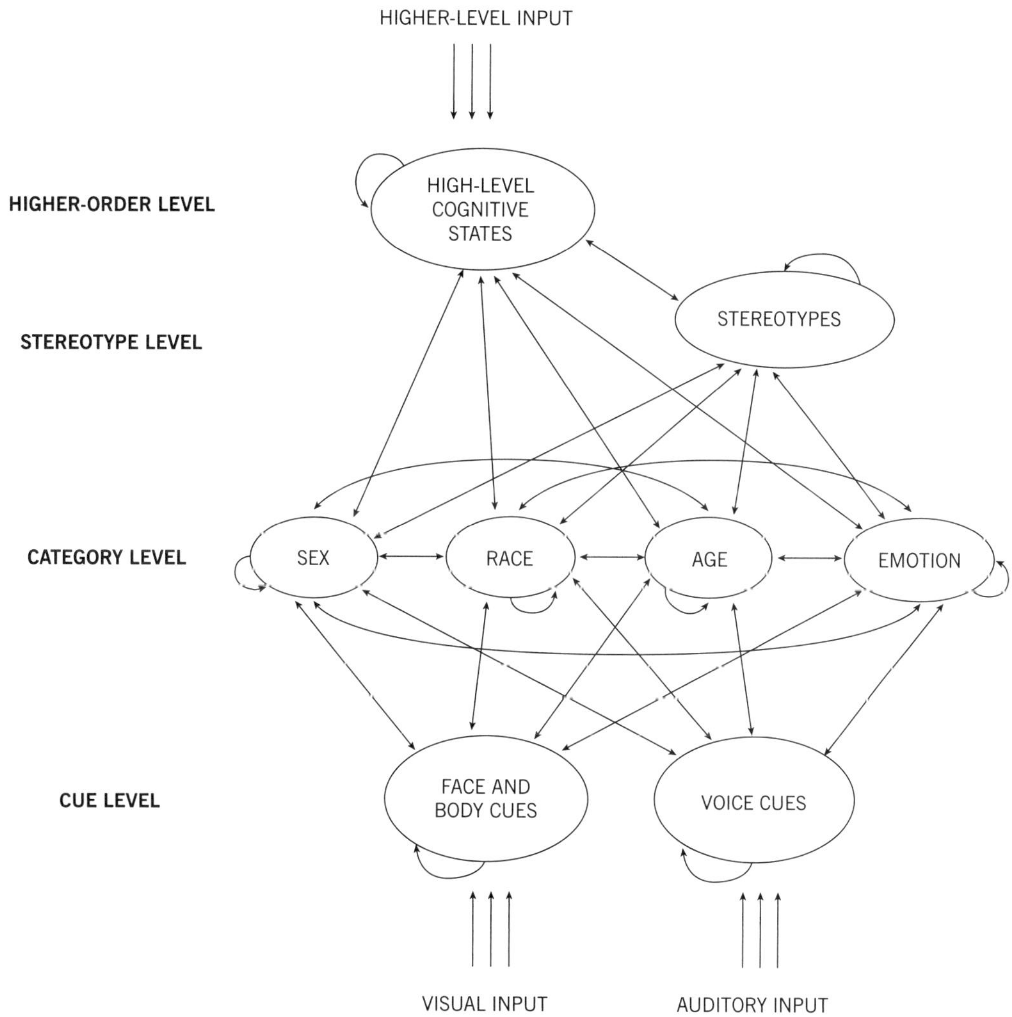

FIGURE 16.2. A general diagram of the dynamic interactive model of person construal. From Freeman and Ambady (2011). Copyright by the American Psychological Association. Reprinted by permission.

hart, Hinton, & McClelland, 1986; Smolensky, 1989; Spivey, 2007), particularly in the context of perceiving other people.

Initially, both bottom-up and top-down inputs stimulate the system (see Figure 16.2). This may include many forms of input, including bottom-up input of another's face, voice, or body, and top-down input from higher-order systems involved in motivations or top-down attention, for example. Every version of the model contains a number of nodes that are typically organized into four levels of processing (corresponding to cues, categories, stereotypes, and high-level cognitive states). At every moment in time, a node has a transient activation level, which can be interpreted as the strength of a tentative hypothesis that the node is represented in the input. After the system is initially stimulated by bottom-up and top-down inputs, activation flows among all nodes at the same time (as a function of their particular connection weights). Note that many connections between the nodes are bidirectional. This results in a dynamic back-and-forth flow of activation among many nodes in the system, leading them gradually to readjust each other's activation more and more as they mutually constrain one another over time. This leads the system to stabilize gradually over time onto an overall pattern of activation that best fits the inputs and maximally satisfies the system's constraints (the inputs and the relationships among nodes). Presumably, we argue, this stable state would correspond to an ultimate perception of another person.

In short, the model assumes that perceptions of other people dynamically evolve over fractions of a second, emerging from the interaction between bottom-up sensory cues and top-down social factors. This renders social categorization to be, in a sense, a gradual process of negotiation between the variety of sensory cues "actually" inherent to a person, and the baggage an individual perceiver brings to the perceptual process.

PUTTING THE "SOCIAL" BACK IN SOCIAL CATEGORIZATION

To illustrate better the dynamics of the model, let us consider an example. It has long been known that race has important relationships with social status. White individuals tend to be stereotyped as having high status, whereas black individuals tend to be stereotyped as having low status. Occupation categories, however, also are associated with status stereotypes: Businesspeople are stereotyped as having high status, whereas janitors are stereotyped as having low status. As such, cues related to occupation might come to activate status stereotypes that then constrain the perception of race, similar to how the surrounding letters in "CAT" and "THE" activated word representations that constrained the perception of the middle letter.

In a previous set of studies, we presented participants with faces generated to have varying level of race content, from white to black, and surrounded those faces by either business or janitor attire (Freeman, Penner, Saperstein, Scheutz, & Ambady, 2011). In Figure 16.1B, for example, we see the same racially ambiguous face surrounded by either business or janitor attire. When participants were asked to categorize the race of these faces, business attire increased the likelihood of a white categorization, whereas janitor attire increased the likelihood of a black categorization. Furthermore, these influences of context were exacerbated as a face's race became more ambiguous. One likely explanation for these effects is that while facial race was being processed, contextual attire cues activated occupation categories in parallel, which in turn began activating status stereotypes. Once active, the stereotypes then constrained categorization by exerting top-down feedback on the race categories with which they happen to be associated. When we implemented this process in a version of our dynamic interactive model, the model's dynamics strongly corroborated these experimental effects.

Figure 16.3 illustrates this specific version of the general model (see Figure 16.2). To illustrate its operations, let us consider the case of the system being presented with a somewhat ambiguous white face with janitor attire. Presenting the system with this stimulus and the task demand of race categorization sets a process into motion in which visual input of the face activates cue nodes and higher-level input of the task demand activates higher-order nodes. The *race task demand* node places excitatory pressure on the *white* and *black* categories, and inhibi-

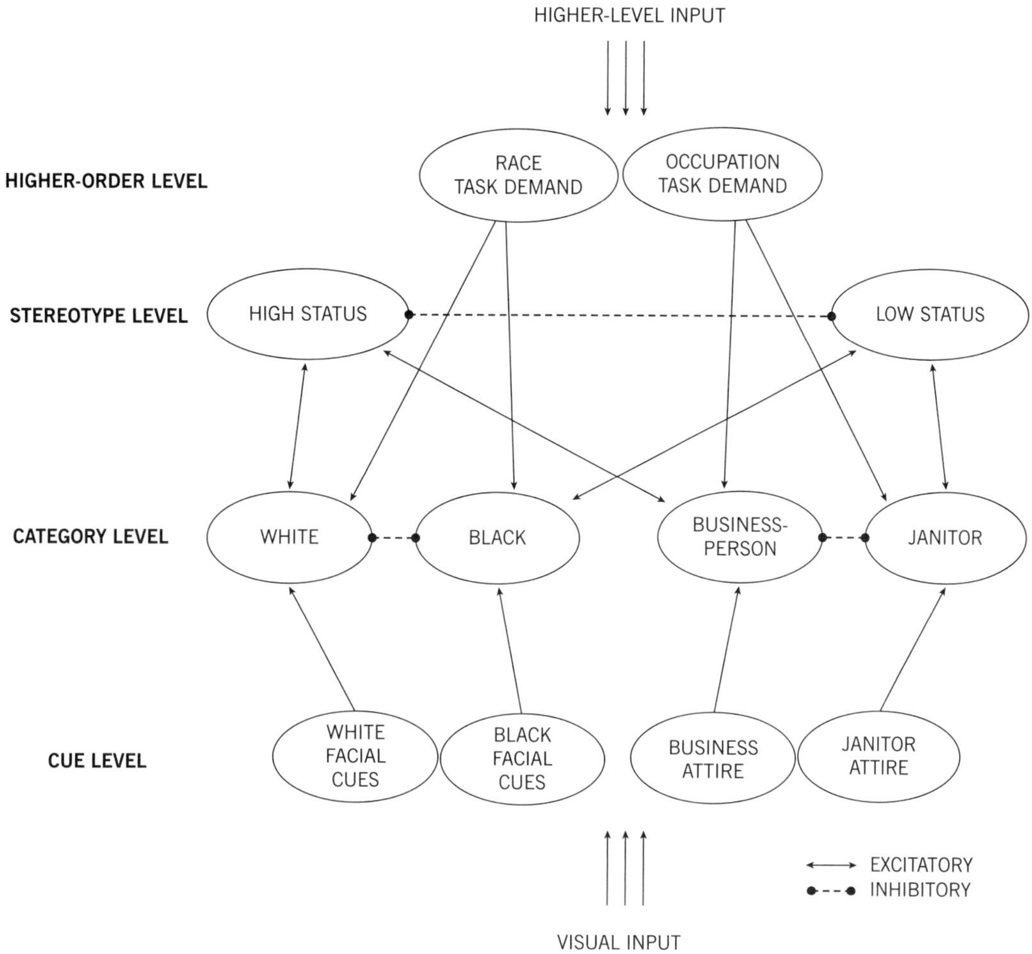

FIGURE 16.3. A specific instantiation of the dynamic interactive model of person construal from Freeman, Penner, Saperstein, Scheutz, and Ambady (2011). Copyright by the Authors. Reprinted by permission.

tory pressure on the *businessperson* and *janitor* categories. This results in the *white* and *black* categories becoming partially active for the particular task. The strongly activated *white facial cues* category excites the *white* category. Now that the *white* and *black* categories are active in parallel, they begin to compete with one another through ongoing, mutual inhibition, and eventually stabilize onto one category (see Freeman et al., 2008; Freeman, Pauker, Apfelbaum, & Ambady, 2010). While this process unfolds, the *white* category puts excitatory pressure on the *high status* stereotype and the *black* category puts excitatory pressure on the *low status* stereotype. Now that the conflicting status stereotypes are also active in parallel, they also begin competing with one another (see Freeman & Ambady, 2009). At the same time, activation of the *janitor attire* node excites the *janitor* category and inhibits the *businessperson* category. Note that the *janitor* category is also inhibited by the *race task demand* node (as this is a race categorization task), so it only gains a small amount of activation. However, that meager amount of activation is sufficient to start putting excitatory pressure on the *low status* stereotype. At this point, the stereotype nodes are being fed activation by both race and occupation categories in an ongoing fashion. Here comes the critical part. Because this is an interactive, recurrent system, while the competition between stereotypes is still resolving, the stereotype nodes also place their own activation pressures back on the category nodes, thereby providing top-down feedback. The result is that the *janitor* category's excitation of the *low status* stereotype winds up exerting excitatory pressure on the *black* category, helping it win against the *white* category.

In some instances, especially when the bottom-up information (i.e., face) is particularly ambiguous, such top-down pressures wouldhave enough strength to make the *black* category more likely to win the race–category competition, thereby driving the system's ultimate categorization responses. In other instances, especially when the bottom-up information is clear-cut, such pressures would not have enough strength to alter responses wholesale. Instead, what occurs is a stronger partial parallel activation of the *black* category (until it gradually decays, succumbing to the *white* category). As a result of stereotypes feeding back into the category competition—even slightly—the activation dynamics of the *black* and *white* categories are altered nevertheless, even though the competition's outcome is not ultimately affected. Computationally, what is happening here is that perceivers' stereotypical expectations are combining with incoming visual information to shape initial categorizations of other people, sometimes wholesale and at other times only temporarily.

Indeed, in a previous set of studies we found that participants' race categorization responses were biased by contextual attire cues, likely due to stereotypes (Freeman et al., 2011). But what about cases where the ultimate response is not biased? In a number of studies, we have used a mouse-tracking technique to open up the categorization process and gain insight into its real-time processing dynamics. This technique allows us to probe further such cases in which the ultimate response does not seem to be particularly biased. In the context of this study, we found that even when participants ultimately categorized a face with janitor attire as white, the process leading up to their response was nevertheless partially biased toward the *black* category (presumably due to the dynamic modulation of stereotypes, triggered by contextual cues). The converse effect held as well. Even when participants ultimately categorized a face with business attire as black, the categorization process was partially biased toward the *white* category. The main mouse-tracking result from this work appears in Figure 16.4.

Participants were presented with a face stimulus and asked to indicate whether the target was black or white by moving the mouse from the bottom-center of the screen to either top corner of the screen (see Figure 16.4). As seen in the figure, before ultimately categorizing a face with janitor attire as white, the mean mouse trajectory was simultaneously and partially attracted to select the black response, continuously across construal. In other words, participants' movements were neither in a discrete pursuit straight to the response associated with bottom-up facial cues (i.e., white) nor in a discrete pursuit straight to the response associated with top-down stereotypes (e.g., black). Instead, the evolving categorization process was always in a weighted combination of both response alternatives, because both bottom-up sensory and top-down social forces were driving the social category dynamics in real time, until partici-

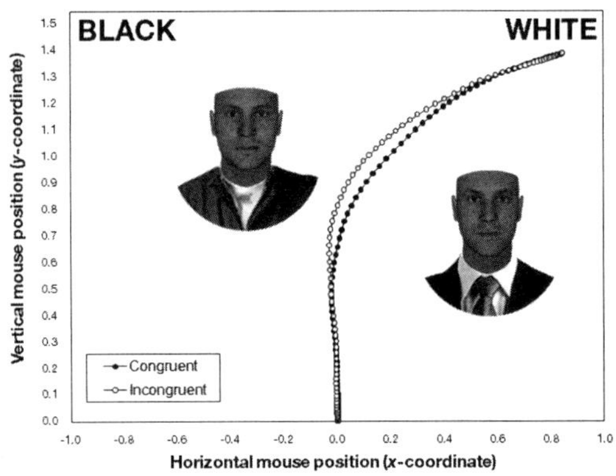

FIGURE 16.4. Main mouse-tracking results. Before ultimately categorizing a face with janitor attire as white, mouse movements exhibited a continuous, partial attraction toward the black category response. A similar attraction effect toward the white category response was observed for cases where faces with business attire were categorized as black. From Freeman, Penner, Saperstein, Scheutz, and Ambady (2011). Copyright by the authors. Reprinted by permission.

pants gradually stabilized onto, in this case, a single, white categorization response.

It is worth noting that because categorizations are compromises between bottom-up and top-down information, the importance of one information source is dependent on the other. Thus, as alluded to in the previous simulation, when perceptual cues are ambiguous and provide only weak information, the bottom-up ambiguity invites strong influences from top-down constraints. Indeed, results from the previous study were consistent with this perspective. We found that as a face's race became increasingly ambiguous, the effects of context and stereotypes became increasingly pronounced; when more ambiguous, perceptions were especially biased by top-down stereotypes and pulled toward the category stereotypically associated with the status cue (Freeman et al., 2011). Thus, there is a tradeoff between bottom-up and top-down influences that is driven by their respective strengths.

Similar principles hold when top-down constraints are weak, thereby inviting strong influences from bottom-up cues. Take, for example, the influences of race categories on sex categorization via stereotypes. A black target will activate stereotypes such as aggressive and athletic, which, due to incidental overlap with the male category, in turn put excitatory pressure on the male category; similarly, an Asian target will activate stereotypes such as docile and communal, which in turn put excitatory pressure on the female category. These top-down pressures from race-triggered stereotype activation could readily bias the sex categorization process, especially when a target's sex is ambiguous (Johnson, Freeman, & Pauker, 2012). However, there are many cases in which such top-down stereotype pressures are weaker. For instance, the *white* category does not have strong associations with sex-related stereotypes; thus, a white target would not induce strong top-down, race-triggered stereotype pressure on sex categorization. In these cases, the top-down constraints on sex categorization would be quite weak, thereby allowing bottom-up cues to be a strong determinant of perceptions (Freeman & Ambady, 2011; Johnson et al., 2012).[1]

Together, what the previous examples illustrate is that initial categorizations of others are, in fact, hardly "initial" at all. They emerge out of feedback loops across a dynamic and interactive person construal system. As automatic and spontaneous as they may be, they are not mere "readouts" of facial features. Instead, they arise out of a complex process shaped by not only bottom-up cues but also the prior knowledge, expectations, and higher-order social cognitive baggage that individual perceivers bring to the table. Specifically, the model assumes that basic social category activation is readily influenced by the very stereotypes and downstream processing it triggers. Not only does activation of the *black* category trigger stereotypes of low-status, for example, but activation of low-status stereotypes influences activation of the *black* category. "Initial" categorizations emerge out of a gradual, dynamic coordination of both sensory factors (e.g., facial cues) and social factors (e.g., stereotypical expectations), ultimately yielding flexible and integrated perceptions of other people.

As described earlier, person perception models in the social literature have tended to focus on high-level impressions and on knowledge about individuals and groups. Models in the cognitive and vision literatures, on the other hand, have described the perceptual mechanisms that permit facial perceptions. A dynamic interactive model might help unify these literatures by describing how the lower-level processing modeled in the cognitive and vision literatures works together with the higher-order processing modeled in the social literature to give rise to person construal. It argues for an intimate and inextricable connection between both the "sensory" and the "social," in which both lower-level sensory and higher-order social factors collaborate in complex ways to give rise to initial categorizations. In such a way, social psychological processes are theoretically permitted to play a larger role in visual construals of other people than has previously been considered.

RELATIONSHIP TO DUAL-PROCESS FRAMEWORKS

In spite of their differences, prior models of person perception, including Fiske and Neuberg's (1990) continuum model, Brewer's (1988) dual-process model, and Kunda and Thagard's (1996) parallel constraint satisfaction model, have all stressed the tension between categorical and individuated styles of processing. The models agree in that both styles of processing are involved in impression formation, but they differ in what priority each contributes to impressions and when various factors may drive their respective contributions. Our model, instead, homes in on perceivers' categorical processing, and aims to understand how particular categories and the stereotypes they trigger become activated in the first place. For example, all three models, as well as Bodenhausen and Macrae's (1998) related model, start with initial categorization. Our model opens up that initial categorization process, well before subsequent person processing and impression formation have had a chance even to begin.

Whereas the previously mentioned models deal with the interplay of individuating information (e.g., he smiled at his friend) and category information (e.g., stereotypes) on forming impressions, our model currently does not aim to account for the accrual of individuating information. Moreover, our model aims to explain basic category and stereotype activation rather than high-level impressions. In the future, however, it would be interesting and valuable to incorporate individuating information into the model, because it could have numerous influences on category and stereotype activation. For now, we can say that once implemented, it would likely function more similarly to Kunda and Thagard's (1996) model than to Fiske and Neuberg's (1990) or Brewer's (1988) model. Hypothetically, individuating information would be processed the moment it is observed and thereafter provide an immediate and parallel constraint on all person construal system processing.

Rather than center on a duality between categorical and individuating information, however, our model centers on a different duality most relevant to person construal: bottom-up sensory versus top-down social cognitive sources of information. Prior person perception models have certainly made the bottom-up versus top-down distinction as well. In such models, however, category knowledge was treated as a top-down biasing structure, whereas individuating/person-based attributes were treated as the bottom-up information sources that build into perceptions (e.g., Brewer, 1988). Instead, our model instead treats category knowledge itself as the perceptual phenomenon of interest; and it views stereotypes and higher-order social cognition as top-down information sources that constrain it, whereas perceptual cues are the bottom-up determinants driving it. Thus, our model deals with the interplay of bottom-up and top-down influences on basic "initial" category and stereotype activations, which in prior models were treated as the top-down influence itself on other phenomena (e.g., impressions).

Such influences in our model are argued to run in parallel with one another, richly interacting via feedback loops produced across a dynamic person construal system. However, it is important to note that there is nothing that distinguishes the inherent nature of bottom-up and top-down information in the model. Rather, it is more appropriate to talk about bottom-up and top-down *effects* on certain representations or levels of processing in the system, rather than the existence of separate bottom-up and top-down *processes*. This is because many excitatory and inhibitory pressures influence (and are influenced by) social category activation, and these arise from complex interactions between lower levels (the cue level) and higher levels (stereotype and higher-order levels) of processing to such an extent that they are difficult to separate as being solely "bottom-up" or "top-down." It is true that the system is initially stimulated by external input that is clearly and unambiguously bottom-up or top-down, with bottom-up input originating from the visual and auditory systems, and top-down input originating from a top-down attentional system or motivational system. However, once the system is initially stimulated by these external bottom-up and top-down inputs, bottom-up and top-down processing become inextricably intertwined.

Take, for example, the effects of status stereotypes on race categorization described earlier. The most proximal mechanism underlying these effects was the accumulated top-down pressures from status stereotypes, which exerted a continuous influence on race categories. But such a top-down effect was set into motion only by the bottom-up processing of contextual attire cues, which activated status stereotypes, which eventually exerted top-down influence on race categories. Thus, while effects in the system can perhaps be described as primarily bottom-up or top-down for descriptive purposes, ultimately bottom-up and top-down processes are in such interaction that it is difficult definitively to tease them apart. The "top-down" influence of status stereotypes only came into being from the "bottom-up" processing of contextual attire cues. Thus, there is an intimate and complicated exchange between the bottom-up and the top-down, between the "sensory" and the "social," that yields ultimate construals. Indeed, we feel that this is not so much a problem as it is a central argument of our framework. A deep coextension exists, we argue, between bottom-up sensory–perceptual and top-down social cognitive processes, in which stable person construals rapidly emerge out of the ongoing interactions between them. And arguably, they are so confounded with one another that attempting to separate them out may not be the most meaningful distinction that research could make (however, see discussion in Freeman & Ambady, 2011, pp. 270–271).

A separate distinction between processes that has given rise to enormous theoretical strides in social psychology has been that of automatic and implicit versus controlled and explicit processes. For example, a variety of social psychological models, including the associative–propositional evaluation (APE) model (Gawronski & Bodenhausen, 2006), the dual-attitude model (Wilson et al., 2000), the systems of evaluation model (SEM; Rydell & McConnell, 2006), and the reflective–impulsive model (RIM; Strack & Deutsch, 2004), posit two at least partially independent processes or systems: one that is associative, implicit, automatic, and/or impulsive, and another that is propositional, explicit, controlled, and/or reflective. In general, the former involves simple associative links that are activated in patterns based on principles of similarity and congruity in a relatively automatic and resource-independent fashion (e.g., similar to a connectionist model). The latter involves higher-order reasoning and controlled, resource-dependent processing, and can often either affirm or deny the former's representations. For example, a spontaneous, implicit negative evaluation of a black target (driven by the former) may be affirmed or denied by one's explicit racial attitudes (driven by the latter). There is considerably more complexity and nuance to each of these models, but common to them all is this general kind of processing division.

Prior models in the person perception literature have dealt with these two processing styles differently. In Fiske and Neuberg's (1990) continuum model, default category- and stereotype-based responding corresponds to more automatic processing, whereas individuated responding (dependent on a perceiver's motivation) corresponds to more controlled processing. In Brewer's (1988) dual-process model, both category- and person-based responding may involve automatic or controlled processing, depending on one's motivation and involvement. In Kunda and Thagard's (1996) model, categorical–stereotypical and individuating information are simultaneously integrated by a single process assumed to be relatively automatic. However, Kunda and Thagard cautioned that impression formation may in many cases involve causal reasoning that recruits additional controlled processing beyond the scope of their model.

Our model is more similar to that of Kunda and Thagard (1996), in that it presumably deals with relatively automatic processing only. This is even more the case with our model than with theirs, however, as the process we model is initial categorization itself, which is widely agreed to be highly automatic (Macrae & Bodenhausen, 2000). Once an initial categorization occurs, however, how the stereotypes it activates then figures into perceivers' impressions and behavior, or is inhibited or controlled, is a separate question receiving considerable debate (Bargh, 1999; Macrae & Bodenhausen, 2000). Despite initial categorization being highly automatic, for example, a number of studies has shown that perceivers' goal states and other preconditions can modulate whether it in fact occurs, rendering it conditionally automatic (Macrae & Bodenhausen, 2000). However, although goals may modulate whether categorizations do or do not occur, it is unclear what their role would be in tampering with the dynamics and outcomes of those categorizations. For example, although perceivers' goals can change whether categorization may occur, if it in fact does occur, can they control whether stereotypes are free to alter basic face processing, biasing it toward a white or black categorization based on contextual cues? Similar to how automatically the word "CAT" is lifted off CAT and "THE" lifted off THE due to readers' stored conceptual knowledge (see Figure 16.1A), it is unclear whether person perceivers would have control over stereotypes' alteration of lower-level perceptual processing. Individual differences in implicit racial prejudice (which presumably influence how strongly racial stereotypes are active; Lepore & Brown, 1997) do appear to influence lower-level perceptual processing (Hugenberg & Bodenhausen, 2004), and this is accounted for in our model (Freeman & Ambady, 2011). Moreover, goals such as task demands certainly play a role in amplifying or attenuating the activation of certain category activations, which is a basic tenet of our model. Future research will need to examine whether more complex goals beyond simple task demands, and other controlled processes, can interact with the relatively automatic person construal system we have modeled to shape basic perceptions. For the time being, we speculate that the answer is "yes," and this may be a very fruitful line for investigation in the future.

CONCLUSION

In summary, the dynamic interactive model of person construal aims to explain the initial category and stereotype activation process—a process that, in extant models in person perception, has formed the starting point for understanding subsequent phenomena. In this process, basic construals of other people rapidly but gradually emerge from an ongoing interaction between bottom-up sensory–perceptual and top-down social cognitive processes. Arguably, they interact to such an extent that it may not be helpful to attempt to tease apart processes as definitively "bottom-up" or "top-down"; instead, it would be more helpful to assess their relative contributions in driving particular effects. That is, we argue that there are not two distinct processes, but only one highly integrative and dynamic process.

The proposed framework should not be seen as competitive with extant models in person perception. Instead, it builds on them with a different level of analysis, zooming in on the initial categorization process itself. In doing so, it connects the higher-order social phenomena more traditionally studied in the person perception and social cognition literatures to basic sensory processes, and argues for their rich coextension in driving the process of construing others. However, many questions remain. How the relatively automatic process of person construal figures in with more controlled processes, and the phenomena richly explored in dual-process frameworks in social psychology, will be extremely important to address in the future. For now, however, by linking the "social" to the "sensory" in such inextricable ways, person construal has arguably been rendered a problem that is not just the province of social psychology to solve, but an exciting collaboration among the cognitive, vision, and neural sciences as well (see Adams, Ambady, Nakayama, & Shimojo, 2011; Balcetis & Lassiter, 2010).

NOTE

1. In virtually all cases, category nodes in instantiations of our model would settle into an attractor state involving only one predominantly active node (e.g., male) within a given dimension (e.g., sex). Because activation is stochastic, even if bottom-up cues are inherently equibiased (e.g., 50% masculine, 50% feminine) and top-down constraints exert equal pressures on both male and female categories, random noise would eventually lead either the male or female category to win the competition. However, the model cannot currently explain more stable categorization responses that are more graded in nature (e.g., biracial/multiracial). Such stable graded category states are being investigated for future instantiations of the model.

ACKNOWLEDGMENTS

Sadly, Nalini Ambady passed away on October 28, 2013. This work was supported by a National Research Service Award fellowship (No. F31-MH092000) from the National Institutes of Health to Jonathan B. Freeman and a National Science Foundation research grant (No. BCS-0435547) to Nalini Ambady.

REFERENCES

Adams, R. B., Ambady, N., Nakayama, K., & Shimojo, S. (2011). *The science of social vision*. New York: Oxford University Press.

Allport, G. W. (1954). *The nature of prejudice*. Oxford, UK: Addison-Wesley.

Balcetis, E., & Dunning, D. (2006). See what you want to see: Motivational influences on visual perception. *Journal of Personality and Social Psychology, 91*, 612–625.

Balcetis, E., & Lassiter, D. (2010). *The social psychology of visual perception*. New York: Psychology Press.

Bar, M. (2004). Visual objects in context. *Nature Reviews Neuroscience, 5*, 617–629.

Bargh, J. A. (1999). The cognitive monster: The case against the controllability of automatic stereotype effects. In S. Chaiken & Y. Trope (Eds.), *Dual-process theories in social psychology* (pp. 361–382). New York: Guilford Press.

Bodenhausen, G. V., & Macrae, C. N. (1998). Stereotype activation and inhibition. In R. S. Wyer, Jr. (Ed.), *Stereotype activation and inhibition* (pp. 1–52). Mahwah, NJ: Erlbaum.

Brewer, M. B. (1988). A dual process model of impression formation. In T. K. Srull & R. S. Wyer (Eds.), *A dual-process model of impression formation: Advances in social cognition* (Vol. 1, pp. 1–36). Hillsdale, NJ: Erlbaum.

Bruce, V., & Young, A. W. (1986). A theoretical perspective for understanding face recognition. *British Journal of Psychology, 77*, 305–327.

Bruner, J. S., & Goodman, C. C. (1947). Value and need as organizing factors in perception. *Journal of Abnormal and Social Psychology, 42*, 33–44.

Calder, A. J., Young, A. W., Perrett, D. I., Etcoff, N. L., & Rowland, D. (1996). Categorical perception of morphed facial expressions. *Visual Cognition, 3*, 81–117.

Devine, P. (1989). Stereotypes and prejudice: Their automatic and controlled components. *Journal of Personality and Social Psychology, 56*, 5–18.

Farah, M. J., Wilson, K. D., Drain, M., & Tanaka, J. N. (1998). What is "special" about face perception? *Psychological Review, 105*, 482–498.

Fiske, S. T., & Neuberg, S. L. (1990). A continuum model of impression formation from category-based to individuating processes: Influences of information and motivation on attention and interpretation. *Advances in Experimental Social Psychology, 23*, 1–74.

Fodor, J. A. (1983). *The modularity of mind*. Cambridge, MA: MIT Press.

Freeman, J. B., & Ambady, N. (2009). Motions of the hand expose the partial and parallel activation of stereotypes. *Psychological Science, 20*, 1183–1188.

Freeman, J. B., & Ambady, N. (2011). A dynamic interactive theory of person construal. *Psychological Review, 118*, 247–279.

Freeman, J. B., Ambady, N., & Holcomb, P. J. (2010). The face-sensitive N170 encodes social category information. *NeuroReport, 21*, 24–28.

Freeman, J. B., Ambady, N., Rule, N. O., & Johnson, K. L. (2008). Will a category cue attract you?: Motor output reveals dynamic competition across person construal. *Journal of Experimental Psychology: General, 137*(4), 673–690.

Freeman, J. B., Pauker, K., Apfelbaum, E. P., & Ambady, N. (2010). Continuous dynamics in the real-time perception of race. *Journal of Experimental Social Psychology, 46*, 179–185.

Freeman, J. B., Penner, A. M., Saperstein, A., Scheutz, M., & Ambady, N. (2011). Looking the part: Social status cues shape race perception. *PLoS ONE, 6*, e25107.

Gawronski, B., & Bodenhausen, G. V. (2006). Associative and propositional processes in evaluation: An integrative review of implicit and explicit attitude change. *Psychological Bulletin, 132*, 692–731.

Gibson, J. J. (1979). *The ecological approach to visual perception*. Boston: Houghton Mifflin.

Gilbert, D. T., & Hixon, J. G. (1991). The trouble of thinking: Activation and application of stereotypic beliefs. *Journal of Personality and Social Psychology, 60*, 509–517.

Grossberg, S. (1980). How does a brain build a cognitive code? *Psychological Review, 87*, 1–51.

Haxby, J. V., Hoffman, E. A., & Gobbini, M. I. (2000). The distributed human neural system for face perception. *Trends in Cognitive Sciences, 4*, 223–233.

Hugenberg, K., & Bodenhausen, G. V. (2004). Ambiguity in social categorization: The role of prejudice and facial affect in race categorization. *Psychological Science, 15*(5), 342–345.

Ito, T. A., & Urland, G. R. (2003). Race and gender on the brain: Electrocortical measures of attention to the race and gender of multiply categorizable individuals. *Journal of Personality and Social Psychology, 85*, 616–626.

Johnson, K. L., & Freeman, J. B. (2010). A "new

look" at person construal: Seeing beyond dominance and discreteness. In E. Balcetis & D. Lassiter (Eds.), *The social psychology of visual perception* (pp. 255–272). New York: Psychology Press.

Johnson, K. L., Freeman, J. B., & Pauker, K. (2012). Race is gendered: How covarying phenotypes and stereotypes bias sex categorization. *Journal of Personality and Social Psychology, 102*, 116–131.

Kunda, Z., & Thagard, P. (1996). Forming impressions from stereotypes, traits, and behaviors: A parallel-constraint-satisfaction theory. *Psychological Review, 103*, 284–308.

Lepore, L., & Brown, R. (1997). Category and stereotype activation: Is prejudice inevitable? *Journal of Personality and Social Psychology, 72*, 275–287.

Macrae, C. N., & Bodenhausen, G. V. (2000). Social cognition: Thinking categorically about others. *Annual Review of Psychology, 51*, 93–120.

Marr, D. (1982). *Vision*. San Francisco: Freeman.

McClelland, J. L. (1991). Stochastic interactive processes and the effect of context on perception. *Cognitive Psychology, 23*, 1–44.

McClelland, J. L., & Rumelhart, D. E. (1981). An interactive activation model of context effects in letter perception: Part 1. An account of basic findings. *Psychological Review, 88*, 375–407.

Pauker, K., Weisbuch, M., Ambady, N., Sommers, S. R., Adams Jr., R. B., & Ivcevic, Z. (2009). Not so black and white: Memory for ambiguous group members. *Journal of Personality and Social Psychology, 96*, 795–810.

Pylyshyn, Z. W. (1984). *Computation and cognition*. Cambridge, MA: MIT Press.

Quinn, K. A., & Macrae, C. N. (2005). Categorizing others: The dynamics of person construal. *Journal of Personality and Social Psychology, 88*(3), 467–479.

Rogers, T. T., & McClelland, J. L. (2004). *Semantic cognition: A parallel distributed processing approach*. Boston: Bradford Books.

Rolls, E. T., & Tovee, M. J. (1995). Sparseness of the neuronal representation of stimuli in the primate temporal visual cortex. *Journal of Neurophysiology, 73*, 713–726.

Rule, N. O., Macrae, C. N., & Ambady, N. (2009). Ambiguous group membership is extracted automatically from faces. *Psychological Science, 20*, 441–443.

Rumelhart, D. E., Hinton, G. E., & McClelland, J. L. (1986). *A general framework for parallel distributed processing*. Cambridge, MA: MIT Press.

Rydell, R. J., & McConnell, A. R. (2006). Understanding implicit and explicit attitude change: A systems of reasoning analysis. *Journal of Personality and Social Psychology, 91*, 995–1008.

Sereno, S. C., & Rayner, K. (2003). Measuring word recognition in reading: Eye movements and event-related potentials. *Trends in Cognitive Sciences, 7*, 489–493.

Smith, P. L., & Ratcliff, R. (2004). Psychology and neurobiology of simple decisions. *Trends in Neurosciences, 27*, 161–168.

Smolensky, P. (1989). Connectionist modeling: Neural computation/mental connections. In L. Nadel, A. Cooper, P. Culicover, & R. M. Harnish (Eds.), *Neural connections, mental computations* (pp. 49–67). Cambridge, MA: MIT Press.

Spivey, M. J. (2007). *The continuity of mind*. New York: Oxford University Press.

Spivey, M. J., & Dale, R. (2006). Continuous dynamics in real-time cognition. *Current Directions in Psychological Science, 15*(5), 207–211.

Strack, F., & Deutsch, R. (2004). Reflective and impulsive determinants of social behavior. *Personality and Social Psychology Review, 8*, 220–247.

Sugase, Y., Yamane, S., Ueno, S., & Kawano, K. (1999). Global and fine information coded by single neurons in the temporal visual cortex. *Nature, 400*, 869–873.

Usher, M., & McClelland, J. L. (2001). The time course of perceptual choice: The leaky, competing accumulator model. *Psychological Review, 108*, 550–592.

CHAPTER 17

Person Perception

Integrating Category- and Individual-Level Information in Face Construal

Kimberly A. Quinn and C. Neil Macrae

Successful social interaction is predicated on the perceiver's ability to understand and predict the behavior of others—a deceptively simple task. From myriad cues—ranging from complex cues such as observed behavior to simple cues such as eye gaze direction and emotional expression (and the inferences that can be drawn from them)—the social perceiver must form a general impression of who the target is and how to interact with him or her. The process becomes even more complicated by the fact that any given individual also belongs to a number of social categories, each of which is associated with stereotypical expectations. Given this challenge, social cognitive psychologists have accorded a central role for social categorization and stereotyping (Allport, 1954; Brewer, 1988; Fiske & Neuberg, 1990). For example, in his seminal analysis of the psychological underpinnings of prejudice, Allport (1954) argued that categorization is not only helpful in streamlining person perception but also inevitable: "The human mind," he asserted, "must think with the aid of categories. . . . Once formed, categories are the basis for normal prejudgment. We cannot possibly avoid this process. Orderly living depends upon it" (p. 20). Stereotypes, not individuated impressions, are assumed to drive the earliest stages of person perception.

In this chapter, our goal is to reopen the question of whether category-level information is indeed the dominant input to person perception, at least in the context of face processing. In so doing, we explore the intersection of category- and individual-level information in face construal. Ultimately, we argue that the cognitive economy that has presumably been served by social categorization at the expense of individuation is better served by a single system characterized by processes that support *both* categorization and individuation.

CATEGORY-LEVEL INFORMATION AS THE DOMINANT INPUT TO PERSON PERCEPTION

Decades after Allport's (1954) assertion about the inevitability of categorization, his influence can be seen not only in theories about prejudice (e.g., Devine, 1989) but also in several influential models of person perception—most notably, Brewer's (1988) dual-process model and Fiske and Neuberg's (1990) continuum model. The models differ in their respective positions on the relationship between stereotyping and individuation. Brewer (1988) assumes that perceivers choose implicitly between stereotyping and individuation, whereas Fiske and Neuberg (1990) give priority to stereotyping and depict individuation as a correction process. Nonetheless, both models assert that some form of categorization is the first and inevitable step in person construal. In Brewer's model, for example, person perception begins with an "identification" phase in which the perceiver automatically places the target along "well-established stimulus dimensions such as gender, age, and skin color" (1988, p. 6)—essentially, a form of "primitive categorization" (Bruner, 1957). Similarly, in Fiske and Neuberg's model, person construal begins with an initial categorization that is "essentially perceptual" (1990, p. 4) and most likely to focus on visual cues (again, sex, race, and age).

The importance accorded to social categorization and its downstream consequence of stereotyping is reflected in two, related hypotheses: (1) Perceivers are more efficient at extracting category-level than individual-level information from social targets; and (2) stereotypes allow perceivers to take mental shortcuts to save time and processing capacity. The first hypothesis is related to the ease with which physical features, particularly in faces, can be used to retrieve relevant information from memory. Quite simply, it is easier to extract category membership from a face than to recognize its owner's identity, in that many social category dimensions (e.g., sex, race, age) are readily apparent in physical features, whereas full-blown identity recognition requires retrieval of nonphysical features (e.g., name, occupation, traits). Evidence for this hypothesis comes from Cloutier, Mason, and Macrae (2005), who demonstrated that three different manipulations of processing difficulty (inversion, blurring, brief presentation) impaired participants' ability to identify familiar celebrities but not to categorize them by sex. This efficiency derives, at least in part, from the fact that even a single feature can support categorization (e.g., Cloutier & Macrae, 2007; Livingstone & Brewer, 2002; Macrae & Martin, 2007) but that identity recognition is heavily reliant on the extraction of configural or holistic information across multiple features (e.g., Maurer, Le Grand, & Mondloch, 2002; Rhodes, Brake, & Atkinson, 1993).

The second hypothesis is related to the requirements of social inference. Generating inferences about a target individual's unique constellation of mental states, goals, and traits should require more attention and processing effort than does the retrieval of already-stored inferences about other members of the target individual's social category. That is, preexisting knowledge structures (i.e., stereotypes) can be used to guide information processing and response generation, especially when other sources of person knowledge are absent, ambiguous, or difficult to acquire (Allport, 1954; Brewer, 1988; Fiske & Neuberg, 1990). Indeed, evidence confirms that stereotype activation and application streamlines most aspects of person perception, including decision making, memorial functioning, attentional processing, and impression formation (for a review, see Quinn, Macrae, & Bodenhausen, 2003). Given these economizing effects, categorical thinking has been characterized as an indispensable cognitive tool in the person perception process (e.g., Gilbert & Hixon, 1991; Macrae, Milne, & Bodenhausen, 1994). That stereotypes further serve a capacity-*saving* function was established by Macrae et al. (1994), who demonstrated that participants who were provided with a social category label to guide their person perception subsequently showed better memory for nonstereotypical information than did participants who were not provided with a label. Sherman, Lee, Bessenoff, and Frost (1998) extended this research to demonstrate that the provision of a social category label enabled participants to direct attention away from stereotype-consistent information and toward not only stereotype-irrelevant information but also to stereotype-*inconsistent* information.

This evidence suggests that given appropriate triggering cues, category-based responding may be the predominant social cognitive outcome at *all* stages of the person perception process. Visual analysis favors the extraction of category-specifying cues, and stereotypes provide attentional and interpretational frameworks to organize relevant information. In this respect, person construal may simply reflect the mind's evolved strategy of imposing a categorical solution on a broad range of problems in perception and cognition (Harnad, 1987).

BEYOND CATEGORICAL INFORMATION: INDIVIDUAL AND IDENTITY

The observations that stereotypes are readily elicited upon perceiving others and "free up" resources for allocation elsewhere (Macrae et al., 1994; Sherman et al., 1998) support the long-standing assertion that stereotype contents are automatically and unavoidably activated during the person perception process (e.g., Allport, 1954; Fiske & Neuberg, 1990). However, the assumption that stereotype activation was automatic and would inevitably color impressions and behavior was challenged by Gilbert and Hixon (1991), who argued that stereotype activation and application were only conditionally automatic—that is, dependent on certain triggering conditions. Gilbert and Hixon demonstrated that mere exposure to a stimulus target (e.g., an Asian woman) was not sufficient to prompt stereotype activation; rather, stereotype activation required attentional resources: Participants who were under cognitive load at the time of exposure to the target showed no evidence of increased stereotype activation. Since this initial demonstration, a host of other factors has been shown to moderate stereotype activation, including perceivers' processing goals (Macrae, Bodenhausen, Milne, Thorn, & Castelli, 1997), self-esteem (Spencer, Fein, Wolfe, Fong, & Dunn, 1998), hormonal fluctuations (Amodio, 2009; Macrae, Alnwick, Milne, & Schloerscheidt, 2002), visual attention (Macrae, Bodenhausen, Milne, & Calvini, 1999), prejudice level (Lepore & Brown, 1997; Moskowitz, Gollwitzer, Wasel, & Schaal, 1999), stereotype control intentions (Sassenberg & Moskowitz, 2005; Stewart & Payne, 2008), and mental imagery (Blair, Ma, & Lenton, 2001), as well as target gaze direction (Macrae, Hood, Milne, Rowe, & Mason, 2002) and context (Castelli, Macrae, Zogmaister, & Arcuri, 2004; Kurzban, Tooby, & Cosmides, 2001; Wittenbrink, Judd, & Park, 2001).

Moreover, several pieces of evidence now indicate that social categorization, like stereotype activation, is not unconditionally automatic. Quinn and Macrae (2005), for example, found that "automatic" sex categorization emerged only when sex was relevant to the task at hand (see also Livingston & Brewer, 2002; Macrae, Quinn, Mason, & Quadflieg, 2005; Wheeler & Fiske, 2005). That social categorization should be only conditionally automatic makes sense, if it is a tool to facilitate the perceiver's ability to form an impression of a social target that can be used to make predictions and guide interactions. Quite simply, person perception can—and should—make use of a wide array of cues beyond social category membership and applicable stereotypes. In processing the faces, bodies, and movements of targets embedded in particular contexts and situations, perceivers are able to glean a wealth of information about both transient and stable target characteristics. Emotional expression, body posture, and eye gaze, for example, all provide insight into a target's context-dependent motives and intentions (for a review, see Macrae & Quadflieg, 2010), and behavior speaks to both transient and chronic dispositions and traits (McCarthy & Skowronski, Chapter 15, this volume). Even facial features allow rapid inferences about personality traits: Targets with "babyface" features (e.g., large eyes, a small nose, thin eyebrows, and a small chin) are perceived as submissive, dependent, naive, and lovable (Berry & McArthur, 1986; Zebrowitz & Montepare, 1992). Some provocative evidence even suggests that perceivers draw trustworthiness inferences on the basis of as little as 33 milliseconds of exposure to an unfamiliar face (see also Willis & Todorov, 2006) and, in some cases, regardless of perceiver goals or intentions (Engell, Haxby, & Todorov, 2007; Winston, Strange, O'Doherty, & Dolan, 2002). More germane to this chapter, person perception often includes the recognition of familiar targets (e.g., friends, colleagues) or at least the recognition that a target is familiar, yet familiarity and identity recognition have received scant attention in social cognitive models of person perception. At best, they have been relegated to the status of outcomes of rather than inputs to person perception.

What are the implications of familiarity and identity recognition for person perception? Social cognitive theorists have long argued that social categorization has privileged status in person perception because it allows the perceiver to draw on stored representations (i.e., stereotypes) to guide expectancies and behavior. However, perceivers also store representations of familiar and known targets. When asked to judge the traits of target individuals from photographs, perceivers' responses continue to be influenced by information previously associated with the faces, even though the precise details have been forgotten (Uleman, Blader, & Todorov, 2005). Similarly, affective person-related knowledge gleaned from minimal information (i.e., reading that someone engages in a disgusting behavior) is spontaneously reactivated when the associated face is encountered again (Todorov, Gobbini, Evans, & Haxby, 2007). In short, familiar individuals trigger the spontaneous activation of biographical knowledge.

On occasion, unfamiliar targets are deemed to be familiar because they resemble friends, family, or celebrities in their appearance or mannerisms. This similarity can lead perceivers to evaluate these targets in line with the people they resemble (e.g., Gawronski & Quinn, 2013; Kraus & Chen, 2010; Verosky & Todorov, 2010) or to ascribe to these targets the same traits, attributes, and characteristics as those of the people they resemble (Chen & Andersen, 1999). For example, when the face of a stranger reminds one of a good friend, traits descriptive of the friend are readily attributed to the unknown other (White & Shapiro, 1987). Physical resemblance to self also influences person perception, such that strangers who resemble the self are rated as more trustworthy (DeBruine, Jones, Little, & Perrett, 2008).

Finally, some targets are encountered on numerous occasions, yet no specific target-related knowledge is acquired (i.e., the woman one sees on the bus every morning). What happens, then, when these familiar yet unknown others are perceived? Perceivers seem to regard perceptually familiar people as more likable than unfamiliar targets (Moreland & Zajonc, 1982), an effect that is likely driven by the misattribution of positive affect elicited by increased perceptual fluency (Winkielman & Cacioppo, 2001). However, recent work also suggests that perceptually familiar individuals may be construed even more stereotypically than unfamiliar others (Smith et al., 2006), perhaps reflecting perceivers' need to make sense of frequently encountered targets.

Thus, it is clear that for familiar targets—and perhaps for unfamiliar targets who are encountered frequently or remind the perceiver of someone—there are stored representations that provide alternatives to categorization-driven stereotypes. In such cases, we would argue that the social categorization would not have privileged status. Particularly with familiar targets, it simply does not seem intuitively reasonable that we would spontaneously process friends and family members in terms of their social category memberships. Given the wealth of individuating information that we have available to us about the traits, attitudes, values, opinions, hobbies, and skills of familiar others—that is, familiarity via experience across multiple occasions and contexts—it certainly seems like it should be more useful to rely on information that we know to be true of the target rather than unverified guesses based on broad generalizations across a group of people.

On a more theoretical level, there are also reasons to argue against the inevitability of social categorization for familiar targets. Any social target can be categorized at multiple levels (Bodenhausen, Macrae, & Sherman, 1999), from superordinate (e.g., "human") to subordinate (e.g., "Leigh"), with many possible levels in between (e.g., "woman"). Each of these levels of categorization is linked with a mental representation that captures both context-free and context-dependent generalities about that particular construal—"stereotypes" about humans, about women, and about an individual named Leigh, for example. Thus, for any individual, the potential exists for "nonsocial" categorization (e.g., animate rather than inanimate, human rather than nonhuman), "social" categorization (i.e., categorization according to socially meaningful dimensions such as sex, race, age), and "individual" categorization (i.e., categorization according to individual identity).

Importantly, however, perceivers have default "entry" or "basic" levels of categorization for classes of targets, and these defaults vary with familiarity and expertise (Jolicoeur, Gluck, & Kosslyn, 1984; Rosch,

Mervis, Gray, Johnson, & Boyes-Braem, 1976). In essence, basic-level categorization maximizes both differentiation between categories and similarity within categories, supporting the ultimate processing goal of cognitive economy (Rosch et al., 1976). In person perception, basic-level categorization may often be characterized by group-level categorization and stereotyping exactly because these forms of processing do provide maximal information with minimal effort. Thus, although group-level categorization might not provide as much within-category family resemblance as individual-level categorization, it would provide much better cue validity when targets are unfamiliar. By definition, perceivers have little if any individuating information about unfamiliar individuals to guide their initial construal, whereas they can draw on informative (if inaccurate) knowledge of relevant groups.

For familiar individuals, however, the basic level of categorization may instead be at the level of the individual rather than the group. Again, categorizing at the level of the individual would serve to maximize within-category family resemblance. In addition, the expertise that perceivers accrue through repeated exposure to, and interaction with, specific individuals has the effect of changing the information that provides the best cue validity. Much of the information that a perceiver might accrue about Leigh, for example, would differentiate her from the category "women"—not only in terms of the ways in which her personality or behavior violate expectations about women, but also in terms of additional information that might be irrelevant to beliefs about women but informative about Leigh. To the extent that stereotype-disconfirming and stereotype-irrelevant information provides the greatest cue validity for making predictions about Leigh, she should be categorized at the level of individual rather than according to her social category. In support of this reasoning, Quinn, Mason, and Macrae (2009) demonstrated that even when social categorization is task-relevant, it does not determine how familiar targets are construed. Although category-based responding may be highly efficient (e.g., Cloutier, Turk, & Macrae, 2007), person perception is nevertheless sufficiently flexible to enable individual-based responses to familiar targets (see also Tanaka, 2001; Turk, Rosenblum, Gazzaniga, & Macrae, 2005). This flexibility, we suggest, derives from the common system that subserves both categorization and individuation—a point to which we return later.

CATEGORY-LEVEL VERSUS IDENTITY-LEVEL CONSTRUAL

Thus far, we have reviewed evidence against the automaticity of social categorization and stereotyping, and argued that models of person perception must incorporate familiarity and identity as inputs rather than relegating them to the status of outcomes. Models from cognitive psychology and neuroscience may be instructive here. Although contemporary models of face processing seek primarily to establish the cognitive and neural underpinnings of identity recognition and are not directly concerned with social categorization, they nonetheless represent attempts to account for *all* of the possible inputs to identity recognition—including social category membership.

The two most influential models of face recognition are Bruce and Young's (1986) functional model and Haxby, Hoffman, and Gobbini's (2000, 2002) distributed neural model. Bruce and Young's (1986) model specifies the cognitive operations underpinning face recognition and posits that qualitatively different operations support the processing of idiosyncratic (i.e., identity specific) and generic (i.e., identity-nonspecific) aspects of faces. Haxby et al.'s (2000, 2002) model similarly distinguishes between the representation of invariant aspects of faces that form the basis of recognition and changeable aspects of faces that facilitate social communication, and specifies the neural substrates of each. Although this might seem to imply that category and identity are separate processes, both models also highlight the importance of a system of cognitive functions (e.g., semantic memory) that works with visual analysis to extract meaning from faces—relevant steps in both categorization and individuation—and Haxby et al.'s model explicitly allows interactivity between component processes. Moreover, "identity-nonspecific" information in the Bruce and Young (1986) model does not necessarily refer to category membership, given that the features denoting sex, race and the like are part of the configuration of features that together denote unique identity. Even if we were to conceptualize identity-nonspecific information as including cues to category membership, debate remains as to whether identity-specific and -nonspecific information are processed independently; indeed, there is now some evidence for the integrated processing of category and identity (e.g., sex and identity: Baudoin & Tiberghien, 2002; Ganel & Goshen-Gottstein, 2002; age and identity: Dagovitch & Ganel, 2010). Thus, social categorization and identity recognition are not completely separable. Instead, social categorization and identity recognition exert mutual influence.

Social Categorization Influences Identity Recognition

One of the most robust findings in face processing is that perceivers are better at recognizing faces from their own racial group than faces from other racial groups—the so-called "own-race bias," "cross-race effect," or "other-race effect" (for a review, see Meissner & Brigham, 2001). Although this bias appears to have a perceptual expertise component (e.g., Kelly et al., 2007), there is now strong evidence that social categorization also plays a critical role in shaping own- and other-race face processing. According to this perspective, the other-race effect emerges because either the coding of race-specifying information (e.g., skin tone) occurs at the expense of individuating information (Levin, 1996, 2000) or the categorization of other-race faces as outgroup members undermines perceivers' motivation to process other-race faces in terms of individual identity (e.g., Hugenberg & Sacco, 2008; Hugenberg, Young, Bernstein, & Sacco, 2010). Much of the evidence for the latter position comes from Hugenberg and colleagues, who have demonstrated that inducing white participants to categorize white faces as outgroup members can lead to poorer recognition of those faces relative to white faces categorized as ingroup members (e.g., Bernstein, Young, & Hugenberg, 2007), presumably because outgroup categorization undermines holistic processing (Hugenberg & Corneille, 2009). Ingroup–outgroup categorization also influences recognition of other-race faces—at least when the context serves to minimize the salience of race categorization (Cassidy, Quinn, & Humphreys, 2011; Hehman, Mania, & Gaertner, 2010) or when encoding favors configural processing (Cassidy, Humphreys, & Quinn, unpublished data). Categorizing other-race faces as ingroup members can also lead to a shift toward greater configural processing (Cassidy, Boutsen, Humphreys, & Quinn, in press; Cassidy et al., 2011, unpublished data)—more akin to the manner in which own-race faces tend to be processed (Rhodes, Brake, Taylor, & Tan, 1989; Sangrigoli & de Schonen, 2004).

Social categorization not only induces general changes in processing and subsequent recognition, but it can also affect how individual features are perceived. Levin and Banaji (2006), for example, demonstrated that categorizing racially ambiguous faces as black or white distorted white participants' perceptions of skin tone. Specifically, when participants were asked to match the skin tone of target faces to reference samples of luminance, they perceived the skin tone of faces labeled as black to be darker than the skin tone of faces labeled as white, even though the faces were matched for skin tone (for a review of evidence about the role of skin tone in face perception, see Maddox, 2004).

Finally, the impact of social categorization on identity recognition may be moderated by other factors known to influence social categorization itself, such as emotional expression. Ackerman et al. (2006), for example, demonstrated that the cross-race effect was reversed when the target faces expressed anger. That is, among white participants, recognition favored own-race over other-race faces when expressions were neutral, but other-race over own-race faces when anger was expressed. Ackerman et al. interpreted their findings according to a functionalist perspective, whereby processing resources are allocated selectively to self-relevant environmental cues—in this case, danger-related stereotypes about racial outgroups that are triggered by threat cues in the environment (e.g., Schaller, Park, & Mueller, 2003).

That categorization influences individuation, on its own, does not provide evidence that the two are subserved by the same rather than different processes. After all, we have reviewed evidence that categorization can proceed on the basis of less information than is required for identity recognition. Categorization may therefore do little more than provide additional input to individuation, rather than being an output of the same set of processes. But if individual-level information can also influence categorization despite being more difficult to extract, then the proposal that the two represent distinct processes becomes less tenable.

Identity Recognition Influences Social Categorization

Just as social categorization has implications for face perception and subsequent identity recognition, so too does identity recognition influence the efficiency of social categorization. Several lines of evidence, for example, are converging on the notion that it is easier to extract categorical information from known versus unknown faces—for example, information such as sex (Bruce, 1986; Rossion, 2002), race (Bruyer, Leclerc, & Quinet, 2004), and age (Bruyer, Lafalize, & Distefano, 1991).

Understanding the emergence of this bidirectional influence has recently received attention in the social cognition literature. The starting point of this research has been the recognition that before a perceiver can recognize a target's unique identity or social category membership (and before the representations associated with these construals can be activated and exert top-down influence), the target's face must first receive basic visual processing. Motivated by theory and evidence from research on vision (e.g., Marr, 1982), as well as evidence that face processing proceeds from the analysis of less complex aspects of faces, such as features, to more complex aspects, such as configural relations among features (e.g., Liu, Harris, & Kanwisher, 2002), social cognitive psychologists have come to recognize processing time as an important moderator of person construal. Ito, Thompson, and Cacioppo (2004), for example, used event-related potentials to track the time course of processing racial ingroup and outgroup faces. Their results demonstrated that faces were distinguished from non-faces approximately 170 milliseconds into processing, that ingroup members were distinguished from (and accorded more attention than) outgroup members at 250 milliseconds, and that evaluative differentiation (which correlated with prejudice level) of ingroup and outgroup faces emerged at 520 milliseconds.

Admittedly, ingroup–outgroup categorization is not *recognition* as conventionally defined, so what are the implications of time course for social categorization and identification, and the ability of individual-level information to influence category-level processing? That is, how are these two processes reflected in the simple-to-complex processing trajectory of visual perception? As we have already noted, social cognitive researchers have long argued for the primacy of categorical thinking, asserting that categorical construal is the most functional level of analysis, because it optimizes information obtained (via stereotypes) against effort expended (e.g., Macrae et al., 1994; Sherman et al., 1998), and that more individuated construals emerge only when perceivers require additional information (e.g., when perceivers are held accountable for their impressions, when targets behave in stereotype-disconfirming ways; Brewer, 1988; Fiske & Neuberg, 1990). Moreover, and as we mentioned previously, it is easier to disrupt identity recognition than social categorization (Cloutier et al., 2005)—presumably because even though categorization can proceed on the basis of a single feature (Brown & Perrett, 1993; Bruce et al., 1993; Cloutier & Macrae, 2007), identity recognition is heavily reliant on the extraction of configural information across multiple features (Leder & Bruce, 2000; Maurer et al., 2002; Rhodes et al., 1993). Together, these arguments and evidence suggest that categorization should emerge earlier in processing.

The time course of categorization versus identification was investigated more directly by Quinn, Mason, and Macrae (2010). Varying the presentation duration of prime faces to capture early versus late processes, they found that for unfamiliar targets, category-based responding (i.e., sex priming) emerged for both earlier and later responses, most likely because the category-relevant information extracted at the earlier time point would not be superseded by identity-relevant information. In contrast, for familiar targets, category-based responding emerged for only earlier responses, ostensibly because the identity-based information extracted at the later time point was sufficient to negate the influence of the category-based information. (See Macrae et al., 2005, and Mason, Cloutier, & Macrae, 2006, for evidence that identity is extracted efficiently from familiar faces, even when the faces are goal-irrelevant and presented in a less-than-optimal inverted orientation.)

INTEGRATING CATEGORY-LEVEL AND INDIVIDUAL-LEVEL INFORMATION: ONE PROCESS OR TWO?

Given the putative functional differences between social categorization and identity recognition (e.g., providing predictions based on generalized stereotypes vs. idiosyncratic attributes), it seems intuitively reasonable to propose that operational differences would underlie the two outcomes. However, categorization and individuation are typically indexed in the social cognitive literature in terms of content rather than process—for example, with categorization indexed as faster responses to or better memory for stereotypical versus nonstereotypical information, and individuation indexed by a *lack* of advantage for stereotypical over nonstereotypical information. These measures reflect the outcomes of categorization versus individuation rather than providing direct access to the processes themselves. Perhaps more critically, both reflect access to semantic representations—albeit representations that depict category-level versus individual-level information (or perhaps group-level vs. individual-level categorization; Bodenhausen et al., 1999). Thus, it is difficult to generate strong conclusions on the basis of the dominant methodological paradigms as to whether categorization and individuation represent a single process with multiple content outputs or two distinct processes.

Nonetheless, regardless of whether the outcome is identity recognition or social categorization, it is undeniable that person perception begins with the visual analysis of the same facial features. In the Bruce and Young (1986) and Haxby et al. (2000, 2002) models, this fact is reflected in the specification of visual analysis and structural encoding as necessary precursors to both identity recognition and social categorization: To evaluate a target according to his or her social group membership (categorization) versus idiosyncratic attributes (individuation), the person must first know who or what the target is. Here, there may appear to be differences, in that categorization can proceed on the basis of single features (e.g., Brown & Perrett, 1993; Bruce et al., 1993; Cloutier et al., 2007) but individuation is supported by the extraction of configurations of features (e.g., Leder & Bruce, 2000; Maurer et al., 2002; Rhodes et al., 1993), and that featural and configural processing are lateralized in separate hemispheres (Mason & Macrae, 2004; Zárate, Stoever, MacLin, & Arms-Chavez, 2008). However, this does not mean that categorization relies solely on featural processing and individuation, on configural processing. Featural information is not lost during configural processing—attention to spatial relationships between *features* is the definition of configural processing—and configural information is extracted from even unfamiliar faces. Configural processing is so entrenched, in fact, that individuals are unable to attend selectively to features even when instructed to do so (Richler, Tanaka, Brown, & Gauthier, 2008).

On the basis that categorization and individuation both prompt access to semantic information (in the form of stereotypes vs. biographical information) and that the same component processes (featural vs. configural processing) are implicated in both, we assert that the early products of person perception (i.e., category-level vs. individual-level construal) are ultimately supported by a common neural architecture (Haxby et al., 2000, 2002). Categorization and individuation, at least at the perceptual level, simply make different demands on parts of the distributed cortical network that subserves person perception (Cloutier et al., 2005; Mason & Macrae, 2004). Both brain imaging (e.g., Dubois et al., 1999; Mason & Macrae, 2004; Rossion, Schiltz, Robaye, Pirenne, & Crommelinck, 2001) and behavioral research (e.g., Baudoin & Tiberghien, 2002; Bruyer et al., 2004; Dagovitch & Ganel, 2010; Ganel & Goshen-Gottstein,

2002; Rossion, 2002) confirm that categorization and identification are integrated in some way during processing. Such a viewpoint is consistent with recent models of object recognition. Tarr and Cheng (2003), for example, have proposed that recognition across all object categories—for example, birds, cars, and *faces*—is supported by a single processing system that is tuned by a combination of experience and instruction. If a single (albeit modular) system is sufficient to recognize all types of objects at varying levels of specificity, it seems reasonable to conclude that categorization and individuation may reflect different social cognitive products of this system.

Our position is also consistent with Freeman and Ambady's (2011) dynamic interactive theory of person construal. According to this theory, person construal emerges gradually "through ongoing cycles of interaction between categories, stereotypes, high-level cognitive states, and the low-level processing of facial, vocal, and bodily cues" (p. 250). A central assumption of the model is that processing involves time-dependent competition between partially active and parallel representations (see also Kunda & Thagard, 1996). Perceptual processing extracts not only features from the targets themselves—for example, face, voice, and posture cues to identity, sex, race, and age—but also features of the processing context (e.g., cues that mark targets as members of contextually rare categories). This processing triggers multiple representations in memory (e.g., stereotypes, representations of similar targets encountered previously, representations of previous encounters with the targets themselves). Meanwhile, representations that were already active when the targets were encountered (e.g., embodied emotional states, self-relevant goals) also contribute to processing. Importantly, this theory accords no special status to either category-level or individual-level information: All representations—categorical, individuated, contextual—compete and over time and settle into a stable state, which often results in a single construal. Whether that construal is categorical or individuated will depend not only on how easily the initial identification can be made (with categorical construal requiring fewer or less complex inputs than individuated construal) but also on the strength of the activated representations (stereotypes vs. stored impressions) activated in memory.

Where Freeman and Ambady (2011) are less clear, however, is in addressing the question of whether categorization and individuation rely on the same or different processes. Our view, akin to the view argued in Kruglanski et al.'s (2003) unimodel of judgment, is that the same processes support both categorization and individuation, albeit perhaps to different extents. Consistent with Bruce and Young's (1986) and Haxby et al.'s (2000, 2002) models of face recognition, and Tarr and Cheng's (2003) discussion of object recognition, we suggest that both categorization and individuation begin with the same inputs (features and configurations derived from visual analysis) and end with the same *kinds* of outcomes (category labels or names, plus the associated semantic representations). The differences, as in the unimodel, are the relative difficulty of extracting the relevant inputs (with categorization tending to be easier than individuation) and the strength and accessibility of the relevant semantic representations (varying as a function of familiarity, goals, etc.).

Moreover, all of these processes—visual analysis, the extraction of featural and configural information, semantic activation—proceed largely automatically. As our review has shown, for example, configural processing occurs involuntarily (Richler et al., 2008) and extremely early in visual analysis (Richler, Mack, Gauthier, & Palmeri, 2009). Even more complex trait judgments (e.g., trustworthiness) appear to happen involuntarily (Engell et al., 2007; Winston et al., 2002) and to require very little visual input (Todorov, Pakrashi, & Oosterhof, 2009). It seems very unlikely that perceivers would be able to engage controlled processing as early as 50 milliseconds into visual analysis, when the processes that enable semantic activation of category and identity information are initiated.

Of course, directed visual processing (Bruce & Young, 1986) can be recruited in the service of current goals, and this processing may lack some of the features of automaticity (e.g., lack of intentionality). For the most part, however, although perceivers can have conscious access to the outcomes of these processes, and certainly must in the case of identity recognition, the extant evidence would suggest that perceivers do not have access to the processes that subserve categorization and individuation/identification. One exception might be cases in which perceivers actively attempt to scan faces for future recognition. Perceivers could, for example, attempt to memorize features, making feature processing intentional. It should be noted, however, that this kind of strategy might shift the "normal" balance between featural and configural processing (Cassidy et al., unpublished data; Fallshore & Schooler, 1995) and might not reflect the same kind of featural processing as that engaged during "normal" face perception. In general, our position is that as long as visual attention is directed toward a face—intentionally or not—then the processes described in this chapter will proceed automatically.

CONCLUSION

In this chapter, we have explored the intersection of category- and individual-level information in person perception and challenged the prevailing assumption that social categorization is necessarily the dominant input to person perception. We have argued that category- and individual-level information contribute to person perception via a single system—that categorization and individuation are merely different products of a single system, relying on different inputs but processed through the same form of visual analysis, promoting access to memorial representations of different strength and with different contents (i.e., stereotypes vs. individuated impressions). This account offers a view of person perception that is equally as oriented toward cognitive economy as previous accounts have been (e.g., Brewer, 1988; Fiske & Neuberg, 1990) but argues that cognitive economy is better served by a single system that promotes greater flexibility and enables the perceiver to construe social targets as efficiently as possible—whether through generalized stereotypes for unfamiliar targets or individuated impressions for familiar targets.

Admittedly, our discussion has considered only a snapshot at the earliest stage of person construal, leaving a number of important questions unanswered. One of these questions centers on the precise relation of categorical information to identity recognition. Indeed, some evidence points to the status of sex in particular as a dimension of identity (e.g., Baudoin & Tiberghien, 2002; cf. Le Gal & Bruce, 2002), and more than two decades ago, Brewer (1988) pointed out that categorical dimensions such as sex exist not only as dimensions for categorization but also as features of the individual. Leigh, for example, can be categorized as a woman, but "female" is also a feature of her identity (see also Bodenhausen et al., 1999). As a result, recognizing the identity of a target may actually preclude inhibiting the categorical features of that target. The possibility that categorical information may be activated in some way even for familiar individuals without "driving" how these individuals are construed (Quinn et al., 2010) deserves exploration.

In addition, we have reviewed the literature on perceivers' responses to briefly presented static images of social targets instead of live, extended social interaction. Given that familiar targets are readily construed in an identity-based manner even at this early stage of processing (Quinn et al., 2009), this would tend to suggest that the later judgmental, memorial, and behavioral effects indicative of categorical thinking (see Macrae & Bodenhausen, 2000) may fail to emerge for these targets. On the other hand, the potential link between individual identity and category-specifying features noted earlier suggests potentially greater complexity in the relationship between earlier and later judgment (see also Kunda, Davies, Adams, & Spencer, 2002). Of interest, therefore, would be work exploring the impact of category-based knowledge structures on the postperceptual operations that shape social cognition when perceivers interact with known others. Research of this kind will contribute to current understanding of how target familiarity and social category membership jointly guide the process and products of person construal.

Finally, we have confined our review and analysis to the earliest stages of person perception, as the perceiver solves the problem of determining what or who the target is. In so doing, we have focused largely on the (conditionally) automatic processes that are engaged when the perceiver first encounters a social target. It remains possible that categorization and individuation represent distinct processes at later stages of person perception, when the perceiver organizes target-relevant information in memory, allocates attention to current processing concerns, and generates target-related inferences. Expectations of consistency, for example, may differ for individual-level versus category-level construal (Hamilton & Sherman, 1996), with implications for the relative complexity and stability of individual versus categorical representations and the processing of representation-consistent versus -inconsistent information.

REFERENCES

Ackerman, J. M., Shapiro, J. R., Neuberg, S. L., Kenrick, D. T., Becker, D. V. Griskevicius, V., et al. (2006). They all look the same to me (unless they're angry). From out-group homogeneity to out-group heterogeneity. *Psychological Science, 17,* 836–840.

Allport, G. W. (1954). *The nature of prejudice.* Cambridge, MA: Addison-Wesley.

Amodio, D. M. (2009). Intergroup anxiety effects on the control of racial stereotypes: A psychneuroendocrine analysis. *Journal of Experimental Social Psychology, 45,* 60–67.

Baudoin, J. Y., & Tiberghien, G. (2002). Sex is a dimension in face recognition. *Journal of Experimental Psychology: Learning, Memory, and Cognition, 28,* 362–365.

Bernstein, M. J., Young, S. G., & Hugenberg, K. (2007). The cross-category effect: Mere social categorization is sufficient to elicit an own-group bias in face recognition. *Psychological Science, 18,* 706–712.

Berry, D. S., & McArthur, L. Z. (1986). Perceiving character in faces: The impact of age-related craniofacial changes on social perception. *Psychological Bulletin, 100,* 3–18.

Blair, I., Ma, J., & Lenton, A. (2001). Imagining stereotypes away: The moderation of automatic stereotypes through mental imagery. *Journal of Personality and Social Psychology, 81,* 828–841.

Bodenhausen, G. V., Macrae, C. N., & Sherman, J. W. (1999). On the dialectics of discrimination: Dual processes in social stereotyping. In S. Chaiken & Y. Trope (Eds.), *Dual-process theories in social psychology* (pp. 271–292). New York: Guilford Press.

Brewer, M. B. (1988). A dual-process model of impression formation. In R. S. Wyer, Jr. & T. K. Srull (Eds.), *Advances in social cognition* (Vol. 1, pp. 1–36). Hillsdale, NJ: Erlbaum.

Brown, E., & Perrett, D. I. (1993). What gives a face its gender? *Perception, 22,* 829–840.

Bruce, V. (1986). Influences of familiarity on the processing of faces. *Perception, 15,* 387–397.

Bruce, V., Burton, A. M., Hanna, E., Healey, P., Mason, O., Coombes, A., et al. (1993). Sex discrimination: How do we tell the difference between male and female faces? *Perception, 22,* 131–152.

Bruce, V., & Young, A. (1986). Understanding face recognition. *British Journal of Psychology, 77,* 305-327.

Bruner, J. S. (1957). On perceptual readiness. *Psychological Review, 64,* 123–152.

Bruyer, R., Lafalize, A., & Distefano, M. (1991). Age decisions on familiar and unfamiliar faces. *Behavioural Processes, 24,* 21–35.

Bruyer, R., Leclerc, S., & Quinet, P. (2004). Ethnic categorization of faces is not independent of face identity. *Perception, 33,* 169–179.

Cassidy, K. D., Boutsen, L., Humphreys, G. W., & Quinn, K. A. (in press). Ingroup categorization affects the structural encoding of other-race faces: Evidence from the N170 event-related potential. *Social Neuroscience.*

Cassidy, K. D., Humphreys, G. W., & Quinn, K. A. (unpublished data). *The influence of ingroup/outgroup categorization on own- and other-race face processing: The moderating role of encoding goals.*

Cassidy, K. D., Quinn, K. A., & Humphreys, G. W. (2011). The influence of ingroup/outgroup categorization on same- and other-race face processing: The moderating role of inter- versus intra-racial context. *Journal of Experimental Social Psychology, 47,* 811–817.

Castelli, L., Macrae, C. N., Zogmaister, C., & Arcuri, L. (2004). A tale of two primes: Contextual limits on stereotype activation. *Social Cognition, 22,* 233–247.

Chen, S., & Andersen, S. M. (1999). Relationships from the past in the present: Significant-other representations and transference in interpersonal life. In M. P. Zanna (Ed.), *Advances in experimental social psychology* (Vol. 31, pp. 123–190). San Diego: Academic Press.

Cloutier, J., & Macrae, C. N. (2007). Who or what are you?: Facial orientation and person construal. *European Journal of Social Psychology, 37,* 1298–1309.

Cloutier, J., Mason, M. F., & Macrae, N. C. (2005). The perceptual determinants of person construal: Reopening the social-cognitive toolbox. *Journal of Personality and Social Psychology, 88,* 885–894.

Cloutier, J., Turk, D. J., & Macrae, C. N. (2007). Extracting variant and invariant information from faces: The neural substrates of gaze detection and sex categorization. *Social Neuroscience, 3,* 69–78.

Dagovitch, Y., & Ganel, T. (2010). Effects of facial identity on age judgments: Evidence from repetition priming. *Experimental Psychology, 57,* 390–397.

DeBruine, L. M., Jones, B. C., Little, A. C., & Perrett, D. I. (2008). Social perception of facial resemblance in humans. *Archives of Sexual Behavior, 37,* 64–77.

Devine, P. G. (1989). Stereotypes and prejudice: Their automatic and controlled components. *Journal of Personality and Social Psychology, 56,* 5–18.

Dubois, S., Rossion, B., Schiltz, C., Bodart, J.-M., Michel, C., Bruyer, R., et al. (1999). Effect of familiarity on the processing of human faces. *NeuroImage, 9,* 278–289.

Engell, A. D., Haxby, J. V., & Todorov, A. (2007). Implicit trustworthiness decisions: Automatic coding of face properties in the human amygdala. *Journal of Cognitive Neuroscience, 19,* 1508–1519.

Fallshore, M. F., & Schooler, J. W. (1995). The verbal vulnerability of perceptual expertise. *Journal of Experimental Psychology: Learning, Memory, and Cognition, 21,* 1608–1623.

Fiske, S. T., & Neuberg, S. L. (1990). A continuum model of impression formation from category-based to individuated processes: Influences of information and motivation on attention and interpretation. In M. P. Zanna (Ed.), *Advances in experimental social psychology* (Vol. 23, pp. 1–74). New York: Academic Press.

Freeman, J. B., & Ambady, N. (2011). A dynamic interactive theory of person construal. *Psychological Review, 118,* 247–279.

Ganel, T., & Goshen-Gottstein, Y. (2002). Perceptual integrality of sex and identity of faces: Further evidence for the single-route hypothesis. *Journal of Experimental Psychology: Human Perception and Performance, 28,* 854–867.

Gawronski, B., & Quinn, K. A. (2013). Guilty by mere similarity: Assimilative effects of facial resemblance on automatic evaluation. *Journal of Experimental Social Psychology, 49,* 120–125.

Gilbert, D. T., & Hixon, J. G. (1991). The trouble of thinking. Activation and application of stereotypic beliefs. *Journal of Personality and Social Psychology, 60,* 509–517.

Hamilton, D., & Sherman, S. (1996). Perceiving persons and groups. *Psychological Review, 103,* 336–355.

Harnad, S. (Ed.). (1987). *Categorical perception: The groundwork of cognition.* New York: Cambridge University Press.

Haxby, J. V., Hoffman, E. A., & Gobbini, M. I. (2000). The distributed neural system for face perception. *Trends in Cognitive Sciences, 4,* 223–233.

Haxby, J. V., Hoffman, E. A., & Gobbini, M. I. (2002). Human neural systems for face recognition and social communication. *Biological Psychiatry, 51,* 59–67.

Hehman, E., Mania, E. W., & Gaertner, S. L. (2010). Where the division lies: Common ingroup identity moderates the cross-race facial-recognition effect. *Journal of Experimental Social Psychology, 46,* 445–448.

Hugenberg, K., & Corneille, O. (2009). Holistic processing is tuned for in-group faces. *Cognitive Science, 33,* 1173–1181.

Hugenberg, K., & Sacco, D. F. (2008). Social categorization and stereotyping: How social categorization biases person perception and face memory. *Social and Personality Psychology Compass, 2,* 1052–1072.

Hugenberg, K., Young, S. G., Bernstein, M. J., & Sacco, D. F. (2010). The categorization–individuation model: An integrative account of the other-race recognition deficit. *Psychological Review, 117,* 1168–1187.

Ito, T. A., Thompson, E., & Cacioppo, J. T. (2004). Tracking the timecourse of social perception: The effects of racial cues on event-related brain potentials. *Personality and Social Psychology Bulletin, 30,* 1267–1280.

Jolicoeur, P., Gluck, M. A., & Kosslyn, S. M. (1984). Pictures and names: Making the connection. *Cognitive Psychology, 16,* 243–275.

Kelly, D. J., Quinn, P. C., Slater, A. M., Lee, K., Ge, L., & Pascalis, O. (2007). The other-race effect develops during infancy: Evidence of perceptual narrowing. *Psychological Science, 18*, 1084–1089.

Kraus, M. W., & Chen, S. (2010). Facial-feature resemblance elicits the transference effect. *Psychological Science, 21*, 518–522.

Kruglanski, A. W., Chun, W. Y., Erb, H. P., Pierro, A., Mannett, L., & Spiegel, S. (2003). A parametric unimodel of human judgment: Integrating dual-process frameworks in social cognition from a single-mode perspective. In J. P. Forgas, K. R. Williams, & W. von Hippel (Eds.), *Social judgments: Implicit and explicit processes* (pp. 137–161). New York Cambridge University Press.

Kunda, Z., Davies, P. G., Adams, B. D., & Spencer, S. J. (2002). The dynamic time course of stereotype activation: Activation, dissipation, and resurrection. *Journal of Personality and Social Psychology, 82*, 283–299.

Kunda, Z., & Thagard, P. (1996). Forming impressions from stereotypes, traits, and behaviors: A parallel-constraint-satisfaction theory. *Psychological Review, 103*, 284–308.

Kurzban, R., Tooby, J., & Cosmides, L. (2001). Can race be erased?: Coalitional computation and social categorization. *Proceedings of the National Academy of Sciences USA, 98*, 15387–15392.

Leder, H., & Bruce, V. (2000). When inverted faces are recognized: The role of configural information in face processing. *The Quarterly Journal of Experimental Psychology: Human Experimental Psychology, 53A*, 513–536.

Le Gal, P. M., & Bruce, V. (2002). Evaluating the independence of sex and expression in judgments of faces. *Perception and Psychophysics, 64*, 230–243.

Lepore, L., & Brown, R. (1997). Category and stereotype activation: Is prejudice inevitable? *Journal of Personality and Social Psychology, 72*, 275–287.

Levin, D. T. (1996). Classifying faces by race: The structure of face categories. *Journal of Experimental Psychology: Learning, Memory, and Cognition, 22*, 1364–1382.

Levin, D. T. (2000). Race as a visual feature: Using visual search and perceptual discrimination tasks to understand face categories and the cross-race recognition deficit. *Journal of Experimental Psychology: General, 129*, 559–574.

Levin, D. T., & Banaji, R. (2006). Distortions in the perceived lightness of faces: The role of race categories. *Journal of Experimental Psychology: General, 135*, 501–512.

Liu, J., Harris, A., & Kanwisher, N. (2002). Stages of processing in face perception: An MEG study. *Nature Neuroscience, 5*, 910–916.

Livingston, R. W., & Brewer, M. B. (2002). What are we really priming?: Cue-based versus category-based processing of facial stimuli. *Journal of Personality and Social Psychology, 82*, 5–18.

Macrae, C. N., Alnwick, K. A., Milne, A. B., & Schloerscheidt, A. M. (2002). Person perception across the menstrual cycle: Hormonal influences on social-cognitive functioning. *Psychological Science, 13*, 532–536.

Macrae, C. N., & Bodenhausen, G. V. (2000). Social cognition: Thinking categorically about others. *Annual Review of Psychology, 51*, 93–120.

Macrae, C. N., Bodenhausen, G. V., Milne, A. B., & Calvini, G. (1999). Seeing more than we can know: Visual attention and category activation. *Journal of Experimental Social Psychology, 35*, 590–602.

Macrae, C. N., Bodenhausen, G. V., Milne, A. B., Thorn, T. M. J., & Castelli, L. (1997). On the activation of social stereotypes: The moderating role of processing objectives. *Journal of Experimental Social Psychology, 33*, 471–489.

Macrae, C. N., Hood, B. M., Milne, A. B., Rowe, A. C., & Mason, M. F. (2002). Are you looking at me?: Eye gaze and person perception. *Psychological Science, 13*, 460–464.

Macrae, C. N., & Martin, D. (2007). A boy primed Sue: Feature-based processing and person construal. *European Journal of Social Psychology, 37*, 793–805.

Macrae, C. N., Milne, A. B., & Bodenhausen, G. V. (1994). Stereotypes as energy-saving devices: A peek inside the cognitive toolbox. *Journal of Personality and Social Psychology, 66*, 37–47.

Macrae, C. N., & Quadflieg, S. (2010). Perceiving people. In S. T. Fiske, D. T. Gilbert, & G. Lindzey (Eds.), *Handbook of social psychology* (Vol. 1, 5th ed., pp. 428–463). Hoboken, NJ: Wiley.

Macrae, C. N., Quinn, K. A., Mason, M. F., & Quadflieg, S. (2005). Understanding others: The face and person construal. *Journal of Personality and Social Psychology, 89*, 686–695.

Maddox, K. B. (2004). Perspectives on racial phenotypicality bias. *Personality and Social Psychology Review, 8*, 383–401.

Marr, D. (1982). *Vision*. San Francisco: Freeman.

Mason, M. F., Cloutier, J., & Macrae, C. N. (2006). On construing others: Category and stereotype activation from facial cues. *Social Cognition, 24*, 540–562.

Mason, M. F., & Macrae, C. N. (2004). Categorizing and individuating others: The neural substrates of person perception. *Journal of Cognitive Neuroscience, 16*, 1785–1795.

Maurer, D., Le Grand, R., & Mondloch, C. J. (2002). The many faces of configural processing. *Trends in Cognitive Sciences, 6*, 255–260.

Meissner, C. A., & Brigham, J. C. (2001). Thirty years of investigating the own-race bias in memory for faces: A meta-analytic review. *Psychology, Public Policy, and Law, 7*, 3–35.

Moreland, L. R., & Zajonc, R. B. (1982). Exposure effects in person perception: Familiarity, similarity, and attraction. *Journal of Experimental Social Psychology, 18*, 395–415.

Moskowitz, G. B., Gollwitzer, P. M., Wasel, W., & Schaal, B. (1999). Preconscious control of stereotype activation through chronic egalitarian goals. *Journal of Personality and Social Psychology, 77*, 167–184.

Quinn, K. A., & Macrae, C. N. (2005). Categorizing others: The dynamics of person construal. *Journal of Personality and Social Psychology, 88*, 467–479.

Quinn, K. A., Macrae, C. N., & Bodenhausen, G. V. (2003). Stereotyping and impression formation. In M. A. Hogg & J. Cooper (Eds.), *Sage handbook of social psychology* (pp. 87–109). Thousand Oaks, CA: Sage.

Quinn, K. A., Mason, M. F., & Macrae, C. N. (2009). Familiarity and person construal: Individuating knowledge moderates the automaticity of category activation. *European Journal of Social Psychology, 39*, 852–861.

Quinn, K. A., Mason, M. F., & Macrae, C. N. (2010). When Arnold is "The Terminator," we no longer see him as a man: The temporal determinants of person perception. *Experimental Psychology, 57*, 27–35.

Rhodes, G., Brake, S., & Atkinson, A. P. (1993). What's lost in inverted faces? *Cognition, 47*, 25–57.

Rhodes, G., Brake, S., Taylor, K., & Tan, S. (1989). Expertise and configural encoding in face recognition. *British Journal of Psychology, 80*, 313–331.

Richler, J. J., Mack, M. L., Gauthier, I., & Palmeri, T. J. (2009). Holistic processing of faces happens at a glance. *Vision Research, 49*, 2856–2861.

Richler, J. J., Tanaka, J. W., Brown, D. D., & Gauthier, I. (2008). Why does selective attention to parts fail in face processing? *Journal of Experimental Psychology: Learning, Memory, and Cognition, 34*, 1356–1368.

Rosch, E., Mervis, C. B., Gray, W., Johnson, D. M., & Boyes-Braem, P. (1976). Basic objects in natural categories. *Cognitive Psychology, 8*, 382–439.

Rossion, B. (2002). Is sex categorization from faces really parallel to face recognition? *Visual Cognition, 9*, 1003–1020.

Rossion, B., Schiltz, C., Robaye, L., Pirenne, D., & Crommelinck, M. (2001). How does the brain discriminate familiar and unfamiliar faces: A PET study of face categorical perception. *Journal of Cognitive Neuroscience, 13*, 1019–1034.

Sangrigoli, S., & de Schonen, S. (2004). Effect of visual experience on face processing: A developmental study of inversion and non-native effects. *Developmental Science, 7*, 74–87.

Sassenberg, K., & Moskowitz, G. B. (2005). Don't stereotype, think different!: Overcoming automatic stereotype activation by mindset priming. *Journal of Experimental Social Psychology, 41*, 506–514.

Schaller, M., Park, J. H., & Mueller, A. (2003). Fear of the dark: Interactive effects of beliefs about danger and ambient darkness on ethnic stereotypes. *Personality and Social Psychology Bulletin, 29*, 637–649.

Sherman, J. W., Lee, A. Y., Bessenoff, G. R., & Frost, L. A. (1998). Stereotype efficiency reconsidered: Encoding flexibility under cognitive load. *Journal of Personality and Social Psychology, 75*, 589–606.

Smith, E. R., Miller, D. A., Maitner, A. T., Crump, S. A., Garcia-Marques, T., & Mackie, D. M. (2006). Familiarity can increase stereotyping. *Journal of Experimental Social Psychology, 42*, 471–478.

Spencer, S. J., Fein, S., Wolfe, C. T., Fong, C., & Dunn, M. (1998). Automatic activation of stereotypes: The role of self-image threat. *Personality and Social Psychology Bulletin, 24*, 1139–1152.

Stewart, B. D., & Payne, B. K. (2008). Bringing automatic stereotyping under control: Implementation intentions as efficient means of thought control. *Personality and Social Psychology Bulletin, 34,* 1332–1345.

Tanaka, J. W. (2001). The entry point of face recognition: Evidence for face expertise. *Journal of Experimental Psychology: General, 130,* 534–543.

Tarr, M. J., & Cheng, Y. D. (2003). Learning to see faces and objects. *Trends in Cognitive Sciences, 7,* 23–30.

Todorov, A., Gobbini, M. I., Evans, K. K., & Haxby, J. V. (2007). Spontaneous retrieval of affective person knowledge in face perception. *Neuropsychologia, 45,* 163–173.

Todorov, A., Pakrashi, M., & Oosterhof, N. N. (2009). Evaluating faces on trustworthiness after minimal time exposure. *Social Cognition, 27,* 813–833.

Turk, D. J., Rosenblum, A. C., Gazzaniga, M. S., & Macrae, C. N. (2005). Seeing John Malkovich: The neural substrates of person categorization. *NeuroImage, 24,* 1147–1153.

Uleman, J. S., Blader, S. L., & Todorov, A. (2005). Implicit impressions. In R. R. Hassin, J. S. Uleman, & J. A. Bargh (Eds.), *The new unconscious* (pp. 362–392). New York: Oxford University Press.

Verosky, S. C., & Todorov, A. (2010). Generalization of affective learning about faces to perceptually similar faces. *Psychological Science, 21,* 779–785.

Wheeler, M. E., & Fiske, S. T. (2005). Controlling racial prejudice. *Psychological Science, 16,* 56–62.

White, G. L., & Shapiro, D. (1987). Don't I know you?: Antecedents and social consequences of perceived familiarity. *Journal of Experimental Social Psychology, 23,* 75–92.

Willis, J., & Todorov, A. (2006). First impressions: Making up your mind after a 100-ms exposure to a face. *Psychological Science, 17,* 592–598.

Winkielman, P., & Cacioppo, J. T. (2001). Mind at ease puts a smile on the face: Psychophysiological evidence that processing facilitation elicits positive affect. *Journal of Personality and Social Psychology, 81,* 989–1000.

Winston, J. S., Strange, B. A., O'Doherty, J., & Dolan, R. J. (2002). Automatic and intentional brain responses during evaluation of trustworthiness of faces. *Nature Neuroscience, 5,* 277–283.

Wittenbrink, B., Judd, C. M., & Park, B. (2001). Spontaneous prejudice in context: Variability in automatically activated attitudes. *Journal of Personality and Social Psychology, 81,* 815–827.

Zárate, M. A., Stoever, C. J., MacLin, M. K., & Arms-Chavez, C. J. (2008). Neurocognitive underpinnings of face perception: Further evidence for distinct person and group perception processes. *Journal of Personality and Social Psychology, 94,* 108–115.

Zebrowitz, L. A., & Montepare, J. M. (1992). Impressions of babyfaced males and females across the lifespan. *Developmental Psychology, 28,* 1143–1152.

CHAPTER 18

Dual-Process Models of Trait Judgments of Self and Others

An Overview and Critique

Stanley B. Klein

This chapter has two objectives. First, I describe research involving trait judgments about the self and others that *can be* interpreted as evidence for a dual-process model. I briefly discuss the findings, and then demonstrate the adequacy of the experimental methods employed and the generality of the results. I conclude that two systems of long-term memory (episodic and semantic) each maintains a functionally independent representation of a person's (self and other) traits, and that their contributions to the trait judgment process can be predicted on the basis of factors such as trait-relevant experience with the person about whom judgments are being made (for reviews, see Klein, 2004; Klein & Gangi, 2010; Klein & Lax, 2010; Klein, Robertson, Gangi, & Loftus, 2008).

I next examine the question of what we believe we are referring to when we employ the term *dual-process*. What constitutes a duality of processes (as opposed to, say, a singularity or a plurality), what comprises the outcome of a process, and so forth? While these concerns might seem more metaphysical than psychological (e.g., Dewey, 1925; James, 1909/1996; Rescher, 1996), I believe that it is a serious mistake to ignore such questions in the pursuit of knowledge. One runs the risk of reducing one's findings and theoretical explications to statements that have legitimate reference primarily to experimental tasks rather than to nature. In short, we need to pay far greater attention to—and a philosophically oriented critique provides us a means for doing so—that to which we believe our findings and conclusions refer.

AN OVERVIEW OF THE DUAL-PROCESS VIEW OF TRAIT KNOWLEDGE ABOUT SELF AND OTHERS

How does a person know that he or she possesses some traits but not others? My research compared two explanations: the *abstraction* view and the *computational* view (summarized in Klein & Loftus, 1993a; Klein et al., 2008). Specifically, the abstraction view maintains that information about one's personality traits is abstracted primarily (though not exclusively; e.g., Klein, Sherman, & Loftus, 1996) from specific behaviors, either as they happen or on the basis of episodic memories of these behaviors. These abstractions are stored in the form of precomputed trait summaries in semantic memory (e.g., Buss & Craik, 1983; Klein & Loftus, 1993a; Klein, Loftus, Trafton, & Fuhrman, 1992; Sherman

& Klein, 1994; Lord, 1993; Sherman, 1996). Trait judgments are made by direct retrieval from this store. When a trait summary is retrieved, trait-consistent episodes are not retrieved along with it (because the information they provide would be redundant; e.g., Klein, Cosmides, Tooby, & Chance, 2002). Trait-consistent episodes are consulted only when retrieval mechanisms fail to access trait summaries (e.g., when a summary does not yet exist for a particular trait; e.g., Klein & Loftus, 1993a; Klein, Loftus, Trafton, et al., 1992).

The computational view, in contrast, assumes there are mechanisms that make trait judgments online by retrieving trait-relevant behaviors from episodic memory and computing their similarity to the trait being judged (e.g., Bower & Gilligan, 1979; Keenan, 1993; Locksley & Lenauer, 1981; Smith & Zárate, 1992). For example, if asked whether I am friendly, I first would search episodic memory for trait-consistent personal episodes (i.e., records of events in which my behavior was friendly). A judgment then would be computed from the episodes retrieved (based, e.g., on how diagnostic they were of friendliness or how fast they could be accessed).

These views carry very different predictions about the need to utilize episodic memories when making trait judgments. If the computational view is correct, then trait-consistent episodes must be retrieved to make a trait judgment. If the abstraction view is correct, then trait-consistent episodes will not be retrieved in making trait judgments, except under certain circumstances (e.g., absence of a summary).

These predictions have been extensively tested through paradigms that take advantage of priming, encoding specificity, encoding variability, patients with specific memory impairments, and several other techniques. Priming results are described below (for converging results using the other methods, see, e.g., Klein, Loftus, & Burton, 1989; Klein & Loftus, 1993a; Klein, Loftus, & Kihlstrom, 1996; Klein, Loftus, & Plog, 1992; Klein, Loftus, Trafton, et al., 1992; Klein, Rozendal, & Cosmides, 2002; Klein, Cosmides, Costabile, & Mei, 2002; Klein, Cosmides, & Costabile, 2003; Klein, Babey, & Sherman, 1997).

Testing for Trait Summaries: The Priming Task

In our priming studies, my colleagues and I presented to each subject many pairs of tasks (task pair members were referred to as the *initial task* and the *target task* to highlight their temporal relation). Each task pairing involved a particular trait adjective (e.g., *stubborn*). The initial task was the potential "prime." The time required to perform the target task was the dependent measure. The independent variable was the nature of the initial task—the prime.

In *one* version of the priming paradigm, the initial task was either a describe task, a control task, or a filler task (other versions are summarized in Klein & Loftus, 1993a). The describe task asked subjects to judge whether the trait adjective was self-descriptive (e.g., "Does this describe you: Stubborn?"). The control task varied depending on the experiment; sometimes it was a define task (e.g., "Think of the definition of the word *stubborn*"), other times it was a request simply to read the adjective presented. Control tasks were shown not to elicit retrieval of trait-relevant behavioral episodes (more about this later). The target task in this version of our priming studies was either the recall task (e.g., "Think of a specific time in which you behaved in stubborn manner") or filler tasks (for details, see Klein & Loftus, 1993a).

If the computational view is correct, then trait-consistent episodes will be activated whenever one is asked to decide whether a trait describes oneself (e.g., by performing the describe task). If trait-consistent episodic memories are activated, then one should be able to retrieve those memories faster (e.g., during performance of a recall target task) after performing a describe task than after performing a control task.

This was not the case: When subjects were asked to recall a specific behavioral incident in which they manifested a particular trait (i.e., the recall target task), those who had initially performed a describe task were no faster than those who had not (e.g., Klein & Loftus, 1990, 1993a, 1993b; Klein et al., 1989; Klein, Loftus, Trafton, et al., 1992; for a recent summary, see Klein et al., 2008). Yet the procedure is known to be sensitive enough to detect episodic priming when it occurs (e.g., Babey, Queller, & Klein, 1998; Klein, Loftus, Trafton, et al., 1992; Schell, Klein, & Babey, 1996; Sherman & Klein, 1994; Sherman, Klein, Laskey, & Wyer, 1998; for experiments showing that this result obtains regardless of how "central" a trait is to one's self-concept, see, Klein, Cosmides, Tooby, & Chance, 2001; Klein & Loftus, 1990, 1993a; Klein, Loftus, Trafton, et al., 1992).

Adequacy of the Definition Control Task

The fact that making a trait judgment did not prime episodic memories of trait-consistent behaviors is consistent with the abstraction view. There is, however, a potential problem with this conclusion. Since the findings described are null, two possible interpretations of the data come to mind (e.g., Greenwald, 1975). First, the failure to find priming may indicate a functional independence between semantic and episodic trait self-knowledge. Second, it may simply reflect limitations in method (e.g., the choice of definition control task). Such concerns were raised early on about our research by both Brown (1993) and Keenan (1993). My colleagues and I subsequently have examined these alternatives, and our findings consistently support the first alternative (e.g., Klein et al., 2008).

First, a little history. Motivating our choice of definition generation as our control task was the assumption that its performance would not involve activation of self-knowledge. Our assumption was based, in part, on the finding that definition generation successfully had been used as a control task in many self-reference effect studies (for review, see Klein & Kihlstrom, 1986; Symons & Johnson, 1997). If definition generation entailed self-referential processing, a define task should prove comparable to self-referential tasks (e.g., a describes task) in its ability to promote good recall. Since this almost never happened—and when it did (e.g., Klein & Kihlstrom, 1986) the reasons were due to specific, theory-based, manipulations of the self-referential task—definition generation seemed an appropriate control task to use in our priming studies.

Although this reasoning seemed plausible, we did not, at least initially, have direct evidence in support of our assumption about the lack of involvement of self-referential processing during word definition. Fortunately, the situation soon changed. In 1992, Klein, Loftus, Trafton, et al. (see also Klein & Loftus, 1993a), demonstrated that, consistent with findings reported elsewhere (e.g., Ganellen & Carver, 1985; Kuiper, 1981; Markus, 1977; Mueller, Thompson, & Dugan, 1986; Klein et al., 1989), trait descriptiveness had reliable effects on the time required to perform initial (i.e., nonprimed) tasks involving trait knowledge of self (e.g., the describe and recall tasks). By contrast, define initial task latencies showed no effect of trait self-descriptiveness. If definition generation *automatically* activates behavioral self-knowledge, and if the time to activate that knowledge is known to vary reliably as a function of its target descriptiveness (self, mother, etc.), it is hard to explain the absence of differential facilitation as a function of trait-descriptiveness in the define initial task condition (for discussion, see Klein & Loftus, 1993c).

Additional support for the appropriateness of the define control task came from the finding that the *pattern* of latencies associated with performance of the self-referential target tasks (describe and recall) was uninfluenced by the initial performance of the define control task (e.g., Klein & Loftus, 1993a; Klein, Loftus, Trafton, et al., 1992; Klein et al., 1997): When response latencies were broken down by trait self-descriptiveness, the pattern of latencies associated with describe and recall when they were the initial task of the pair were virtually identical to the patterns obtained when they were performed *following* performance of the define task (i.e., when they served as target tasks). The same outcomes obtained when the task referent was changed from self to other. That is, the presence or absence of the define task had no effect on the pattern of response latencies found with self-referential task performance.

In other studies we used different control tasks and obtained the same results as studies employing the define task. For example, Klein et al. (1997) replaced the definition generation with a task that only required participants to read silently the trait word presented. The *read* task functioned identically to the define control task.

Converging Evidence for a Functional Independence

A considerable proportion of our published work on trait self-judgments has been devoted to explicating conditions under which priming will and will not be found. Specifically, my colleagues and I do not maintain that episodic and semantic trait knowledge are totally separate, noninteracting systems. Rather, we assumed the relation is one of *functional independence*. To say that two memory systems are functionally independent does not mean they have nothing to do with one another or that they are completely separate. Rather, as Tulving (1983, p. 66) puts it, functional independence means that "one system can operate independently of the other, though not necessarily as efficiently as it could with the support of the other intact system."

Our functional independence hypothesis was not based exclusively on findings from the priming paradigm. As we observed (Klein & Loftus, 1993a, p. 15), "the findings from any one paradigm are open to multiple interpretations and vulnerable to the charge that they reflect more the idiosyncrasies of the methodology used than the variables of interest." Accordingly, my colleagues and I complemented our priming studies with results from studies using other methodologies.

For example, Klein, Loftus, and Plog (1992) made use of the phenomenon of transfer-appropriate processing (e.g., Roediger & Blaxton, 1987; Roediger, Weldon, & Challis, 1989) in a study of recognition memory for traits, to show that different processes are involved in accessing the two types of knowledge. Klein et al. (1989, Experiment 4) applied the principle of encoding variability (e.g., Bower, 1972; Martin, 1971) in a study of recall for traits, and found that the type of information made available when making trait judgments is different from that made available when retrieving trait-relevant behaviors. And Klein et al. (1997) presented evidence from Dunn and Kirsner's (1988) technique of reversed association to demonstrate that trait judgments and behavioral retrieval are mediated by functionally independent memory systems.

Another line of evidence for the functional independence of semantic and episodic self-knowledge comes from patients with neurological disabilities. Klein and Loftus (1993a; see also Klein & Kihlstrom, 1998) proposed that patients suffering from various forms of episodic amnesia would provide a particularly effective method for examining the respective contributions of episodic and semantic memory to the creation of trait self-knowledge. This is because such patients often experience highly selective memory loss, typically displaying relatively intact semantic memory, with impaired access to episodic memory (e.g., Cermak, 1984; Moscovitch, Yaschyshyn, Ziegler, & Nadel, 2000; Parkin, 1987; Tulving, 1995). Accordingly, tests of trait knowledge can be conducted in these patients with assurance that episodic memory for traits is not involved.

If semantic memory contains personality trait summaries, patients should be able to know what they are like despite being unable to recall the particular experiences from which that knowledge was derived. There are neuropsychological data from five patients: K. C. (Tulving, 1993), W. J. (Klein, Loftus, & Kihlstrom, 1996), and D. B. (Klein, Rozendal, et al., 2002), all of whom suffer from varying degrees (partial to total) of episodic amnesia; R. J. (Klein, Chan, & Loftus, 1999; Klein, Cosmides, Costabile, & Mei, 2002; Klein, Cosmides, Murray, & Tooby, 2004), who is autistic; and K. R. (Klein, Cosmides, & Costabile, 2003) who has Alzheimer's dementia. The results of these case studies can be summarized as follows:

1. Retrieving trait summaries does not depend on accessing episodic memories. Accurate trait judgments can be made by amnesic individuals—even people who cannot retrieve *any* episodic memories (e.g., K. C., D. B.).[1]
2. That K. C. knows his postmorbid personality (but not his premorbid personality) suggests that trait summaries can be updated without accessing episodic memories.
3. Intact retrieval of personality trait summaries can occur despite Alzheimer's dementia so severe that it impairs access to knowledge about many semantic domains (K. R.).
4. D. B. and R. J. have intact knowledge

of their own personality traits, yet they show impairments in other domains of semantic knowledge (personal history; general history; facts about animals, foods, objects; etc.). This is a dissociation *between* domains within semantic memory. This suggests that trait self-knowledge is a functionally isolable subsystem within semantic memory.

5. D. B. knows his own personality traits but not his daughter's. This suggests that knowledge about one's own traits is stored separately from knowledge of other people's traits (the same conclusion is evidenced from data from R. J. and K. R.).

Beyond Functional Independence

Our research also has identified conditions in which episodic and semantic trait knowledge are *functionally dependent* (e.g., Babey et al., 1998; Klein, Cosmides, Tooby, et al., 2001, 2002). For example, Klein, Cosmides, Tooby, et al. (2002) have argued that an excellent package of speed plus accuracy can be engineered into a decision system by *jointly* activating a trait summary and episodic memories inconsistent with it. Trait summaries allow fast access to relevant information. But a trait summary (e.g., "I am usually friendly") gives information about behavior under "average" circumstances. It does not tell you under what circumstances a behavior deviates from average. In deciding how to behave, one is always facing a particular situation.

Thus, a generalization is most useful when its scope is *delimited*—when it is accompanied by information specifying those situations in which it does not apply. Episodic memories that are inconsistent with a generalization can serve this function, because they encode specific situations in which the generalization fails to predict the outcome. To make judgments that are both fast and accurate, judgment procedures should be designed to search for summary information in semantic memory and, on retrieving it, also search for episodic memories that are inconsistent with that summary—ones that place boundary conditions on the summary's scope (see also Schank, 1982). Thus, there is a function to maintaining trait-relevant episodic memories, even after a semantic summary has been formed: Memories of behavioral episodes can provide boundary conditions on the scope of generalizations.

The *scope* hypothesis was tested in a series of experiments on trait self-judgments using a variant of the priming paradigm described earlier. Klein, Cosmides, Tooby, et al. (2001, 2002) showed that when a trait summary is retrieved, trait-inconsistent behavioral episodes are retrieved along with it (this was found regardless of whether the person being judged was self or other). More specifically, the time it took subjects to recall a trait-inconsistent episode was faster following a describe task than following a control task. In other words, asking a subject whether he or she is kind coactivates memories of episodes in which that person did something unkind (and vice versa). Consistent with the scope hypothesis, inconsistent episodes are primed when a trait summary has been retrieved. When a trait summary is absent, trait-consistent episodes are primed. This makes sense: In the absence of a trait summary, episodes are the only information one has on which to base a judgment. (Note that when talking about episodic trait knowledge, we do not restrict the content of recollection to dispositional acts that have been directly experienced. An episodic recollection also can include memory of third party reports—that is, information about a person's character dispositions conveyed by others.)

The Mental Representation of Trait Knowledge about Other Persons

My colleagues and I also have argued that the same model (termed the *mixed model*) of trait judgments can be extended to describe the mental representation of trait knowledge about others (e.g., Babey, 1998; Babey et al., 1998; Klein & Loftus, 1993a; Klein, Loftus, Trafton, et al., 1992; Klein et al., 2008; Sherman & Klein, 1994; Sherman, 1996; Sherman et al., 1998). According to our model, one's representation of a person's traits (self or other) varies with the amount of experience one has had with that person. If the amount of experience is not sufficient to support abstraction, then trait knowledge will be represented only at the level of behavioral memories. Trait judgments about the person, therefore, must be based on behavioral memories (i.e., evidence in episodic memory). However, as the amount of experience becomes sufficiently large, trait knowledge is increasingly likely to be abstracted and represented in summary form. When this happens, trait judgments may be made by directly accessing the appropriate semantic memory representation (i.e., a trait summary). Thus, the model proposes that the more knowledge one has about a person's behavior, the more likely one is to have formed summary representations and the less likely one is to base judgments of that person on memories of specific behavioral episodes (for similar views, see Anderson, 1989; Park, 1986).

A series of studies by Klein and Loftus and their colleagues has provided evidence consistent with their model (Babey et al., 1998; Klein & Loftus, 1993a; Klein, Loftus, Trafton, et al., 1992, Experiment 1; Sherman & Klein, 1994). In one study (Klein, Loftus, Trafton, et al., 1992; Experiment 1), in which the target persons were the subjects' mothers, subjects first completed a series of priming trials, then rated each stimulus trait for the degree to which it described their mothers. Klein, Loftus, Trafton, et al. found no evidence that a describe task facilitated retrieval of trait-consistent behavioral episodes when the trait in question was highly descriptive of one's mother. However, they found considerable evidence of facilitation when traits were rated medium in mother-descriptiveness. To explain these findings, they (see also Klein, Cosmides, Tooby, & Chance, 2002; Klein & Loftus, 1993a; Klein et al., 2008) proposed that traits rated highly descriptive of another person are those that he or she has manifested most often, and are hence those for which subjects have observed a relatively large number of behaviors. Accordingly, highly descriptive traits are likely to be those for which subjects have created a semantic memory representation—a trait summary—that can be accessed to perform the describe task. Because memories of trait-consistent behavioral episodes would not be activated, the describe task would be no more beneficial than a define task to the subsequent performance of a recall task.

In contrast, medium-descriptive traits are likely to be those for which subjects have observed fewer behavioral exemplars. This means it is less likely that subjects will have a memory in the form of a trait summary. In the absence of a trait summary, subjects would have to retrieve trait-relevant behavioral knowledge from episodic memory to make descriptiveness judgments. Consequently, a describe task would be more beneficial than a define task in performing a subsequent recall task, and one would observe faster retrieval of trait-consistent episodes following a describe task. (The reason for assuming that retrieval will be biased toward trait-consistent behaviors follows from research showing that people rely on "positive test" strategies in many tasks [e.g., Klayman & Ha, 1987; Wason, 1968], including when answering questions about the trait characteristics of others: They are more likely to search memory for examples of the trait being judged than for examples of its opposite [e.g., Devine, Hirt, & Gehrke, 1990; Fong & Markus, 1982; Snyder & Cantor, 1979).

Thus, consistent with the predictions of the Klein, Loftus, Trafton, et al. (1992) model, for judgments about well-known others (e.g., one's mother), trait-consistent behavioral episodes appear to be required when the trait being judged is medium in mother-descriptiveness, but not when the trait being judged is highly descriptive of the mother (clear prediction cannot be made for low-descriptive traits; Klein, Loftus, Trafton, et al., 1992; Klein & Loftus, 1993a; Klein et al., 2001).

It is important to note that these same considerations apply to the self. While it is difficult to find situations in which we have not had sufficient trait-relevant behavioral experience to form a semantic abstraction, such circumstances can be arranged. Under such conditions, the pattern of response latencies conforms to the predictions of the mixed model (e.g., Klein & Loftus, 1993a; Klein, Loftus, Trafton, et al., 1992; but see Klein, Sherman, et al., 1996, for an important caveat).

A Summary: The Mixed Model—Predicting When Trait Judgments Activate Episodic or Semantic Memory

I have argued that this pattern of findings is best accounted for by a mixed exemplar–abstraction model of trait knowledge. According to this model, one's mental representation of a person's traits should vary with the amount of trait-relevant experience one has had with that person. If the amount of experience is not sufficient to support abstraction, then trait knowledge will be represented only at the level of behavioral exemplars (i.e., episodic memory). But as the amount of experience becomes sufficiently large, trait knowledge is increasingly likely to be abstracted and represented in summary form in semantic memory.

For trait judgments, then, the type of memory-based knowledge retrieved depends on the amount of trait-relevant experience in memory. Behavioral exemplars will be retrieved from episodic memory primarily when experience is low, and an appropriate semantic summary is therefore not available. However, if summary trait knowledge is available, our research suggests that it will be retrieved in favor of behavioral exemplars (see also Anderson, 1989; Carlston, 1980). In fact, once a summary representation has been formed, episodic recollection of the specific exemplars that led to that representation appear to play little or no part in the trait judgment process: Recall task latencies are unaffected by performance of an initial describe task (and vice versa) when the amount of trait-relevant experience is large (for an exception to this rule, see the section titled "Beyond Functional Independence").

It is beyond the scope of this chapter to discuss in detail the various contexts and conditions that lead a person making a trait judgment (about either self or other) to be more or less likely to utilize episodic memory versus semantic memory. There are, however, a number of recent papers that provide a comprehensive summary of relevant findings for readers who are interested (e.g., Klein & Lax, 2010; Klein et al., 2008). The evidence suggests that judgments about both self and others (which show strong overlap in the mechanisms involved in making trait attributions) are similarly affected by a number of factors, for example, the amount of trait-relevant behavioral experience (e.g., Klein et al., 2001; Klein & Loftus, 1993c; Klein, Sherman, et al., 1996; Sherman & Klein, 1994; Sherman, 1996), the personal relevance (i.e., how descriptive is the trait of Person *X*?) of the trait being judged (e.g., Klein et al., 1997; Klein & Loftus, 1993a; Klein, Loftus, Trafton, et al., 1992), judgment context (e.g., Klein & Loftus, 1993a, 1993b; Klein, Sherman, et al., 1996); and comparison person–group (e.g., Babey, 1998; Sherman et al., 1998). Each of these factors has been found to make substantial contributions to the memorial route taken in the act of making a trait judgment.[2]

In summary, Klein, Loftus, and colleagues' mixed model—the finding that semantic trait knowledge (of self and other) is represented and accessed separately from episodic knowledge of trait-relevant behaviors—is based on a *convergence* of findings from a number of sources. Although it is not difficult to generate alternative explanations for findings from a single experimental procedure, it becomes increasingly difficult to do so when experiments using different dependent measures (e.g., response latency, recall, recognition), different control tasks (e.g., definition generation, read-only), and different participant populations (e.g., normal, amnesic, autistic, dementia) yield the same findings.

ON PROCESS: WHAT'S IN A WORD?

When reading about dual-process models in psychological research, one notes that much effort is devoted to explaining the experimental setup and interpreting results. Considerably less time, however, is devoted to discussing and clarifying the notion of *process* per se, despite the fact that this is a primary construct motivating experimental design and used to frame interpretation of outcomes. And, a lack of clarity in the constructs used ultimately leads to a lack of clarity in the questions posed, and therefore to a lack of clarity in the design of the experiments supposed to provide an answer to those questions.

So, what do psychologists mean when we use the term *process*? To what do our empirical and theoretical findings refer? As mentioned, explicit discussion of the focal assumption of *process* seldom is found in treatments of *psychological process*, a term accorded considerable causal efficacy in the workings of the mind (as the present volume attests).

To cut to the chase, the nature of *process*, as used in psychology, consists primarily of assumptions (often tacit) uninformed by a historically rich philosophical treatment that has struggled to specify both its properties and its differences from other conceptualizations about nature (e.g., Rescher, 1996).

While I do not presume that philosophical debate sheds definitive light on *process*, I do believe that appreciation of philosophical analysis and insights is warranted. Otherwise we risk "reference without a clear referent." Moreover, we unintentionally inherit a host of well-defined and investigated, but perhaps unaccommodating, assumptions about the term we adopt.

In a deep sense, the notion of *process* is a metaphysical construct, invoked as a way of conceptualizing the nature of reality. In traditional metaphysics, *process* views of nature are contrasted with *substance*-based models (e.g., Bergson, 1911; Dewey, 1925; James, 1909/1996; Rescher, 1996, 2000; Whitehead, 1929). The latter assume that reality ultimately is reducible to *metaphysical simples* of physical substance (i.e., objects or things whose posited nature varies with the sophistication of our measuring devices, conceptual abilities, and the questions we are able to ask). In ancient Greece, for example, the primacy of substance was thought to be atom-like particles (e.g., Democritus) traveling through the void (for extensive treatment, see Aristotle's *Metaphysics*, which held substance to be the primary constituent of reality, possessing properties such as quality, quantity, and relation). In the 20th century, following great strides in our conceptual and methodological understanding, a host of subatomic "entities" has superseded atoms as the building blocks of the universe (protons, neutrons, neutrinos, etc.).

In contrast to *substance* metaphysics, which has dominated the philosophical and scientific landscape for more than 2,000 years (e.g., Rescher, 1996), *process* metaphysics, whose beginnings can be traced to fragments of the writings of Heraclitus (e.g., Geldard, 2000), has left less of an imprint on Western thought. Writing some 2,500 year ago, Heraclitus argued that time and change are the primary categories of understanding, and that process, accordingly, should be seen as the favored category of ontological description. A process philosopher is therefore someone for whom properties such as temporality, change, novelty, and activity are metaphysically fundamental. As Rescher (1996) puts it:

> A process is a coordinated group of changes in the complexion of reality, an organized family of *occurrences* that are systematically linked to one another either causally or functionally. It is emphatically *not* a change in or of an individual thing, but can simply relate to some aspect of the general "condition of things." A process consists in an integrated series of connected developments unfolding in conjoint coordination in line with a definite program. Processes are coordinated with occurrences or events: Processes always involve various events, and events exist only in and through processes. (p. 38, emphasis added)

As an overarching theory of reality, the process philosopher posits that macro-processes organize sub- (i.e., micro) processes into a larger whole. Accordingly, a process-oriented approach to reality is one that takes seriously the idea of events and their *constant* evolution toward a greater (and often more organized and positive) product.

Despite early contributions from Heraclitus and Leibniz, process philosophy did not begin to flourish until the revolutionary contributions of Charles Darwin, whose evolutionary principles provided a clear organic instantiation of the ideas of novelty, growth, and change. Not surprisingly, many aspects of process philosophy are hospitable to a scientific research agenda (change, adaptation, spatial and temporal relations). Others, however, are less congenial to "current" scientific practice (e.g., Klein, 2012).

For instance, processes are ongoing and constantly changing, albeit at varying rates (e.g., Gendlin, 1962). Science, in contrast, is most comfortable trying to immobilize change in the form of abstract, timeless laws and equations (e.g., Rescher, 1996; Spencer Brown, 1957; there are, of course, notable exceptions—particularly the increasing reliance on differential equations to capture the dynamics of the natural world). In this regard, the work of substance philosophers is more in tune with many scientific endeavors.

By definition, a process is something that continually is evolving and undergoing (often novel) alterations both in its structures and products. Such mutability may be an accurate reflection of nature, but it carries with it the clear implication that processes, by definition, are not blessed with inherent stability and therefore are not easily captured by the fixed abstractions characteristic of nondynamic mathematical formalizations (e.g.,

$F = ma$ or $E = mc^2$). Entities, for the process philosopher, constantly are in flux, and attempts to capture that movement by codification into a fixed system ultimately is an exercise in the futility. Transience is the key. Thus, psychologists who posit dual-process models of behavior or cognition are, by definition, engaged in an illusive enterprise—since the referents of their models are, of conceptual necessity, ephemeral.

Processes also are goal oriented (e.g., Rescher, 1996; Whitehead, 1929). In that sense, they reintroduce a way of thinking that has been anathema to scientific theory for at least several hundred years—teleology. Do psychologists really want to embrace ultimate purpose as a cornerstone of their attempts to make sense of the evolution and workings of the brain/mind? Perhaps they do. But this is a commitment that should not be taken lightly. One needs to be aware of the assumptions and presumptions one implicitly adopts when taking a particular theoretical stance. And *process* is such a stance.

Another issue arising from a process orientation to model construction is the risk it raises of a potentially infinite concatenation of micro- or subprocesses composing the macro-process of theoretical interest. Making matters more difficult still, these micro-processes also are in a continual state of flux, making it hard to pin down exactly where in its constant metamorphosis a particular process currently resides. Where does one subprocess end and the next one begin? Process, as a metaphysical stance on the ultimate constituents of reality, does not admit to arbitrary cutoffs. In psychology, we often draw our lines at points of theoretical or methodological convenience–interest. But this is an external imposition on process, a socially consensual fiat that reduces process to a selected subset of the *whole*—that is, the macro-process.

Moreover, how many subprocesses are causally relevant to any specific experimental outcome? In this chapter I have discussed the role of two sub-"processes" that participate in the trait judgment process—those based on the operation of episodic and semantic memory. But memory is not a unitary thing (according to the process view, it is not a *thing* at all!). Rather, it entails a host of sub-subprocesses, including the usual suspects (e.g., encoding, storage, and retrieval), as well as an abundance of other, less well-examined but critically relevant, memory operations (self-reflection, agency, personal ownership, etc.; Klein, German, Cosmides, & Gabriel, 2004). And each of these sub-subprocesses is, in turn influenced by related, causally efficacious, sub-sub-subprocesses, and so on. So, in what sense are we dealing with a *dual*-process model of any*thing*?

To summarize, in adopting terminology from process metaphysics, we inadvertently assume responsibility for a host of theoretical commitments that may compromise our ability to delineate the relatively clear-cut processes we assume are involved in mental operations of interest (or at least, we make it very hard to convincingly demonstrate we can do so). And those processes, if involved, would not be involved (at least in a numerically identical sense) for very long, since process philosophy assumes continual development and change (e.g., Rescher, 2000). I suggest that if psychologists had an appreciation for the logical specification of the terminology they so readily adopt, they might not be so glib in its use. Of course, one could simply ignore what philosophy has to say and continue with "business as usual" or adopt a purely operationalist stance (note, logical positivism has not been widely embraced during the past 50 years!). But sweeping these issue under the metaphysical rug and hoping for the best in doing so is to widen, not lessen, the gap between "reality in itself" and our subjective realizations of its nature.

Thus, the notion of *dual-process* models of mental function can be sustained only if one is willing to *ignore* (1) the necessarily transient nature of the phenomenon under investigation; (2) the potential infinity of sub- or micro-processes that comprise a specific macro-process selected for study; (3) the fact that the beginnings and endings of processes do not necessarily respect boundaries we establish (boundaries often motivated by methodological convenience); (4) the fact that we are adopting a metaphysical stance that is antithetical to a substance-based interpretation of "reality"; (5) the fact that an assumption of process *duality* likely is a myth of convenience; that according to process metaphysics, it is likely that "reality" is based on a *plurality* of processes (e.g., James, 1909/1996; Klein, 2012); (6) the fact that all processes are goal oriented and therefore teleological; (7) the fact that the ostensible outcome of *a* process is multi-realizable; that a potentially infinite set of processes can lead to the same outcome at any arbitrarily selected cutoff point; and, most important, (8) holism (i.e., living systems are continuous processes rather than combinations of discreet components). By treating mental operations in the latter, piecemeal (i.e., reductionist and substantivist) fashion, we inadvertently obfuscate the nature of the "reality" we seek to explicate.

If the reader is comfortable with these conditions (and I assume some of the conditions would not be any cause for concern), then all is well. But—and this is important—it is crucial that the investigator adopting a term or construct be clear about what conceptual demands that adoption entails.

It might seem to the reader that I am placing undue emphasis on what might be seen as mere "semantics." After all, "*process* is just a word—we all know what we mean when we use it!" But by adopting the term *process*, we tacitly (and in most cases unintentionally) take on the theoretical and metaphysical commitments that come with the term. And this, I suggest, is something that many of us would not knowingly be willing to do.

I personally believe than many of principles of process philosophy are good ways to think about the reality (e.g., constant change, novelty, coherence, holism, purposive; e.g., Klein, 2012), but I am not ready to accord this philosophical position ascendency over a subtantialist interpretation of nature. And that is what I am doing—whether or not I intend to do so—when I use the term *process* to describe models or theories. It may turn out that Heraclitus, Leibniz, Bergson, Whitehead, and others were correct to assume that reality conforms to the tenets of process metaphysics. But I do not think, at least at this still-early stage in the development of our science, it advisable to take strong (largely tacit) stands on whether the entities of our inquiries are best seen as substance or process.

The debate over *metaphysical simples* (i.e., the ultimate constituents of nature) is a live one. And, despite psychology's reliance on substantive concepts, a few researchers have proposed process-oriented models that actually adhere closely to philosophical tenets. Gendlin (1962), for example, has shown how one can, by including process-oriented assumptions, generate a dynamic and empirically fruitful exploration of personality that avoids much of the inevitable stasis of substantivist-based models of dispositional character. However, I do not think at this point that psychology needs to shackle itself with a particular theoretical position—the debate, I believe, will culminate in a compromise, finding a place for both substance and process in our ontology.

A Systems Approach

So, what to do? My preference would be to distance psychology from any real (or perceived) allegiance to a particular metaphysical stance (substantive or processural) and instead adopt terminology from *systems* philosophy to describe our interests in multiple routes to specific outcomes. This move certainly is not free of metaphysical commitments, but it is far less beholden to a particular metaphysics, particularly one that *demands* a choice between substance and process (Rescher, 1996). Indeed, the systems approach accommodates *both* substance and process. Equally important, it does not take a stand with regard to which is accorded primacy.

What is a *system*? A system can be defined primarily with respect to its *functionality* rather than with respect to a specific *ontology*. From an evolutionary perspective, a system consists of those component parts—and their coordinated interactions—that are necessary to accomplish a specific adaptive task. As an example, the circulatory system consists of many components (e.g., a heart, a vascular network, valves, the lungs)—that is, *things* that *act* (i.e., both substance and process) in a precise and coordinated way to accomplish an adaptive task: transporting energetically important material to and from the host in which the system resides. The functional identity of each part is defined with respect to the job it performs within the system that evolved to realize this adaptive function. Thus, despite the ability to contract rhythmically, the heart is not a pump unless there is fluid to transport and a mechanism for its delivery. It becomes a pump in the context of a system whose function is to ensure the movement of blood through the body.

From this perspective, a trait judgment system can be viewed as a coadapted relation between components whose joint efforts are required to perform certain adaptive functions. These components include obvious things such as storage in autobiographical memory, belief in the personal ownership of one's memories (Klein & Nichols, 2012), and the ability to retrieve those memories when requested. But the system is not limited to those components. For an organism to behave "more appropriately" (i.e., more adaptively) at a later time because of experiences at an earlier time, it must be equipped with mechanisms that not only retrieve ontogenetically acquired information but also use this information to make decisions and drive behavior. Moreover, because decision mechanisms, or rules often differ in what information they require, different sets of decision rules will activate different retrieval systems and may access different datasets. Without engines that can search for and retrieve the right information, supplying it to the right decision rule at the right time, an organ designed to store ontogenetically acquired information would be a pointless appendage (e.g., Klein, Cosmides, Tooby, et al., 2002). Seen in this way, there may be no such thing as "trait judgment" per se. Instead, there may be a large number of systems, each associated with a particular set of trait judgment machinery and armed with a particular goal for making the judgment.

A systems approach to dual-aspect models in psychology has the advantage of being freed of unwanted assumptions that follow from embracing a process philosophy. It also fits comfortably into the increasingly popular *systems approach* to the human sciences. This approach has wide appeal both in biology (e.g., Kitano, 2002; Palsson, 2006; von Bertalanffy, 1968) and psychology. With regard to psychology, the systems approach is used to analyze and conceptualize everything from systems of cognition (e.g., Foster & Jelicic, 1999; Schacter & Tulving, 1994) to anatomical mappings of the brain (e.g., Uttal, 2009) to neural dynamics (e.g., Kelso & Engstrom, 2006; Nunez, 2010).

In summary, rather than talk about dual *process*, we may be better served by talking and thinking about the dual or multiple *systems* that mediate observed behavior. In so doing we remain agnostic with regard to a particular (and, depending on one's favored interpretation of nature, contentious) set of metaphysical assumptions, which, if explicitly considered, likely would prompt more questions than answers. A systems approach, by contrast, is *relatively* free of metaphysical handcuffs and has the additional advantage of being widely adopted as a way of conceptualizing behavior in both physical and psychological domains.

The words we use to describe our theories and explicate our findings *do* (or, at least, *should*!) matter. They carry with them conceptual commitments we may not intend or endorse. The sooner we recognize this, the greater our progress will be toward the worthy goal of interdisciplinary communication—toward building a community of scientists and academics that truly is convergent, interactive, and collaborative across domains.

NOTES

1. Prior to presenting our neurological casework, it is important to address the question of whether these participants, despite suffering episodic amnesia, were able to access memory for lived events (albeit unconsciously), which could implicitly have influenced their semantic judgments. I have two responses. First, in terms of definitions, episodic memory is held to be the conscious recollection of past personal events (e.g., Klein, Cosmides, Tooby, et al., 2002; Wheeler, Stuss, & Tulving, 1997). Accordingly, the notion of unconscious episodic influence on semantic judgments is clearly at odds with the meaning of the term *episodic memory* as it currently is used in the literature.

   However, one could reasonably adopt the position that exemplars (e.g., Hintzman, 1986), though not consciously available for verbal report, nonetheless are active at a subconscious level when a semantic decision is requested. Aware of this concern, my colleagues and I (e.g., Klein & Loftus, 1993a; Klein et al., 1989) have devoted a substantial amount of our research (consisting of multiple methods—for example, priming techniques, transfer appropriate processing, the method of reversed association; e.g., Klein, Loftus, & Plog, 1992; Klein et al., 1997) to show that episodically based self-knowledge is not activated (consciously or unconsciously) when participants perform semantic judgments about the self (e.g., Klein, 2004; Klein et al., 2008).

2. Of course, the memorial representations of trait knowledge about self and other—and their subsequent use during trait judgment tasks—are not identical in all respects (e.g., Klein, Sherman, & Loftus, 1996; Klein, Cosmides, Tooby, et al., 2002; Klein & Lax, 2010; Klein, Rozendal, et al., 2002). However, most differences found are contingent on anticipated variations in factors such as the amount of trait-relevant experience one has of the target person a (self or other) and the type of context in which the judgment occurs (e.g., Babey, 1998; Klein & Sherman, 1994; Klein & Loftus, 1993a; Sherman et al., 1988). One unanticipated difference is the finding that trait self-knowledge and trait knowledge of others may be subserved by different, dissociable systems with semantic memory (for review and evidence, see Klein & Lax, 2010).

REFERENCES

Anderson, N. H. (1989). Functional memory and on-line attribution. In J. N. Bassili (Ed.), *On-line cognition in person perception* (pp. 175–220). Hillsdale, NJ: Erlbaum.

Babey, S. H. (1998). *Intergroup effects in the mental representation of stereotypes*. Unpublished doctoral dissertation, University of California at Santa Barbara, Santa Barbara, CA.

Babey, S. H., Queller, S., & Klein, S. B. (1998). The role of expectancy violating behaviors in the representation of trait knowledge: A summary-plus-exception model of social memory. *Social Cognition, 16*, 287–339.

Bergson, H. (1911). *Creative evolution*. London: Macmillan.

Bower, G. H. (1972). Perceptual groups as coding units in immediate memory. *Psychonomic Science, 27*, 217–219.

Bower, G. H., & Gilligan, S. G. (1979). Remembering information related to one's self. *Journal of Research in Personality, 13*, 420–432.

Brown, N. R. (1993). Response times, retrieval strategies, and the investigation of autobiographical memory. In T. K. Srull & R. S. Wyer (Eds.), *Advances in social cognition* (Vol. 5, pp. 61–68). Hillsdale, NJ: Erlbaum.

Buss, D. M., & Craik, K. H. (1983). The act frequency approach to personality. *Psychological Review, 90*, 105–126.

Carlston, D. E. (1980). Events, inferences, and impression formation. In R. Hastie, T. M. Ostrom, E. B. Ebbesen, R. S. Wyer, D. L. Hamilton, & D. E. Carlston (Eds.), *Person memory: The cognitive basis of social perception* (pp. 89–119). Hillsdale, NJ: Erlbaum.

Cermak, L. S. (1984). The episodic–semantic memory distinction in amnesia. In L. R. Squire & N. Butters (Eds.), *Neuropsychology of memory* (pp. 45–54). New York: Guilford Press.

Devine, P. G., Hirt, E. R., & Gehrke, E. M. (1990). Diagnostic and confirmation strategies in trait hypothesis testing. *Journal of Personality and Social Psychology, 58*, 952–963.

Dewey, J. (1925). *Experience and nature*. Chicago: Open Press.

Dunn, J. C., & Kirsner, K. (1988). Discovering functionally independent mental processes: The principle of reversed association. *Psychological Rreview, 95*, 91–101.

Fong, G. T., & Marcus, H. (1982). Self-schemas and judgments about others. *Social Cognition, 1*, 191–204.

Foster, J. K., & Jelicic, M. (1999). *Memory: Systems, process, or function?* New York: Oxford University Press.

Ganellen, R. J., & Carver, C. S. (1985). Why does self-reference promote incidental encoding? *Journal of Experimental Social Psychology, 21*, 284–300.

Geldard, R. (2000). *Remembering Heraclitus*. New York: Lindisfarne Books.

Gendlin, E. (1962). *Experiencing and the creation of meaning: A philosophical and psychological approach to the subjective*. Evanston, IL: Northwestern University Press.

Greenwald, A. G. (1975). Consequences of prejudice against the null hypothesis. *Psychological Bulletin, 82*, 1–20.

Hintzman, D. L. (1986). "Schema abstraction" in a multitrace memory model. *Psychological Review, 93*, 411–428.

James, W. (1996). *A pluralistic universe*. Lincoln: University of Nebraska Press. (Original work published 1909)

Keenan, J. M. (1993). An exemplar model can explain Klein and Loftus' results. In T. K. Srull & R. S. Wyer (Eds.), *Advances in social cognition* (Vol. 5, pp. 69–77). Hillsdale, NJ: Erlbaum.

Kelso, J. A. S., & Engstrom, D. A. (2006). *The complementary nature.* Cambridge, MA: MIT Press.

Kitano, H. (2002). Computational systems biology. *Nature, 420,* 206–210.

Klayman, J., & Ha, Y. (1987). Confirmation, disconfirmation, and information in hypothesis testing. *Psychological Review, 94,* 211–228.

Klein, S. B. (2004). The cognitive neuroscience of knowing one's self. In M. S. Gazzaniga (Ed.), *The cognitive neurosciences* (Vol. 3, pp. 1077–1089). Cambridge, MA: MIT Press.

Klein, S. B. (2012). The self and its brain. *Social Cognition, 30,* 474–518.

Klein, S. B., Babey, S. H., & Sherman, J. W. (1997). The functional independence of trait and behavioral self-knowledge: Methodological considerations and new empirical findings. *Social Cognition, 15,* 183–203.

Klein, S. B., Chan, R. L., & Loftus, J. (1999). Independence of episodic and semantic self-knowledge: The case from autism. *Social Cognition, 17,* 413–436.

Klein, S. B., Cosmides, L., & Costabile, K. A. (2003). Preserved knowledge of self in a case of Alzheimer's dementia. *Social Cognition, 21,* 157–165.

Klein, S. B., Cosmides, L., Costabile, K. A., & Mei, L. (2002). Is there something special about the self?: A neuropsychological case study. *Journal of Research in Personality, 36,* 490–506.

Klein, S. B., Cosmides, L., Murray, E. R., & Tooby, J. (2004). On the acquisition of knowledge about personality traits: Does learning about the self engage different mechanisms than learning about others. *Social Cognition, 22,* 367–390.

Klein, S. B., Cosmides, L., Tooby, J., & Chance, S. (2001). Priming exceptions: A test of the scope hypothesis in naturalistic trait judgments. *Social Cognition, 19,* 443–468.

Klein, S. B., Cosmides, L., Tooby, J., & Chance, S. (2002). Decisions and the evolution of memory: Multiple systems, multiple functions. *Psychological Review, 109,* 306–329.

Klein, S. B., & Gangi, C. E. (2010). The multiplicity of self: Neuropsychological evidence and its implications for the self as a construct in psychological research. *The Year in Cognitive Neuroscience 2010: Annals of the New York Academy of Sciences, 1191,* 1–15.

Klein, S. B., German, T. P., Cosmides, L., & Gabriel, R. (2004). A theory of autobiographical memory: Necessary components and disorders resulting from their loss. *Social Cognition, 22,* 460–490.

Klein, S. B., & Kihlstrom, J. F. (1986). Elaboration, organization, and the self-reference effect in memory. *Journal of Experimental Psychology: General, 115,* 26–38.

Klein, S. B., & Kihlstrom, J. F. (1998). On bridging the gap between social–personality psychology and neuropsychology. *Personality and Social Psychology Review, 2,* 228–242.

Klein, S. B., & Lax, M. L. (2010). The unanticipated resilience of trait self-knowledge in the face of neural damage. *Memory, 18,* 918–948.

Klein, S. B., & Loftus, J. (1990). The role of abstract and exemplar-based knowledge in self-judgments: Implications for a cognitive model of the self. In T. K. Srull & R. S. Wyer (Eds.), *Advances in social cognition* (Vol. 3, pp. 131–139). Hillsdale, NJ: Erlbaum.

Klein, S. B., & Loftus, J. (1993a). The mental representation of trait and autobiographical knowledge about the self. In T. K. Srull & R. S. Wyer (Eds.), *Advances in social cognition* (Vol. 5, pp. 1–49). Hillsdale, NJ: Erlbaum.

Klein., S. B., & Loftus, J. (1993b). Behavioral experience and trait judgments about the self. *Personality and Social Psychology Bulletin, 19,* 740–745.

Klein, S. B., & Loftus, J. (1993c). Some lingering self-doubts: Reply to commentaries. In T. K. Srull & R. S. Wyer (Eds.), *Advances in social cognition* (Vol. 5, pp. 171–180). Hillsdale, NJ: Erlbaum.

Klein, S. B., Loftus, J., & Burton, H. A. (1989). Two self-reference effects: The importance of distinguishing between self-descriptiveness judgments and autobiographical retrieval in self-referent encoding. *Journal of Personality and Social Psychology, 56,* 853–865.

Klein, S. B., Loftus, J., & Kihlstrom, J. F. (1996). Self-knowledge of an amnesic patient: Toward a neuropsychology of personality and social psychology. *Journal of Experimental Psychology: General, 125,* 250–260.

Klein, S. B., Loftus, J., & Plog, A. E. (1992). Trait judgments about the self: Evidence from the encoding specificity paradigm. *Personality and Social Psychology Bulletin, 18,* 730–735.

Klein, S. B., Loftus, J., Trafton, R. G., &

Fuhrman, R. W. (1992). The use of exemplars and abstractions in trait judgments: A model of trait knowledge about the self and others. *Journal of Personality and Social Psychology, 63*, 739–753.

Klein, S. B., & Nichols, S. (2012). Memory and the sense of personal identity. *Mind, 121*, 677–702.

Klein, S. B., Robertson, T. E., Gangi, C. E., & Loftus, J. (2008). The functional independence of trait self-knowledge: Commentary on Sakaki (2007). *Memory, 16*, 556–565.

Klein, S. B., Rozendal, K., & Cosmides, L. (2002). A social-cognitive neuroscience analysis of the self. *Social Cognition, 20*, 105–135.

Klein, S. B., Sherman, J. W., & Loftus, J. (1996). The role of episodic and semantic memory in the development of trait self-knowledge. *Social Cognition, 14*, 277–291.

Kuiper, N. A. (1981). Convergent evidence for the self as a prototype: The "inverted-U RT effect" for self and other judgments. *Personality and Social Psychology Bulletin, 7*, 438–443.

Locksley, A., & Lenauer, M. (1981). Considerations for a theory of self-inference processes. In N. Cantor & J. F. Kihlstrom (Eds.), *Personality, cognition, and social interaction* (pp. 263–277). Hillsdale, NJ: Erlbaum.

Lord, C. G. (1993). The "social self" component of trait knowledge about the self. In T. K. Srull & R. S. Wyer (Eds.), *Advances in social cognition* (Vol. 5, pp. 91–100). Hillsdale, NJ: Erlbaum.

Markus, H. (1977). Self-schemata and processing information about the self. *Journal of Personality and Social Psychology, 35*, 63–78.

Martin, E. (1971). Verbal learning theory and independent retrieval phenomena. *Psychological Review, 78*, 314–332.

Moscovitch, M., Yaschyshyn, T., Ziegler, M., & Nadel, L. (2000). Remote episodic memory and retrograde amnesia: Was Endel Tulving right all along? In E. Tulving (Ed.), *Memory, consciousness, and the brain: The Tallinn conference* (pp. 331–345). Philadelphia: Psychology Press.

Mueller, J. H., Thompson, W. B., & Dugan, K. (1986). Trait distinctiveness and accessibility in the self-schema. *Personality and Social Psychology Bulletin, 12*, 81–89.

Nunez, P. L. (2010). *Brain, mind, and the structure of reality*. New York: Oxford University Press.

Palsson, B. O. (2006). *Systems biology: Properties of reconstructed networks*. New York: Cambridge University Press.

Park, B. (1986). A method for studying the development of impressions of real people. *Journal of Personality and Social Psychology, 51*, 907–917.

Parkin, A. J. (1987). *Memory and amnesia*. New York: Blackwell.

Rescher, N. (1996). *Process metaphysics*. Albany: State University of New York Press.

Rescher, N. (2000). *Process philosophy: A survey of basic issues*. Pittsburgh: University of Pittsburgh Press.

Roediger, H. L., & Blaxton, T. A. (1987). Effects of varying modality, surface features, and retention interval on priming in word-fragment completion. *Memory and Cognition, 15*, 379–388.

Roediger, H. L., Weldon, M. S., & Challis, B. H. (1989). Explaining dissociations between implicit and explicit measures of retention: A processing account. In H. L. Roediger & F. I. M. Craik (Eds.), *Varieties of memory and consciousness: Essays in honour of Endel Tulving* (pp. 3–41). Hillsdale, NJ: Erlbaum.

Schacter, D. L., & Tulving, E. (Eds.). (1994). *Memory systems 1994*. Cambridge, MA: MIT Press.

Schank, R. C. (1982). *Dynamic memory: A theory of reminding and learning in computers and people*. New York: Cambridge University Press.

Schell, T. L., Klein, S. B., & Babey, S. H. (1996). Testing a hierarchical model of self-knowledge. *Psychological Science, 7*, 170–173.

Sherman, J. W. (1996). Development and mental representation of stereotypes. *Journal of Personality and Social Psychology, 70*, 1126–1141.

Sherman, J. W., & Klein, S. B. (1994). Development and representation of personality impressions. *Journal of Personality and Social Psychology, 67*, 972–983.

Sherman, J. W., Klein, S. B., Laskey, A., & Wyer, N. A. (1998). Intergroup bias in group judgment processes: The role of behavioral memories. *Journal of Experimental Social Psychology, 34*, 51–65.

Smith, E. R., & Zárate, M. A. (1992). Exemplar-based models of social judgment. *Psychological Review, 99*, 3–21.

Snyder, M., & Cantor, N. (1979). Testing hypotheses about other people: The use of historical knowledge. *Journal of Experimental Social Psychology, 15*, 330–342.

Spencer Brown, G. (1957). *Probability and scientific inference*. London: Longmans, Green & Company.

Symons, C. S., & Johnson, B. T. (1997). The self-reference effect in memory: A meta-analysis. *Psychological Bulletin, 121*, 371–394.

Tulving, E. (1983). *Elements of episodic memory*. New York: Oxford University Press.

Tulving, E. (1993). Self-knowledge of an amnesic individual is represented abstractly. In T. K. Srull & R. S. Wyer (Eds.), *Advances in social cognition* (Vol. 5, pp. 147–156). Hillsdale, NJ: Erlbaum.

Tulving, E. (1995). Organization of memory: Quo vadis? In M. S. Gazzaniga (Ed.), *The cognitive neurosciences* (pp. 839–853). Cambridge, MA: MIT Press.

Uttal, W. R. (2009). *Distributed neural systems: Beyond the new phrenology*. Cornwall-on-Hudson, NY: Sloan.

von Bertalanffy, L. (1968). *General system theory: Foundations, development, applications*. New York: Braziller.

Wason, P. C. (1968). Reasoning about a rule. *Quarterly Journal of Experimental Psychology, 20*, 273–281.

Wheeler, M. A., Stuss, D. T., & Tulving, E. (1997). Toward a theory of episodic memory: The frontal lobes and autonoetic consciousness. *Psychological Bulletin, 121*, 331–354.

Whitehead, A. N. (1929). *Process and reality*. New York: Macmillan.

CHAPTER 19

Automaticity, Control, and the Social Brain

Robert P. Spunt and Matthew D. Lieberman

The social world is good at keeping the human brain busy, posing cognitive challenges that are complex, frequent, and enormously important to our well-being. In fact, the computational demands of the social world may be the principal reason why the human brain has evolved to its present form and function relative to other primates (Dunbar, 1993). Importantly, the human brain is often able to make sense of the social world without making the conscious mind do too much work. This is because many of its processes are automatically initiated by the presence of relevant social stimuli and run to completion without much, if any, conscious intervention (Bargh & Chartrand, 1999; Gilbert, Pelham, & Krull, 1988). Not surprisingly, then, the idea that mental processes vary in their level of automaticity has had a powerful influence on theories of social cognition (Chaiken & Trope, 1999).

In the past two decades, the rapid development of methods for peering into the working human brain has made it possible to study the operation of the brain as it confronts and reflects on social information. As a result, we now know a great deal about the neuroanatomical correlates of social cognition. Although automaticity and control have been invoked to describe the operation of the social brain (cf. Lieberman, Gaunt, Gilbert, & Trope, 2002; Lieberman, 2007; Morris & Mason, 2009), there appears to be no consensus regarding what these constructs mean in terms of brain function or how they should be investigated using the methods of social neuroscience (but see Satpute & Lieberman, 2006). Hence, we begin this chapter by broadly considering how the construct of automaticity should be understood and investigated in social neuroscience. Next, we narrow our focus to social neuroscience research, to a fundamental topic in social cognition, in which questions of automaticity have historically had a large influence: causal attribution of observed behavior. Such research has identified two large-scale systems in the human brain that are reliably associated with dissociable functions in the causal attribution of behavior: the so-called mirror neuron and mentalizing systems. Now that these systems have been identified, social neuroscience has reached a point that questions about the automaticity of social causal attribution can be tackled by investigating the operating characteristics of the brain systems with which that process is reliably associated. Based on existing research, we propose an identification–attribution (I-A) model of these two systems' contributions to the causal explanation of behavior, with the mirror neuron system supporting relatively automatic behavior identification and the mentalizing system supporting relatively controlled social causal inference. After introducing the model, we evaluate existing evidence regarding the operating characteristics of these two systems. Finally, we consider directions for future research.

NEURAL AUTOMATICITY

What do the constructs of automaticity and control mean in terms of the social brain? Figure 19.1 depicts what could be called the *categorical framework*, so named because it treats automaticity and control as separate processing categories that can each be described by a set of operating characteristics. *Automatic processes* are those that operate unconsciously, inefficiently, unintentionally, and in a manner incapable of being controlled, while *controlled processes* are those that do not possess these characteristics. The position of the arrows on the brain image in Figure 19.1 illustrates the conflation of bottom-up (i.e., stimulus-driven) processing in the brain with automaticity, and top-down (i.e., goal-driven) processing in the brain with control.

The categorical framework, although intuitive and in many cases useful, glosses over a great deal of complexity. Here, we follow Bargh (1989, 1994) in advocating a multidimensional framework in which the automaticity profile of a neurocognitive process is described in terms of a set of partially orthogonal dimensions. These dimensions are *awareness*, *efficiency*, *intentionality*, and *controllability*. In the first part of this section, we define these dimensions and identify methods for investigating them in the brain (Table 19.1). Following this, we conclude the section by proposing that claims regarding neural automaticity should include a specification of the conditions of operation.

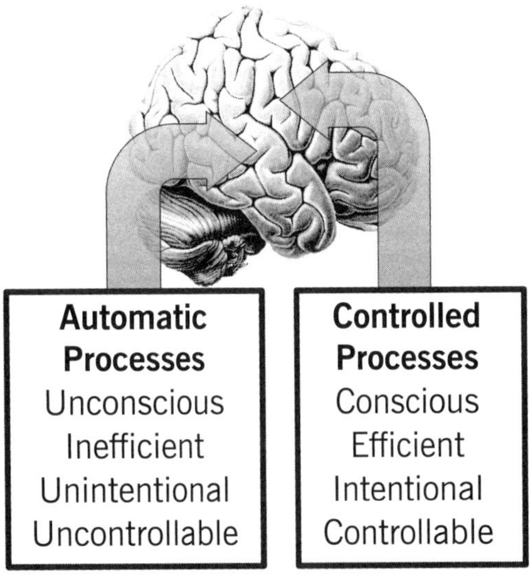

FIGURE 19.1. The categorical view of automaticity and control in the brain.

Awareness

Awareness, often used synonymously with *consciousness,* refers to the extent to which the subject is phenomenally aware of the stimulus that initiates a process, the operation of the process itself, and/or the output of the process. What does it mean to say that a person has awareness of a neural process? In the current state of the psychological and brain sciences, this is more a metaphysical question than a scientific one. However, from a methodological perspective one can establish operation *without* awareness by testing whether subliminal stimulus variation impacts neural activity. In terms of experimental design, the logic is identical to behavioral studies employing subliminal primes (Bargh & Chartrand, 2000). Yet unlike behavioral studies, the researcher is not dependent on measuring a behavioral outcome (e.g., response latency, recall) to establish that the subliminal stimulus induced a nonconscious process. Instead, measures of brain activity can be used to establish nonconscious processing. For example, numerous functional magnetic resonance imaging (fMRI) studies have now observed amygdala sensitivity to variation in the emotional expression (Whalen et al., 1998) or value (Morris, Ohman, & Dolan, 1999) of faces presented subliminally. On the basis of such data, one can conclude that some component of face processing in the amygdala *can* occur in the absence of awareness. However, this does not permit the conclusion that face processing in the amygdala is *always* automatic or that other functions associated with the amygdala are automatic (more on this later).

TABLE 19.1. Four Dimensions of Neural Automaticity: Definitions and Methods of Investigation

Dimension	Definition	Methods
Awareness	The extent to which the subject is phenomenally aware of the stimulus, process, and/or response	1. Subliminal stimulus variation (e.g., Whalen et al., 1998) 2. Induce and measure implicit versus explicit learning (e.g., Foerde et al., 2006)
Efficiency	The extent to which a process can run to completion quickly and in the absence of effort and/or attention	1. Dual-task paradigms (e.g., Poldrack, 2006) 2. Task-irrelevant stimulus variation (e.g., Winston et al., 2002) 3. High-resolution measurement of response timing (e.g., Van Berkum et al., 2009)
Intention	The extent to which a process is initiated by an explicit intention to do so	1. Manipulate processing goal (e.g., Hesse et al., 2008) 2. Manipulate processing demand (i.e., difficulty/load) (e.g., McKiernan et al., 2003)
Control	The extent to which an ongoing process can be altered by an explicit intention to do so	Initiate process of interest, then induce goal to alter processing (e.g., Ochsner et al., 2002)

Another method for tapping process awareness involves establishing a disconnect between self-reported behavioral intentions and a neural process known to be associated with the intended behavior. To the extent that such a disconnect is observed, one can conclude that the subject is unaware of the neural process. Using this logic, researchers have suggested that the formation of movement intentions operates unconsciously insofar as neural activity associated with the production of movements actually precedes participants' self-reported decision to move (Desmurget & Sirigu, 2009). Using a similar logic, work from our group has shown in several studies that neural processes at work during the consumption of persuasive messages do a better job of predicting participants' ensuing behavior than do participants' own self-reported intentions to engage in those behaviors (Falk, Berkman, Mann, Harrison, & Lieberman, 2010; Falk, Berkman, Whalen, & Lieberman, 2011). On the flip side, claims that a neural process is available to awareness can be supported by observations of tight coupling between self-reported phenomenal states (e.g., frustration) and a neural process (e.g., the neural response to errors; Spunt, Lieberman, Cohen, & Eisenberger, 2012). These studies suggest that in addition to the use of subliminal stimulus variation, the careful assessment of (self-reported) phenomenal experience can be used to make claims about processing (un)awareness.

Efficiency

The *efficiency* of a neurocognitive process can be defined as the extent to which it can be executed quickly and in the absence of attention. Phenomenologically, efficient processes are fast and effortless (e.g., recognizing a familiar face), whereas less efficient processes are slow and effortful (e.g., mentally computing the product of 42 and 79). Importantly, efficient processing is not the same as *spontaneous* processing. Spontaneity simply means that a process will be engaged even in the absence of an external stimulus to do so (e.g., the instruction to multiply 42 and 79). Hence, a process that begins spontaneously need not operate efficiently.

The principal method for studying processing efficiency is the dual-task paradigm, in which the researcher gives the subject a primary task known to engage the process of interest and simultaneously varies either the presence or difficulty of a secondary task (often called a manipulation of "cognitive load"). When a dual-task paradigm is employed in a behavioral study, questions about efficiency can only be answered if both tasks produce measurable behavioral outcomes that validly reflect successful engagement of the primary and secondary processes. When such outcomes are available, one can confirm that cognitive load was successfully induced (by examining performance of the secondary task) and assess the extent to which it affects performance on the primary task. If performance on the primary task is unaffected by load, one can infer that the process associated with the primary task is efficient.

Dual-task paradigms can be used to study neural efficiency by engaging the neural process of interest in a primary task, while simultaneously varying either the presence or difficulty of a secondary task. However, when measuring brain activity, one is no longer dependent on observations of performance variability, since variability in the neural response is now a (more) direct measure of the process of interest. Hence, primary tasks that do not produce a behavioral outcome, such as supraliminal stimulus manipulations, can be used to study neural efficiency (e.g., Pessoa, McKenna, Gutierrez, & Ungerleider, 2002). However, it should be emphasized that in order for a supraliminal stimulus manipulation to provide evidence of neural efficiency, it must be paired with a cognitively demanding secondary task, so that strategic stimulus processing can be ruled out as an alternative explanation. Moreover, we note that to categorize such a paradigm as "dual-task" is perhaps a misnomer, since passive stimulus perception is not a "task" in the traditional sense. Hence, it may be more appropriate to characterize this type paradigm as involving "task-independent stimulus variation."

Using dual-task paradigms in neuroimaging experiments is not without its problems (Satpute & Lieberman, 2006). Perhaps the most significant problem occurs when the primary and secondary tasks have overlapping neural correlates. When they do, a region whose level of activity is unaffected by the introduction of the secondary task may demonstrate such an effect not because of efficient operation in the primary task but because of its involvement in the secondary task. Hence, it is important in studies of neural efficiency to establish that regions demonstrating evidence of efficient operation are not associated with performance of the secondary task (e.g., in an independent localizer scan and/or by reference to meta-analytic evidence). Moreover, while it is the case that neural efficiency can be studied using the neural response alone as the outcome of interest, having behavioral indices of efficient operation (e.g., accuracy, response latency) can help constrain interpretation of such effects (as in Foerde, Knowlton, & Poldrack, 2006). For instance, a region that responds with equal magnitude to a particular stimulus category (e.g., faces) regardless of level of load is consistent with efficient processing. However, if its response is correlated with some behavioral outcome (e.g., postscan recall) only in conditions of low load, then this can be used to infer inefficient processing.

Processing efficiency is often defined in terms of the speed with which the process can be completed. Studies using fMRI are somewhat ill equipped to study processing speed, because the measured signal is dependent on the relatively slow hemodynamic response to neural activity, hence offering temporal resolutions on the order of seconds. Instead, researchers interested in the speed of the neural response must turn to techniques such as electroencephalography (EEG) and magnetoencephalography (MEG), which provide temporal resolution on the order of milliseconds. Using such techniques, researchers have, for instance, shed light on efficient processing of action-related language in the brain's motor system (for a review, see Hauk, Shtyrov, & Pulvermüller, 2008).

Intentionality and Controllability

The dimensions of intentionality and controllability are closely linked and are discussed together here. Whereas the *intentionality* of a mental process regards the extent to which its initiation depends on the presence of an explicit intention to initiate it, *controllability* refers to the extent to which the course of a process can be altered (i.e., modulated or terminated) after it has begun. Methodologically, we consider two ways in which the intentionality of a region's operation can be investigated. The first involves manipulating the subject's goal while presenting no stimulation. Using such a method, researchers have, for example, demonstrating that visual cortices of the brain are subject to intentional control insofar as they activate when subjects intentionally engage in visual imagery (for a review, see Kossyln, Ganis, & Thompson, 2001). A second method involves manipulating the subject's goal while either holding stimulation constant (e.g., Spunt, Falk, & Lieberman, 2010) or crossing the goal manipulation with a stimulus manipulation (e.g., Winston, Strange, O'Doherty, & Dolan, 2002; Spunt & Lieberman, 2012b).

To investigate controllability, the researcher must first induce the process of interest (e.g., a negative emotional response to an aversive stimulus), then manipulate the presence of a goal to in some way alter the process (e.g., diminish the negative emotional response by reappraising the stimulus; Ochsner, Bunge, Gross, & Gabrieli, 2002). This method allows the researcher to assess the dynamic interaction of bottom-up (i.e., stimulus-driven) and top-down (i.e., goal-driven) psychological processes. In order to do so, studies employing this method typically proceed by identifying a region (or set of regions) as implementing the top-down process (e.g., searching the brain for regions associated with the presence and/or successful execution of the control goal) and a region (or set of regions) whose association with the bottom-up process is affected by the presence and/or successful execution of the control goal. Furthermore, these studies can employ a variety of connectivity analyses to determine whether activation of the region identified as "controller" exhibits dynamic changes in activity that track goal-dependent changes in activation of the region(s) identified as "target" (Lieberman, 2011).

When the process to be controlled is initiated by presentation of a stimulus, researchers should be careful in interpreting goal-dependent changes in neural processing of the stimulus (Pessoa, Kastner, & Ungerleider, 2003). This is because these changes could be caused by a direct influence of the controller region(s) on the target region(s) or by an indirect path in which the controller region(s) produce shifts in spatial attention that ultimately alter the bottom-up inputs to target regions (Posner, 1980). This issue can be at least partially addressed by tracking eye movements (e.g., Dalton et al., 2005). Yet even when spatial attention is confirmed by eye-tracking data, it remains possible that the controller has an influence not by directly altering the target but by altering inputs to the target.

Neural Automaticity Is Conditional

It is important to emphasize that claims about automaticity should regard specific functions of regions rather than the regions themselves. For instance, consider the case of the amygdala, often invoked as a paradigmatic example of neural automaticity. Although some studies have shown that this region responds to subliminally presented threat cues (e.g., Morris et al., 1999), other work suggests that the automatic response of the amygdala to such cues is dependent on the presence of sufficient attention to the sensory modality in which such cues are presented (e.g., Pessoa et al., 2002). For example, Mothes-Lasch, Mentzel, Miltner, and Straube (2011) simultaneously presented threatening auditory cues (angry or neutral voices) and neutral visual stimuli (cross or circle) to subjects and manipulated whether they judged the gender of the speaker or the type of visual symbol. Replicating previous research, the amygdala robustly responded when participants attended to the voice during the gender judgment task. However, this effect was extinguished when attention was instead directed toward the visual modality in the symbol judgment task. Studies such as this one suggest a conditional view of automaticity in the amygdala that be phrased as *When a threat cue is present in a sensory modality to which attention is being directed, the amygdala can detect it even in the absence of explicit awareness.* In addition, such statements might also include the method used to measure the amygdala response insofar as different methods capture the response at different timescales (cf. Luo et al., 2010).

Thus, in addition to the multidimensional approach presented earlier, it is important to recognize that neural automaticity is *conditional* (Bargh, 1989). This is because regions do not operate in isolation but are part and parcel of distributed functional networks that are constantly being modulated by changes in the internal and external environment (Pessoa, 2008). Even holding the region constant, function can vary dramatically depending on the conditions under which it is engaged (Poldrack, 2006). In addition, it is likely the case that even when holding the region and function constant, the automaticity profile may be conditional. These considerations must be kept in mind when using the construct of automaticity to talk about and study the working brain.

Of course, we note that anatomy-based variables can be useful for informing theories about the operating characteristics of neural processes. One such variable is the distance from the sensory periphery. This concept is helpful insofar as regions that are closer to the sensory periphery (e.g., visual cortices) are probably more likely to exhibit high levels of automaticity than are regions more distant from the sensory periphery (e.g., prefrontal areas). Another such variable is the connectivity profile of a brain region. To the extent that a region has extensive connectivity with the rest of the brain, it is more likely to operate in different ways depending on conditions of its operation (Pessoa, 2008).

BRAIN SYSTEMS FOR THE CAUSAL EXPLANATION OF BEHAVIOR

Given the many demands placed on the brain by the social world, our discussion of the existing social neuroscience research pertaining to automaticity is limited to just one of its demands: explaining the behavior of others. The causal explanation of behavior has a long history in social psychology, studied primarily under the name of attribution theory (Heider, 1958; Jones & Harris, 1965). Moreover, the distinction between automaticity and control has had a strong influence on attribution theories, producing several dual-process models of the attributional inference (Gilbert, 1989; Trope, 1986; Lieberman et al., 2002). Although there are notable differences among existing models, they generally agree that attributional inferences are the result of an initial stage in which stimulus input about behavior is automatically identified, and a subsequent stage in which the identified behavior is attributed to an inferred social cause, using processes that are at least partially dependent on control. Importantly, these models are of the dual-process ilk in two ways. One, they specify two dissociable processes: identification and attribution. Two, they specify two dissociable operating characteristics of these processes: automaticity and control.[1] In this section, we start with the former, which predicts that identification and attributional processes will rely on dissociable neural processes.

What does it mean for an observer to identify another person's behavior? From the perspective of attribution theory, the output of the identification process must produce a representation that is attribution-relevant, that is, capable of being explained in terms of the actor's underlying disposition (Jones & Harris, 1965). From the perspective of perception, behavior identification entails extracting from the complex and ever-changing inflow of sensory input an understanding of *what* it is that the other person is doing with his or her body, that is, his or her motor intention. Social neuroscience suggests that in order for an observer to understand what *another person* is doing with his or her body, the observer may use some of the same processes involved in using *his or her own* body. Not surprisingly, a distributed set of regions in the human brain reliably responds when individuals produce motor actions such as grasping. What may be more surprising is that many of these same regions are active when individuals merely watch other people producing similar motor actions. This set of regions has come to be known as the human *mirror neuron system* (MNS; Figure 19.2A; Rizzolatti & Craighero, 2004), and canonically includes dorsal and ventral regions of the premotor cortex (dPMC and vPMC) and a region of the parietal cortex in the rostral inferior parietal lobule (IPL) extending into the intraparietal sulcus (IPS).[2] The concept of a mirror neuron is based on studies of single-cell activity in the macaque brain, which have mapped neurons responding similarly to the production and perception of motor actions. To summarize this rather large and influential body of animal research, it appears that collectively these "mirror neurons" evidence a rapid neural process of translating sensory input about another person's motor action (e.g., the sight of a hand moving toward a cup of coffee) into a representation of the action's goal (the person is going to grip the cup; Gallese, Fadiga, Fogassi, & Rizzolatti,

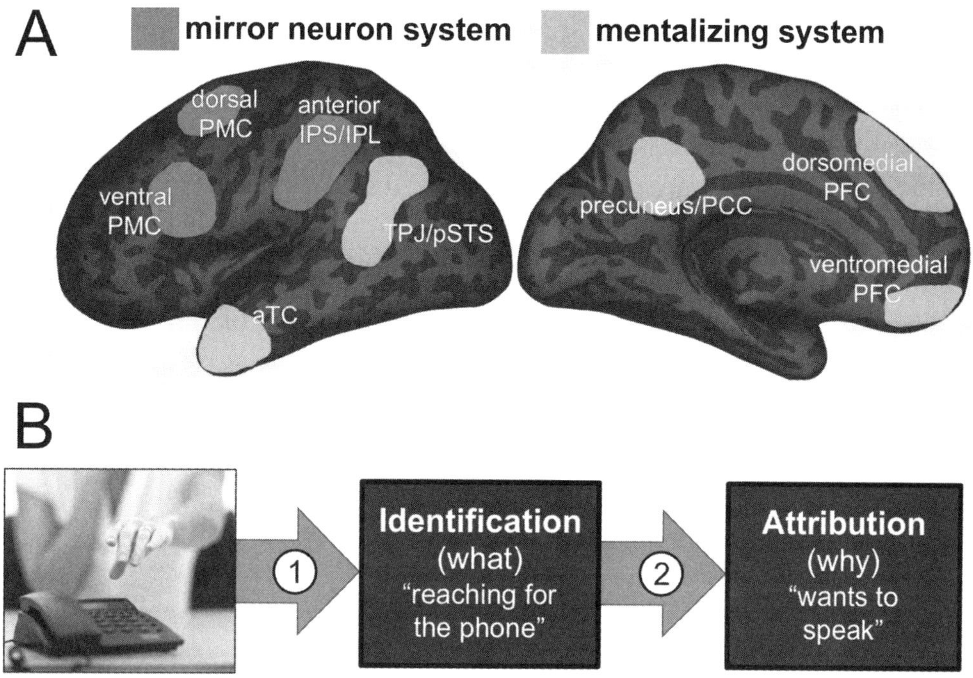

FIGURE 19.2. (A) Two brain systems involved in social cognition. PMC, premotor cortex; IPS, intraparietal sulcus; IPL, inferior parietal lobule; aTC, anterior temporal cortex; TPJ, temporoparietal junction; pSTS, posterior superior temporal sulcus; PCC, posterior cingulate cortex; PFC, prefrontal cortex. (B) The identification–attribution model of MNS and MZS contributions to understanding observed behaviors. The MNS is hypothesized to contribute primarily to identifying observed motor behaviors (Path 1), while the MZS is hypothesized to contribute primarily to attributing identified behaviors to inferred social causes (Path 2).

1996) and the intended outcome of reaching that goal (the person is going to raise the cup to his or her mouth, Fogassi et al., 2005). Neuroimaging studies suggest that similar processes are at work in the human MNS (Zacks et al., 2001; Iacoboni et al., 2005; Hamilton & Grafton, 2006, 2008; de Lange, Spronk, Willems, Toni, & Bekkering, 2008).

Imagine seeing a man reach for glass of scotch at 10:00 A.M. Your friend asks you, "Why is he doing it?" and you answer, "In order to take a drink." Your rather unsatisfactory conclusion is a verbalization of the hypothesized contribution of the MNS to action understanding (Iacoboni et al., 2005; Gallese, 2007). Although this answer is technically and grammatically correct, it is most assuredly not the kind of answer your friend was looking for. If Fritz Heider were alive today, he might say that the MNS ends at the beginning of an inferential process that concludes not with observable actions but with unobservable entities such as motive, belief, character, and context. Inferring these kinds of entities—mental states, traits, and social context—is referred to as an act of *mentalizing* (Frith & Frith, 2006). Within social neuroscience, the discovery of mirror neurons is rivaled in importance by the discovery of a collection of regions in the human brain that reliably activate when individuals are prompted to think about the mental states of others (Frith & Frith, 2006; Saxe, 2006). This *mentalizing system* (MZS; Figure 19.2A) canonically includes the dorsomedial prefrontal cortex (dmPFC), an area of the medial parietal cortex spanning the precuneus and posterior cingulate cortex (PC/PCC), the temporoparietal junction at the posterior end of the superior temporal sulcus (TPJ/pSTS), and the anterior temporal cortex (aTC). Although the earliest work on the MZS primarily relied on either verbal descriptions or abstract depictions of human behavior, more recent work has demonstrated that the MZS does come online to make sense of observed actions (Grèzes, Frith, & Passingham, 2004; Brass, Schmitt, Spengler, & Gergely, 2007; de Lange et al., 2008).

On the basis of this prior work, we have tested an I-A model of MNS and MZS contributions to social cognition, in which the MNS supports the identification of observed motor behaviors (Path 1 in Figure 19.2B), while the MZS supports the process of inferring the social causes that explain identified behaviors (Path 2 in Figure 19.2B). Put another way, the MNS makes sense of what a body is doing so that the MZS can use that information to make sense of what is going on in the person's mind. To explicitly investigate the I-A model we have developed a general method called the *why/how paradigm* (Spunt et al., 2010; Spunt, Satpute, & Lieberman, 2011). The paradigm is simple: Participants are shown a behavioral stimulus (e.g., a video clip or description of a familiar, goal-directed action) and on different trials are induced to think of one important part of *how* the behavior is occurring or one plausible reason explaining *why* the behavior is occurring. This is a face-valid manipulation of identification and attribution goals, and features high ecological validity, using natural language to induce spontaneous, open-ended social cognition. Given that the task is a goal manipulation, it permits using the same stimuli in both conditions. This feature makes it feasible to use highly complex and naturalistic social stimuli, and offers the possibility of teasing part bottom-up stimulus effects from top-down goal-driven effects.

A recent study (Spunt & Lieberman, 2012a; Figure 19.3) illustrates well the use of the *why/how paradigm* to test the I-A model. While undergoing fMRI, healthy volunteers were presented with familiar human actions either by video or text and were asked either to identify *how* (identification goal) or to infer *why* (attribution goal). Identification and attribution goals strongly distinguished activity in the MNS and MZS, respectively, and these effects were present regardless of whether the behavior was presented in a video or text. However, some areas of the MNS showed a strong preference for behaviors presented in a video as opposed to in text, and this effect was present regardless of the observer's explicit goal. This suggests that the MNS may translate sensory information about behavior into meaningful motor acts, even when the observer's explicit goal is not to identify motor acts but to make causal attributions. Moreover, it suggests that the MNS may not be critically involved in making attributional inferences when such inferences are made from behaviors described in text. This is because, when actions are *observed*, sensory input about action must be identified in meaningful ways in order for attributional processing to begin. In support of this, we found that areas of the MNS and MZS were functionally coupled, but only when participants made attributions about *observed* behaviors. In contrast, when attributions were made for verbal descriptions of behaviors, such a functional coupling was not observed, a finding consistent with the proposition that only during action *perception* does the MZS depend on the MNS for the identification of behavior. This study, along with others from our group (Spunt et al., 2011; Spunt & Lieberman, 2012b), provides strong support for the I-A model of the functions of the MNS and MZS in social inference.

AUTOMATICITY PROFILES OF THE MNS AND MZS

If we watch someone perform a familiar action, it is as if we literally *see* what they are doing in a psychological sense. When we see someone reaching for a glass of water, the characterization as "reaching" comes to us as a given. We do not experience the act in terms of its complex physical kinematics. By the time we notice it, it is already infused with psychological interpretation. This psychological perception does not feel like it is based on any sort of information processing at all; it is, in a sense, given to us prior to any sort of cognitive elaboration. Of course, on the basis of such perceptions we can explicitly verbalize an understanding of the person's likely state of mind, such as his or her motives, beliefs, and personal character. Correspondent with this phenomenological

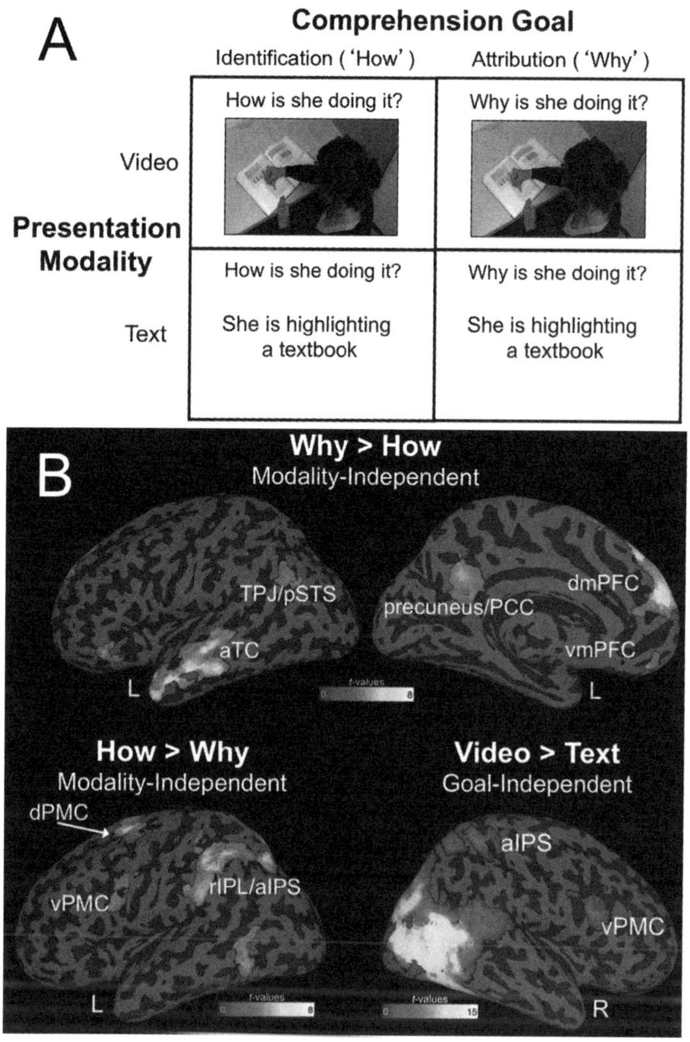

FIGURE 19.3. (A) The experimental design used in Spunt and Lieberman (2012a) and discussed in the text. (B) Regions recruited by the identification and attribution goals regardless of presentation modality, and regions recruited by the presence of an action in a video (compared to an action described in text) regardless of the observer's explicit comprehension goal. vPMC, ventral premotor cortex; dPMC, dorsal premotor cortex; aIPS, anterior intraparietal sulcus; rIPL, rostral inferior parietal lobule; aTC, anterior temporal cortex; TPJ, temporoparietal junction; pSTS, posterior superior temporal sulcus; PCC, posterior cingulate cortex; dmPFC, dorsomedial prefrontal cortex; vmPFC, ventromedial prefrontal cortex.

description, it is tempting to assume that that the MNS operates automatically, while the MZS operates under relatively more control. In the previous section, we presented evidence associating the MNS with the *identification* of perceived behavior and the MZS with the *attribution* of such perceptions to inferred causes. In this section, we evaluate the case for automaticity and control in the MNS and the MZS, respectively. As we earlier tried to make clear, the categorical view of automaticity and control ought to be supplanted by a multidimensional view that describes neurocognition not as either automatic or controlled but as having a potentially complex and conditional automaticity profile. Therefore, we review existing social neuroscience evidence regarding the operating characteristics of the MNS and MZS in order to make some preliminary proposals regarding their automaticity profiles. We make no claim to comprehensiveness, and in order to narrow our scope we primarily focus on studies using fMRI.

Theoretical treatments of the MNS have often included the proposition that the system operates automatically (Gallese, 2003, 2007, 2009; Coricelli, 2005; Iacoboni et al., 2005; Keysers & Gazzola, 2006). However, this proposition has received very little empirical testing. To our knowledge, no study has explicitly examined the operating characteristics of mirror neurons in the macaque brain. In that animal research, the best evidence that might be marshaled for the automaticity claim seems to be the rapidity with which these neurons respond during action observation. However, the speed of response is not typically analyzed; moreover, speed is only one part of the *efficiency* dimension of automaticity. To establish efficiency, it would be necessary to load the monkey with a secondary task, while simultaneously presenting actions. Hence, we believe that on the basis of the monkey studies alone, there is only limited evidence for automaticity, and such evidence applies to only one dimension (efficiency) of automaticity. Moreover, it is unknown to what extent the efficiency of this response is dependent on explicit attention to the action stimulus. Insofar as monkeys require extensive training in order to participate in these experiments, it seems likely that appropriate attentional control is a condition of the efficient response of macaque mirror neurons.

In humans, the automaticity claim has received relatively more attention (selected studies are listed in Table 19.2). In an influential study attempting to investigate this claim, Iacoboni and colleagues (2005) had participants watch actions that either did or did not feature a context that suggested the action's intention. Some participants were also given the explicit goal to infer the action's intention, while others were simply instructed to watch passively. Contextualized actions elicited increased activation in the right vPMC, and this effect did not interact with the goal manipulation. This finding was used to support the claim that the right vPMC automatically encodes the physical contact of an action in the service of understanding that action's intention. In terms of the multidimensional framework articulated earlier (and summarized in Table 19.1), this claim to automaticity seems to primarily regard the *efficiency* with which the right vPMC encodes the stimulus manipulation. However, in order for a stimulus manipulation to provide evidence of efficient operation, it must be paired with a manipulation of attentional load that is unrelated to the stimulus manipulation. The explicit goal to infer intention, insofar as it is directly (and purposefully) related to the stimulus manipulation, is not an appropriate induction of attentional load. Therefore, though the result from Iacoboni et al. (2005) is consistent with efficient operation, it does not demonstrate it and in fact did not even test it.

Two studies have used dual-task paradigms explicitly to investigate the efficiency of the MNS response during action observation. Chong, Williams, Cunnington, and Mattingley (2008) presented videos of moving hands, stationary hands, or random dot motion to participants and simultaneously manipulated the difficulty of a secondary visual discrimination task (visual load) that was superimposed onto the videos. Increasing visual load attenuated the response of left posterior inferior frontal gyrus (pIFG; pars triangularis) only during hand observation, a finding consistent with nonefficient operation of this region during action observation. However, it is useful to note that this region of the IFG is more anterior than is typically observed in studies of action observation and imitation (for a meta-analysis, see Caspers, Zilles, Laird, & Eickhoff, 2010). In a recent study (Spunt & Lieberman, 2013), we simultaneously manipulated participants' comprehension goal and their level of memory load while they watched videos of goal-directed actions. Compared to a fixation baseline, action observation elicited activation in bilateral vPMC, left dPMC, and left anterior IPS that was unaffected by level of memory load. To our knowledge, this is the most direct evidence yet for an efficient response of the MNS to actions.

Although Iacoboni and colleagues (2005) did not find support for the controllability claim, several other studies have. Indeed,

TABLE 19.2. Selected fMRI Studies Germane to the Automaticity Profile of the Mirror Neuron System (MNS) Response during Action Observation

Study	Method	Findings	Implications
Iacoboni et al. (1999)	Manipulated presence of goal to imitate observed actions	Imitation goal increased activation in left pIFG and aIPS	Some MNS areas are controllable
Iacoboni et al. (2005)	Manipulated (1) presence of context in observed actions and (2) presence of goal to infer action intention	Presence of context increased activation in right vPMC regardless of observer goal	Context senstivity in some MNS areas is spontaneous
Chong et al. (2008)	Manipulated visual load during observation of moving hands, stationary hands, or dot motion	Load decreased left pIFG activation only during hand observation	Some MNS areas operate nonefficiently under visual load
Hesse et al. (2008)	Manipulated attention to the means or the end of observed actions	Attention to means (relative to end) increased activation in bilateral aIPS/rIPL and right vPMC/pIFG	Some MNS areas are controllable
Spunt et al. (2011)	Manipulated presence of goal to verbally identify observed actions	Relative to passive observation, active identification increased activation in right pIFG and rIPL and left aIPS	Some MNS areas are controllable
Spunt & Lieberman (2012b)	Manipulated (1) attention to how or why actions are performed and (2) presentation modality (text vs. video)	Attention to how increased activation in left vPMC, dPMC, and aIPS/rIPL regardless of presentation modality	Some MNS areas are controllable and can be intentionally operated
Spunt & Lieberman (2013)	Manipulated (1) processing goal and (2) memory load during action observation	Load did not affect activation of bilateral vPMC and left dPMC and aIPS for any processing goal	Some MNS areas operate efficiently under memory load

Note. aIPS, anterior intraparietal sulcus; dPMC/vPMC, dorsal/ventral premotor cortex; dPMS; pIFG, posterior inferior frontal gyrus; rIPL, rostral inferior parietal lobule.

years earlier, Iacoboni and colleagues (1999) showed that the goal to imitate rather than passively observe actions enhanced activation in the MNS. Later on, Hesse, Sparing, and Fink (2008) presented videos of hand actions while participants judged either aspects of the action's means or its outcome. Compared to attending to the outcome of the action, attention to means produced significantly more activation in the MNS. Similarly, Spunt et al. (2011) showed that during action observation, the goal to verbally identify rather than passively observe enhanced activation in several regions of the MNS. These findings are corroborated by the previously reviewed work from our group (Spunt & Lieberman, 2012a, 2012b), which similarly demonstrates that attention to *how* an action is performed enhances MNS activation more than attention to *why* the same action was performed. Indeed, even in the absence of observable actions, as when an action is merely described (Spunt et al., 2010), attention to *how* strongly engages regions consistent with the MNS, demonstrating that this system can be intentionally operated. These studies strongly undermine the notion that the MNS always operates automatically. However, we do not argue that the MNS is a controlled system. Rather, in line with the dimensional–conditional approach to automaticity outlined earlier, we believe that claims to automaticity in the MNS should specify both dimensions and conditions of operation.

Discourse about the MZS often claims that this system relies on controlled processing (for a review, see Lieberman, 2010). However, as with the MNS, the operating characteristics of the MZS have received somewhat limited empirical investigation (selected studies are listed in Table 19.3). The majority of research on the MZS, insofar as it uses explicit goal manipulations to induce the representation of mental states (for reviews, see Carrington & Bailey, 2009; Van Overwalle & Baetens, 2009), can be said to firmly establish that MZS operation *is* indeed subject to intentional control. Indeed, it has been suggested that in the context of action observation, some areas of the MZS may not only be subject to control but also may themselves exert control over other regions (Spengler, Cramon, & Brass, 2009). In a recent study, we further investigated the controlled operating characteristics of the MZS. It has been suggested that the central component of controlled processing is working memory, which allows for online maintenance and serial manipulation of mental representations. Hence, one method for establishing controlled processing in the MZS is to determine whether it operates like a working memory system for social cognition. The most common method for investigating working memory is parametrically manipulating the amount of information to be held in mind. However, studies of working memory have almost exclusively investigated the maintenance and manipulation of nonsocial information, such as numbers and sensorimotor representations. In a recent study (Meyer, Spunt, Berkman, Taylor, & Lieberman, 2012), we developed a paradigm for investigating the online maintenance and manipulation of *social* representations, or *social working memory*. While undergoing fMRI, participants were asked to rank two, three, or four of their friends on a trait dimension (e.g., generosity) during a 6-second delay period. At the end of the period, they made a rank judgment (e.g., Is Rebecca the second most generous?) that could be coded as accurate or inaccurate based on ratings collected from the participant prior to the fMRI study. When they accurately ranked their friends, regions of the MZS, in particular the dmPFC, PCC/PC, and TPJ, demonstrated parametric increases in activity as a function of the number of friends to be ranked. This strongly suggests that regions of the MZS can be *intentionally* operated in a top-down fashion to manage increasing social cognitive demands. This converges with other studies showing that the dmPFC shows enhanced activation for more difficult mental state inferences (Jenkins & Mitchell, 2010) and in individuals who evidence greater degrees of mentalizing while playing a competitive game (Coricelli & Nagel, 2009).

Several studies have used either task-irrelevant stimulus manipulations or dual-task paradigms to evaluate the efficiency of MZS operation during the processing of social information. Several studies have used task-irrelevant stimulus manipulations to demonstrate that, for example, descriptions of behavior that are strongly associated with personality traits (i.e., are trait-diagnostic) elicit activation in areas of the MZS even when participants do not explicitly have the goal of making trait inferences (Mitchell, Cloutier, Banaji, & Macrae, 2006; Ma, Vandekerckhove, Overwalle, Seurinck, & Fias, 2011). Yet these studies only provide information about the *spontaneity* of MZS activation during social information processing. In order to provide information about *efficiency*, the manipulation (stimulus or goal) intended to produce MZS activation must be paired with a manipulation of the difficulty of a secondary task. To our knowledge, only two studies have successfully employed this method. In one, den Ouden, Frith, Frith, and Blakemore (2005) presented participants with written scenarios manipulated to induce mentalizing while simultaneously manipulating the presence of a secondary visual judgment task. Although the dmPFC was associated with mentalizing when participants were not under attentional load, this association was extinguished by the induction of load. In a previously discussed study from our group (Spunt & Lieberman, 2013), we used a dual-task paradigm to investigate the efficiency of the MZS during action observation. We factorially manipulated participants' comprehension goal (using the why/how paradigm

TABLE 19.3. Selected fMRI Studies Germane to the Automaticity Profile of the Mentalizing System (MZS) during Social Cognition

Study	Method	Findings	Implications
den Ouden et al. (2005)	Manipulated presence of (1) mentalizing judgments and (2) attentional load	Presence of attentional load extinguished dmPFC association with mentalizing judgments	Some MZS areas operate nonefficiently under attentional load
Mitchell et al. (2006)	Manipulated (1) trait diagnosticity of behavioral descriptions and (2) goal to form an impression or attend to the trial sequence	dmPFC activity distinguished diagnostic from nondiagnostic behaviors only when subjects had the sequencing goal	Some MZS areas spontaneously activate for trait-diagnostic behavioral descriptions
Coricelli & Nagel (2009)	Measured level of strategic mental state reasoning in a game where personal outcomes depend on others' choices	Individuals evidencing higher levels of mental state reasoning showed increased dmPFC and vmPFC activation	Some MZS areas are sensitive to amount of mentalizing across individuals
Spengler et al. (2009)	Subjects performed both a mentalizing task and a separate task demanding inhibition of automatic imitation	Mentalizing and imitation-inhibition tasks recruited common areas of mPFC and right TPJ	Some MZS areas are involved in control over automatic imitation
Jenkins & Mitchell (2010)	Subjects inferred characters' beliefs or preferences from scenarios that differed in the certainty with which such inferences could be made	Uncertain (ambiguous) mental state inferences increased dmPFC activation regardless of type of mental state	Some MZS areas track difficulty of mental state inferences
Ma et al. (2011)	Manipulated (1) trait diagnosticity of behavioral descriptions and (2) goal to passively read or actively infer trait	Trait-diagnostic descriptions activated dmPFC, left TPJ, and bilateral aTC in both the passive and active tasks	Some MZS areas spontaneously activate for trait-diagnostic behavioral descriptions
Wagner et al. (2011)	Manipulated social content in photographs while subjects made mentalizing-irrelevant judgments	Photographs of social scenes increased activation in the MZS; this effect was stronger for high trait empathizers	Spontaneous activation of MZS to social stimuli shows individual differences
Rameson et al. (2011)	Measured empathy for emotionally expressive actors viewed either under memory load or with the instruction to actively empathize	dmPFC activation was reduced under load; trait empathy was associated with mPFC activation only under load	Efficient activation of MZS under memory load shows individual differences
Meyer et al. (2012)	Manipulated mentalizing demands by having subjects rank either 2, 3, or 4 friends on a trait dimension	Increasing mentalizing demands increased activation in dmPFC, PCC/PC, and left TPJ	Some MZS areas are sensitive to increasing mentalizing demands
Spunt & Lieberman (2013)	Manipulated (1) mentalizing goal and (2) level of memory load during action observation	Increasing memory load extinguished assocation of dmPFC and left aTC with mentalizing goal	Some MZS areas operate nonefficiently under memory load

Note. aTC, anterior temporal cortex; dmPFC/vmPFC, dorsomedial/ventromedial prefrontal cortex; PC, precuneus; PCC, posterior cingulate cortex; TPJ, temporoparietal junction.

described earlier) and their level of memory load during the observation of goal-directed actions. Whereas several regions of the MNS showed a load-independent response to the actions, suggesting efficient operation, two regions of the MZS, namely, the dmPFC and the left aTC, showed a response that was strongly modulated by load only when participants had the goal to understand the actor's motives (that is, in the *why* condition). This suggests that under some conditions, the MZS can be intentionally operated upon, and that this operation is dependent on the availability of attentional resources.

Although some areas of the MZS may be critically involved in the online control of social cognition, several studies have shown that that MZS activation can be driven by stimulus variation in the absence of an explicit goal to infer mental states (Mitchell et al., 2006; Brass et al., 2007; Ma et al., 2011; Wagner, Dal Cin, Sargent, Kelley, & Heatherton, 2011; Wheatley, Milleville, & Martin, 2007), a feature that suggests efficient processing. For example, Wagner et al. (2011) had participants undergo fMRI while categorizing a series of images as containing animals, vegetables, or minerals. As a group, they observed increased MZS activation in response to photographs of humans (category: animal) compared to photographs of nonhuman animals, vegetables, or minerals. Insofar as this activation was task-irrelevant, this suggests efficient processing. Moreover, they found that individuals reporting higher levels of trait empathy exhibiting enhanced task-irrelevant activation of the MZS. As described earlier, this captures not the efficiency but the spontaneity of MZS activation. In order to capture the former dimension, the difficulty of the task-irrelevant judgment could have been manipulated to see whether the level of spontaneous MZS activation was unaffected by increasing attentional load. In a recent study, members of our group observed a similar effect in the MZS while also manipulating load. Rameson, Morelli, and Lieberman (2011) used fMRI to investigate efficiency of MZS during the perception of contextualized emotional displays. Participants viewed photographs of targets expressing emotions with one of two instructions: (1) empathize with the target or (2) watch while holding in mind an 8-digit number (an induction of cognitive load). Consistent with inefficient operation, several regions of the MZS were strongly deactivated by the induction of load. However, consistent with individual differences in efficient operation, reports of trait empathy were associated with MZS activation to the photographs when individuals were under cognitive load. High trait empathizers produced similar levels of MZS activity with and without the cognitive load. As with the MNS, these studies suggest the importance of a multidimensional and conditional view of automaticity in the MZS. Moreover, they suggest that an important condition on MZS automaticity may be individual differences in social expertise.

Summary

In this section, we have reviewed social neuroscience evidence regarding the operating characteristics of the MNS and MZS during action observation and social cognition (summarized in Tables 19.2 and 19.3). We first considered the claim that the MNS operates automatically, and concluded that while there *is* some evidence to suggest that the MNS operates *efficiently* (e.g., Iacoboni et al., 2005; Spunt & Lieberman, 2013), there is also plenty of evidence demonstrating that its operation is subject to online control (e.g., Iacoboni et al., 1999; Hesse et al., 2008; Spunt et al., 2010; Spunt & Lieberman, 2012a, 2012b). Next, we considered the claim that the MZS is a controlled processing system. Regarding this claim, there is strong evidence supporting the claim that the MZS is indeed subject to online control and may even operate in a manner that adapts to the processing demands of the task at hand (e.g., Meyer et al., 2012). Several researchers have attempted to demonstrate that the MZS operates *efficiently* in the presence of relevant social stimuli; however, a close examination of these methods shows that most claims to *efficiency* in the MZS are based on *only* the demonstration of spontaneous (i.e., task-irrelevant) activation (e.g., Mitchell et al., 2006; Brass et al., 2007; Wagner et al., 2011). This raises a point that is worth repeating: Spontaneous operation by itself does not constitute a demonstration of efficient operation. To our knowledge, the only study to test directly the efficiency claim actually showed inefficient operation of two core regions of the MZS (Spunt & Lieberman, 2013). The review further underscores the utility of a dimensional–conditional approach to neural automaticity that acknowledges multiple dimensions of operation that may be sensitive to the context (i.e., condition) of operation. Moreover, it highlights the need to scrutinize carefully the methods used to investigate the operating characteristics of a neural process.

CONCLUSION

In writing this chapter we had two basic motivations. One, we sought to apply the multidimensional framework of automaticity (Bargh, 1994) to social neuroscience research examining the operating characteristics of social information processing in the brain. We believe this provides a useful framework within which to make claims regarding the operating characteristics of neural processes. Moreover, we believe it underscores the utility of social neuroscience studies for testing hypotheses regarding the operating characteristics of the mental processes that are near and dear to social psychologists. One of these processes—the causal explanation of behavior—motivated the second part of this chapter, which was to critically evaluate the automaticity profiles of two brain systems known to be involved in this process. Overall, we believe our analysis emphasizes the necessity of conditional statements regarding the automaticity of a brain system. The methods of social neuroscience can shed light on the nature of automaticity and control in social cognition by allowing psychological scientists to characterize the operating characteristics of the brain systems known to support social cognition. In so doing, the goals should not be to reify a neural process as automatic but to identify the conditions under which it does (or does not) demonstrate characteristics of automatic operation. In other words, the critical question should not be *whether* the social brain operates automatically; rather, the critical question should be *when* and *for whom* it operates automatically.

NOTES

1. We recognize the the two most influential attributional process models, Trope's identification–inference model (Trope, 1986) and Gilbert's characterization–correction model (Gilbert et al., 1988) disagree regarding the automaticity profile of attributional processing. Whereas in Trope's model the attribution process is described by a single controlled process, Gilbert's model decomposes the attributional process into a sequence of two steps: automatic attribution to disposition (in line with work on spontaneous trait inference; cf. Uleman, Saribay, & Gonzalez, 2008) followed by controlled correction of the attribution based on additional information (e.g., situational information).
2. Given that single neurons exhibiting production–perception "mirroring" have not been identified in the canonical areas of the human MNS (but see Mukamel, Ekstrom, Kaplan, Iacoboni, & Fried, 2010, for a study identifying them in other areas), some researchers prefer alternative labels such as the *mirror system,* the *motor resonance system,* or the *action observation network.*

REFERENCES

Bargh, J. (1989). Conditional automaticity: Varieties of automatic influence in social perception and cognition. In J. Uleman & J. Bargh (Eds.), *Unintended thought* (pp. 3–51). New York: Guilford Press.

Bargh, J. A. (1994). The four horsemen of automaticity: Awareness, intention, efficiency, and control in social cognition. In R. S. Wyer, Jr. & T. K. Srull (Eds.), *Handbook of social cognition* (2nd ed., pp. 1–40). Hillsdale, NJ: Erlbaum.

Bargh, J. A., & Chartrand, T. L. (1999). The unbearable automaticity of being. *American Psychologist, 54*(7), 462–479.

Bargh, J. A., & Chartrand, T. L. (2000). The mind in the middle: A practical guide to priming and automaticity research. In H. Reis & C. Judd (Eds.), *Handbook of research methods in social and personality psychology* (pp. 253–285). New York: Cambridge University Press.

Brass, M., Schmitt, R. M., Spengler, S., & Gergely, G. (2007). Investigating action understanding: Inferential processes versus action simulation. *Current Biology, 17*(24), 2117–2121.

Carrington, S. J., & Bailey, A. J. (2009). Are there theory of mind regions in the brain?: A review of the neuroimaging literature. *Human Brain Mapping, 30*(8), 2313–2335.

Caspers, S., Zilles, K., Laird, A. R., & Eickhoff, S. B. (2010). ALE meta-analysis of action observation and imitation in the human brain. *NeuroImage, 50*(3), 1148–1167.

Chaiken, S., & Trope, Y. (Eds.). (1999). *Dual-process theories in social psychology.* New York: Guilford Press.

Chong, T. T.-J., Williams, M. A., Cunnington, R., & Mattingley, J. B. (2008). Selective attention modulates inferior frontal gyrus activity during action observation. *NeuroImage, 40*(1), 298–307.

Coricelli, G. (2005). Two-levels of mental states attribution: From automaticity to voluntariness. *Neuropsychologia, 43,* 294–500.

Coricelli, G., & Nagel, R. (2009). Neural correlates of depth of strategic reasoning in medial prefrontal cortex. *Proceedings of the National Academy of Sciences, 106*(23), 9163–9168.

Dalton, K. M., Nacewicz, B. M., Johnstone, T., Schaefer, H. S., Gernsbacher, M. A., Goldsmith, H. H., et al. (2005). Gaze fixation and the neural circuitry of face processing in autism. *Nature Neuroscience, 8*(4), 519–526.

de Lange, F. P., Spronk, M., Willems, R. M., Toni, I., & Bekkering, H. (2008). Complementary systems for understanding action intentions. *Current Biology, 18*(6), 454–457.

den Ouden, H. E. M., Frith, U., Frith, C., & Blakemore, S.-J. (2005). Thinking about intentions. *NeuroImage, 28*(4), 787–796.

Desmurget, M., & Sirigu, A. (2009). A parietal–premotor network for movement intention and motor awareness. *Trends in Cognitive Sciences, 13*(10), 411–419.

Dunbar, R. I. M. (1993). Coevolution of neocortical size, group size and language in humans. *Behavioral and Brain Sciences, 16*(4), 681–693.

Falk, E. B., Berkman, E. T., Mann, T., Harrison, B., & Lieberman, M. D. (2010). Predicting persuasion-induced behavior change from the brain. *Journal of Neuroscience, 30*(25), 8421–8424.

Falk, E. B., Berkman, E. T., Whalen, D., & Lieberman, M. D. (2011). Neural activity during health messaging predicts reductions in smoking above and beyond self-report. *Health Psychology, 30*(2), 177–185.

Foerde, K., Knowlton, B. J., & Poldrack, R. A. (2006). Modulation of competing memory systems by distraction. *Proceedings of the National Academy of Sciences USA, 103*(31), 11778–11783.

Fogassi, L., Ferrari, P. F., Gesierich, B., Rozzi, S., Chersi, F., & Rizzolatti, G. (2005). Parietal lobe: from action organization to intention understanding. *Science, 308*(5722), 662–667.

Frith, C. D., & Frith, U. (2006). The neural basis of mentalizing. *Neuron, 50*(4), 531–534.

Gallese, V. (2003). The manifold nature of interpersonal relations: The quest for a common mechanism. *Philosophical Transactions of the Royal Society of London B: Biological Sciences, 358*(1431), 517–528.

Gallese, V. (2007). Before and below "theory of mind": Embodied simulation and the neural correlates of social cognition. *Philosophical Transactions of the Royal Society of London B: Biological Sciences, 362*(1480), 659–669.

Gallese, V. (2009). Motor abstraction: A neuroscientific account of how action goals and intentions are mapped and understood. *Psychological Research, 73*(4), 486–498.

Gallese, V., Fadiga, L., Fogassi, L., & Rizzolatti, G. (1996). Action recognition in the premotor cortex. *Brain, 119*(2), 593–609.

Gilbert, D. (1989). Thinking lightly about others: Automatic components of the social inference process. In J. Uleman & J. Bargh (Eds.), *Unintended thought* (pp. 189–212). New York: Guilford Press.

Gilbert, D., Pelham, B., & Krull, D. (1988). On cognitive busyness: When person perceivers meet persons perceived. *Journal of Personality and Social Psychology, 54*(5), 733–740.

Grèzes, J., Frith, C., & Passingham, R. E. (2004). Brain mechanisms for inferring deceit in the actions of others. *Journal of Neuroscience, 24*(24), 5500–5505.

Hamilton, A. F. de C., & Grafton, S. T. (2006). Goal representation in human anterior intraparietal sulcus. *Journal of Neuroscience, 26*(4), 1133–1137.

Hamilton, A. F. de C., & Grafton, S. T. (2008). Action outcomes are represented in human inferior frontoparietal cortex. *Cerebral Cortex, 18*(5), 1160–1168.

Hauk, O., Shtyrov, Y., & Pulvermüller, F. (2008). The time course of action and action-word comprehension in the human brain as revealed by neurophysiology. *Journal of Physiology (Paris), 102*(1–3), 50–58.

Heider, F. (1958). *The psychology of interpersonal relations.* New York: Wiley.

Hesse, M., Sparing, R., & Fink, G. (2008). End or means—The "what" and "how" of observed intentional actions. *Journal of Cognitive Neuroscience*, *21*(4), 776–790.

Iacoboni, M., Molnar-Szakacs, I., Gallese, V., Buccino, G., Mazziotta, J. C., & Rizzolatti, G. (2005). Grasping the intentions of others with one's own mirror neuron system. *PLoS Biology*, *3*(3), 529–535.

Iacoboni, M., Woods, R. P., Brass, M., Bekkering, H., Mazziotta, J. C., & Rizzolatti, G. (1999). Cortical mechanisms of human imitation. *Science*, *286*(5449), 2526–2528.

Jenkins, A., & Mitchell, J. (2010). Mentalizing under uncertainty: Dissociated neural responses to ambiguous and unambiguous mental state inferences. *Cerebral Cortex*, *20*, 404–410.

Jones, E., & Harris, V. (1965). From acts to dispositions: The attribution process in person perception. In L. Berkowitz (Ed.), *Advances in experimental social psycholgoy* (Vol. 2, pp. 219–266). San Diego: Academic Press.

Jones, E., & Harris, V. (1967). The attribution of attitudes. *Journal of Experimental Social Psychology*, *3*(1), 1–24.

Keysers, C., & Gazzola, V. (2006). Towards a unifying neural theory of social cognition. *Progress in Brain Research*, *156*, 379–401.

Kosslyn, S. M., Ganis, G., & Thompson, W. L. (2001). Neural foundations of imagery. *Nature Reviews Neuroscience*, *2*(9), 635–642.

Lieberman, M. (2010). Social cognitive neuroscience. In S. Fiske, D. Gilbert, & G. Lindzey (Eds.), *Handbook of social psychology* (5th ed., pp. 143–193). New York: McGraw-Hill.

Lieberman, M. (2011). Why symbolic processing of affect can disrupt negative affect: Social cognitive and affective neuroscience investigations. In A. Todorov, S. Fiske, & D. Prentice (Eds.), *Social neuroscience: Toward understanding the underpinnings of the social mind* (pp. 188–209). New York: Oxford University Press.

Lieberman, M. D. (2007). The X-and C-systems: The neural basis of automatic and controlled social cognition. In E. Harmon-Jones & P. Winkielman (Eds.), *Fundamentals of social neuroscience* (pp. 290–315). New York: Guilford Press.

Lieberman, M., Gaunt, R., Gilbert, D., & Trope, Y. (2002). Reflection and reflexion: A social cognitive neuroscience approach to attributional inference. *Advances in Experimental Social Psychology*, *34*, 199–249.

Luo, Q., Holroyd, T., Majestic, C., Cheng, X., Schechter, J., & Blair, R. J. (2010). Emotional automaticity is a matter of timing. *The Journal of Neuroscience*, *30*(17), 5825–5829.

Ma, N., Vandekerckhove, M., Overwalle, F. V., Seurinck, R., & Fias, W. (2011). Spontaneous and intentional trait inferences recruit a common mentalizing network to a different degree: Spontaneous inferences activate only its core areas. *Social Neuroscience*, *6*(2), 123–138.

McKiernan, K. A., Kaufman, J. N., Kucera-Thompson, J., & Binder, J. R. (2003). A parametric manipulation of factors affecting task-induced deactivation in functional neuroimaging. *Journal of Cognitive Neuroscience*, *15*(3), 394–408.

Meyer, M. L., Spunt, R. P., Berkman, E. T., Taylor, S. E., & Lieberman, M. D. (2012). Evidence for social working memory from a parametric functional MRI study. *Proceedings of the National Academy of Sciences*, *109*(6), 1883–1888.

Mitchell, J., Cloutier, J., Banaji, M., & Macrae, C. (2006). Medial prefrontal dissociations during processing of trait diagnostic and nondiagnostic person information. *Social Cognitive and Affective Neuroscience*, *1*(1), 49–55.

Morris, J. S., Ohman, A., & Dolan, R. J. (1999). A subcortical pathway to the right amygdala mediating "unseen" fear. *Proceedings of the National Academy of Sciences USA*, *96*(4), 1680–1685.

Morris, M. W., & Mason, M. F. (2009). Intentionality in intuitive versus analytic processing: insights from social cognitive neuroscience. *Psychological Inquiry*, *20*(1), 58–65.

Mothes-Lasch, M., Mentzel, H. J., Miltner, W. H. R., & Straube, T. (2011). Visual attention modulates brain activation to angry voices. *The Journal of Neuroscience*, *31*(26), 9594–9598.

Mukamel, R., Ekstrom, A. D., Kaplan, J., Iacoboni, M., & Fried, I. (2010). Single-Neuron Responses in Humans during Execution and Observation of Actions. *Current Biology*, *20*(8), 750–756.

Ochsner, K. N., Bunge, S. A., Gross, J. J., & Gabrieli, J. D. E. (2002). Rethinking feelings: An fMRI study of the cognitive regulation of emotion. *Journal of Cognitive Neuroscience*, *14*(8), 1215–1229.

Pessoa, L. (2008). On the relationship between emotion and cognition. *Nature Reviews Neuroscience*, *9*(2), 148–158.

Pessoa, L., Kastner, S., & Ungerleider, L. G. (2003). Neuroimaging studies of attention: from modulation of sensory processing to top-down control. *The Journal of Neuroscience, 23*(10), 3990–3998.

Pessoa, L., McKenna, M., Gutierrez, E., & Ungerleider, L. G. (2002). Neural processing of emotional faces requires attention. *Proceedings of the National Academy of Sciences USA, 99*(17), 11458–11463.

Poldrack, R. (2006). Can cognitive processes be inferred from neuroimaging data? *Trends in Cognitive Sciences, 10*(2), 59–63.

Posner, M. I. (1980). Orienting of attention. *Quarterly Journal of Experimental Psychology, 32*(1), 3–25.

Rameson, L. T., Morelli, S. A., & Lieberman, M. D. (2011). The neural correlates of empathy: Experience, automaticity, and prosocial behavior. *Journal of Cognitive Neuroscience, 24*(1), 235–245.

Rizzolatti, G., & Craighero, L. (2004). The mirror-neuron system. *Annual Review of Neuroscience, 27*, 169–192.

Satpute, A. B., & Lieberman, M. D. (2006). Integrating automatic and controlled processes into neurocognitive models of social cognition. *Brain Research, 1079*(1), 86–97.

Saxe, R. (2006). Uniquely human social cognition. *Current Opinion in Neurobiology, 16*(2), 235–239.

Spengler, S., Cramon, D. Y. V., & Brass, M. (2009). Control of shared representations relies on key processes involved in mental state attribution. *Human Brain Mapping, 30*(11), 3704–3718.

Spunt, R. P., Falk, E. B., & Lieberman, M. D. (2010). Dissociable neural systems support retrieval of how and why action knowledge. *Psychological Science, 21*(11), 1593–1598.

Spunt, R. P., & Lieberman, M. D. (2012a). An integrative model of the neural systems supporting the comprehension of observed emotional behavior. *NeuroImage, 59*, 3050–3059.

Spunt, R. P., & Lieberman, M. D. (2012b). Dissociating modality-specific and supramodal neural systems for action understanding. *Journal of Neuroscience, 32*(10), 3575–3583.

Spunt, R. P., & Lieberman, M. D. (2013). The busy social brain: Evidence for automaticity and control in the neural systems supporting social cognition and action understanding. *Psychological Science, 24*(1), 80–86.

Spunt, R. P., Lieberman, M. D., Cohen, J. R., & Eisenberger, N. I. (2012). The phenomenology of error processing: The dorsal ACC response to stop-signal errors tracks reports of negative affect. *Journal of Cognitive Neuroscience, 24*(8), 1753–1765.

Spunt, R. P., Satpute, A. B., & Lieberman, M. D. (2011). Identifying the what, why, and how of an observed action: An fMRI study of mentalizing and mechanizing during action observation. *Journal of Cognitive Neuroscience, 23*(1), 63–74.

Trope, Y. (1986). Identification and inferential processes in dispositional attribution. *Psychological Review, 93*(3), 239–257.

Uleman, J., Saribay, S., & Gonzalez, C. (2008). Spontaneous inferences, implicit impressions, and implicit theories. *Annual Reviews of Psychology, 59*, 329–360.

Van Berkum, J. J. A., Holleman, B., Nieuwland, M., Otten, M., & Murre, J. (2009). Right or Wrong? The Brain's Fast Response to Morally Objectionable Statements. *Psychological Science, 20*(9), 1092–1099.

Van Overwalle, F., & Baetens, K. (2009). Understanding others' actions and goals by mirror and mentalizing systems: A meta-analysis. *NeuroImage, 48*, 564–584.

Wagner, D. D., Dal Cin, S., Sargent, J. D., Kelley, W. M., & Heatherton, T. F. (2011). Spontaneous action representation in smokers when watching movie characters smoke. *Journal of Neuroscience, 31*(3), 894–898.

Whalen, P. J., Rauch, S. L., Etcoff, N. L., McInerney, S. C., Lee, M. B., & Jenike, M. A. (1998). Masked presentations of emotional facial expressions modulate amygdala activity without explicit knowledge. *The Journal of Neuroscience, 18*(1), 411–418.

Wheatley, T., Milleville, S., & Martin, A. (2007). Understanding animate agents: Distinct roles for the social network and mirror system. *Psychological Science, 18*(6), 469–474.

Winston, J. S., Strange, B. A., O'Doherty, J., & Dolan, R. J. (2002). Automatic and intentional brain responses during evaluation of trustworthiness of faces. *Nature Neuroscience, 5*(3), 277–283.

Zacks, J. M., Braver, T. S., Sheridan, M. A., Donaldson, D. I., Snyder, A. Z., Ollinger, J. M., et al. (2001). Human brain activity time-locked to perceptual event boundaries. *Nature Neuroscience, 4*(6), 651–655.

PART VI

THINKING AND REASONING

CHAPTER 20

The Human Unconscious

A Functional Perspective

Ran R. Hassin and Asael Y. Sklar

Dual-process theories have many advantages. They divide the world into two categories (e.g., systems, types of processes), and two is a quantity that our minds can easily grasp. They usually tell simple, intuitively compelling stories: There are good and bad guys. Conscious and unconscious. Systematic and heuristic. Rule-based and associationist. Hot versus cool. Slow and fast. Importantly, dual-process models have had a very productive career in the young history of experimental psychology. As the success of the first edition of this volume shows, they have inspired generations of scientists interested in higher level cognition and have led to many important discoveries about our minds. It is with great sadness, then, that we report that we do not have a dual-process theory to propose here.

We are interested in what it means to be human—that is, in the mental functions that make us who we are. Mammals, not reptiles. Great apes, not monkeys. Humans, not chimps. We suspect that there are many such functions, but here we focus on one type that seems very intuitive: functions that require human consciousness (as far as we know, other animals do not have the kind of consciousness that we have). Examined from this perspective, our experimental approach in the last decade might look weird at the outset: We examined high-level functions that are performed by *non*conscious processes. This approach should have allowed us to map the functional limitations of nonconscious processes, thereby providing hints about where we should look for the unique functions of consciousness. Examined from this perspective, our project was not very successful. Papers from various laboratories around the world, including ours, made it clear that many functions that were traditionally assumed to be uniquely conscious can take place nonconsciously. One brick after another, the wall that separates conscious from nonconscious processes has shrunk. We feel it was a very informative shrinkage.

In this chapter we take this shrinkage seriously.

Using it as our point of departure we suggest a simple idea, one that is even simpler than a dual-process theory: It divides the world into *one* category, not two. Our idea is also simpler in that it focuses on just one of the attributes that have been associated with dual-process models, namely, conscious awareness. We suggest that every fundamental, basic-level cognitive function can occur nonconsciously. In other words, we propose that there is no fundamental cognitive function that, strictly speaking, requires consciousness.

If our theory of mind is more or less intact, then your head is currently in one of two positions. You either furrow your eyebrows, murmuring to yourself, *they cannot be serious,* or else you shake your head from one side to the other, telling yourself, in disbelief, *they cannot be serious.*[1] After all, there are so many functions that obviously require consciousness that it does not even take a second to come up with a set of five. You can get a dozen in less than a minute, which is better than the amazing deals proposed by Dunkin' Donuts. Just to give you a flavor, here is taste of our donuts:

- *Planning.* Whether it is parenting, going on vacation, or simply eating dinner, we spend quite a lot of time consciously planning our next moves, those that we think will come after them, and those that actually come after them. Is the timing good for having children, or shall we wait until after the postdoc (tenure, world recognition, Nobel prize)? Where shall we go after spending 4 nights in London? Is Paris the best, or is it Rome? Shall we fly or take the train? And what's for dinner tonight? Salad, organic steaks and fresh fruits, healthy all around, or something that the children actually eat, like chicken fingers and fries. Not healthy maybe, but edible for all.
- *Goal pursuit.* Goal pursuit includes planning, of course, but it encompasses much more. When we choose to write a chapter and sit to stare the screen, we need to know how well we do. Does a paragraph count as a good morning's work? How about one sentence? Shall we close the door, or simply go home? Is it time for a radical change in plans? In other words, goal pursuit also includes choices between means; monitoring the environment for feedback, the processing of this feedback and, accordingly, the flexible change of plans.
- *Self-control.* Everyone who has ever had a weakness—and who hasn't?—must have experienced conscious difficulties in overcoming it. From alcohol to donuts, and from sex with interns to taking the day off, the challenge is identical: How do we overcome temptations and follow the route suggested by our high-level goals? We must have the type of consciousness we have in order to do so, no? Can dogs pass the famous Mischelian marshmallow test? Can they really give up one bone now for two later?
- *Culture.* Some animals can pursue goals and may even have rudimentary plans and self-control. Certainly some chimps can. But, by and large, animals do not have culture. As far as we know, they do not have literature, classical music, and pop culture. No Picassos, Einsteins, or Lady Gagas. No God. *Homo sapiens* is the only species (that we know of) that has a generative language and systematic formal systems that handle abstract, symbolic computations (e.g., math). Yes, after months of training, Herb Terrace's chimps learned abstract numbers and could utter a few hundred signs, but they could not *really* talk, and they could not add and subtract; they couldn't *really* do math (Terrace, Petitto, Sanders, & Bever, 1979).

  If conscious chimps cannot read or do math, can our unconscious processes do so?
- *Thinking.* Here we are, sitting in our office, staring at the screen and thinking thoughts. Conscious thoughts, needless to say. Some are about the chapter we are writing, but others (most?) are not. We consciously develop an idea of how to begin a long-due chapter for a great edited book. We consciously think where to go from this beginning. We consciously weigh the strength of the argument (and, oh, by the way, we consciously think: *Is it time for coffee already?*). Thoughts must be conscious, mustn't they? After all, we sit here and type thoughts . . . that come our mind as they come . . . some are almost ready, well phrased . . . and sometimes the argument seem to hold. Sometimes our fingers seem to be thinking for us—but where is the conscious thought behind our fingers?

This is a set of just five examples, and we could easily expand it as much as you would like. In all likelihood you, the reader, can immediately add a few functions that we did not not list (we beg you: do it; write them down and come back to them later; otherwise they won't let you read this chapter quietly). After all, consciousness appears to be causally involved in many processes, virtually all of the time. It therefore seems to be a necessary requirement for many of the functions that make us human, with all our faults and advantages.

Before we go on, let us just put one fear to rest. Our argument does not imply that consciousness does not make a difference. That it does not affect our lives. That whether you are your wakeful, conscious, cheerful, lovely self, or a zombie bereft of any phenomenology, does not matter. In all likelihood, it does. We cannot be easily dismissed as epiphenomenologists, who argue that consciousness has no causal relationship with mental and physical reality. How and why it interacts with reality is, at least for us, one of the most fascinating questions scientists of the mind ask themselves in the beginning of this new millennium.

So we are not epiphenomenologists. What are we, then?

INITIAL POSITION AND DEFINITIONS

The principle we propose is very simple: Unconscious processes can carry out every fundamental, basic-level function that conscious processes can perform. In a recent paper on this topic, Hassin (2013) paraphrased President Obama's 2008 slogan "Yes we can," and referred to our approach as "Yes It Can," or YIC. In that sense, our unconscious processes are like the 2008 candidate Barack Obama, who coined the slogan "Yes we can." An important implication of YIC is that a scientific answer to the mystery of consciousness would not be in the form of *Consciousness is necessary for F*, where *F* is a fundamental cognitive function.

As we note later in the chapter, the fact that a function can occur nonconsciously does not mean that it will always occur nonconsciously (Bargh, 1994). We then suggest a number of factors that can alter the likelihood that a process would be performed nonconsciously. If conditions are met, the function will be performed nonconsciously. If not, it will either be performed consciously or not at all. We will end the chapter by succinctly discussing some implications of our theorizing to the question with which we opened this chapter: What is it that consciousness gives us that makes us who we are?

Why would we even begin to think that YIC is a reasonable stance? We can see at least two good reasons. First, consciousness is notoriously limited in its processing capacity (Baars & Ave, 1997; Baddeley, 2007; Kahneman, 1973). Like any other precious resource, we simply have very little of it. Even reading this simple sentence captures most of your consciousness (or did we *catch your* mind wandering?). So while you read this, what happens to your goals (*find a new computer*), plans (*find out how to prepare* coq au vin *for dinner*), your political grievances (*wait until you have a government like ours if nothing comes easily to mind*), solving mysteries (*so how does the mind work, after all?*), goals (*vacation on Long Island*), plans (*movie tonight?*), and so forth? What happens to all of this mental hustle and bustle when you read a simple sentence?

One possible answer is *nothing, zero, zilch*. When a topic is out of your conscious sight, it is also out of your mind. No consciousness, no progress. Given the number of mental chores in our mental to-do list, however, this does not seem like the most efficient and advantageous arrangement. It will be much better for you if, when you read this chapter, you can also work on other issues that require your attention. This *argument from resources* gives initial credence to YIC.

Second, consciousness as we experience it today seems to be a recent development in the evolution of our species (Dennett, 1996; Reber, 1992; Rozin, Sprague, & Epstein, 1976). It is hard to imagine our consciousness without the kind of language that we have at our disposal, without our evolved system of formal, abstract mental representations (not to mention the iPhone). If what we believe we know about the speed of evolutionary changes is correct[2], then it seems unlikely that much of our mind/brain is dedicated to consciousness. Thus, if there is a fundamental cognitive function that you need at your disposal, it had better function nonconsciously. This *argument from evolution* gives YIC some added face-value validity.

But cognitive scientists are not easily swayed by arguments. In the end, we always say that it is an empirical question. Can you, or can you not, make plans for cooking *coq au vin* without knowing that you do? Can you, or can you not, add the prices of coffee, a muffin, and a side of bacon without consciously going through the arithmetic motions?

Cognitive scientists like data, and our approach in this chapter is to give you data. We review developments in cognitive and social psychology, as well as in motivational psychology and the cognitive neurosciences. These developments, we argue, support YIC. Unfortunately, arguments and data, even when both are strong, are not proof. Unlike our linear algebra professor, at the end of this chapter we will not be able to declare triumphantly: Q.E.D. (*quod erat demonstrandum,* that which was to be demonstrated). But it seems to us that the argument we make is not weak, and that the method we propose is rather generic. We believe, then, that our arguments and data suggest that YIC is a possibility worthy of your consideration. And, yes, even the function of consciousness you harbor right now—and you must, because everyone we talk to has his or her pet function of consciousness—can occur without awareness.

A few definitions are in order before we go on. We use the term *cognition* in a broad sense that includes not only the processes that traditionally fall under the category of "cognition," but also those that are often referred to as "motivation" and "emotion." We use the adjective *high-level* to describe processes that are postperceptual and involve complex considerations and cognitive control. Sometimes examples can do a better job than definitions (Wittgenstein, 1963), so here is a partial list: inhibition, shifting, working memory (WM), inferences, causal reasoning, attribution, metaphor comprehension, narrative construction, and logic. Last, cognitive functions vary in their fundamentality, that is, in how inherent they are to normal cognitive functioning, and in their level of abstractness (Rosch, Mervis, Gray, Johnson, & Boyes-Braem, 1976). YIC, as we have proposed it, concerns fundamental, basic-level functions. The fact that we lack taxonomies of cognitive functions renders this definition somewhat vague but we suspect that even without accepted taxonomies these issues are quite consensual. Thus, for example, we are likely to agree that the function of combining emotional cues (e.g., vocal and facial) is more fundamental than the function that maps a certain sound to a keypress. Likewise, the function of inhibiting unnecessary materials from WM seems more basic level than that of deleting from WM recent information about one's annoying aunt Nitza. We therefore use the term *fundamental function* as shorthand for *fundamental, basic-level function.*

Last, it is important to distinguish between *subliminal perception/priming* and *unconscious cognition* (see Bargh & Morsella, 2008). In investigating subliminal priming, one attempts to find out the extent to which nonconsciously perceived stimuli can be processed, while mapping their possible effects (for recent reviews, see Kouider & Dehaene, 2007; Van den Bussche, Van den Noortgate, & Reynvoet, 2009). Scientists who study unconscious cognition examine unconscious processes without limiting themselves to subliminality: Awareness of the relevant processes and/or their products is the main issue here (for recent overviews, see Bargh, 2007; Gawronski & Payne, 2010; Hassin, Uleman, & Bargh, 2005). The evidence that is reviewed here comes from both lines of research.

ADOPTING A FUNCTIONAL STANCE

There are intellectual discussions within the cognitive sciences that stand to gain much from adopting a functional stance—a stance that grounds the study of cognition in an understanding of cognitive functions (Marr, 1982). What is a cognitive function? One identifies a cognitive function of a process *P* when one gives a teleological answer to the question *What is it that P does?* Here are a few examples. One function of memory is to store information for later use. One function of self-control is to overcome temptations, and one function of fear is to focus our attention on fear-eliciting objects.[3]

Why should one adopt a functional stance? One answer would be that the cognitive sciences are functional in nature: They are *about* understanding the functions of the mind/brain, and how they are implemented (Marr, 1982). While we think that adopting a functional approach is a good move in the cognitive sciences in general, for our current discussion it has an additional advantage: It does not allow us to commit the frequent mistake of confounding a functional characterization of a mental process with a description of its characteristics. To take just one example, if one is interested in emotion regulation, one needs to offer a functional definition of it (e.g., emotion regulation is the function that takes an emotional mental state *X* and turns it into *Y*). Whether or not the processes that implement this function are necessarily conscious (and/or intentional and/or effortful, etc.) is an empirical question, not a definitional one. In other words, one cannot include these characteristics in the definition of the function one studies, unless one wants to restrict oneself to a specific subset. Here, then, we adopt a functional approach to the study of unconscious processes.

In the following sections we describe recent advances in the cognitive sciences vis-à-vis the functional abilities of nonconscious processes. And here is a spoiler: The reviews will suggest that functions that were traditionally assumed to require consciousness do not, strictly speaking, require consciousness.

EXECUTIVE FUNCTIONS

Executive functions are cognitive functions that regulate other cognitive functions, and they are commonly associated with self-control (or "willpower") and the prefrontal cortex (Miyake & Friedman, 2012). Importantly, executive functions are often thought of as being closely associated with (or even requiring) conscious processing (e.g., Baars, 2002; Dehaene & Naccache, 2001). Our review in this section focuses on two functions that have relatively precise operational definitions and have been studied extensively vis-à vis conscious awareness: inhibition and shifting.

Inhibition

The executive function *inhibition* is the "ability to deliberately inhibit dominant, automatic, or prepotent responses when necessary" (Miyake et al., 2000, p. 57). Many cognitive tasks rely on inhibition, including celebrity tasks such as the Stroop (Stroop, 1935) and the stop-signal (Logan, 1994). A recent account has even suggested that inhibition is closely linked to a general factor that explains variance shared by other executive functions (Miyake & Friedman, 2012).

In recent years Victor Lamme, Simon van Gaal, and their colleagues have repeatedly shown that inhibition can be triggered by subliminal stimuli (Wokke, van Gaal, Scholte, Ridderinkhof, & Lamme, 2011; van Gaal, Ridderinkhof, Fahrenfort, Scholte, & Lamme, 2008; van Gaal, Ridderinkhof, Van den Wildenberg, & Lamme, 2009; for a review see van Gaal, de Lange, & Cohen, 2012). In one of their first experiments, participants engaged in a go/no-go task in which they were asked to respond rapidly to a target, and to withhold responses if a no-go stimulus had been presented before the target (van Gaal et al., 2008). Critically, on some trials this no-go stimulus was weakly masked and therefore conscious, whereas on others it was strongly masked and therefore subliminal. The results show that the subliminal priming of a no-go stimulus increased the likelihood of withholding responses, and that it increased reaction times to responses that were not withheld. These results have been extended by showing that subliminally triggered inhibition is correlated with activity in the prefrontal cortex (van Gaal et al., 2008), that the magnitude of unconscious inhibition is correlated with participants' ability to consciously inhibit responses (van Gaal et al., 2009), and that subliminally triggered inhibition does not rely on a strong preexisting association between the no-go signal and inhibition (Wokke et al., 2011). Taken together, these data allow us to conclude that inhibition does not require consciousness.

Shifting

Defined as "shifting back and forth between multiple tasks, operations, or mental sets" (Miyake et al., 2000, p. 55), and associated with various task-switching paradigms, *shifting* is an executive function that has been studied quite extensively vis-à-vis conscious awareness. To examine nonconscious shifting, researchers use a modified task-switching paradigm. In a "regular" task-switching experiment there are cues that indicate whether to perform Task A or Task B. In the modified version, the task cues are preceded by subliminal primes. The prime may be either identical to the task cue (e.g., both signal participants to perform Task A; congruent trials) or different (e.g., the prime signals Task B, whereas the task cue signals Task A; incongruent trials). Results from this paradigm show that participants are slower to respond on incongruent (vs. congruent) trials (Mattler, 2003), and that subliminal primes lead to activation in brain areas that are associated with the task that they prime (Lau & Passingham, 2007). Later studies used various paradigms that allowed for a wider generalization and yielded similar results (Reuss, Kiesel, Kunde, & Hommel, 2011; Zhou & Davis, 2012). Considered together, these results strongly suggest that shifting does not require conscious awareness.

And a Bit More . . .

Our choice of executive functions was one of convenience; inhibition and shifting are not only central executive functions, but they have also been studied extensively in relation to nonconscious processing. But is it possible that researchers are "looking under the lamppost," and that we cannot generalize from these examples to executive functions more generally? A thorough discussion of the structure of executive functions is well beyond the scope of this chapter.[4] But to take one concrete example, Miyake and colleagues (2000) propose that there are three main executive functions: inhibition, shifting, and updating and monitoring of WM representations. Can the latter operate outside of conscious awareness, too?

Our lab's work on implicit WM suggests that the answer is positive (Hassin, Bargh, Engell, & McCulloch, 2009). To examine implicit WM Hassin et al. developed a paradigm in which small disks that are either empty (bagel-shaped) or full appear one at a time in various locations on a computer screen. Participants' task is to respond with one key press if a disk is empty and another key press if the disk is full. The disks appear in sequences of five, separated by a fixation square. In Pattern sequences, the locations of the disks create a pattern (e.g., a zigzag). In the Broken Pattern condition, the locations of first four disks are identical to those of pattern sequences, but the fifth disk breaks the patterns. Pattern and Broken Pattern sequences are equally probable, so the likelihood of a "pattern move" from the fourth to the fifth disk is identical to the likelihood of a "broken pattern" move. Hence "simple" implicit learning across sequences cannot help performance in this task.

Extracting the patterns and gaining from them requires active maintenance of ordered information (the locations of disks), context-relevant updating of information (with incoming disks), and goal-relevant computations (i.e., pattern extraction and anticipation formation). The extracted information is immediately available to control behavior and cognition, in the service of current goals (of being fast and accurate). These functions are traditionally associated with WM (Hassin, 2005), yet across a set of five experiments that used various probing techniques we failed to find any evidence of awareness.

These data, then, strongly suggest that monitoring and updating can occur outside of conscious awareness. Yet, we want to mention here two limitations of this research. First, we did not use subliminal stimuli, that is, the disks themselves were visible (for a study that does use subliminal stimuli, see Soto, Mäntylä, & Silvanto, 2011). Second, while our task requires some forms of monitoring and updating, it falls short of meeting all of the functions described by Miyake and colleagues (2000). Personally, we see no a priori reason to assume that the latter processes do not occur nonconsciously, but this is an open empirical question.

GOAL PURSUIT

Intuitively, goal pursuit seems to involve quite a bit of conscious processing: from the first stages of goal adoption (should one pursue a career in architecture or become an actor?) to means selection (MIT or Harvard?) to monitoring progress (how good was my exhibition in PS1?) and correction (go back to the drawing board) to overcoming obstacles (appeal decision of the MOMA curator) and reevaluation (maybe fatherhood, after all?). It is hardly surprising, then, that goal pursuit traditionally was assumed to be a consciously controlled process (Ajzen, 1991; Bandura, 1986; Deci & Ryan, 1985; Locke & Latham, 1990).

Research on automatic goal pursuit, however, suggests that goal pursuit is not necessarily conscious. In one of the first empirical papers on the subject, Bargh, Gollwitzer, Lee-Chai, Barndollar, and Trötschel (2001) used word search tasks to prime the goal of cooperation. In this priming technique, participants were asked to find a list of words in a matrix of letters. In the experimental condition, many of these words were cooperation-related. In the control condition the primes were replaced by goal-neutral words. Participants then went on to play a commons resource dilemma, in what was allegedly a separate, unrelated experiment. The results showed that participants who had been primed with the goal of cooperation cooperated more than those who had not been primed. Yet they did not consciously realize that a goal had been primed, or that they were more committed to cooperation.

Using various priming methods, psychologists have primed goals such as solving puzzles, achievement, obtaining sex, and impression formation. In some of these studies, the goals were primed subliminally (see Bijleveld, Custers, & Aarts, 2011; Fishbach, Friedman, & Kruglanski, 2003). In others, evidence for unawareness comes from debriefings in which participants' phenomenology was thoroughly examined. A vast majority of these studies failed to find differences in goal-related phenomenology between participants in the priming and control conditions. In other words, while motivation priming is strong enough to affect behavior, it does not seem to affect subjective reports (for recent reviews, see Custers & Aarts, 2010; Dijksterhuis & Aarts, 2010; Fishbach & Ferguson, 2007). In light of this research, it seems safe to suggest that one goal can be activated nonconsciously, and that it can then go on to be pursued outside of conscious awareness.

But we rarely pursue only one goal at a time. Think of yourself now: You read this chapter hoping (we hope) that it will help you to obtain a goal. You are also a scientist (maybe), with publication, mentoring, and teaching goals. You are likely to have a few goals related to your roles as a family member (e.g., mother, son, sibling, nephew), and you may have other goals such as losing weight, having fun, and preserving the environment, to mention just a few. The upshot of this clearly is that at any given point in time we pursue multiple goals, and some of them compete for our attention. If we cannot handle goal conflict nonconsciously, our consciousness is likely to be flooded with conflicts it needs to resolve.

Recently Tali Kleiman and I demonstrated that goal conflicts can occur outside of conscious awareness (Kleiman & Hassin, 2011). In one set of studies we primed a cooperation goal in the context of a commons resource dilemma in which the dominant goal is competition (selfishness; Brewer & Kramer, 1986; Fehr & Fischbacher, 2003). Since cooperation is the nondominant goal, priming it should increase the conflict between these goals. Indirect markers of conflict (i.e., variability in repeated decisions, increase in reaction times and arousal) showed that, indeed, priming resulted in increased conflict. Yet, across six experiments we failed to detect differences in explicit measures of conflict. One of the experiments used a trial-by-trial assessment of conflict, yet failed in documenting it too. A mini-meta analysis of all the experiments in this set, with 233 participants, still did not provide evidence for changes in phenomenology.

CONCEPTUAL INFORMATION INTEGRATION (AND MORE)

Integrating and manipulating abstract units of meaning (e.g., numbers, words, objects) is a set of cognitive functions that is widely considered to require consciousness (Baars, 2002, 2005; Baumeister & Masicampo, 2010; Greenwald, 1992; Morewedge & Kahneman, 2010). Two recent studies that used subliminal presentations considerably challenged this view.[5] In the first, participants were instructed to compute the sum and average of supraliminally presented sets of four numbers (e.g., 7, 4, 3, 2; Van Opstal, de Lange, & Dehaene, 2011). Unbeknownst to them, the target sets were preceded by subliminally primed sets (e.g., 9, 6, 5, 8). The results showed that the sum and average of the subliminally primed sets affected the responses to the target sets, thereby providing evidence for the integration of numbers. The nature of the task did not allow the authors to argue for nonconscious arithmetic computations, but we review evidence for arithmetic later in this section.

The second paper provides evidence for the semantic integration of multiple objects in a visual scene (Mudrik, Breska, Lamy, & Deouell, 2011). In this study participants were presented with pictures that were masked by continuous flash suppression (CFS), which consists of a presentation of a target stimulus to one eye and a simultaneous presentation of rapidly changing masks to the other eye. The rapidly changing masks dominate awareness until the target breaks into consciousness (Costello, Jiang, Baartman, McGlennen, & He, 2009; Jiang, Costello, & He, 2007; Yang, Zald, & Blake, 2007). Importantly, this suppression may last seconds, thereby allowing prolonged cognitive processing (Tsuchiya & Koch, 2005). Participants in this study were asked to press a button as soon as they saw the pictures or any parts of them. Thus, the dependent variable was how long it takes a stimulus to break suppression and appear in consciousness. The results showed that incongruent pictures (e.g., a person shooting a tennis racket out of a bow) broke suppression before congruent pictures (e.g., a person shooting an arrow out of a bow). Put differently, incongruent pictures appeared in consciousness before congruent pictures. Note that in order to differentiate between congruent and incongruent pictures, participants had to identify at least two objects (e.g., the racket and the bow) and combine these two units of meaning into one (incongruent) whole.

The evidence from these two articles, then, suggests that abstract units of meaning can be integrated without consciousness, thereby challenging the modal view, which holds that conscious awareness is a necessary condition for performing this function.

Two recent sets of experiments significantly extend these initial results by providing evidence for nonconscious reading of multiple-word expressions and for nonconscious arithmetic (Sklar et al., 2012). In the first series, participants were presented with multiple-word expressions that were masked by CFS. The expressions could be either semantically consistent (e.g., *John made coffee*) or not (e.g., *John ironed coffee*). Participants were asked to press a button as soon as they saw verbal stimuli or any parts of them (e.g., a letter), and the duration of suppression from awareness served as the dependent variable. The results clearly showed that semantically inconsistent word combinations broke suppression faster than semantically consistent expressions. In another study in this set, Sklar et al. used affective value of verbal expressions to examine word integration. In this set of experiments, Sklar et al. compared the subliminal processing of short verbal expressions with affective tones that ranged from being very negative (e.g., baby in the oven, concentration camp) to neutral (e.g., parking lot), to mildly positive (e.g., ironed shirt). The dependent variable was again suppression duration, or how long it takes stimuli to break suppression and appear in consciousness. The results clearly showed that affective value of verbal expressions affects suppression duration, such that the more negative an expression is the faster it breaks suppression. They therefore suggest that multiple words were integrated into verbal expressions outside of conscious awareness.

In the second series of studies (Sklar et al., 2012), CFS-masked arithmetic problems (e.g., 9 – 3 – 2 =) were presented to participants, followed by supraliminal presentation of a target number (e.g., 4). Participants were asked to name the target numbers, and Sklar et al. measured how long it took them to begin pronunciation. There were two conditions. In the compatible condition, the target was the solution to the primed problem (e.g., subliminal 9 – 3 – 1 was followed by supraliminal 5), whereas in the incompatible condition it was not (e.g., the target was 6). The result of a series of experiments showed that compatibility made a difference: Participants were quicker in the compatible condition. These results strongly suggest that the problems were solved, and objective and subjective measures assured that there was no awareness of the primes.

To conclude, while early evidence might have suggested that consciousness is necessary for integrating abstract units of meaning, recent evidence seem to challenge this view significantly by providing evidence for the integration of numbers, words, and visual objects (for more functions, see Hassin, 2013).

IS THAT ALL?

The functions we have reviewed are but a small fraction of the functions of our high-level cognitive processes. They are meant to exemplify a principle and a way of conducting our science, rather than an exhaustive list of the functions that operate nonconsciously (according to our best data to date). The point we want to make is simple: When one adopts a functional stance, examining high-level cognition through the lenses of the functions it performs, one can conceptually and empirically dissociate the functions and their characteristics. Adopting this view quickly reveals that a host of functions that were traditionally associated with conscious awareness can also occur nonconsciously.

The argument that nonconscious processes have *the ability* to perform a function *F* does not imply that they will always (or even frequently) do so, however. It is a statement about what these processes *can* do, not about what they *actually* do. To learn more about the actualities, one has to ask *when* can one expect nonconscious processes to perform *F*. In the case of scientists, the likelihood of producing a great paper increases with their basic abilities, motivation, and experience. Here we propose to treat nonconscious processes the same way we treat scientists: with careful attention to details. Specifically, we suggest that abilities, motivation, and experience determine whether a certain function will or will not occur nonconsciously *at a given point in time.*

Ability

People who are good at math can compute without calculators what the rest of us can hardly do with calculators. People who are good self-controllers can inhibit impulses that, uninhibited, may ruin the careers of others, and those with good analytic skills get SAT scores that make us all look like fools. Executive functions and WM capacity are known to be important determinants of high-level conscious cognitive processes (Conway & Kane, 2005; Redick, Heitz, & Engle, 2007; Ricks, Turley-Ames, & Wiley, 2007). Generally speaking, those of us with large WM capacity do better than those with smaller capacity. Is it reasonable to expect that there is a nonconscious parallel to these kinds of processes, one that determine the abilities of nonconscious processes?

Recent research suggests that there might be. As reviewed earlier in more detail, we have recently shown that WM can operate outside of conscious awareness (Hassin, Bargh, Engell, et al., 2009; Hassin, 2005), and a number of laboratories have shown that executive functions can operate nonconsciously (see the earlier section, "Executive Functions"; also see Hassin, Bargh, & Zimerman, 2009; Soto et al., 2011). It seems to us that it is reasonable to assume that there are individual differences in the capacity for high-level, nonconscious processes of this sort, and that variation in implicit WM capacity and nonconscious executive functions would be determinants of high-level, nonconscious processes.

Motivation

Evidence for the role of motivation (and needs) in the processing of subliminal stimuli has begun to emerge in the area of subliminal persuasion. To take just one example, priming a certain brand of drink leads to increased drinking of this brand, but only if subjects have the relevant need, that is, if they are thirsty (Karremans, Stroebe, & Claus, 2006; see also Bermeitinger et al., 2009; Strahan, Spencer, & Zanna, 2002). In our laboratory we used goal priming to examine similar issues: We have shown that achievement priming increases the likelihood that subliminal primes will affect choice (Milyavsky, Hassin, & Schul, 2012).

Given the important role of motivation in human behavior more generally, we see no reason to suspect that motivation is not a key determinant of nonconscious processes. Hence, we suggest that one needs to motivate the unconscious to perform tasks, in the same way that one needs to motivate consciousness to engage in effortful processing.

Experience

The vast automatization literature (Bargh, 1994; Kahneman & Treisman, 1984; Schneider & Shiffrin, 1977) suggests that the more automatic a process becomes, the more likely it is to occur effortlessly and nonconsciously (e.g., Barrouillet & Fayol, 1998). One implication of these findings is that there are *developmental trajectories* in the capabilities of the unconscious, a result that has two implications for the current discussion. First, it suggests that at different points in life, our nonconscious processes can perform different functions. Second, given that different individuals are exposed to different environments and develop different skills, one should expect *individual differences* in the capabilities of nonconscious processes. To the best of our knowledge, there is very little data on the subject.

Generally speaking, then, YIC holds that every fundamental, basic-level cognitive function that one can perform consciously in one's head, one will also be able to perform nonconsciously in one's head, given that one has the relevant ability, motivation, and experience. For example, in state-of-the-art techniques such as CFS we can present subliminal stimuli for up to 2 seconds. YIC holds, then, that given enough motivation, every arithmetic function that one can do consciously in 2 seconds one will be able to do under CFS.

ON CONSCIOUSNESS

So at last we get to discuss the implications of our view and review for the scientific understanding of the functions of consciousness. In the introduction we mentioned that we are not epiphenomenologists; that is, we are not arguing that consciousness does not make a difference, that it lacks any causal powers. Here is a basic intuition we believe all of us share: Some of us would be willing to dye our hair orange for $500, would require $1,000 for complete body waxing, would eat cockroaches for $20,000, and would be willing to consider losing a finger for $1,000,000. Healthy normal people, under normal circumstances (who don't need the money to save the life of their child, etc.), would never agree to lose their consciousness. In other words, even if nonconscious processes can perform every fundamental, basic-level cognitive function, we would not give up our phenomenology. It seems to us that we would be completely different creatures without it, and maybe we are wrong, but we prefer the creatures we are right now.

One interesting question is why do we have the feeling? Another is how is it that consciousness makes a difference, and to what? (If it does, we must note that we view this assertion as a hypothesis. Until proven wrong, though, we are sticking to it.)

YIC holds that every fundamental, basic-level cognitive function that can be carried out consciously can also be carried out nonconsciously. But the ways in which these functions are achieved—their implementation—may be different. In other words, nonconscious (vs. conscious) functions may use different algorithms, different representations, and different recruitment of brain networks. This postulation should not be taken to imply a dual-process model. We do not propose that there are two different and distinct mind/brain systems—one conscious, the other not—that perform (the same) cognitive functions independently of each other. Conscious awareness, rather, is seen here as a contingent property of fundamental functions (or of stages of their implementation). Yet given the differences we mentioned earlier, it is entirely possible (and sometimes even likely) that conscious processes will play out differently than nonconscious ones. The following example conveys some of these intuitions.

Imagine, for example, that you are interviewing for your dream academic job. The chair of the department turns out to be a little weird. Before you leave her office, she tells you that the department has voted, and that their decision appears on her computer screen. She then excuses herself, and you are left in her office, alone, and her screen basically stares at you. In one possible scenario, the message *THE JOB IS ALL YOURS* is flashed subliminally (assume, for the sake of argument, that people can read short sentences even if they are presented subliminally). In the other scenario, the message is simply there, on the screen, for you to see. We contend that it is unlikely that the two messages will have the same effect. Yes, as scientists, we may be able to show that you have an elevated galvanic skin response (GSR) in response to the subliminal message, but not to a scrambled version of it (ALL JOB THE YOURS); that you will be happier after nonconsciously reading the message (treating yourself, perhaps, to a donut) than after the scrambled one; and so forth. But only in one scenario would you leave the room ecstatic, and only in one scenario would you spend the afternoon daydreaming about how to decorate your office in William James hall. Only in one scenario would you be so engrossed in fantasizing that you would accidentally bump into a woman, offer her coffee as compensation, tell her enthusiastically about your new job, and find yourself, 5 hours later, agreeing to accept her offer and come work under her at the White House. Only in one scenario, would you find yourself a year later, after your President loses the election, without an academic job, thinking about what to do in life.

So even if one assumes that both messages are read and understood, whether or not reading is accompanied by conscious awareness is likely to play out differently.

Another source of differences between conscious and nonconscious processes has to do with the conditions that enable their operation. In a previous section we discussed three factors that determine the likelihood that a nonconscious process will kick in: experience, motivation, and ability. Suppose a function F begins operating nonconsciously when experience reaches a level of E_j; motivation, a level of M_j; and ability, A_j. Suppose, furthermore, that for the same function to run consciously, it requires motivation M_i, where $M_i > M_j$, and ability A_i, where $A_i < A_j$. In this hypothetical example, $F_{\text{conscious}}$ will differ from $F_{\text{nonconscious}}$, simply because they will run in different situations.

You may object by arguing that, really, $F_{\text{conscious}}$ and $F_{\text{nonconscious}}$ are similar here. And you may have a point. But note that the fate of a creature without phenomenology will be different than that of a creature with phenomenology, thereby suggesting that having a phenomenology makes a difference.

Another objection to YIC may hold that, with all due respect to nonconscious processes, the great works of culture (broadly defined to include everything from Picasso to Einstein to Eminem) require consciousness. This objection is not confined to great works of art; it also applies to more mundane contributions such as letters to the *New York Times*, a caring e-mail to a friend, a fun note left on your spouse's pillow, or a joke one makes at a party. There are two points we wish to make here. First, note that all of these works of art require nonconscious processes. Take nonconscious processes away and you are left with . . . what? This point is often overlooked: Without the hard work of nonconscious processes, consciousness would have very little to work with. While you can imagine completely nonconscious contributions (e.g., this sentence has not been planned or thought of before it is actually typed), it is much more difficult to imagine these contributions without nonconscious processes.

Second, ask yourself why you are so certain that consciousness is a necessary prerequisite for the creation of complex cultural works such as paintings and scientific theories. Do we have data to support it? The answer, we believe, is negative. True, we know of no scientific theory that was developed by a person in a vegetative state. Similarly, we know of no theory developed by animals with consciousness that is very different than our own, say chimps. But note that being in a vegetative state involves much more than losing consciousness, and there are many differences between chimps and us, not just in the structure of phenomenology. To answer the question of whether Picasso could have painted a Picasso without being aware of it, we must have Picasso devoid of consciousness, and only consciousness. We do not yet posses the technology that allows us to knock down consciousness, and only consciousness; hence, this experiment cannot be conducted. Given the intricacies of the human mind, we are not optimistic about the feasibility of developing such a technique.

CODA: BACK TO DUAL-PROCESS MODELS

This is a book about dual processes, but we offered no dual-process model. Yet we believe that the current contribution is relevant to our theories of the mind in general, and to dual-process models in particular. In various guises, the dichotomy between conscious and nonconscious processes (implicit vs. explicit, etc.) is central to many dual-process models. Even when it is not explicitly stated, it often lurks in the back of the minds of authors and readers alike. Using a functional approach, this chapter calls for a reevaluation of the default (if often tacit) assumption that associates high-level cognitive processes and conscious awareness. Defaults are very powerful in our lives. They shape how we see and think about the world. They are often very helpful, chopping through uncertainty to provide us with a comprehensible view of the world. One cannot imagine efficient cognitive processes without defaults. Yet defaults do not come without a price: They direct our conceptual attention, and resources, toward certain avenues, while leading us to ignore others. They help us make leaps that are not always justifiable. They conceal truths. Changing defaults has the potential of releasing constraints from our exploration space and shedding new light on existing data and theories. We hope that the tools we propose here—YIC and the functional approach—will help us reexamine our defaults, leading to improved understanding of the unconscious mind and the functions of consciousness.

NOTES

1. Well, there is always a third option: that you are basically emotionless, flatly telling yourself, yawning, "Oh, no, not this topic again." If this is the case, then it is time for you to move on. We'll be talking about unconscious processes and consciousness for the next 10 pages or so.
2. Relatively recent work on genetics and epigenetics may suggest that this view should be updated (Jablonka & Lamb, 2005).
3. These definitions *are meant as demonstrations* of the stance; they are not meant to be exhaustive.
4. But see Miyake et al. (2000) and Miyake and Friedman (2012).
5. Evidence with nonsubliminal stimuli is abundant, yet, naturally, it is less conclusive in terms of access to consciousness. Unfortunately, reviewing this evidence is beyond the scope of this chapter. To give readers a taste, it includes inferences (Uleman, Adil Saribay, & Gonzalez, 2008), integration of information during decision making (Dijksterhuis, Bos, Nordgren, & Van Baaren, 2006), and insight formation (Metcalfe & Wiebe, 1987; Metcalfe, 1986). For relatively recent overviews see Dijksterhuis (2010), Bargh (2007), and Hassin, Uleman, and Bargh (2005).

REFERENCES

Ajzen, I. (1991). The theory of planned behavior. *Organizational Behavior and Human Decision Processes*, *50*, 179–211.

Baars, B. J. (2002). The conscious access hypothesis: Origins and recent evidence. *Trends in Cognitive Sciences*, *6*(1), 47–52.

Baars, B. J. (2005). Global workspace theory of consciousness: Toward a cognitive neuroscience of human experience. *Progress in Brain Research*, *150*, 45–53.

Baars, B. J., & Ave, D. (1997). Global workspace theory, a rigorous scientific theory of consciousness. *Journal of Consciousness Studies*, *4*(4), 292–309.

Baddeley, A. (2007). *Working memory, thought, and action*. New York: Oxford University Press.

Bandura, A. (1986). *Social foundations of thought and action: A social cognitive theory*. Upper Saddle River, NJ: Prentice Hall.

Bargh, J. A. (1994). The four horsemen of automaticity: Awareness, intention, efficiency, and control in social cognition. In R. S. Wyer, Jr. & T. K. Srull (Eds.), *Handbook of social cognition* (2nd ed., pp. 1–40). Hillsdale, NJ: Erlbaum.

Bargh, J. A. (Ed.). (2007). *Social psychology and the unconscious: The automaticity of higher mental processes*. New York: Psychology Press.

Bargh, J. A., Gollwitzer, P. M., Lee-Chai, A., Barndollar, K., & Trötschel, R. (2001). The automated will: Nonconscious activation and pursuit of behavioral goals. *Journal of Personality and Social Psychology*, *81*(6), 1014–1027.

Bargh, J. A., & Morsella, E. (2008). The unconscious mind. *Perspectives on Psychological Science*, *3*(1), 73–79.

Barrouillet, P., & Fayol, M. (1998). From algorithmic computing to direct retrieval: Evidence from number and alphabetic arithmetic in children and adults. *Memory and Cognition*, *26*(2), 355–368.

Baumeister, R. F., & Masicampo, E. J. (2010). Conscious thought is for facilitating social and cultural interactions: how mental simulations serve the animal–culture interface. *Psychological Review, 117*(3), 945–971.

Bermeitinger, C., Goelz, R., Johr, N., Neumann, M., Ecker, U. K. H., & Doerr, R. (2009). The hidden persuaders break into the tired brain. *Journal of Experimental Social Psychology, 45*(2), 320–326.

Bijleveld, E., Custers, R., & Aarts, H. (2011). Once the money is in sight: Distinctive effects of conscious and unconscious rewards on task performance. *Journal of Experimental Social Psychology, 47*(4), 865–869.

Brewer, M. B., & Kramer, R. M. (1986). Choice behavior in social dilemmas: Effects of social identity, group size, and decision framing. *Journal of Personality and Social Psychology, 50*(3), 543–549.

Conway, A., & Kane, M. (2005). Working memory span tasks: A methodological review and user's guide. *Psychonomic Bulletin and Review, 12*(5), 769–786.

Costello, P., Jiang, Y., Baartman, B., McGlennen, K., & He, S. (2009). Semantic and subword priming during binocular suppression. *Consciousness and Cognition, 18*(2), 375–382.

Custers, R., & Aarts, H. (2010). The unconscious will: How the pursuit of goals operates outside of conscious awareness. *Science, 329*(5987), 47–50.

Deci, E. L., & Ryan, R. M. (1985). The general causality orientations scale: Self-determination in personality. *Journal of Research in Personality, 19*(2), 109–134.

Dehaene, S., & Naccache, L. (2001). Towards a cognitive neuroscience of consciousness: Basic evidence and a workspace framework. *Cognition, 79*(1–2), 1–37.

Dennett, D. C. D. (1996). *Darwin's dangerous idea: Evolution and the meanings of life*. New York: Simon & Schuster.

Dijksterhuis, A., & Aarts, H. (2010). Goals, attention, and (un)consciousness. *Annual Review of Psychology, 61*, 467–490.

Dijksterhuis, A., Bos, M. W., Nordgren, L. F., & Van Baaren, R. B. (2006). On making the right choice: The deliberation-without-attention effect. *Science, 311*(5763), 1005–1007.

Dijksterhuis, A. P. (2010). Automaticity and the unconscious. In S. T. Fiske, D. T. Gilbert, & G. Lindzey (Eds.), *Handbook of social psychology* (5th ed., pp. 228–267). New York: Wiley.

Fehr, E., & Fischbacher, U. (2003). The nature of human altruism. *Nature, 425*(6960), 785–791.

Fishbach, A., & Ferguson, M. J. M. (2007). The goal construct in social psychology. In A. W. Kruglanski & E. T. Higgins (Eds.), *Social psychology: Handbook of basic principles* (2nd ed., pp. 490–515). New York: Guilford Press.

Fishbach, A., Friedman, R. S., & Kruglanski, A. W. (2003). Leading us not unto temptation: Momentary allurements elicit overriding goal activation. *Journal of Personality and Social Psychology, 84*(2), 296–309.

Gawronski, B., & Payne, B. K. (2010). *Handbook of implicit social cognition: Measurement, theory, and applications*. New York: Guilford Press.

Greenwald, A. G. (1992). New Look 3: Unconscious cognition reclaimed. *American Psychologist, 47*(6), 766–779.

Hassin, R. R. (2005). Non-conscious control and implicit working memory. In R. R. Hassin, J. S. Uleman, & J. A. Bargh (Eds.), *The new unconscious* (pp. 196–225). New York: Oxford University Press.

Hassin, R. R. (2013). Yes it can: On the functional abilities of the human unconscious. *Perspectives on Psychological Science, 8*(2), 195–207.

Hassin, R. R., Bargh, J. A., Engell, A. D., & McCulloch, K. C. (2009). Implicit working memory. *Consciousness and Cognition, 18*(3), 665–678.

Hassin, R. R., Bargh, J. A., & Zimerman, S. (2009). Automatic and flexible: The case of non-conscious goal pursuit. *Social Cognition, 27*(1), 20–36.

Hassin, R. R., Uleman, J. S., & Bargh, J. A. (2005). *The new unconscious*. New York: Oxford University Press.

Jablonka, E., & Lamb, M. J. (2005). *Evolution in four dimensions: Genetic, epigenetic, behavioral, and symbolic variation in the history of life*. Cambridge, MA: MIT Press.

Jiang, Y., Costello, P., & He, S. (2007). Processing of invisible stimuli: advantage of upright faces and recognizable words in overcoming interocular suppression. *Psychological Science, 18*(4), 349–355.

Kahneman, D. (1973). *Attention and effort*. Englewood Cliffs, NJ: Prentice Hall.

Kahneman, D., & Treisman, A. (1984). Changing views of attention and automaticity?. In R. Parasuraman & D. Davies (Eds.), *Varieties of attention?* (pp. 29–61). New York: Academic Press.

Karremans, J. C., Stroebe, W., & Claus, J. (2006). Beyond Vicary's fantasies: The impact of subliminal priming and brand choice. *Jour-*

nal of Experimental Social Psychology, 42(6), 792–798.

Kleiman, T., & Hassin, R. R. (2011). Nonconscious goal conflicts. *Journal of Experimental Social Psychology, 47*(3), 521–532.

Kouider, S., & Dehaene, S. (2007). Levels of processing during non-conscious perception: A critical review of visual masking. *Philosophical transactions of the Royal Society of London B: Biological Sciences, 362*(1481), 857–875.

Lau, H. C., & Passingham, R. E. (2007). Unconscious activation of the cognitive control system in the human prefrontal cortex. *Journal of Neuroscience, 27*(21), 5805–5811.

Locke, E. A., & Latham, G. P. (1990). *A theory of goal setting & task performance.* Englewood Cliffs, NJ: Prentice Hall.

Logan, G. D. (1994). On the ability to inhibit thought and action: A users' guide to the stop signal paradigm. In D. Dagenbach & T. H. Carr (Eds.), *Inhibitory processes in attention, memory, and language* (pp. 189–239). San Diego: Academic Press.

Marr, D. (1982). *Vision: A computational investigation into the human representation and processing of visual information.* San Francisco: Freeman.

Mattler, U. (2003). Priming of mental operations by masked stimuli. *Perception and Psychophysics, 65*(2), 167–187.

Metcalfe, J. (1986). Feeling of knowing in memory and problem solving. *Journal of Experimental Psychology: Learning, Memory and Cognition, 12*(2), 288–294.

Metcalfe, J., & Wiebe, D. (1987). Intuition in insight and noninsight problem solving. *Memory and Cognition, 15*(3), 238–246.

Milyavsky, M., Hassin, R. R., & Schul, Y. (2012). Guess what?: Implicit motivation boosts the influence of subliminal information on choice. *Consciousness and Cognition, 21*(3), 1232–1241.

Miyake, A., & Friedman, N. P. (2012). The nature and organization of individual differences in executive functions: Four general conclusions. *Current Directions in Psychological Science, 21*(1), 8–14.

Miyake, A., Friedman, N. P., Emerson, M. J., Witzki, A. H., Howerter, A., & Wager, T. D. (2000). The unity and diversity of executive functions and their contributions to complex "Frontal Lobe" tasks: A latent variable analysis. *Cognitive Psychology, 41*(1), 49–100.

Morewedge, C. K., & Kahneman, D. (2010). Associative processes in intuitive judgment. *Trends in Cognitive Sciences, 14*(10), 435–440.

Mudrik, L., Breska, A., Lamy, D., & Deouell, L. Y. (2011). Integration without awareness: expanding the limits of unconscious processing. *Psychological Science, 22*(6), 764–770.

Reber, A. S. (1992). The cognitive unconscious: An evolutionary perspective. *Consciousness and Cognition, 1,* 93–133.

Redick, T. S., Heitz, R. P., & Engle, R. W. (2007). Working memory capacity and inhibition: Cognitive and social consequences. In D. S. Gorfein & C. M. MacLeod (Eds.), *Inhibition in cognition* (pp. 125–142). Washington, DC: American Psychological Association.

Reuss, H., Kiesel, A., Kunde, W., & Hommel, B. (2011). Unconscious activation of task sets. *Consciousness and Cognition, 20*(3), 556–567.

Ricks, T., Turley-Ames, K., & Wiley, J. (2007). Effects of working memory capacity on mental set due to domain knowledge. *Memory and Cognition, 35*(6), 1456–1462.

Rosch, E., Mervis, C. B., Gray, W. D., Johnson, D. M., & Boyes-Braem, P. (1976). Basic objects in natural categories. *Cognitive Psychology, 8*(3), 382–439.

Rozin, P., Sprague, J. M., & Epstein, A. N. (1976). The evolution of intelligence and access to the cognitive unconscious. In J. M. Sprague & A. N. Epstein (Eds.), *Progress in psychobiology and physiological psychology* (Vol. 6, pp. 245–280). San Diego: Academic Press.

Schneider, W., & Shiffrin, R. M. (1977). Controlled and automatic human information processing: I. Detection, search, and attention. *Psychological Review, 84*(1), 1–66.

Sklar, A. Y., Levi, N., Goldstein, A., Mandel, R., Maril, A., & Hassin, R. R. (2012). Reading and doing arithmetic nonconsciously. *Proceedings of the National Academy of Sciences, 109*(48), 19614–19619.

Soto, D., Mäntylä, T., & Silvanto, J. (2011). Working memory without consciousness. *Current Biology, 21*(22), 912–913.

Strahan, E. J., Spencer, S. J., & Zanna, M. P. (2002). Subliminal priming and persuasion: Striking while the iron is hot. *Journal of Experimental Social Psychology, 38*(6), 556–568.

Stroop, J. (1935). Studies of interference in serial verbal reactions. *Journal of Experimental Psychology: General, 18,* 643–662.

Terrace, H., Petitto, L., Sanders, R., & Bever, T. (1979). Can an ape create a sentence?. *Science*, *206*, 891–902.

Tsuchiya, N., & Koch, C. (2005). Continuous flash suppression reduces negative afterimages. *Nature Neuroscience*, *8*(8), 1096–1101.

Uleman, J. S., Adil Saribay, S., & Gonzalez, C. M. (2008). Spontaneous inferences, implicit impressions, and implicit theories. *Annual Review of Psychology*, *59*, 329–360.

Van den Bussche, E., Van den Noortgate, W., & Reynvoet, B. (2009). Mechanisms of masked priming: A meta-analysis. *Psychological Bulletin*, *135*(3), 452–477.

van Gaal, S., De Lange, F. P., & Cohen, M. X. (2012). The role of consciousness in cognitive control and decision making. *Frontiers in Human Neuroscience*, *6*, 121.

van Gaal, S., Ridderinkhof, K. R., Fahrenfort, J. J., Scholte, H. S., & Lamme, V. A. (2008). Frontal cortex mediates unconsciously triggered inhibitory control. *Journal of Neuroscience*, *28*(32), 8053–8062.

van Gaal, S., Ridderinkhof, K. R., Van den Wildenberg, W. P. M., & Lamme, V. A. (2009). Dissociating consciousness from inhibitory control: Evidence for unconsciously triggered response inhibition in the stop-signal task. *Journal of Experimental Psychology: Human Perception and Performance*, *35*(4), 1129–1139.

Van Opstal, F., De Lange, F. P., & Dehaene, S. (2011). Rapid parallel semantic processing of numbers without awareness. *Cognition*, *120*(1), 136–147.

Wittgenstein, L. (1963). *Philosophical investigations* (G. Anscombe, Trans.). New York: Macmillan.

Wokke, M. E., van Gaal, S., Scholte, H. S., Ridderinkhof, K. R., & Lamme, V. A. (2011). The flexible nature of unconscious cognition. *PloS ONE*, *6*(9), e25729.

Yang, E., Zald, D. H., & Blake, R. (2007). Fearful expressions gain preferential access to awareness during continuous flash suppression. *Emotion*, *7*(4), 882–886.

Zhou, F. A., & Davis, G. (2012). Unconscious priming of task sets: The role of spatial attention. *Attention, Perception, and Psychophysics*, *74*(1), 105–114.

CHAPTER 21

Metacognitive Processes and Subjective Experiences

Rainer Greifeneder and Norbert Schwarz

Proponents of theories of judgment commonly assume that people give more weight to information they consider reliable, diagnostic, and relevant to the task at hand than to information they consider unreliable, nondiagnostic or irrelevant. This empirically well-supported assumption implies that people evaluate the available information (object-level thoughts) with respect to its reliability, diagnosticity for the target, and relevance for the judgment (meta-level thoughts)–and that the outcome of such meta-level assessments can enhance, impair, or reverse the impact of the object-level thoughts. How people form these meta-level assessments is the topic of theorizing and research in metacognition, which studies how people think about their own thinking. In this chapter we review key lessons from metacognitive research, with a focus on social judgment, and discuss them in the context of dual-process models (for overviews of metacognitive work in other domains, see Dunlosky & Metcalfe, 2008; Koriat, 2007). It highlights that metacognitive assessments can be based on declarative as well as experiential information and can involve inference processes that vary widely in the cognitive and motivational resources they demand.

Early dual-process models in social psychology (Chaiken, 1980; Petty & Cacioppo, 1986) emphasized that processing can be more or less resource-intensive and related this distinction to a continuum from low-elaboration processing to high-elaboration processing, often referred to as heuristic versus systematic or peripheral versus central route processing (for recent reviews, see Chaiken & Ledgerwood, 2012; Petty & Briñol, 2012). More recent dual-process models introduced additional distinctions, drawing on an increased understanding of the role of automaticity in information processing (Andersen, Moskowitz, Blair, & Nosek, 2007; Spunt & Lieberman, Chapter 19, and Forscher & Devine, Chapter 31, this volume). The metacognitive research we review has not been designed to have a bearing on different criteria of automaticity, and has mostly attended to variables that are affected by, or influence, processing opportunity, ability, and motivation. Other dual-process models emphasize the distinction between associative and rule-based or propositional processing (e.g., Gawronski & Bodenhausen, 2006; Strack & Deutsch, 2004, 2012). Like any other evaluation, metacognitive evaluations of one's own thoughts involve propositional reasoning and can therefore occur, per definition, only in a propositional mode. The declarative and experiential inputs on which they draw are the output of associative processes that determine the content that comes to mind and the feelings of ease or difficulty that accompany it. What the propositional evaluation looks like—for instance, how many propositions relevant to the assessment are taken into account—is again a function of elaboration or, more generally, processing intensity (e.g., Gawronski & Bodenhausen, 2006). From this perspective, the opportunity, ability, and motivation to engage in resource-intensive processing play a key role across different dual-process frameworks; it is this commonality on which we focus in what follows.

PREVIEW

In this first section we introduce basic concepts of metacognition; we illustrate how metacognitive judgment can draw on declarative as well as experiential information, and how each source of information can serve as input into low-intensity as well as high-intensity processing. We conceptualize the use of experiential information in terms of feelings-as-information theory (Schwarz, 2012; Schwarz & Clore, 1983, 2007) and focus on the role of "cognitive feelings" (Clore, 1992), which here are metacognitive experiences of ease or difficulty that accompany the thought process.

Next, we ask whether cognitive feelings exert more influence under conditions of low-intensity or of high-intensity processing. While the majority of the available empirical evidence suggests that metacognitive experiences are more likely to be relied on in conditions of low-intensity processing, the picture is more complex, depending on the specific meta-level thoughts on which cognitive feelings are brought to bear.

Finally, we address the reverse causal pathway and ask whether different cognitive feelings are differentially likely to prompt low-intensity versus high-intensity processing. We close with some caveats and issues for future research.

METACOGNITION: THINKING ABOUT ONE'S THOUGHTS

Metacognition research distinguishes primary, object-level thoughts about a target of judgment from secondary, meta-level thoughts about one's own primary thoughts. Some of these meta-level thoughts pertain to one's cognitive performance; they include whether one has understood some information correctly (judgments of comprehension), whether one is likely to remember it when needed (judgments of learning), whether one "really" knows something even though one cannot retrieve it at the moment (feelings of knowing), and many related issues (for extensive reviews, see Dunlosky & Metcalfe, 2008; Koriat, 2007). These assessments are central to the very idea of metacognition—thinking about one's own thinking. Other meta-level assessments pertain to attributes of the object-level information one considers, such as whether the information is internally consistent, likely to be true, or relevant to the task (for reviews, see Petty, Briñol, Tormala, & Wegener, 2007; Schwarz, in press). These assessments can pertain to self-generated information as well as information provided by others. While the latter case is less obviously an instance of thoughts about one's own thoughts than the former, the difference is only a matter of degree. To evaluate information from extraneous sources, it has to be mentally represented first, thus becoming part of one's own thinking. More important, assessments of external information rely heavily on assessments of one's own thoughts about the external information, including, for example, whether one can trust one's own interpretation of it, whether it is compatible with other things one believes, and so on. In what follows, we highlight this common component and treat assessments of reliability, diagnosticity, and relevance as metacognitive, independent of whether they pertain to self-generated thoughts or externally presented information. Both kinds of assessments can be made in a more or less resource-demanding manner and on the basis of declarative or experiential inputs. We illustrate this with different strategies for assessing an attribute of particular interest to social psychologists, namely, the likely truth of a belief.

Declarative and Experiential Information in Truth Perceptions

Information that is considered valid and reliable exerts more influence on judgment and behavior, independent of whether the information is recalled from memory or received from someone else. In making these assessments, people attend to a limited set of criteria, usually a subset of what might be considered the "Big Five" of truth assessment. In what follows, we review research suggesting that each of these "Big Five" can be formed based on either declarative or experiential inputs.

One criterion is *social consensus*: If many people believe it, then there is probably something to it (Festinger, 1954). Accordingly, people are more confident in their beliefs when the beliefs are shared by others (e.g., Newcomb, 1943; Visser & Mirabile, 2004), are more likely to endorse a message when many others have done so before them (Cialdini, 2009), and trust their memories of an event more when others remember it in similar ways (e.g., Ross, Buehler, & Karr, 1998). Conversely, perceiving dissent reliably undermines message acceptance, which makes reports on real or fabricated controversies an efficient strategy for swaying public opinion (Lewandowsky, Ecker, Seifert, Schwarz, & Cook, 2012). To assess the extent of consensus, one can draw on declarative information by consulting survey data or asking friends, potentially weighting one's friends' opinions by their expertise. Alternatively, one may simply rely on how "familiar" the belief feels. Because one is more frequently exposed to widely shared beliefs than to highly idiosyncratic ones, the apparent familiarity of a belief provides a (fallible) experiential indicator of its popularity. Hence, the mere repetition of a belief can increase perceived social consensus even when all repetitions come from the same, single source, making a single repetitive voice sound like a chorus (Weaver, Garcia, Schwarz, & Miller, 2007).

A second criterion is whether the belief is *consistent* with other things one believes. This can be assessed analytically by checking the information against other knowledge, which requires motivation and cognitive resources, as observed in many studies in the tradition of cognitive response approaches to persuasion (Petty, Ostrom, & Brock, 1981). A less demanding indicator is again provided by one's metacognitive experiences and affective responses. Information that is inconsistent with one's beliefs is processed less fluently (Winkielman, Huber, Kavanagh, & Schwarz, 2012) and elicits negative feelings (Festinger, 1957), an assumption shared by many theories of cognitive consistency (Abelson et al., 1968; Gawronski & Strack, 2012). Accordingly, declarative as well as experiential inputs can indicate whether a given proposition is consistent with other things one believes.

A third criterion is that a given piece of information is also more likely to be accepted as true when it fits a broader story that lends *coherence* to its individual elements, as observed in basic research on mental models (for a review, see Johnson-Laird, 2012) and extensive analyses of jury decision making (Pennington & Hastie, 1992, 1993). Coherence can be determined through a systematic analysis of the relationships between different pieces of declarative information. Alternatively, it can be assessed by attending to one's processing experience: Coherent stories are easier to process than stories with internal contradictions (Johnson-Laird, 2012), which makes ease of processing an (imperfect) indicator of coherence. Indeed, people draw on their fluency experience when they evaluate how well things "go together" (Topolinski, 2012), as observed in judgments of semantic coherence (Topolinski & Strack, 2008, 2009), and syllogistic reasoning (Morsanyi & Handley, 2012).

Fourth, people's confidence in a belief increases with the *amount of supporting evidence*. The extent of support can be assessed by an external search, as in a scientific literature review, or by recall of pertinent information from memory; in either case, a larger amount of supportive declarative information increases confidence. Alternatively, support can be gauged from how *easy* it is to find supportive evidence—the more evidence there is, the easier it should be to find some (either in memory or the literature). In turn, the easier it is, the more evidence is likely available. This lay theory is at the heart of Tversky and Kahneman's (1973) availability heuristic. Because it is easier to find or generate a few rather than many pieces of supporting information, the factual recall of information, and pertaining cognitive experiences, result in opposing inferences. On the one hand, reliance on declarative information results in higher confidence the more supporting evidence one retrieves; on the other hand, reliance on experiential information results in lower confidence, because the difficulty associated with finding many pieces of supporting evidence suggests that there are not many (Schwarz et al., 1991; for reviews, see Schwarz, 1998, 2004). Accordingly, people have less confidence in their beliefs after attempting to generate many rather than few supporting arguments (Haddock, Rothman, Reber, & Schwarz, 1999; Tormala, Petty, & Briñol, 2002). Similarly, people perceive information provided by a job applicant as less credible after mustering many reasons for why this person has told the truth, but as more credible after mustering many reasons for why this person was lying (Ask, Greifeneder, & Reinhard, 2012). In each case, because recalling many instances is difficult, people seem to conclude that the respective amount of supporting object-level thoughts is low, thus not supporting the account in question.

Finally, the likelihood that a belief is accepted as true increases with the perceived credibility and expertise of its source (for reviews, see Eagly & Chaiken, 1993; Petty & Cacioppo, 1986). As decades of persuasion research illustrate, evaluations of *source credibility* can be based on declarative information that bears, for example, on the communicator's education, achievement, or institutional affiliation; alternatively, credibility judgments can be based on experiential information. For example, repeated exposure to pictures of a face makes the face seem more familiar, resulting in judgments of higher honesty and sincerity (Brown, Brown, & Zoccoli, 2002). Similarly, the mere repetition of a name can make an unknown name seem familiar, making its bearer "famous overnight" (Jacoby, Kelley, Brown, & Jasechko, 1989; Jacoby, Woloshyn, & Kelley, 1989), which may also result in an increase in perceived expertise.

As the example of truth assessment illustrates, metacognitive judgments can be based on declarative as well as experiential information. Moreover, it can involve high-intensity and low-intensity processing, in that truth judgments can be formed either with effort or in a lean and fast fashion. The previous review of findings may have created the impression that reliance on experiential information and low-intensity processing go together, while declarative information and high-intensity processing team up. Though appealing in its simplicity, the picture is more complex, because declarative pieces of information are also at the heart of many simple heuristics that are relied on when processing intensity is low (e.g., a babyfaced person is trusted; Zebrowitz & Montepare, 1992), and experiential information has also been shown to be critical when processing intensity is high (e.g., Wänke & Bless, 2000). Hence, source of information and type of processing are not to be equated (but also they may not be orthogonal, as reflected in the research reviewed later).

In the case of truth judgments, fluently processed information enjoys an advantage over disfluently processed information: It seems to be more popular; to be backed-up by more extensive supporting evidence; and to be more consistent with one's own beliefs, more coherent, and more likely to come from a credible source. All these perceptions reflect underlying lay theories that link specific cognitive experiences with (subjective perceptions of) real-world characteristics. For instance, because widely shared beliefs are encountered more often than highly idiosyncratic ones (a real-world characteristic), they are perceived as more familiar (cognitive experience)—in turn, apparent familiarity of a belief may provide an experiential indicator of its popularity. Note that such lay theories turn the factual link between real-world characteristics and subjective experiences upside down, drawing inferences from the consequent (e.g., familiarity) to the antecedent (e.g., popularity). Such proceeding is legitimate when the link between antecedent and consequent is bidirectionally true, but potentially misleading in all other cases. If these other cases constitute the majority, fluency will be a fallible cue for truth. Having said this, it is important to keep in mind that the same argument pertains to lay theories that build on declarative information. Though fallible, reliance on experiential information may therefore prove to be a reliable source of information in meta-level thought, likely as reliable as heuristic reliance on declarative information (see also Greifeneder, Bless, & Scholl, 2013; Herzog & Hertwig, 2013).

Cognitive Feelings as a Source of Information

The subjective experience of ease or difficulty arises from the dynamics of one's own information processing at the object level and is inherently metacognitive. At the most basic level the experience conveys that what one does is easy or difficult, which informs judgments of effort. People infer, for example, that preparing a lunch roll takes more time and skill when the recipe is printed in a difficult rather than an easy to read font (Song & Schwarz, 2008b), thus mistaking the difficulty of reading as indicative of the difficulty of doing. In addition, easy processing feels more pleasant than difficult processing, as reflected in self-reports and physiological measures of affect (e.g., Winkielman & Cacioppo, 2001). This affective experience, in turn, informs judgments of preference, beauty, and related attributes (Reber, Winkielman, & Schwarz, 1998; for a review, see Reber, Schwarz, & Winkielman, 2004).

Going beyond these global effort and affect dimensions, people form more specific inferences from their metacognitive experiences by drawing on applicable lay theories of mental processes. For instance, as noted in the preceding discussion of truth judgments, people infer that information is more familiar, more internally coherent, or more consistent with their beliefs when information processing is easy. In the case of truth judgments, the application of different lay theories converges on the same conclusion: If it is easy to process, it is probably true, independent of the specific criterion considered. This is presumably why fluently processed messages are more persuasive and "sticky" than disfluent messages. In other cases, however, different lay theories lead to diverging conclusions from the same experience, depending on which of many potentially applicable theories is brought to mind by the task at hand. For example, people who find it difficult to remember many details of an event conclude that the event happened long ago when asked about its date, but when asked how much attention they paid to it at the time conclude that it was not particularly important to them–whereas either of these factors can explain their poor memory, they have different downstream implications for related judgments (for a review, see Schwarz, 2010). Thus, the numerous variables that can influence ease of processing give rise to a broad range of lay theories that guide individuals' inferences from metacognitive experiences, which renders these inferences highly malleable. Which lay theory is brought to bear is likely a function of the lay theory's applicability and accessibility, and may in turn be guided by experiential information.

Fluency experiences may be caused by the judgmental target (and are therefore inherent) or be due to sources unrelated to the judgmental target (and therefore incidental). Unfortunately, individuals are often more sensitive to the experience than to its source and frequently misread processing experiences that arise from incidental variables as bearing on attributes of what they are thinking about. Such incidental influences are well-documented in the literature. For instance, people infer product preferences from easy- versus difficult-to-read print fonts (e.g., Novemsky, Dhar, Schwarz, & Simonson, 2007), essay quality from differentially legible handwriting (Greifeneder et al., 2010; Greifeneder, Zelt, Seele, Bottenberg, & Alt, 2012), truth from rhyming (e.g., McGlone & Tofighbakhsh, 2000) and from high or low figure–ground contrast (e.g., Reber & Schwarz, 1999), risk from ease of pronunciation (e.g., Song & Schwarz, 2009), or concept usability from ease or difficulty of sentence unscrambling (Greifeneder & Bless, 2010). Most variables that can facilitate or impair perceptual and conceptual processing may constitute a source of incidental influence (for a review, see Alter & Oppenheimer, 2009), unless there is reason to discredit the source. Indeed, people do *not* rely on their metacognitive experiences as a source of information when their representativeness of the target or relevance to the task at hand is called into question (for a review, see Greifeneder, Bless, & Pham, 2011). Accordingly, attributing difficulty of recall to the influence of allegedly distracting background music (Schwarz et al., 1991), or realizing that it may simply result from a difficult-to-read print font (Novemsky et al., 2007), eliminates the otherwise observed influence of processing fluency. Conversely, experiencing a feeling despite opposing influences increases its perceived informational value; for example, finding recall easy despite allegedly distracting music enhances the impact of the accessibility experience (Schwarz et al., 1991). In short, the use of metacognitive experiences as a source of information follows the principles of feelings-as-information theory, which was initially developed to account for the influence of moods and emotions (for an integrative review, see Schwarz, 2012).

DO COGNITIVE FEELINGS EXERT MORE INFLUENCE UNDER LOW-INTENSITY OR HIGH-INTENSITY PROCESSING?

Many dual-process theories of persuasion share the assumption that relatively effortful high-intensity processing requires motivation, ability, and opportunity (Chaiken & Ledgerwood, 2012; Eagly & Chaiken, 1993; Petty & Briñol, 2012; Petty & Cacioppo, 1986). Decades of research indicate that recipients are more likely to elaborate on the content of a message when the issue is important; when their cognitive ability is high; and when their opportunity is unconstrained by time pressure, fatigue, and related variables; conversely, they are more likely to rely on heuristic cues when issue relevance, ability, and/or opportunity are low. This work further indicated that most inputs can influence judgment under both low-intensity and high-intensity processing, although in differential ways. When an issue is of high personal relevance, for example, recipients process consensus information analytically, and pay attention to attributes such as sample size, giving the information more weight when based on a larger sample; in contrast, when the issue is of low personal relevance, they think less about the inputs and use consensus information as a heuristic cue, making its impact independent of sample size (see Eagly & Chaiken, 1993). Notably, it is the same input, but it is used differently depending on low-intensity or high-intensity processing. Similarly, the source of a message may serve as a heuristic cue when processing motivation or ability is low, or as an argument that is taken into consideration during message elaboration when processing motivation and ability are high, resulting in differential message representations and judgments (Petty & Cacioppo, 1986). The same regularities apply to the use of metacognitive experiences and other feelings as a source of information.

Pitting Thought Content against Processing Experience

To date, researchers interested in the differential use of cognitive feelings under low-intensity versus high-intensity processing have primarily relied on an experimental paradigm introduced by Schwarz and colleagues (1991) that pits accessible thought content against metacognitive experiences. Participants are asked to recall either few or many instances of an event or behavior, or to generate few or many arguments for or against a proposition. What constitutes "few" or "many" thoughts in this paradigm is determined in a pretest that asks participants to list as many instances or arguments as come to mind; the modal number of thoughts listed in the pretest minus (or plus) 50% is the number of thoughts requested in the "few" (or "many") condition. This creates a situation in which listing few thoughts is experienced as easy, whereas listing many thoughts is experienced as difficult, thus setting the stage for exploring the relative contribution of thought content (declarative information) and cognitive feelings (experiential information) that accompany its generation. At present, the vast majority of the available evidence indicates that low-intensity processing fosters reliance on cognitive feelings at the expense of accessible content, whereas high-intensity processing attenuates reliance on cognitive feelings (for a review, see Greifeneder, Bless, et al., 2011). However, some noteworthy exceptions high light that declarative content, as well as cognitive feelings, can also serve as input in the respective "other" processing mode under specific conditions. We address both sets of findings in turn and identify the conditions under which each one is likely to hold.

Low-Intensity Processing Increases Reliance on Cognitive Feelings

Processing Motivation

Rothman and Schwarz (1998) asked men to retrieve few (easy) or many (difficulty) behaviors that can increase or decrease their risk of heart disease. To test the role of processing motivation they drew on the *personal relevance* of the topic by assessing participants' family history of heart disease and by framing the task in terms of either one's own personal risk or the risk for an average American. If high processing motivation fosters processing of thought content, participants with a family history of heart disease who think about their own behavior should elaborate on the behaviors they listed; they should therefore see themselves as being at higher risk after listing many rather than few risk-increasing behaviors and at lower risk after listing many rather than few risk-decreasing behaviors. In contrast, participants without a family history, or participants who were asked to think about others, should find the task less relevant. If low personal relevance fosters reliance on the ease with which the respective behaviors came to mind, the otherwise observed pattern should be observed. Because recalling many behaviors (of any kind) is difficult, they should infer that they rarely engage in them, resulting in lower judgments of risk after recalling many rather than few examples of their own risk-increasing behaviors and higher judgments of risk after recalling many rather than few examples of their own risk-decreasing behaviors. The results were consistent with these predictions. When the task pertained to the personal behaviors and their own risk, men with a family history of heart disease relied on the content of recall, whereas men without a family history relied on experienced ease of recall; but when the task pertained to the behaviors and risk of an average person, all relied on ease of recall. Both effects presumably reflect that low personal relevance decreases processing intensity, giving an advantage to experiential information of high immediacy. Conceptual replications of these findings were reported by Broemer (2004), Grayson and Schwarz (1999), Greifeneder (2007), and Haddock (2002), among others.

Other manipulations of processing motivation converge with these findings. Aarts and Dijksterhuis (1999, Experiment 2) manipulated participants' *accuracy motivation* through instructions and found that only participants with low accuracy motivation relied on their ease-of-retrieval experiences in making frequency estimates (see also Greifeneder, 2007, Experiment 1). Greifeneder and colleagues tested the role of *uncertainty* in individuals' use of ease versus content of retrieval as a basis of judgment. As predicted, they found that cognitive experiences influenced judgments and behaviors under conditions of certainty, which fosters low-intensity processing, but not under conditions of uncertainty, which usually motivates high-intensity processing (Greifeneder, Müller, Stahlberg, Van den Bos, & Bless, 2011a, 2011b; Müller, Greifeneder, Stahlberg, Van den Bos, & Bless, 2010; see also Janssen, Müller, & Greifeneder, 2011).

Complementing these findings, Florack and Zoabi (2003) assessed participants' need for cognition, an individual-difference variable that distinguishes people who are differentially likely to engage spontaneously in high-intensity processing. They found that individuals low in need for cognition relied more on their cognitive feelings than did individuals high in need for cognition, who relied on accessible content.

Processing Opportunity

Further highlighting the link between low-intensity processing and reliance on cognitive feelings, Greifeneder and Bless (2007) manipulated participants' processing capacity through a secondary task. They consistently found that participants under high cognitive load relied on the ease with which they could bring behaviors or arguments to mind, whereas participants under low cognitive load drew on the thought content they had generated. Complementing these judgment effects, they also observed important differences in response time: High-load participants, who based their judgments on their cognitive feelings, were equally fast after generating few or many arguments; in contrast, low-load participants, who based their judgments on accessible content, took longer to arrive at a judgment after generating many rather than few arguments (see also Koriat & Levy-Sadot, 1999). This pattern reflects that the more inputs are considered, the more time high-intensity processing takes, which is not the case for the summary information provided by one's cognitive feelings, which serve as input under conditions of low-intensity processing.

Throughout, these studies indicate that reliance on the subjective experience of ease or difficulty of recall or thought generation increases with decreasing processing motivation, ability or opportunity, that is, in conditions of low-intensity processing.

High-Intensity Processing Increases Reliance on Cognitive Feelings

In contrast, a second line of work suggests the opposite conclusion, namely, that cognitive feelings are more likely to influence judgments under conditions of *high* processing motivation. A crucial difference between these lines of work is the judgment on which the feeling is brought to bear. In the previous studies, target judgments are explicitly or implicitly presumed to be mediated by the inferred amount of existing information (e.g., Schwarz et al., 1991). However, the same cognitive experiences can also influence individuals' confidence in their own thoughts, as initially shown by Haddock and colleagues (1999; Haddock, Rothman, & Schwarz, 1996): Generating many arguments in favor of one's opinion is difficult and undermines one's confidence in one's own thoughts. Not surprisingly, such shifts in confidence and related measures of attitude strength have downstream consequences for other judgments.

Most importantly, people give more weight to information they are confident about than to information they are less confident about, as noted in our discussion of metacognitive truth assessments. Research in the tradition of dual-process models of persuasion showed that such assessments of information quality are more likely under conditions of high processing motivation, ability, and opportunity (Chen & Chaiken, 1999; Petty & Cacioppo, 1986). Likewise, other dual-mode models, such as the associative–propositional evaluation model (Gawronski & Bodenhausen, 2006), hold that more propositions are considered with increasing levels of processing intensity. This provides a pathway in which the initial metacognitive experience influences one's trust in one's own thoughts, which can subsequently feed into other judgments to which these thoughts are relevant.

Drawing initial attention to this possibility, Wänke and Bless (2000) observed that ease-of-retrieval experiences had more impact under conditions of high motivation than under conditions of low motivation, in contrast to what earlier work would have predicted. This was the case when motivation was operationalized via need for cognition or by instructing participants to report accurate (high motivation) versus spontaneous reactions (low motivation). Similarly, Tormala and colleagues (2002) found that ease-of-retrieval experiences influenced the evaluation of an examination policy in conditions of high, but not low, processing motivation, again operationalized through need for cognition or an accountability manipulation. Relatedly, Hirt, Kardes, and Markman (2004) observed more reliance on cognitive feelings as information among participants with high rather than low need for structure (Webster & Kruglanski, 1994). These findings are compatible with the assumption that participants brought their metacognitive experiences to bear on their own thought, giving their own thoughts more weight when ease of recall or thought generation suggested that they could have confidence in what they were thinking. Such metacognitive evaluations of one's own thoughts have recently been integrated into dual-process models of persuasion (Briñol & Petty, 2009), where they are assumed to serve different roles under different processing conditions, as is the case for any other source of information.

Summary

The reviewed evidence reiterates a central theme of research on metacognitive experiences: Their meaning is context sensitive, and what people infer from a given experience depends on which of many potentially applicable lay theories is brought to mind (Schwarz, 2010). Finding it difficult to recall many behaviors that increase one's risk of heart disease may suggest, for example, that one's risk is low (a judgment consistent with Tversky and Kahneman's, 1973, availability heuristic) or that one lacks expertise in this domain (or else the task would not be that hard). In the former case, the experience is brought to bear on the frequency of the focal behavior itself, which is more likely under conditions of low-intensity processing; in the latter case, the experience is brought to bear on the diagnosticity of one's own thoughts, which figures more prominently under conditions of high-intensity processing. While this distinction organizes the reviewed findings, it is important to note that the influence of metacognitive experiences on one's thought confidence is itself very often an effect of low-intensity processing, as discussed earlier. If so, the increased impact of metacognitive experiences under high-intensity processing may merely be a downstream effect of initial low-intensity processing during the evaluation of one's own thoughts. Future research may fruitfully address these complexities, preferably by extending the range of fluency manipulations beyond the recall and thought-generation tasks used in the great majority of the currently available work.

DO COGNITIVE FEELINGS INFLUENCE THE LIKELIHOOD OF LOW-INTENSITY VERSUS HIGH-INTENSITY PROCESSING?

Dual-process models of persuasion generally share the assumption that people are more likely to engage in effortful content processing when their motivation, ability, and opportunity to do so are high. *Ceteris paribus,* processing motivation is higher when people encounter a potential problem that needs attention than when they cruise along in a benign context. Feelings-as-information theory holds that affective and cognitive feelings play an important role in this process by providing information about one's current situation, which guides the choice of subsequent processing strategy (Schwarz, 1990, 2012). Feelings that provide a problem signal foster vigilance and the adoption of a detail-oriented, bottom-up processing style, which is usually adaptive. In contrast, feelings that characterize the situation as benign are not, by themselves, associated with particular processing requirements. They foster reliance on preexisting knowledge structures and top-down processing, *unless* goals or task demands require otherwise (Bless & Schwarz, 1999). Studies bearing on the influence of moods and emotions on processing style are consistent with these assumptions (for a review, see Schwarz & Clore, 2007). Here, we focus on the role of metacognitive experiences.

As our review of metacognitive truth assessments illustrated, fluently processed information is more likely to be accepted at face value than disfluently processed information. Not surprisingly, such metacognitive truth assessments influence how much people scrutinize information: When disfluent processing suggests that something may be wrong, the details receive more attention, and distortions are more likely to be noticed. For example, when asked, "How many animals of each kind did Moses take on the Ark?" most people answer "two," despite knowing that the biblical actor was Noah, not Moses. But as Song and Schwarz (2008a) observed, merely presenting the question in a difficult-to-read print font can reduce the error rate from 88% (when the question is printed in Arial) to 53% (when the question is printed in gray Brush Script). However, the same manipulation reduces correct answers to the question "Which country is famous for cuckoo clocks and pocket knives?" (Switzerland). In both cases, disfluency due to the print font discourages reliance on the first thing that comes to mind, which improves performance when the spontaneous association is misleading (the Moses question), but impairs performance when the spontaneous association is correct (the Switzerland question). Similarly, Alter, Oppenheimer, Epley, and Eyre (2007) reported that disfluency improved performance on a variety of tasks, including syllogistic reasoning and logical problem solving, by increasing the likelihood of more effortful processing. For the same reason, difficult-to-read material is also better remembered, presumably because it received more detailed attention at encoding (Diemand-Yauman, Oppenheimer, & Vaughan, 2011). Finally, Greifeneder and Bless (2010) reported that fluent prime activation led to assimilation, but disfluent prime activation led to contrast in a standard Donald-paradigm, presumably because fluency tags the accessible prime with a go or use signal, whereas disfluency serves as a stop signal.

As these examples illustrate, disfluency is likely to trigger high-intensity processing, presumably because it flags the material for closer scrutiny. This improves performance on tasks that benefit from closer scrutiny but impairs performance on tasks that benefit from reliance on less effortful judgment strategies. We hasten to add, however, that the driving force is presumably not fluency or disfluency per se, but the meaning of the experience in context (Schwarz, 2010). In contexts in which people learn, for example, that fluently processed information is likely to be false (e.g., Unkelbach, 2007), the otherwise observed relationship should be reversed. In addition, fluent processing feels good, and positive affect itself makes elaborative processing and high attention to detail less likely (Schwarz, 1990, 2002). Hence, both the informational value of (dis)fluency and the accompanying affect are likely to foster high-intensity processing under disfluency, and future research may fruitfully attempt to determine their relative contributions.

CODA

People think about their own thinking and evaluate their primary object-level thoughts on a variety of dimensions, including reliability, truth, diagnosticity for a specific target, or relevance for a specific judgment. Such meta-level assessments can be formed in a relatively lean and fast fashion (here referred to as *low-intensity processing*), or in a more capacity-demanding slower fashion (here referred to as *high-intensity processing*). Moreover, these assessments can be based on declarative or experiential information. This chapter has reviewed many links between the two kinds of processing and the two sources of information, sketching a complex picture in which cognitive feelings play a critical role. Importantly, the way cognitive feelings are used as information, or channel subsequent information processing, depends on the interpretation of the feeling in the respective contexts. One of the challenges lying ahead will be to understand further what guides interpretation, thereby adding additional complexity to metacognition.

REFERENCES

Aarts, H., & Dijksterhuis, A. (1999). How often did I do it?: Experienced ease of retrieval and frequency estimates of past behavior. *Acta Psychologica, 103*, 77–89.

Abelson, R. P., Aronson, E., McGuire, W. J., Newcomb, T. M., Rosenberg, M. J., & Tannenbaum, P. H. (Eds.). (1968). *Theories of cognitive consistency: A sourcebook*. Chicago: Rand-McNally.

Alter, A. L., & Oppenheimer, D. M. (2009). Uniting the tribes of fluency to form a metacognitive nation. *Personality and Social Psychology Review, 13*, 219–235.

Alter, A. L., Oppenheimer, D. M., Epley, N., & Eyre, R. N. (2007). Overcoming intuition: Metacognitive difficulty activates analytic reasoning. *Journal of Experimental Psychology: General, 136*, 569–576.

Andersen, S. M., Moskowitz, G. B., Blair, I. V., & Nosek, B. (2007). Feelings and phenomenal experiences. In A. W. Kruglanski & E. T. Higgins (Eds.), *Social psychology: Handbook of basic principles* (2nd ed., pp. 138–175). New York: Guilford Press.

Ask, K., Greifeneder, R., & Reinhard, M. A. (2012). On the ease of (dis)believing: The role of accessibility experiences in credibility judgments. *Applied Cognitive Psychology, 26*, 779–784.

Bless, H., & Schwarz, N. (1999). Sufficient and necessary conditions in dual-mode models: The case of mood and information processing. In S. Chaiken & Y. Trope (Eds.), *Dual-process theories in social psychology* (pp. 423–440). New York: Guilford Press.

Briñol, P., & Petty, R. (2009). Persuasion: Insights from the self-validation hypothesis. In *Advances in experimental social psychology* (Vol. 41, pp. 69–118). San Diego: Academic Press.

Broemer, P. (2004). Ease of imagination moderates reactions to differently framed health messages. *European Journal of Social Psychology, 34*, 103–119.

Brown, A. S., Brown, L. A., & Zoccoli, S. L. (2002). Repetition-based credibility enhancement of unfamiliar faces. *The American Journal of Psychology, 115*, 199–209.

Chaiken, S. (1980). Heuristic versus systematic information processing and the use of source versus message cues in persuasion. *Journal of Personality and Social Psychology, 39*, 752–766.

Chaiken, S., & Ledgerwood, A. (2012). A theory of heuristic and systematic information processing. In P. A. Van Lange, A. W. Kruglanski & E. Higgins (Eds.), *Handbook of theories of social psychology* (pp. 246–266). Thousand Oaks, CA: Sage.

Chen, S., & Chaiken, S. (1999). The heuristic–systematic model in its broader context. In S. Chaiken & Y. Trope (Eds.), *Dual-process theories in social psychology* (pp. 73–96). New York: Guilford Press.

Cialdini, R. B. (2009). *Influence: Science and practice*. Boston: Pearson.

Clore, G. L. (1992). Cognitive phenomenology: Feelings and the construction of judgment. In L. L. Martin & A. Tesser (Eds.), *The construction of social judgments* (pp. 133–163). Hillsdale, NJ: Erlbaum.

Diemand-Yauman, C., Oppenheimer, D. M., & Vaughan, E. B. (2011). Fortune favors the bold (and the italicized): Effects of disfluency on educational outcomes. *Cognition, 118*, 114–118.

Dunlosky, J., & Metcalfe, J. (2008). *Metacognition*. Thousand Oaks, CA: Sage.

Eagly, A. H., & Chaiken, S. (1993). *The psychology of attitudes*. Fort Worth, TX: Harcourt Brace Jovanovich.

Festinger, L. (1954). A theory of social comparison processes. *Human Relations, 7*, 117–140.

Festinger, L. (1957). *A theory of cognitive dissonance*. Stanford, CA: Standford University Press.

Florack, A., & Zoabi, H. (2003). Risikoverhalten bei Aktiengeschäften: Wenn Anleger nachdenklich werden [Risk behavior in share transactions: When investors think about reasons]. *Zeitschrift für Sozialpsychologie, 34*, 65–78.

Gawronski, B., & Bodenhausen, G. V. (2006). Associative and propositional processes in evaluation: An integrative review of implicit and explicit attitude change. *Psychological Bulletin, 132*, 692–731.

Gawronski, B., & Strack, F. (Eds.). (2012). *Cognitive consistency: A fundamental principle in social cognition*. New York: Guilford Press.

Grayson, C. E., & Schwarz, N. (1999). Beliefs influence information processing strategies: Declarative and experiential information in risk assessment. *Social Cognition, 17*, 1–18.

Greifeneder, R. (2007). *Reliance on accessibility experiences in judgment and decision making*. Lengerich: Pabst Science.

Greifeneder, R., Alt, A., Bottenberg, K., Seele, T., Zelt, S., & Wagener, D. (2010). On writing legibly: Processing fluency systematically biases evaluations of handwritten material. *Social Psychological and Personality Science, 1*, 230–237.

Greifeneder, R., & Bless, H. (2007). Relying on accessible content versus accessibility experiences: The case of processing capacity. *Social Cognition, 25*, 853–881.

Greifeneder, R., & Bless, H. (2010). The fate of activated information in impression formation: Fluency of concept activation moderates the emergence of assimilation versus contrast. *British Journal of Social Psychology, 49*, 405–414.

Greifeneder, R., Bless, H., & Pham, M. T. (2011). When do people rely on affective and cognitive feelings in judgment?: A review. *Personality and Social Psychology Review, 15*, 107–141.

Greifeneder, R., Bless, H., & Scholl, S. (2013). About swift defaults and sophisticated safety nets: A process perspective on fl uency's validity in judgment. In C. Unkelbach & R. Greifeneder (Eds.), *The experience of thinking: How the fluency of mental processes influences cognition and behavior* (pp. 220–233). Hove, UK: Psychology Press.

Greifeneder, R., Müller, P., Stahlberg, D., Van den Bos, K., & Bless, H. (2011a). Beyond procedure's content: Cognitive subjective experiences in procedural justice judgments. *Experimental Psychology, 58*, 341–352.

Greifeneder, R., Müller, P., Stahlberg, D., Van den Bos, K., & Bless, H. (2011b). Guiding trustful behavior: The role of accessible content and accessibility experiences. *Journal of Behavioral Decision Making, 24*, 498–514.

Greifeneder, R., Zelt, S., Seele, T., Bottenberg, K., & Alt, A. (2012). Towards a better understanding of the legibility bias in performance assessments: The case of gender-based inferences. *British Journal of Educational Psychology, 82*, 361–374.

Haddock, G. (2002). It's easy to like or dislike Tony Blair: Accessibility experiences and the favourability of attitude judgments. *British Journal of Psychology, 93*, 257–267.

Haddock, G., Rothman, A. J., Reber, R., & Schwarz, N. (1999). Forming judgments of attitude certainty, intensity, and importance: The role of subjective experiences. *Personality and Social Psychology Bulletin, 25*, 771–782.

Haddock, G., Rothman, A. J., & Schwarz, N. (1996). Are (some) reports of attitude strength context dependent? *Canadian Journal of Behavioural Science, 28*, 313–316.

Herzog, S. M., & Hertwig, R. (2013). The ecological validity of fluency. In C. Unkelbach & R. Greifeneder (Eds.), *The experience of thinking: How the fluency of mental processes influences cognition and behavior* (pp. 190–219). Hove, UK: Psychology Press.

Hirt, E. R., Kardes, F. R., & Markman, K. D. (2004). Activating a mental simulation mindset through generation of alternatives: Implications for debiasing in related and unrelated domains. *Journal of Experimental Social Psychology, 40*, 374–383.

Jacoby, L. L., Kelley, C. M., Brown, J., & Jasechko, J. (1989). Becoming famous overnight: Limits of the ability to avoid unconscious influences of the past. *Journal of Personality and Social Psychology, 56*, 326–338.

Jacoby, L. L., Woloshyn, V., & Kelley, C. (1989). Becoming famous without being recognized: Unconscious influences of memory produced by dividing attention. *Journal of Experimental Psychology: General, 118*, 115–125.

Janssen, J., Müller, P., & Greifeneder, R. (2011). Cognitive processes in procedural justice judgments. The role of ease-of-retrieval, uncertainty, and experience. *Journal of Organizational Behavior, 32*, 726–750.

Johnson-Laird, P. N. (2012). Mental models and consistency. In B. Gawronski & F. Strack (Eds.), *Cognitive consistency: A fundamental principle in social cognition* (pp. 225–243). New York: Guilford Press.

Koriat, A. (2007). Metacognition and consciousness. In P. D. Zelazo, M. Moscovitch, & E. Thompson (Eds.), *The Cambridge handbook of consciousness* (pp. 289–326). New York: Cambridge University Press.

Koriat, A., & Levy-Sadot, R. (1999). Processes underlying metacognitive judgments: Information-based and experience-based monitoring of one's own knowledge. In S. Chaiken & Y. Trope (Eds.), *Dual-process theories in social psychology* (pp. 483–502). New York: Guilford Press.

Lewandowsky, S., Ecker, U. K., Seifert, C. M., Schwarz, N., & Cook, J. (2012). Misinformation and its correction continued influence and successful debiasing. *Psychological Science in the Public Interest, 13*, 106–131.

McGlone, M. S., & Tofighbakhsh, J. (2000). Birds of a feather flock conjointly (?): Rhyme as reason in aphorisms. *Psychological Science, 11*, 424–428.

Morsanyi, K., & Handley, S. J. (2012). Logic feels so good—I like it!: Evidence for intuitive detection of logicality in syllogistic reasoning. *Journal of Experimental Psychology: Learning Memory and Cognition, 38*, 596–616.

Müller, P., Greifeneder, R., Stahlberg, D., Van den Bos, K., & Bless, H. (2010). Shaping cooperation behavior: The role of accessibility experiences. *European Journal of Social Psychology, 40*, 178–187.

Newcomb, T. M. (1943). *Personality and social change*. New York: Holt, Rinehart & Winston.

Novemsky, N., Dhar, R., Schwarz, N., & Simonson, I. (2007). Preference fluency in choice. *Journal of Marketing Research, 54*, 347–356.

Pennington, N., & Hastie, R. (1992). Explaining the evidence: Tests of the story model for juror decision making. *Journal of Personality and Social Psychology, 62*, 189–206.

Pennington, N., & Hastie, R. (1993). The story model for juror decision making. In R. Hastie (Ed.), *Inside the juror* (pp. 192–223). New York: Cambridge University Press.

Petty, R., & Briñol, P. (2012). The elaboriation likelihood model. In P. A. Van Lange, A. W. Kruglanski, & E. Higgins (Eds.), *Handbook of theories of social psychology* (pp. 224–245). Thousand Oaks, CA: Sage.

Petty, R., Briñol, P., Tormala, Z. L., & Wegener, D. (2007). The role of meta-cognition in social psychology. In E. T. Higgins & A. W. Kruglanski (Eds.), *Social psychology: A handbook of basic principles* (2nd ed., pp. 254–284). New York: Guilford Press.

Petty, R. E., & Cacioppo, J. T. (1986). The elaboration likelihood model of persuasion. In L. Berkowitz (Ed.), *Advances in experimental social psychology* (Vol. 19, pp. 123–205). New York: Academic Press.

Petty, R. E., Ostrom, T. M., & Brock, T. C. (Eds.). (1981). *Cognitive responses in persuasion*. Hillsdale, NJ: Erlbaum.

Reber, R., & Schwarz, N. (1999). Effects of perceptual fluency on judgments of truth. *Consciousness and Cognition: An International Journal, 8*, 338–342.

Reber, R., Schwarz, N., & Winkielman, P. (2004). Processing fluency and aesthetic pleasure: Is beauty in the perceiver's processing experience? *Personality and Social Psychology Review, 8*, 364–382.

Reber, R., Winkielman, P., & Schwarz, N. (1998). Effects of perceptual fluency on affective judgments. *Psychological Science, 9*, 45–48.

Ross, M., Buehler, R., & Karr, J. W. (1998). Assessing the accuracy of conflicting autobiographical memories. *Memory and Cognition, 26*, 1233–1244.

Rothman, A. J., & Schwarz, N. (1998). Constructing perceptions of vulnerability: Personal relevance and the use of experiential information in health judgments. *Personality and Social Psychology Bulletin, 24*, 1053–1064.

Schwarz, N. (1990). Feelings as information: Informational and motivational functions of affective states. In E. T. Higgins & R. M. Sorrentino (Eds.), *Handbook of motivation and cognition: Foundations of social behavior* (Vol. 2, pp. 527–561). New York: Guilford Press.

Schwarz, N. (1998). Accessible content and accessibility experiences: The interplay of declarative and experiential information in judgment. *Personality and Social Psychology Review, 2*, 87–99.

Schwarz, N. (2002). Situated cognition and the wisdom in feelings: Cognitive tuning. In L. F. Barrett & P. Salovey (Eds.), *The wisdom in feeling: Psychological processes in emotional intelligence* (pp. 144–166). New York: Guilford Press.

Schwarz, N. (2004). Metacognitive experiences in consumer judgment and decision making. *Journal of Consumer Psychology, 14*, 332–348.

Schwarz, N. (2010). Meaning in context: Metacognitive experiences. In L. F. Barrett, B. Mesquita, & E. Smith (Eds.), *The mind in context* (pp. 105–125). New York: Guilford Press.

Schwarz, N. (2012). Feelings-as-information theory. In P. A. Van Lange, A. W. Kruglanski, & E. Higgins (Eds.), *Handbook of theories of social psychology* (pp. 289–308). Thousand Oaks, CA: Sage.

Schwarz, N. (in press). Metacognition. In M. Mikulincer & P. R. Shaver (Eds.), *APA handbook of personality and social psychology: Atti Vol. 1 Attitudes and social cognition*. Washington, DC: American Psychological Association.

Schwarz, N., Bless, H., Strack, F., Klumpp, G., Rittenauer-Schatka, H., & Simons, A. (1991). Ease of retrieval as information: Another look at the availability heuristic. *Journal of Personality and Social Psychology, 61*, 195–202.

Schwarz, N., & Clore, G. L. (1983). Mood, misattribution, and judgment of well-being: Informative and directive functions of affective states. *Journal of Personality and Social Psychology, 45*, 513–523.

Schwarz, N., & Clore, G. L. (2007). Feelings and phenomenal experiences. In A. W. Kruglanski & E. T. Higgins (Eds.), *Social psychology: Handbook of basic principles* (2nd ed., pp. 385–407). New York: Guilford Press.

Song, H., & Schwarz, N. (2008a). Fluency and the detection of misleading questions: Low processing fluency attenuates the Moses illusion. *Social Cognition, 26*, 791–799.

Song, H., & Schwarz, N. (2008b). If it's hard to read, it's hard to do. *Psychological Science, 19*, 986–988.

Song, H., & Schwarz, N. (2009). If it's difficult to pronounce, it must be risky: Fluency, familiarity, and risk perception. *Psychological Science, 20*, 135–138.

Strack, F., & Deutsch, R. (2004). Reflective and impulsive determinants of social behavior. *Personality and Social Psychology Review, 8*, 220–247.

Strack, F., & Deutsch, R. (2012). A theory of impulse and reflection. In P. A. Van Lange, A. W. Kruglanski, & E. Higgins (Eds.), *Handbook of theories of social psychology* (pp. 97–117). Thousand Oaks, CA: Sage.

Topolinski, S. (2012). Nonpropositional consistency. In B. Gawronski & F. Strack (Eds.), *Cognitive consistency: A fundamental principle in social cognition* (pp. 112–131). New York: Guilford Press.

Topolinski, S., & Strack, F. (2008). Where there's a will—there's no intuition. The unintentional basis of semantic coherence judgments. *Journal of Memory and Language, 58*, 1032–1048.

Topolinski, S., & Strack, F. (2009). The architecture of intuition: Fluency and affect determine intuitive judgments of semantic and visual coherence and judgments of grammaticality in artificial grammar learning. *Journal of Experimental Psychology: General, 138*, 39–63.

Tormala, Z. L., Petty, R. E., & Briñol, P. (2002). Ease of retrieval effects in persuasion: A self-validation analysis. *Personality and Social Psychology Bulletin, 28*, 1700–1712.

Tversky, A., & Kahneman, D. (1973). Availability: A heuristic for judging frequency and probability. *Cognitive Psychology, 5*, 207–232.

Unkelbach, C. (2007). Reversing the truth effect: Learning the interpretation of processing fluency in judgments of truth. *Journal of Experimental Psychology: Learning, Memory and Cognition, 33*, 219–230.

Visser, P. S., & Mirabile, R. R. (2004). Attitudes in the social context: The impact of social network composition on individual-level attitude strength. *Journal of Personality and Social Psychology, 87*, 779–795.

Wänke, M., & Bless, H. (2000). The effects of subjective ease of retrieval on attitudinal judgments: The moderating role of processing motivation. In H. Bless & J. P. Forgas (Eds.), *The message within: The role of subjective experience in social cognition and behavior* (pp. 143–161). Philadelphia: Psychology Press.

Weaver, K., Garcia, S. M., Schwarz, N., & Miller, D. T. (2007). Inferring the popularity of an opinion from its familiarity: A repetitive voice can sound like a chorus. *Journal of Personality and Social Psychology, 92*, 821–833.

Webster, D. M., & Kruglanski, A. W. (1994). Individual differences in need for cognitive closure. *Journal of Personality and Social Psychology, 67*, 1049–1062.

Winkielman, P., & Cacioppo, J. T. (2001). Mind at ease puts a smile on the face: Psychophysiological evidence that processing facilitation elicits positive affect. *Journal of Personality and Social Psychology, 81*, 989–1000.

Winkielman, P., Huber, D. E., Kavanagh, L., & Schwarz, N. (2012). Fluency of consistency: When thoughts fit nicely and flow smoothly. In B. Gawronski & F. Strack (Eds.), *Cognitive consistency: A fundamental principle in social cognition* (pp. 89–111). New York: Guilford Press.

Zebrowitz, L. A., & Montepare, J. M. (1992). Impressions of babyfaced individuals across the life span. *Developmental Psychology, 28*, 1143–1143.

CHAPTER 22

Same or Different?

How Similarity versus Dissimilarity Focus Shapes Social Information Processing

Thomas Mussweiler

Same or different? This simple question pervades much of human thinking. In fact, it seems that whenever humans process information, whenever they are confronted with a given stimulus set, they spontaneously extract similarity—often without intent or effort (Markman & Gentner, 2005). Even children as young as 4.5 months extract basic similarity from perceptual input (Baillargeon, 1993). Clearly, similarity is one of the basic building blocks of human cognition. In line with this notion, psychological theorizing and research have excelled in demonstrating just how central similarity is in human information processing. Indeed, similarity critically shapes many basic elements of human cognition, such as memory (Hintzman, 1986), categorization (Medin & Schaffer, 1978), problem solving (Reed, Ernst, & Banerji, 1974), and decision making (Kahneman & Miller, 1986; Medin, Goldstone, & Markman, 1995). These examples attest that, indeed, the "sense of sameness is the very keel and backbone of our thinking," as William James (1890/1950, p. 459) put it.

Similarity, however, not only serves as the keel of our thinking but also as the backbone of our social behavior. Clearly, similarity is one of the fundamental constituents of human social interaction. Humans are not only attracted to similar others (Byrne, 1997) and—as a consequence—are primarily surrounded by others of similar age, ethnicity, gender, education, attitudes, and interests (McPherson, Smith-Lovin, & Cook, 2001), but they also behave in fundamentally different ways when interacting with similar versus dissimilar others (Brewer, 1979; Deaux, 1996): They are, for example, more likely to model the behavior of (Hilmert, Kulik, & Christenfeld, 2006), allocate resources to (Tajfel, Billig, Bundy, & Flament, 1971), reward the positive behavior of (Chen & Li, 2009), and punish norm violations against (Bernhard, Fischbacher, & Fehr, 2006) similar than dissimilar others.

As this short sampler of research on similarity processing attests, similarity is a fundamental feature that is spontaneously and effortlessly extracted from a given stimulus configuration. In light of the resulting omnipresence of similarity information, it seems only natural to assume that—once extracted—similarity critically influences subsequent information processing. This possibility is captured by the notion that much of social information processing critically depends on whether judges focus on similarities or differences.

MECHANISMS OF SIMILARITY VERSUS DISSIMILARITY TESTING

More specifically, these alternative informational foci on similarities versus differences correspond to two facets of the same social-cognitive mechanism. When processing information about their social world, humans often seek specific knowledge that helps them with the task at hand. Obtaining such knowledge is often achieved by mechanisms of hypothesis testing in which judges relate their stored knowledge regarding the target to the judgmental task at hand (Trope & Liberman, 1996). Such hypothesis-testing processes are often selective, in that they focus on a single hypothesis that is then evaluated against a specific criterion (Sanbonmatsu, Posavac, Kardes, & Mantel, 1998; see also Klayman & Ha, 1987; Trope & Liberman, 1996). Rather than engaging in an exhaustive comparative test of all plausible hypotheses, judges often limit themselves to the test of a single focal hypothesis. Similarity—in light of its central role in human information processing more generally—is one essential factor that informs social information processors about which specific hypothesis they may test.

With respect to the similarity of a given set of stimuli, two basic hypotheses can be distinguished. Judges can either test the possibility that the target stimuli are similar or they can test the possibility that the target stimuli are dissimilar. Which of these hypotheses is tested depends on the perceived overall similarity of the target stimuli. According to the selective accessibility model (Mussweiler, 2003), as an initial step of information processing, judges engage in a quick holistic assessment of the stimuli at hand (Smith, Shoben, & Rips, 1974), in which they briefly consider a small number of salient features (e.g., category membership, salient characteristics) to determine whether the given stimuli are generally similar or dissimilar. The outcome of this screening is a broad assessment of similarity. Although such an assessment by itself is too general to be used as the basis for most tasks at hand, it is sufficient to determine the specific nature of the hypothesis that is then being tested. The hypothesis-testing mechanism thus focuses on the possibility that is suggested by the initial holistic assessment. If this assessment indicates that the given stimuli are generally similar to one another, judges engage in a process of similarity testing and further test the hypothesis that the stimuli are indeed similar. If the initial assessment indicates that the given stimuli are dissimilar from one another, however, judges engage in a process of dissimilarity testing and further test the hypothesis that the stimuli are indeed dissimilar.

The literature on hypothesis testing further suggests that once a hypothesis is selected, it is often tested by focusing on hypothesis-consistent evidence (Klayman & Ha, 1987; Snyder & Swann, 1978; Trope & Bassok, 1982; Trope & Liberman, 1996). This suggests that if judges engage in similarity testing, they will do so by selectively searching for knowledge indicating that the given stimuli are indeed similar. By the same token, if judges engage in dissimilarity testing, then they do so by selectively searching for knowledge indicating that the given stimuli are indeed dissimilar. This selectivity in the acquisition of judgment-relevant knowledge has clear informational consequences. The mechanism of similarity testing selectively increases the accessibility of evidence indicating similarity, whereas dissimilarity testing selectively increases the accessibility of evidence indicating dissimilarity. This selective accessibility effect constitutes the core informational consequence of similarity versus dissimilarity testing.

To the extent that information that was rendered selectively accessible forms the basis for subsequent judgments, feelings, and behaviors, these psychological reactions reflect the implications of this information. If evidence indicating similarity forms the basis, then judgments, feelings, and behaviors are assimilated toward the standard. If evidence indicating dissimilarity forms the basis, then judgments, feelings, and behaviors are contrasted away from the standard. This suggests that the default consequence of similarity testing is assimilation, whereas dissimilarity testing typically leads to contrast.

According to this description, the selective accessibility mechanism may at first sight appear to be a fairly deliberate, conscious, and elaborate process. And, in fact, situations in which judges deliberately seek judgment-relevant information are likely to involve selective accessibility mechanisms in which judges are consciously aware of at least some of the individual components. As we will see in the remainder of this chapter, however, the selective accessibility mechanisms of similarity and dissimilarity testing constitute ubiquitous mechanisms of social information processing that are frequently, if not continuously, engaged. As is true for other psychological mechanisms humans frequently engage in (Bargh, 1997; Smith, 1994), selective accessibility mechanisms are likely to become proceduralized (Mussweiler, 2003) so that they unfold automatically—that is, without intent or awareness and absorbing little processing capacity. Such automatic selective accessibility mechanisms are also likely to blur the boundaries between the individual processing components.

CONSEQUENCES OF SIMILARITY VERSUS DISSIMILARITY TESTING

The intimate link between similarity testing and assimilation on the one hand, and dissimilarity testing and contrast on the other is illustrated by a host of empirical findings demonstrating that (1) inducing judges to focus on similarities leads to assimilation, whereas inducing them to focus on differences leads to contrast, and (2) assimilation is accompanied by a generalized focus on similarities, whereas contrast is accompanied by a focus on differences.

The first direct support for this notion stems from a social comparison study in which judges were induced to engage in either similarity testing or dissimilarity testing before comparing themselves to a given social standard (Mussweiler, 2001). This study used a procedural priming logic to induce the respective foci on similarities versus differences. Before engaging in the critical social comparison, participants compared two pictures and listed either all the similarities or all the differences they could find between them. Doing so sets participants' minds on either of these two alternative processing styles, so that they applied the primed informational focus to the subsequent social comparison. Participants who focused on similarities between the two pictures also focused on similarities between themselves and the standard person. Those who focused on differences between the two pictures also focused on differences between themselves and the standard person. The results of this study demonstrated that how the social comparison influenced participants' self-evaluations depended on the induced informational focus. Judges who were primed to focus on similarities and therefore to engage in similarity testing assimilated self-evaluations toward the standard. Judges who were primed to focus on differences and therefore to engage in dissimilarity testing contrasted self-evaluations away from the standard. Following this initial study, a host of findings has demonstrated that procedurally priming judges to engage in similarity versus dissimilarity testing yields assimilative versus contrastive consequences across a variety of judgmental, affective, and behavioral outcome variables. Judges induced to engage in similarity testing not only assimilate judgments about their own characteristics to a given social standard (Mussweiler, 2001; Mussweiler, Rüter, & Epstude, 2004a), but they also assimilate judgments about others to a given performance standard (Damisch, Mussweiler, & Plessner, 2006), a given trait concept (Mussweiler & Damisch, 2008) or an activated stereotype (Corcoran, Hundhammer, & Mussweiler, 2009). In much the same way, affective and behavioral reactions are shaped by induced foci on similarities versus differences. Participants who are procedurally primed to engage in similarity testing assimilate their affective reactions to those of others and are therefore prone to emotional contagion effects (Epstude & Mussweiler, 2009). They also assimilate their performance behavior more to a given standard (Bittner, 2011; Crusius & Mussweiler, 2012; Haddock, Macrae, & Fleck, 2002). In all these cases, participants engaging in dissimilarity testing show contrast in their judgmental, affective, and behavioral reactions.

These findings demonstrate an intimate link between similarity testing and assimilation on the one hand, and dissimilarity testing and contrast on the other hand. Further support for this notion comes from studies demonstrating that assimilation and contrast are accompanied by traces of similarity and dissimilarity testing. In one study, for example, participants who were asked to evaluate their own athletic abilities were confronted with either moderate or extreme comparison standards of athletic ability (Mussweiler et al., 2004a). For example, participants were confronted with either the moderately low standard Bill Clinton or with the extremely low standard Pope John Paul. They then evaluated a number of core athletic abilities, such as the number of sit-ups they could perform and the time they needed to run 100 meters. Consistent with evidence in the social judgment literature (Herr, 1986), participants assimilated their self-evaluations to the moderate standards and contrasted them away from the extreme standards. Subsequent to these assimilative and contrastive comparisons, we assessed participants' focus on similarities versus dissimilarities. To do so, participants worked on a picture comparison task that was similar to the one previously applied to *induce* a focus on similarities versus differences (Mussweiler, 2001). This time, however, the task was used to *assess* these alternative informational foci. Specifically, participants were asked to compare two pictures and to indicate how similar these pictures were. Results demonstrate that participants rated both pictures as more similar after comparing themselves with a moderate rather than an extreme social comparison standard. That is, assimilation was accompanied by a general informational focus on similarities, whereas judgmental contrast was accompanied by a general focus on differences (see also Mussweiler & Damisch, 2008).

Taken together, these findings demonstrate that the alternative informational foci on similarities versus dissimilarities are closely associated with assimilative and contrastive context effects on judgment, affect, and behavior. Inducing participants to focus on similarities versus differences determines whether they assimilate their judgments, feelings, and behaviors toward context stimuli or contrast away from them. Vice versa, assimilating toward the context induces participants to focus on similarities, whereas contrasting away from the context induces them to focus on differences. This intimate link between assimilation versus contrast on the one hand, and similarity versus dissimilarity focus on the other, suggests that assimilative and contrastive context effects are produced by the two alternative selective accessibility mechanisms of similarity and dissimilarity testing.

CHARACTERISTICS OF SIMILARITY VERSUS DISSIMILARITY TESTING

The two alternative mechanisms of similarity and dissimilarity testing draw on the same cognitive architecture and involve the same submechanisms of hypothesis testing and accessibility. No matter whether judges test for similarity or dissimilarity, they selectively seek hypothesis-consistent knowledge, and their subsequent psychological reactions are led by the information that was selectively rendered accessible during this hypothesis test. Similarity and dissimilarity testing differ not in the basic cognitive processes they involve, but only in the concrete hypothesis that is put to a test. These two alternative mechanisms are therefore best described as twins rather than rivals. They involve the same submechanisms, draw on the same representations, and, consequently, also share many characteristics.

One characteristic that is of particular importance for social-cognitive mechanisms is their automatic versus controlled nature. Classic conceptualizations of automaticity in social cognition (Bargh, 1994) differentiate among four aspects: intention, awareness, efficiency, and control. In light of their apparent mechanistic kinship, similarity and dissimilarity testing obtain similar scores on all these four accounts. Specifically, both mechanisms are often carried out without intention or awareness, both are highly efficient, and both are difficult to control.

Similarity and dissimilarity testing are often carried out spontaneously, that is, without the intention to engage in these mechanisms. Typically, the mere coaccessibility (Kruglanski & Mayseless, 1990) of a set of stimuli is sufficient to trigger similarity or dissimilarity testing. In fact, much of the research described in this chapter captures conditions in which judges spontaneously engage in similarity or dissimilarity testing merely because a set of stimuli happened to be on the judges' mind at the same time. For example, merely activating a social comparison standard while participants engage in self-evaluative judgments (Mussweiler, Rüter, & Epstude, 2004b) is sufficient to induce participants to engage in similarity versus dissimilarity testing, as is apparent from the signature assimilative versus contrastive consequence of both mechanisms.

Furthermore, similarity and dissimilarity testing are often carried out outside of judges' awareness. In fact, traces of both mechanisms become apparent even if participants are not aware of the stimuli that enter into the respective mechanisms. For example, the assimilative versus contrastive judgmental consequences of similarity versus dissimilarity testing social comparisons occur even if the respective social comparison standards are presented outside of participants' awareness (Mussweiler et al., 2004b). Furthermore, the informational consequences of similarity testing, namely, selective accessibility, are apparent even if comparison standards are presented subliminally (Mussweiler & Englich, 2005). Presupposing that participants are unlikely to be aware of how they process information of which they remain unaware in the first place, this evidence suggests that similarity and dissimilarity testing are often carried out outside of awareness.

As a consequence of this lack of awareness (Strack & Hannover, 1996; Wilson & Brekke, 1994), similarity and dissimilarity testing are difficult to control. In fact, the consequences of both mechanisms often prevail even if the stimuli involved in similarity and dissimilarity testing are clearly unlikely to yield valuable information for the judgment at hand. The most striking example of this tendency is provided by research on the anchoring heuristic (Tversky & Kahneman, 1974), which constitutes one example of the judgmental consequences of similarity testing (Mussweiler & Strack, 2000; Strack & Mussweiler, 1997). In fact, anchoring effects occur even if the anchor values are determined at random and therefore clearly do not constitute helpful information. In much the same way, similarity and dissimilarity testing consequences hold even if the critical stimuli have little informational value. Social comparison standards, for example, influence self-evaluations even if they are so extreme that they clearly do not provide valuable information about the self (Mussweiler et al., 2004a). This suggests that the consequences of similarity and dissimilarity testing are indeed difficult to control.

Both similarity and dissimilarity testing therefore appear to fulfill basic criteria for automatic processes. This is generally also the case for the fourth criterion of efficiency. Given the spontaneity and frequency with which similarity and dissimilarity testing are carried out, they are also likely to be highly efficient. In fact, because both mechanisms allow judges to focus on a subset of judgment-relevant knowledge, they increase the efficiency of information processing (Mussweiler & Epstude, 2009). Nevertheless, there is reason to believe that similarity testing is even more efficient than dissimilarity testing. This is the case, because a focus on similarities appears to be inherent in early stages of any comparison, no matter whether it later focuses on similarities or differences. When considering two stimuli vis-à-vis one another, judges typically start out by considering fundamental ways in which the two are similar. It has been suggested that such an initial focus on similarities is engaged during comparison, because it helps to establish a shared relational structure among stimulus features of the target and the standard (Gentner & Markman, 1994, 1997; Medin, Goldstone, & Gentner, 1993; Ritov, 2000). Consistent with this notion of an initial similarity focus, it has been demonstrated that similar features play a particularly prominent role during comparison (Srull & Gaelick, 1983; Tversky, 1977). Thus, in most comparison situations, judges initially focus on similarities between the target and the standard. Because of this initial focus on similarities, focusing on differences in later comparison stages involves a task switch. This is not the case if judges keep their initial focus on similarities. In this respect, dissimilarity testing is more likely to involve performance-impeding task-switching costs (Meiran, 1996) than similarity testing. As a consequence, similarity testing is likely to require fewer processing resources. In addition, similarity testing is more likely to allow judges to substitute target information that is missing or difficult to obtain with information about the comparison standard (Medin et al., 1993), a mechanisms that has been described as *information transfer* (Mussweiler & Epstude, 2009). In fact, the more similar the target and standard, the more likely the information transfer (Sarason et al., 1991). This suggests that similarity testing may allow judges to consider less information about the target stimulus, because they are more likely to substitute information with readily available information about the comparison standard. For these reasons, similarity testing is likely to be more efficient than dissimilarity testing. In line with this reasoning, recent research demonstrates that participants who were induced to engage in similarity testing searched for less target information and were therefore more efficient in a comparative judgment task than participants who were induced to engage in dissimilarity testing (Corcoran, Epstude, Damisch, & Mussweiler, 2011).

A second characteristic of similarity testing is that it entails lower levels of uncertainty than dissimilarity testing. This is again the case because information transfer—the use of easily accessible standard knowledge for missing target knowledge—is more readily carried out during similarity rather than dissimilarity testing. But why does information transfer reduce judgmental uncertainty? To answer this question, one has to examine what kind of standard knowledge humans spontaneously use during judgment. Oftentimes, they use so-called routine standards (i.e., standards about which they have abundant information available) that they have frequently used in the past (Mussweiler & Rüter, 2003; Rüter & Mussweiler, 2005), and the use of which holds important efficiency advantages (Corcoran & Mussweiler, 2009). In social judgment, the self constitutes such a routine standard. When judging others, judges therefore often rely on information about themselves (Dunning & Hayes, 1996). Doing so simplifies their judgment remarkably. Rather than arduously search for judgment-relevant knowledge about a judgmental target they know very little about (e.g., a stranger), judges simply rely on the rich and readily accessible information about the standard (i.e., the self). During information processing, accessible standard information may therefore be used as a proxy for inaccessible target information. Such information transfer is likely to reduce uncertainty. This is the case, because judges are more certain about the rich and well-known information they have about a routinely used comparison standard than about the scarce and potentially novel information they have about a target about which they have rarely thought. In social judgment, for example, judges have richer and more reliable information about the self than about any other person (Kihlstrom & Cantor, 1984). Using this more reliable information about the self as a proxy for unreliable information about another person is likely to reduce the uncertainty associated with judging this person. The same holds for nonsocial judgments. The uncertainty that is associated with judging a novel target (e.g., a novel cell phone) is likely to be reduced to the extent that judges rely on the rich and reliable information they have about a potential routine standard (e.g., their own cell phones) (Mussweiler & Posten, 2012). This reasoning suggests that the mechanism that is more likely to entail information transfer, namely, similarity testing, is also likely to reduce judgmental uncertainty more substantially. This possibility is in line with a recent set of studies (Posten & Mussweiler, in preparation) demonstrating that judges who were induced to engage in similarity testing in a series of judgment tasks indicated more certainty about and bet more fictitious money on the correctness of their judgments than participants who were induced to engage in dissimilarity testing.

Taken together, this research suggests that similarity and dissimilarity testing share many core characteristics. Specifically, both mechanisms often unfold automatically—in an efficient manner, without intention and awareness. At the same time, and despite the overall similarity of both mechanisms, similarity testing differs from dissimilarity testing in at least two important ways. First, similarity testing allows for more efficient information processing than does dissimilarity testing. Second, similarity testing entails lower levels of uncertainty than dissimilarity testing. These two advantages relate to two of the biggest challenges humans face in information processing. Humans as cognitive misers (Taylor, 1981) are often overwhelmed by the multiplicity and complexity of tasks they have to master. As a consequence, they often have to rely on those mechanisms that allow them to process information efficiently. Humans also often experience as aversive the uncertainty that is inherent in many of the judgments they make (Whalen, 1998) and are motivated to reduce it. Similarity testing deals with both of these challenges and is therefore more likely to constitute the default processing strategy.

ANTECEDENTS OF SIMILARITY VERSUS DISSIMILARITY TESTING

In light of these similarities and differences between both processing mechanisms, understanding the antecedents of similarity and dissimilarity testing assumes particular importance. When do humans focus on similarities when processing incoming information, and when do they focus on differences? Research to date has identified a series of antecedents that influence which of these two alternative mechanisms unfolds. These antecedents relate to characteristics of the stimuli that are being processed, as well as to characteristics of the physical, psychological, and social context of information processing.

The most obvious class of antecedents certainly is related to characteristics of the critical stimuli that are being processed. In fact, it seems only natural to assume that judges are more likely to focus on similarities when processing stimuli that to start with are more similar. In line with this general notion, ample evidence demonstrates that the assimilative consequences of similarity testing are indeed more likely to occur for stimuli that, for example, share a distinct characteristic (Brown, Novick, Lord, & Richards, 1992), belong to the same category (Brewer & Weber, 1994; Mussweiler & Bodenhausen, 2002), and are close on the judgmental dimension itself (Mussweiler et al., 2004a) or on a related dimension (Lockwood & Kunda, 1997; for a more detailed review, see Mussweiler, 2003).

In addition to these characteristics of the processed stimuli themselves, factors characterizing the physical, psychological, and social context in which information processing takes place have also been found to influence whether judges focus on similarities or differences. With respect to the physical context, for example, it has been demonstrated that ambient physical warmth fosters a focus on similarities and therefore similarity testing with its ensuing consequences (IJzerman & Semin, 2009; Steinmetz & Mussweiler, 2011). In line with this possibility, recent research suggests that physical warmth and interpersonal similarity are intimately linked. Experiencing physical warmth, for example, fosters the perception of social proximity: Participants holding a warm beverage see themselves as closer to another person than participants holding a cold beverage (IJzerman & Semin, 2009). In light of the fact that social proximity is in turn closely related to similarity, this finding suggests that warmth may induce similarity testing. The results of a recent set of studies (Steinmetz & Mussweiler, 2011) support this possibility and demonstrate that participants who process information in a warm rather than in a cold setting see a given stimulus set as more similar and assimilate their self-evaluations more toward a given social comparison standard. Warm physical contexts therefore appear to trigger similarity testing.

Similar influences on the operation of similarity versus dissimilarity testing have been described for distinct psychological contexts. In particular, specific information-processing styles, as well as specific bodily experiences, have been suggested to foster similarity versus dissimilarity testing. With regard to processing styles, it has been suggested that participants who process information with a more global processing style that focuses on the overall stimulus configuration are more likely to engage in similarity testing, whereas participants who process information with a more local processing style that focuses on details are more likely to engage in dissimilarity testing (Förster, 2009). As a consequence of this connection, the operation of similarity versus dissimilarity testing is also indirectly fostered by those factors that induce judges to engage more in global versus local processing, such as temporal distance, regulatory focus, or motivational orientations (Förster, 2009; Kuschel, Förster, & Denzler, 2010). In addition to these influences of specific processing styles, similarity versus dissimilarity testing can also be directly triggered by specific proprioceptive experiences that have become associated with and therefore constitute embodied substrates of similarity. In fact, just as physically leaning forward induces judges to think more ahead (Miles, Karpinska, Lumsden, & Macrae, 2010), physically performing converging arm movements that bring both arms together induces judges to see stimuli as more similar and to assimilate to a given social standard (Steinmetz & Mussweiler, 2013).

Finally, characteristics of the social context may induce similarity versus dissimilarity testing. One particularly important social context variable is interpersonal trust versus distrust, two core elements of humans' social life that shape each and every social interaction. In situations that are characterized by trust, people typically rely on routine information-processing strategies. In contrast, a state of distrust signals a potentially harmful environment and fosters the use of nonroutine strategies. This fundamental processing difference for trust versus distrust is apparent on different levels of information processing. On the most basic level of semantic activation, for example, distrust fosters the spontaneous activation of incongruent (Schul, Mayo, & Burnstein, 2004) and remote (Mayer & Mussweiler, 2011) associations. On higher levels of information processing, distrust enhances cognitive flexibility and creativity (Mayer & Mussweiler, 2011), leads to the generation of counterscenarios (Schul, Burnstein, & Bardi, 1996), and reduces the correspondence bias (Fein, Hilton, & Miller, 1990). These findings demonstrate that distrust induces people to deviate from their default ways of information processing. Applying this basic insight to the interplay of similarity and dissimilarity testing suggests that judges may deviate from the default processing strategy of similarity testing and engage in dissimilarity testing under distrust. In line with this possibility, it has been demonstrated that distrust indeed induces judges to see stimuli as less similar and to show less of the assimilative judgmental effects that are the signature of similarity testing (Posten & Mussweiler, 2013). These findings demonstrate that the operation of similarity versus dissimilarity testing depends on a core social context variable such as trust versus distrust.

On a more abstract level, these findings also suggest that whether similarity or dissimilarity testing is engaged depends on whether—for whatever reason—judges rely on their routine ways of information processing. Whenever judges leave their beaten tracks of social thinking, they are likely also to deviate from their routine to engage in similarity testing. Distrust constitutes an important social context variable that pushes judges toward the nonroutine mechanism of dissimilarity testing (Posten & Mussweiler, 2013). Distrust, however, is clearly not the only variable that signals potentially harmful environments and therefore induces judges to engage in nonroutine information processing. Negative mood, for example, serves similar signaling functions and has been shown to make judges process information more thoroughly and therefore in less routine ways (Schwarz, 1990, 1998). This suggests that humans may be more likely to engage in dissimilarity testing if they are in a negative mood. Furthermore, dissimilarity testing as the more capacity-consuming processing alternative (Corcoran et al., 2011) is more likely to be engaged if judges have the processing capacities available that this nonroutine mechanism requires. Whenever judges' processing capacities are drained because they are tired (Bodenhausen, 1990), depleted (Baumeister, Bratslavsky, Muraven, & Tice, 1998), or busy doing something else (Bargh, 1982; Wickens, 1976), they are likely to resort to the routine mechanism of similarity testing. In line with this possibility, the assimilative effects that constitute the signature consequence of similarity testing are more likely to occur under such suboptimal processing conditions (e.g., Bodenhausen, 1990; Bodenhausen & Lichtenstein, 1987; Martin, Seta, & Crelia, 1990).

Taken together, these findings demonstrate that the interplay of similarity and dissimilarity testing is shaped by the physical, psychological, and social context of information processing. Because similarity testing is the default mechanism that allows for more efficient information processing, it is more likely to operate if conditions that foster routine information processing are in place.

UBIQUITY OF SIMILARITY VERSUS DISSIMILARITY TESTING

Similarity and dissimilarity testing constitute ubiquitous mechanisms in social information processing. Not only do induced foci on similarities versus differences yield assimilative versus contrastive effects across a variety of judgmental, affective, and behavioral paradigms, these respective foci also appear to be spontaneously activated whenever the pertinent conditions are met. Merely putting participants in a physical context with warm ambient temperatures (Steinmetz & Mussweiler, 2011) or in a social context that is characterized by trust (Posten & Mussweiler, 2013), for example, is sufficient to make them focus more on similarities in an unrelated stimulus set. As a consequence, their psychological reactions show the assimilative consequences that are the signature of similarity testing. The diverse nature of antecedents that have been identified to induce a similarity versus dissimilarity focus suggests that these foci are omnipresent in human social information processing. If similarity is indeed the "keel and backbone of our thinking" (James, 1890/1950, p. 459) and if similarity is indeed spontaneously and effortlessly extracted from any stimulus set (Markman & Gentner, 2005), it is likely to feed into any instance of social information processing. In line with this general proposition, the research described in this chapter suggests that the two alternative mechanisms of similarity versus dissimilarity testing contribute to many of the core phenomena of social psychological research.

REFERENCES

Baillargeon, R. (1993). The object concept revisited: New directions in the investigation of infants' physical knowledge. In C. E. Granrud (Ed.), *Visual perception and cognition in infancy* (pp. 265–315). Hillsdale, NJ: Erlbaum.

Bargh, J. A. (1982). Attention and automaticity in the processing of self-relevant information. *Journal of Personality and Social Psychology, 43*, 425–436.

Bargh, J. A. (1994). The four horsemen of automaticity: Awareness, intention, efficiency, and control in social cognition. In R. S. Wyer & T. K. Srull (Eds.), *Handbook of social cognition, Vol. 1: Basic processes* (2nd ed., pp. 1–40). Hillsdale, NJ: Erlbaum.

Bargh, J. A. (1997). The automaticity of everyday life. In R. S. Wyer (Ed.), *Advances in social cognition* (Vol. 10, pp. 1–61). Mahwah, NJ: Erlbaum.

Baumeister, R. F., Bratslavsky, E., Muraven, M., & Tice, D. M. (1998). Ego depletion: Is the active self a limited resource? *Journal of Personality and Social Psychology, 74*, 1252–1265.

Bernhard, H., Fischbacher, U., & Fehr, E. (2006). Parochial altruism in humans. *Nature, 442*, 912–915.

Bittner, J. V. (2011). Implicit processing goals combine with explicit goal standards to motivate performance through underlying comparison processes. *European Journal of Social Psychology, 41*, 210–219.

Bodenhausen, G. V. (1990). Stereotypes as judgmental heuristics: Evidence of circadian variations in discrimination. *Psychological Science, 1*, 319–322.

Bodenhausen, G. V., & Lichtenstein, M. (1987). Social stereotypes and information-processing strategies: The impact of task complexity. *Journal of Personality and Social Psychology, 52*, 871–880.

Brewer, M. B. (1979). In-group bias in the minimal intergroup situation: A cognitive-motivational analysis. *Psychological Bulletin, 86*, 307–324.

Brewer, M. B., & Weber, J. G. (1994). Self-evaluation effects of interpersonal versus intergroup social comparison. *Journal of Personality and Social Psychology, 66*, 268–275.

Brown, J. D., Novick, N. J., Lord, K. A., & Richards, J. M. (1992). When Gulliver travels: Social context, psychological closeness, and self-appraisals. *Journal of Personality and Social Psychology, 62*, 717–727.

Byrne, D. (1997). An overview (and underview) of research and theory within the attraction paradigm. *Journal of Social and Personal Relationships, 14*, 417–431.

Chen, Y., & Li, S. X. (2009). Group identity and social preferences. *American Economic Review, 99*, 431–457.

Corcoran, K., Epstude, K., Damisch, L., & Mussweiler, T. (2011). Fast similarities: Efficiency advantages of similarity-focused comparisons. *Journal of Experimental Psychology: Learning, Memory, and Cognition, 37*, 1280–1286.

Corcoran, K., Hundhammer, T., & Mussweiler, T. (2009). A tool for thought!: When comparative thinking reduces stereotyping effects. *Journal of Experimental Social Psychology, 45*, 1008–1011.

Corcoran, K., & Mussweiler, T. (2009). The efficiency of social comparisons with routine standards. *Social Cognition, 27*, 939–948.

Crusius, J., & Mussweiler, T. (2012). To achieve or not to achieve?: Comparative mindsets elicit assimilation and contrast in goal priming. *European Journal of Social Psychology, 42*, 780–788.

Damisch, L., Mussweiler, T., & Plessner, H. (2006). Olympic medals as fruits of comparison?: Assimilation and contrast in sequential performance judgments. *Journal of Experimental Psychology: Applied, 12*, 166–178.

Deaux, K. (1996). Social identification. In E. T. Higgins & A. W. Kruglanski (Eds.), *Social psychology: Handbook of basic principles* (pp. 777–798). New York: Guilford Press.

Dunning, D., & Hayes, A. F. (1996). Evidence for egocentric comparison in social judgment. *Journal of Personality and Social Psychology, 71*, 213–229.

Epstude, K., & Mussweiler, T. (2009). What you feel is how you compare: How comparisons influence the social induction of affect. *Emotion, 9*, 1–14.

Fein, S., Hilton, J. L., & Miller, D. T. (1990). Suspicion of ulterior motivation and the correspondence bias. *Journal of Personality and Social Psychology, 58*, 753–764.

Förster, J. (2009). Relations between perceptual and conceptual scope: How global versus local processing fits a focus on similarity versus dissimilarity. *Journal of Experimental Psychology: General, 138*, 88–111.

Gentner, D., & Markman, A. B. (1994). Structural alignment in comparison: No difference without similarity. *Psychological Science, 5*, 152–158.

Gentner, D., & Markman, A. B. (1997). Structure mapping in analogy and similarity. *American Psychologist, 52*, 45–56.

Haddock, G., Macrae, C. N., & Fleck, S. (2002). Syrian science and smart supermodels: On the when and how of perception–behavior effects. *Social Cognition, 20*, 4691–4479.

Herr, P. M. (1986). Consequences of priming: Judgment and behavior. *Journal of Personality and Social Psychology, 51*, 1106–1115.

Hilmert, C. J., Kulik, J. A., & Christenfeld, N. J. S. (2006). Positive and negative opinion modeling: The influence of another's similarity and dissimilarity. *Journal of Personality and Social Psychology, 90*, 440–452.

Hintzman, D. L. (1986). "Schema abstraction" in a multiple-trace memory model. *Psychological Review, 93*, 411–428.

IJzerman, H., & Semin, G. R. (2009). The thermometer of social relations: Mapping social proximity on temperature. *Psychological Science, 20*, 1214–1220.

James, W. (1950). *The principles of psychology*. Oxford, UK: Dover. (Original work published 1890)

Kahneman, D., & Miller, D. T. (1986). Norm theory: Comparing reality to its alternatives. *Psychological Review, 93*, 136–153.

Kihlstrom, J. F., & Cantor, N. (1984). Mental representations of the self. In L. Berkowitz (Ed.), *Advances in experimental social psychology* (Vol. 17, pp. 1–48). San Diego: Academic Press.

Klayman, J., & Ha, Y. (1987). Confirmation, disconfirmation, and information in hypothesis testing. *Psychological Review, 94*, 211–228.

Kruglanski, A. W., & Mayseless, O. (1990). Classic and current social comparison research: Expanding the perspective. *Psychological Bulletin, 108*, 195–208.

Kuschel, S., Förster, J., & Denzler, M. (2010). Going beyond information given: How approach versus avoidance cues influence access to higher order information. *Social Psychological and Personality Science, 1*, 4–11.

Lockwood, P., & Kunda, Z. (1997). Superstars and me: Predicting the impact of role models on the self. *Journal of Personality and Social Psychology, 73*, 91–103.

Markman, A. B., & Gentner, D. (2005). Nonintentional similarity processing. In R. R. Hassin, J. S. Uleman, & J. A. Bargh (Eds.), *The new unconscious* (pp. 107–137). New York: Oxford University Press.

Martin, L. L., Seta, J. J., & Crelia, R. A. (1990). Assimilation and contrast as a function of people's willingness and ability to expend effort in forming an impression. *Journal of Personality and Social Psychology, 59*, 27–37.

Mayer, J., & Mussweiler, T. (2011). Suspicious spirits, flexible minds: When distrust enhances creativity. *Journal of Personality and Social Psychology, 101*, 1262–1277.

McPherson, M., Smith-Lovin, L., & Cook, J. M. (2001). Birds of a feather: Homophily in social networks. *Annual Review of Sociology, 27*, 415–444.

Medin, D. L., Goldstone, R. L., & Gentner, D. (1993). Respects for similarity. *Psychological Review, 100*, 254–278.

Medin, D. L., Goldstone, R. L., & Markman, A. B. (1995). Comparison and choice: Relations between similarity processes and decision processes. *Psychonomic Bulletin & Review, 2*, 1–19.

Medin, D. L., & Schaffer, M. M. (1978). Context theory of classification learning. *Psychological Review, 85*, 207–238.

Meiran, N. (1996). Reconfiguration of processing mode prior to task performance. *Journal of Experimental Psychology: Learning, Memory, and Cognition, 22*, 1423–1442.

Miles, L. K., Karpinska, K., Lumsden, J., & Macrae, C. N. (2010). The meandering mind: Vection and mental time travel. *PLoS ONE, 5*, e10825.

Mussweiler, T. (2001). "Seek and ye shall find": Antecedents of assimilation and contrast in social comparison. *European Journal of Social Psychology, 31*, 499–509.

Mussweiler, T. (2003). Comparison processes in social judgment: Mechanisms and consequences. *Psychological Review, 110*, 472–489.

Mussweiler, T., & Bodenhausen, G. V. (2002). I know you are, but what am I?: Self-evaluative consequences of judging in-group and outgroup members. *Journal of Personality and Social Psychology, 82*, 19–32.

Mussweiler, T., & Damisch, L. (2008). Going back to Donald: How comparisons shape judgmental priming effects. *Journal of Personality and Social Psychology, 95*, 1295–1315.

Mussweiler, T., & Englich, B. (2005). Subliminal anchoring: Judgmental consequences and underlying mechanisms. *Organizational Behavior and Human Decision Processes, 98*, 133–143.

Mussweiler, T., & Epstude, K. (2009). Relatively fast!: Efficiency advantages of comparative thinking. *Journal of Experimental Psychology: General, 138*, 1–21.

Mussweiler, T., & Posten, A.-C. (2012). Relatively certain! Comparative thinking reduces uncertainty. *Cognition, 122*, 236–240.

Mussweiler, T., & Rüter, K. (2003). What friends are for! The use of routine standards in social comparison. *Journal of Personality and Social Psychology, 85*, 467–481.

Mussweiler, T., Rüter, K., & Epstude, K. (2004a). The ups and downs of social comparison: Mechanisms of assimilation and contrast. *Journal of Personality and Social Psychology, 87*, 832–844.

Mussweiler, T., Rüter, K., & Epstude, K. (2004b). The man who wasn't there: Subliminal social comparison standards influence self-evaluation. *Journal of Experimental Social Psychology, 40*, 689–696.

Mussweiler, T., & Strack, F. (2000). The use of category and exemplar knowledge in the solution of anchoring tasks. *Journal of Personality and Social Psychology, 78*, 1038–1052.

Posten, A.-C., & Mussweiler, T. (in preparation). *That certain something! Focusing on similarities reduces judgmental uncertainty.*

Posten, A.-C., & Mussweiler, T. (2013). When distrust frees your mind: The stereotype-reducing effects of distrust. *Journal of Personality and Social Psychology, 105*, 567–584.

Reed, S. K., Ernst, G. W., & Banerji, R. (1974). The role of analogy in transfer between similar problem states. *Cognitive Psychology, 6*, 436–450.

Ritov, I. (2000). The role of expectations in comparisons. *Psychological Review, 107*, 345–357.

Rüter, K., & Mussweiler, T. (2005). Bonds of friendship: Comparative self-evaluations evoke the use of routine standards. *Social Cognition, 23*, 137–160.

Sanbonmatsu, D. M., Posavac, S. S., Kardes, F. R., & Mantel, S. P. (1998). Selective hypothesis testing. *Psychonomic Bulletin & Review, 5*, 197–220.

Sarason, B. R., Pierce, G. R., Shearin, E. N., Sarason, I. G., Waltz, J. A., & Poppe, L. (1991). Perceived social support and working models of self and actual others. *Journal of Personality and Social Psychology, 60*, 273–287.

Schul, Y., Burnstein, E., & Bardi, A. (1996). Dealing with deceptions that are difficult to detect: Encoding and judgment as a function of preparing to receive invalid information. *Journal of Experimental Social Psychology, 32*, 228–253.

Schul, Y., Mayo, R., & Burnstein, E. (2004). Encoding under trust and distrust: The spontaneous activation of incongruent cognitions. *Journal of Personality and Social Psychology, 86*, 668–679.

Schwarz, N. (1990). Feelings as information: Informational and motivational functions of affective states. In E. Tory Higgins & R. M. Sorrentino (Eds.), *Handbook of motivation and cognition: Foundations of social behavior* (Vol. 2, pp. 527–561). New York: Guilford Press.

Schwarz, N. (1998). Warmer and more social: Recent developments in cognitive social psychology. *Annual Review of Sociology, 24*, 239–264.

Smith, E. E., Shoben, E. J., & Rips, L. J. (1974). Structure and process in semantic memory: A featural model for semantic decisions. *Psychological Review, 81*, 214–241.

Smith, E. R. (1994). Procedural knowledge and processing strategies in social cognition. In R. S. Wyer & T. K. Srull (Eds.), *Handbook of social cognition: Vol. 1.: Basic processes* (2nd ed., pp. 99–151). Hillsdale, NJ: Erlbaum.

Snyder, M., & Swann, W. B. (1978). Hypothesis-testing processes in social interaction. *Journal of Personality and Social Psychology, 36,* 1202–1212.

Srull, T. K., & Gaelick, L. (1983). General principles and individual differences in the self as a habitual reference point: An examination of self–other judgments of similarity. *Social Cognition, 2,* 108–121.

Steinmetz, J., & Mussweiler, T. (2011). Breaking the ice: How physical warmth shapes social comparison consequences. *Journal of Experimental Social Psychology, 47,* 1025–1028.

Steinmetz, J., & Mussweiler, T. (2013). *Hands together: How moving your arms affects self-evaluation.* Unpublished manuscript.

Strack, F., & Hannover, B. (1996). Awareness of influence as a precondition for implementing correctional goals. In P. M. Gollwitzer & J. A. Bargh (Eds.), *The psychology of action: Linking cognition and motivation to behavior* (pp. 579–596). New York: Guilford Press.

Strack, F., & Mussweiler, T. (1997). Explaining the enigmatic anchoring effect: Mechanisms of selective accessibility. *Journal of Personality and Social Psychology, 73,* 437–446.

Tajfel, H., Billig, M. G., Bundy, R. P., & Flament, C. (1971). Social categorization and intergroup behaviour. *European Journal of Social Psychology, 1,* 149–178.

Taylor, S. E. (1981). The interface of cognitive and social psychology. In J. H. Harvey (Ed.), *Cognition, social behavior, and the environment* (pp. 189–211). Hillsdale, NJ: Erlbaum.

Trope, Y., & Bassok, M. (1982). Confirmatory and diagnosing strategies in social information gathering. *Journal of Personality and Social Psychology, 43,* 22–34.

Trope, Y., & Liberman, A. (1996). Social hypothesis testing: Cognitive and motivational mechanisms. In E. T. Higgins & A. W. Kruglanski (Eds.), *Social psychology: Handbook of basic principles* (pp. 239–270). New York: Guilford Press.

Tversky, A. (1977). Features of similarity. *Psychological Review, 84,* 327–352.

Tversky, A., & Kahneman, D. (1974). Judgment under uncertainty: Heuristics and biases. *Science, 185,* 1124–1131.

Whalen, P. J. (1998). Fear, vigilance, and ambiguity: Initial neuroimaging studies of the human amygdala. *Current Directions in Psychological Science, 7,* 177–188.

Wickens, C. D. (1976). The effects of divided attention on information processing in manual tracking. *Journal of Experimental Psychology: Human Perception and Performance, 2,* 1–13.

Wilson, T. D., & Brekke, N. (1994). Mental contamination and mental correction: Unwanted influences on judgments and evaluations. *Psychological Bulletin, 116,* 117–142.

CHAPTER 23

Visual versus Verbal Thinking and Dual-Process Moral Cognition

Elinor Amit, Sara Gottlieb, and Joshua D. Greene

Moral judgments are not produced by a unified "moral faculty." Instead, they are influenced by a combination of automatic emotional responses and controlled cognitive processes with distinctive cognitive profiles (Cushman, Young, & Hauser, 2006; Greene, Morelli, Lowenberg, Nystrom, & Cohen, 2008; Moore, Clark, & Kane, 2008; Paxton, Ungar, & Greene, 2011) and neural substrates (Greene, Sommerville, Nystrom, Darley, & Cohen, 2001; Greene, Nystrom, Engell, Darley, & Cohen, 2004; Mendez, Anderson, & Shapira, 2005; Koenigs et al., 2007; Ciaramelli, Muccioli, Ladavas, & Di Pellegrino, 2007). This dual-process framework (Shiffrin & Schneider, 1977; Sloman, 1996; Loewenstein, 1996; Chaiken & Trope, 1999; Metcalfe & Mischel, 1999; Lieberman, Gaunt, Gilbert, & Trope, 2002; Stanovich & West, 2000; Kahneman, 2003, 2011) answers some questions while raising many others, including the following: What triggers the automatic emotional responses that influence our moral judgments? What accounts for the variability in these "gut reactions," both from person to person and situation to situation? Parallel questions arise concerning the influence of controlled cognition on moral judgment. In this chapter, we address these questions, focusing on the role of domain-general cognitive processes. More specifically, we consider the respective influences of *visual* and *verbal* thinking on moral judgment.

First, we briefly review the most relevant literature on automatic versus controlled processes in moral judgment and decision making. Next, we discuss the distinctive features of visual versus verbal processing, then present a set of related hypotheses concerning the respective influences of visual and verbal thinking on moral judgment, followed by evidence indicating a special connection between visual imagery and deontological moral judgment. We also consider a possible relationship between visual and verbal cognition on the one hand, and the primary and secondary emotion distinction on the other. Finally, we conclude with some speculative thoughts concerning the relationships among the various cognitive distinctions discussed in this chapter.

MORAL DILEMMAS AND DUAL-PROCESS MORAL COGNITION

We and others have used moral dilemmas in experiments aimed at breaking moral judgment down into component processes. (Early examples include Greene et al., 2001, 2004, 2008; Mendez et al., 2005; Koenigs et al., 2007; Ciaramelli et al., 2007; Cushman et al., 2006. Earlier work examined moral dilemmas, but without a dual-process framework: Petrinovich, O'Neill, & Jorgensen, 1993, Mikhail, 2000). This is a useful strategy given that moral dilemmas tend to erupt at the fault lines between competing cognitive processes (Cushman & Greene, 2012). On a philosophical level, these dilemmas capture the pervasive tension between the rights of the individual and the greater good (Greene, 2007; Paxton, Bruni, & Greene, 2013). On a cognitive level, they reveal the dual-process structure of moral cognition. For example, in the classic *footbridge* dilemma (Thomson, 1985), one can save five lives by pushing an innocent person into the path of a runaway trolley. Here, *deontological* judgments favoring the rights of the individual ("It's wrong to push the man, even if it saves more lives") are preferentially supported by automatic emotional responses (Greene et al., 2001; Mendez et al., 2005; Koenigs et al., 2007; Ciaramelli et al., 2007), while *utilitarian* (or *consequentialist*) judgments favoring the greater good ("Better to push and save more lives") are preferentially supported by controlled cognitive processes (Greene et al., 2004, 2008).

Before moving on, we wish to clarify our use of the potentially misleading word *cognitive*. It sometimes refers to a class of psychological processes to be contrasted with more emotional or affective processes, as in the journal *Social Cognitive and Affective Neuroscience*. At other times, *cognitive* refers more broadly to psychological process that may be characterized in terms of information processing (i.e., all psychological processes), as in the journal *Trends in Cognitive Sciences*, which covers research in all areas of psychology including emotion/affect. Emotions are "cognitive" in the second sense but not the first. Here we avoid the more narrow use of *cognitive*, which we regard as a relic from a time when psychologists failed to appreciate the information-processing nature of emotions. When we wish to distinguish automatic emotional responses from the more controlled processes on the opposite side of our dual-process framework, we refer to the latter as *controlled* processes or *controlled cognitive* processes, with no implication that emotions are not "cognitive" in the broader, information-processing sense. Likewise, we recognize that not all automatic processes are emotional, as in, for example, early visual processing.

The distinction between automatic and controlled processes is familiar enough, but it is used by different researchers to contrast different clusters of characteristics. Along with the core automatic–controlled distinction, researchers often distinguish between processes that are fast versus slow, unconscious versus conscious, implicit versus explicit, effortless versus effortful, intuitive versus reflective, more emotional versus less emotional, and those that require minimal versus substantial use of central cognitive resources (Evans, 2008; Kahneman, 2003). In the context of moral judgment, we believe that all of these distinctions apply, but with some caveats. In our view—indeed, in any sensible view of moral psychology—automatic and controlled processes interact, which makes teasing apart their respective contributions challenging. Controlled, conscious, reflective processes may bring to light new information (e.g., through explicit reasoning) or highlight old information (e.g., through heightened attention or willful acts of imagination). These private mental acts may then trigger automatic emotional responses. For example, one might respond to an imagined scene much as one would respond to the scene itself. But in the case of the imagined scene the response is triggered automatically by an endogenous controlled cognitive process rather than by an external stimulus. (See Cushman, Gray, Gaffey, & Mendes, 2012, described below.) Having had such a response, one might become consciously aware of the response, if not the complete chain of cognitive events that triggered it. One might reflect on that response, deliberate about it, and ultimately override its action tendency. Thus, when it comes to complex judgments and decisions, it may be rare for a behavioral response to be purely automatic, and it may be impossible for a behavioral response to be purely controlled: Controlled cognitive processes must have something more automatic on which to operate (Miller & Cohen, 2001). Nevertheless, it may be possible to identify distinctive influences of automatic and controlled processes on moral judgment, as we explain below.

Initial evidence for our dual-process theory of moral judgment came from functional magnetic resonance imaging (fMRI) studies demonstrating the engagement of brain regions associated with emotion and social cognition in response to "personal" dilemmas such as the footbridge case (Greene et al., 2001, 2004; Schaich Borg, Hynes, Van Horn, Grafton, & Sinnott-Armstrong, 2006). These regions include the ventromedial prefrontal cortex (vmPFC) and the amygdala. A study of patients with frontotemporal dementia (FTD), which produces "emotional blunting," provided more direct causal evidence for the connection between emotional responses and deontological judgment (Mendez et al., 2005). Here, patients with FTD, relative to control subjects/patients, were three times more likely to favor pushing the man off the footbridge in the name of the greater good. Subsequent studies examining patients with vmPFC damage underscored this point, showing that patients with such emotion-related damage make more utilitarian judgments (Koenigs et al., 2007; Ciaramelli et al., 2007; Moretto, Ladavas, Mattioli, & di Pellegrino, 2010; Thomas, Croft, & Tranel, 2011). Likewise, a positive emotion induction can increase utilitarian judgment, counteracting the negative emotional response to pushing the man (Valedesolo & DeSteno, 2006), though this does not work for all positive emotions (Strohminger, Lewis, & Meyer, 2011). Other studies have linked deontological judgment to heightened physiological responses (Moretto et al., 2010; Navarrete, McDonald, Mott, & Asher, 2012, Cushman et al., 2012) and normal conscious access to one's emotional states, as compared to individuals with degrees of alexithymia (Koven, 2011). On a molecular level, deontological judgment is increased by citalopram, a selective serotonin reuptake inhibitor (SSRI) that, in the short-term, heightens certain kinds of emotional responses by increasing the availability of serotonin (Crockett, Clark, Hauser, & Robbins, 2010). Conversely, deontological judgment can be reduced by the anti-anxiety drug lorazepam (Perkins et al., 2012).

On the other side of the dual-process equation, many studies associate utilitarian judgments favoring the greater good with the engagement of controlled cognition. Brain regions associated with cognitive control, most notably parts of dorsolateral PFC, exhibit increased activity when people make utilitarian judgments (Greene et al., 2004). More recent behavioral studies implicate controlled cognition by showing that cognitive load selectively interferes with utilitarian judgment (Greene et al., 2008, Trémolière, Neys, & Bonnefon, 2012), that utilitarian judgment increases with deliberation time (Suter & Hertwig, 2011), and that utilitarian judgment can be increased by inducing a more reflective mindset (Paxton et al., 2011). Other correlational studies associate utilitarian judgment with increased "need for cognition" (Bartels, 2008) and (for some instances of utilitarian judgment) working memory capacity (Moore et al., 2008). Some have argued that utilitarian judgments in response to moral dilemmas reflect an absence of concern about doing harm rather than a moral concern for the greater good. Most notably, Bartels and Pizzaro (2011) found that utilitarian judgments are positively related to various antisocial personality characteristics, including psychopathy and Machiavellianism. However, more recent evidence (Conway & Gawronski, 2013) generated using the "process dissociation" procedure (Jacoby, 1991) casts doubt on this view by distinguishing lack of concern about harming people (what one might call "un-deontology") from positive utilitarian moral concerns. Conway and Gawronski (2013) show that deontological and utilitarian motivations are distinct moral motivations with distinct cognitive profiles, consistent with the dual-process theory described earlier: Subjects with stronger deontological inclinations tend to be higher in empathic concern, and deontological inclinations are selectively increased by an empathy manipulation. In contrast, subjects with stronger utilitarian inclinations tend to be higher in "need for cognition" (Cacioppo & Petty, 1982), and utilitarian inclinations are selectively decreased by cognitive load.

THE NOT SPECIFICALLY MORAL DOMAIN

For centuries philosophers and folk psychologists have referred to a "moral sense" or "moral faculty," an idea that retains proponents today (Mikhail 2000, 2011; Hauser, 2006). As noted earlier, a strong form of psychological faculty for morality has been ruled out, as moral judgment involves the operations of distinct and often competing cognitive systems. The mere "involvement" of diverse cognitive systems does not, by itself, challenge the idea of a core "moral faculty." People who respond to moral questions must, at the very least, rely on auditory or visual cognition to receive information about the question at hand. Likewise, moral judges must use their capacities for language, memory, motor responding, and so forth, in familiar and routine ways. But the dual-process theory outlined earlier poses a deeper challenge to theories positing a unified moral faculty. If we are correct, it is not just that multiple systems are "involved." Instead, different cognitive systems underwrite different kinds of moral values. In other words, moral cognition is fractured in a deep way.

Much of the idea of a "moral faculty" might be retained if these distinct cognitive systems were dedicated specifically to moral judgment, but we have already seen evidence that they are not. For example, we know that various forms of cognitive load interfere specifically with utilitarian moral judgment (Greene et al., 2008; Trémolière et al., 2012; Conway & Gawronski, 2013). The concurrent tasks used in these load paradigms have nothing to do with morality (e.g., hitting a button when a certain number appears) Thus, these cognitive load experiments show that moral judgment depends, at least to some extent, on domain-general processing. More to the point, these studies show that *specific kinds* of moral judgment *depend preferentially* on domain-general processing. In other words, the role that controlled cognition plays in moral judgment is not merely like the role that auditory processing plays in hearing about moral dilemmas.

We have seen similar evidence on the emotional side. Once again, positive emotions (more specifically, "mirth") can have a distinctive influence on moral judgment (Valdesolo & DeSteno, 2006), indicating that moral emotions exist in an affective space that is shared with emotional responses that are not naturally regarded as "moral." This should come as no surprise given that moral considerations must be weighed against other considerations that are not necessarily moral, a capability that would appear to require a "common currency" for moral and nonmoral values (Chib, Rangel, Shimojo, & O'Doherty, 2009). The most direct evidence for this idea comes from Shenhav and Greene (2010), who conducted an fMRI study in which they varied the magnitude and probability of morally salient outcomes. For example, abandoning one drowning person might enable one to save five others with a probability of 50%, or 20 others with a probability of 40%, and so on. They provided evidence that moral judgments such as these rely on domain-general valuation mechanisms, ones that also represent and integrate information about probability and magnitude in nonmoral contexts, such as self-interested economic decision making (Knutson, Taylor, Kaufman, Peterson, & Glover, 2005). Thus, core representations of value in moral judgment are probably not representations of *moral* value per se, but simply value in a more generic sense. Furthermore, it seems that emotional responses, such as the negative response to pushing the man off the footbridge, depend in surprising ways on how our brains represent actions: People are more likely to approve of using a person as a trolley-stopper if, instead of pushing the man directly off the footbridge, one hits a switch that drops him through a trap door (Cushman et al., 2006; Greene et al., 2009).

The foregoing discussion indicates that a lot of moral thinking is not specifically moral thinking: Moral judgment depends in substantive ways on cognitive systems that perform rather general (not specifically moral) functions. This naturally prompts the question: What other kinds of not specifically moral thinking have distinctive influences on moral judgment? Here we consider the respective contributions of *visual* and *verbal* thinking to moral judgment. We begin with a discussion of distinctive features of visual and verbal thinking.

THE ADAPTIVE DESIGN OF INFORMATION PROCESSING: VISUAL VERSUS VERBAL

Pictures are concrete representations that in nearly all cases[1] physically resemble their referent objects. They are *analog* representations (Goodman, 1976). In contrast, words in nearly all cases[2] represent more abstractly and bear more arbitrary relations to their referents. Words are *digital* representations that comprise a finite set of discrete units.

Words typically correspond to categories and refer to a broad range of concrete objects (Glaser, 1992; Paivio, 1986). Consider, for example, visual and verbal representations of a chair or the concept "chair." A picture of a chair will typically represent some specific chair, with a specific number of legs, adjoined at specific angles, etc. But the word *chair* is far more general.There is effectively an infinite number of ways in which one can draw a chair, or even a kitchen chair, or a red kitchen chair with four legs. Words are, once again, more abstract.

One of the most influential theories concerning differences in the processing of pictures and words is the dual-coding theory (DCT, Paivio, 1986). According to DCT, there are two separate representation systems. One is specialized for representing information conveyed by spatial, nonverbal stimuli, and the other is specialized for representing information conveyed verbally. Words are initially represented by the verbal system, and scenes and pictures are initially represented by the nonverbal or imagery system. In subsequent processing, each stimulus can be coded by the other system as well—hence the possibility of dual coding. The theory does not posit mutually exclusive processing of words and pictures: Each stimulus can be encoded and processed by each of the two systems. The major explanatory variable in the theory is the imaginability of the input. Pictures are readily imaginable. Concrete words are also easily imaginable; therefore, such words are likely to be encoded by the image system as well as the verbal system. In contrast, abstract words are likely to be encoded by the verbal system only. This difference explains the superiority in memory of concrete over abstract words, and, often, of pictures over words.

The concrete–abstract distinction in dual coding theory is relevant, but, in our view, it does not map perfectly onto the distinction between pictures and words. According to DCT, in principle, words can be as concrete as pictures (although pictures cannot be as abstract as some words). When concreteness (or abstractness) is comparable, processing is comparable according to dual coding theory. In our view, words are always more abstract than pictures; therefore, we expect to see some reliable differences between them. Concrete words, such as the word *table*, and pictures, such as an outline drawing of a table, are close relatives in dual coding theory. Both stimuli are dual-coded by both systems. Consequently, comparable performance is expected with such stimuli. In our view, there is an inevitable difference in concreteness–abstractness between the word *table* and the picture of a table, even though both items are highly imaginable. The reason is that the word *table* encompasses a larger category (innumerable individual tables), while a picture of a table represents a specific table. As a result, pictures are categorized better than words (including concrete, readily imaginable words), are less potent primes, are rendered less accurate by incidental changes, and impart a sense of proximity. All of these features go beyond those posited by the dual coding theory.

Amit, Algom, and Trope (2009) have related this difference in abstractness between visual and verbal representations to another important cognitive dimension, that of *psychological distance* (Trope & Liberman, 2010). They hypothesize that people preferentially represent items that are psychologically proximal (either spatially, temporally, or socially) in visual format and preferentially represent psychologically distal items in verbal format. This preference exists in two ways: as a tendency to represent some items visually and other items verbally, and as a processing advantage when items are represented in the preferred manner. This medium–distance hypothesis builds on construal-level theory (CLT; Trope & Liberman, 2010), according to which people prefer to represent information more abstractly when they are more distant from the target of thought.

There are two accounts for this medium–distance association. The first account is *functional*: Because words are relatively abstract, they capture the essential properties of an item, those that are likely to remain constant across changes in location, or context more generally. For example, a chair's visual appearance varies depending on lighting, the angle from which it is viewed, and whether or not it has been repainted. Yet it remains the same chair, and, conveniently, may be referred to by the same word, *chair,* or by the same phrase, "Dana's favorite chair." After the chair is repainted, the picture may be out of date, but the word applies as well as ever. The second account of the medium–distance association is *perceptual*: Pictures are subject to perceptual analyses akin to those performed on the objects themselves (Glaser, 1992; Stenberg, 2006; see also, DeLoache, Pierroutsakos, Uttal, Rosengren, & Gottlieb, 1998; DeLoache, Pierroutsakos, & Uttal, 2003). For the most part (e.g., outside of astronomy), perception occurs only in the presence of the perceived object. Without the object present, there is nothing for photons to bounce off of, nothing to emit pressure waves or airborne molecules, and therefore nothing to impinge on our sensory surfaces and engage our perceptual faculties. Perception, then, presupposes proximity. And because pictures are perceived more or less as objects are perceived, they, too, convey a feeling of proximity. Words, in contrast, need not convey proximity. On the contrary, one of the most useful aspects of language is that it allows us to communicate and think about things that are not present. Thus, visual perceptions present objects as "here and now," whether or not they are, while words specialize in conveying information across space and time.

Thus, two related rationales—one functional and the other perceptual—invite the hypothesis that visual representations are associated with proximity, while verbal representations are associated with distance.

Recent research supports this medium–distance hypothesis (Amit, Algom, & Trope, 2009). In one experiment, participants viewed two items (e.g., an apple, a chair) either verbally or pictorially, and in apparently "distal" and "proximal" locations within a depth illusion. As predicted, participants were faster to identify pictures of objects when they were near rather than distant, but they were faster to identify words denoting those objects when they were distant rather than near. Other experiments that manipulated temporal distance (using ancient vs. modern objects; e.g., a cart vs. a car) and social distance (using domestic vs. foreign objects; e.g., a dollar vs. a euro) found similar results. Furthermore, the same pattern of results was obtained with other cognitive tasks, such as speeded categorization, selective attention (Amit, Algom, & Trope, 2009), and memory (Amit, Rim, Halbeisen, Algom, & Trope, in preparation; Amit, Algom, Trope, & Liberman, 2008). Here, we hypothesize that the association between medium (visual vs. verbal) and distance has implications for emotional responses and evaluations. Our theory begins with the idea that proximal objects–events tend to be more emotionally salient. This principle makes functional sense. Emotions are ultimately for *doing*, not just feeling, and events that are "here and now" are more likely to require an immediate response. For example, Mobbs et al. (2007) found that as a threat becomes spatially closer, brain activity shifts from the vmPFC to the periaqueductal gray, indicating a shift from general evaluative representation ("common currency") to preparation for defensive behavior. A further step connects visual representation to emotion by way of proximity: If you hear the word *lion,* you may need to act, but you may also simply be overhearing an idle conversation about lions. In contrast, if you see a lion, the odds that you need to act, or at least be on guard, are much higher. (Of course, you could be at the zoo. But zoos are recent inventions, unlike conversations.)

This argument is consistent with Kensinger and Schacter's (2006) account of the difference between pictures and words in eliciting emotional reactions, with corresponding lateralization in the amygdala.

> The specificity of the right-amygdala response (to pictures and not to words) and the generality of the left-amygdala response (to both stimulus types) may reflect their respective roles in automatic processing (perhaps more likely to occur for pictures than for words) versus elaborative, associative, or conceptual processing (which may occur for both pictures and words . . .). The latter interpretation would be consistent with recent evidence indicating that left-lateralized amygdala activity tends to be elicited across a wider range of tasks than is right-lateralized amygdala activity. (p. 121).

Consistent with this dissociation, other research indicates that visual representations, as compared to verbal representations, are more emotionally salient (Holmes & Mathews, 2005; Holmes, Mathews, Dalgleish, & Mackintosh, 2006; Holmes, Mathews, Mackintosh, & Dalgleish, 2008;

Kensinger & Schacter, 2006; De Houwer & Hermans, 1994). For example, Holmes and Mathews (2005) asked participants to read ambiguous event descriptions that were eventually resolved in a negative direction. They were asked either to imagine the situation or to focus on the meaning of the words. Holmes and Matthews found that state anxiety increased significantly over time for those in the group given imagery instructions, but not for those asked to focus on the verbal meaning. Similarly, in another study, Holmes et al. (2008), presented picture–caption pairs to participants and instructed them to produce either an image or a verbal sentence, and to integrate each picture with its caption (experimental blocks alternated between negative or benign meaning combinations). Compared with the verbal condition, state anxiety scores in the imagery group increased more across negative combination blocks, but decreased across benign blocks. Reported liking for pictures, when displayed alone at the beginning and end of the experiment, decreased for pictures that had been in negative (rather than benign) combinations, and this difference was significantly greater in the imagery group. Finally, De Houwer and Hermans (1994) used a word–picture affective Stroop task and found that emotional pictures, but not words, produced interference effects. Furthermore, naming times were shorter for negative pictures, but not for negative words. The authors concluded that pictures have privileged access to emotional information. This makes sense from an evolutionary perspective given that visual information has been triggering emotional responses for millions of years, while language is a relatively recent evolutionary development.

In summary, there is evidence that visual representations, relative to verbal representations, are more emotionally salient. This may be because things that are perceived visually—especially historically, but also today—are more likely to be "here and now" and to demand an immediate response. In contrast, verbal representations appear to have a "comparative advantage" when it comes to representing things that are distal and more abstract, and are therefore less likely to demand an immediate response.

VISUAL THINKING, VERBAL THINKING, AND MORAL JUDGMENT: SOME CONVERGENT HYPOTHESES

We may now integrate the foregoing discussion of dual-process moral cognition with the foregoing discussion of visual and verbal cognition. Putting these together suggests the following line of reasoning: If deontological moral judgments are preferentially supported by emotional responses, and visual imagery facilitates emotional responses, then perhaps visual imagery preferentially supports deontological judgments. Likewise, if utilitarian judgments are preferentially supported by less emotional forms of thinking, and if verbal processing facilitates responses that are less emotional (more abstract, distanced), then perhaps verbal processing may preferentially support utilitarian judgments.

These hypotheses are, in fact, also suggested by a related line of reasoning, emanating from cognitive neuroscience: Many of the brain regions most consistently engaged by moral judgment (Greene et al., 2001; Greene, 2009) are part of the "default network" (Gusnard & Raichle, 2001). According to one theory of default network function (Buckner, Andrews-Hanna, & Schacter, 2008), it is responsible for generating mental simulations of events that are not "here and now," such as events that are in the past, in the future, or in the minds of others. In light of this, one might suppose that moral dilemmas (and especially those that are most emotionally engaging) elicit increased activity in the default network as people imagine the events described in the dilemma, events such as a runaway trolley headed toward five innocent people and oneself reluctantly pushing an innocent person in front of that trolley in the hope of stopping it. Moreover, one might suppose that such mental simulations trigger emotional responses that guide moral judgments, such as the judgment that it is wrong to push the man off the footbridge. Finally, one might suppose that such simulations are in part *sensory* simulations, complete with visual imagery, and that this imagery plays a key role in triggering the aforementioned emotional responses.

If we are correct, such responses are not necessarily triggered by mental stimulations. On the contrary, insofar as mental simulations of events are emotionally salient, it is because the events themselves are, or would be, even more emotionally salient. This hypothesis is supported by recent work by Cushman et al. (2012), who took physiological recordings from subjects while they physically simulated violent actions in the lab (e.g., smashing someone's realistic-looking false leg with a hammer). Subjects experienced heightened physiological responses (peripheral vasoconstriction) when performing these pseudoviolent actions, as compared to performing physically similar actions that are not pseudoviolent (e.g., hammering a nail), and to observing others perform the same pseudoviolent actions. Critically, for our present purposes, the strength of these physiological responses was positively correlated with deontological responses to hypothetical moral dilemmas, suggesting that emotional responses to mentally simulated violence are related to emotional responses to actual violence. (This assumes, of course, that Cushman et al.'s physical simulations of violence produce reactions similar to those produced by actual violence. See also experiments combining virtual reality and physiological recordings; Navarrete et al., 2012).

Yet another rationale for this hypothesis follows from CLT (Liberman & Trope, 2008; Trope & Liberman, 2010). Once again, according to CLT, objects and events may be represented (construed) at multiple levels of abstraction. (See also action identification theory; Vallacher & Wegner, 1985). High-level construals are relatively abstract, reflecting overarching goals ("I'm moving to a new house"). Low-level construals, in contrast, are relatively concrete, reflecting the means employed to achieve overarching goals ("I'm loading boxes into a truck"). If, as suggested earlier, words are more abstract representations than pictures, then words and pictures may respectively map onto high and low levels of construal (Amit, Algom, & Trope, 2009; Amit, Algom, Trope, & Liberman, 2009). Indeed, the former researchers have shown that verbal representations facilitate more abstract, high-level construals, while visual representations facilitate more concrete, low-level construals. For example, participants in one experiment organized items associated with a camping trip into groups. In one condition, the items were presented as words. In the other condition, they were presented as pictures. When the items were presented as words, participants grouped them into a smaller number of more abstract categories. When the items were presented as pictures, participants grouped them into a larger number of more concrete categories.

Notably, utilitarian judgments give precedence to ends ("Better to save more lives . . ."). Deontological judgments, in contrast, famously give precedence to concerns about means ("But it's simply wrong to kill an innocent person, even for a good cause"). This suggests that utilitarian judgments may be facilitated by high-level construals, while deontological judgments may be facilitated by low-level construals.

Putting the foregoing ideas together suggests yet another line of reasoning that leads to our central prediction: Visual imagery is inherently concrete, depicting specific objects, actions, and other events. When one visualizes a purposeful action, the means employed to achieve the desired end will most likely be visualized in a concrete way. For example, if one visualizes someone baking bread, one is very likely to visualize the tools used to bake the bread (rolling pin, oven, etc.). Thus, we hypothesize that visual imagery naturally facilitates low-level construals of actions, whereby the means to the end of the action is represented as a concrete chain of physical events. And, thus, by highlighting the concrete means by which ends are achieved, visual imagery facilitates deontological moral judgments (at least in contexts in which the harmful action is a means to a greater good, as in the case of pushing the man off the footbridge). Along parallel lines, we hypothesize that verbal processing facilitates more abstract representations, and that these more abstract representations promote higher-level construals that emphasize the ends to be achieved over the means used to achieve them. Thus, according to this hypothesis, verbal thinking will facilitate utilitarian judgment.

Thus, we have three related rationales—from dual-process moral cognition, from the cognitive neuroscience of the default network, and from CLT—all pointing toward the same hypotheses: Visual thinking facilitates deontological moral judgment, and verbal thinking facilitates utilitarian judgment.

VISUAL IMAGERY AND MORAL JUDGMENT: EVIDENCE

We have conducted three experiments that test these ideas (Amit & Greene, 2012). In the first of these, we employed a measure of visual versus verbal cognitive style adapted from Kraemer, Rosenberg, and Thompson-Schill (2009). Subjects completed two matched working memory tasks, one visual and the other verbal. In the visual version, subjects saw a target shape, then had to identify one of two subsequently presented shapes as having more attributes in common with the target. In the verbal version, the visual attributes were replaced by words (e.g., *striped, red*). The visual and verbal tasks were matched for difficulty. Our index of cognitive style (visual vs. verbal) was the difference in accuracy between the visual and verbal versions of the working memory task. After completing the memory tasks, subjects responded to a set of moral dilemmas, including the footbridge dilemma, along with other, similar "high-conflict personal" dilemmas (Koenigs et al., 2007) in which one can kill one person in order to save the lives of several others. As predicted, we found that participants with relatively higher visual scores, indicating a more visual cognitive style, made more deontological judgments. That is, they were less approving of violating the rights of one person in order to produce a greater good for others.

In our second experiment we used an experimental manipulation to test for a causal relationship between cognitive style and moral judgment. In each experimental trial, the participant read a moral dilemma and deliberated while engaging in a 2-back working memory task (Kirchner, 1958). In the visual version, subjects saw a series of shapes (e.g., triangle, circle) and were asked to indicate by button press whether the present shape was identical to the shape presented two items previously. In the verbal version, visual shapes were replaced by words naming shapes. Thus, subjects were exposed to either visual interference or verbal interference while making moral judgments. We also included a no-interference control condition. As predicted, visual interference made judgments more utilitarian, both in comparison to verbal interference and no interference. Given what we know about the role of emotion in deontological judgment (discussed earlier), this suggests that visual imagery plays a role in triggering the emotional responses that drive deontological judgments. We note that we did not observe a parallel effect with verbal interference. That is, verbal interference did not decrease utilitarian judgment, despite our prediction, and despite the fact that other forms of cognitive load have this effect (Greene et al., 2008, Trémolière et al., 2012).

A third experiment examined more closely the contents of these morally salient visualizations. A natural hypothesis is that visual imagery preferentially supports deontological judgment, because people tend to visualize the harm caused as a means more than harm to be avoided as an end. For example, in the footbridge dilemma, people tend to visualize the harm to the person who is pushed more than they visualize the harm that will befall the five other people if nothing is done. We tested this hypothesis using self-reports concerning the contents of people's visual imagery. In a between-subjects design, people responded to either the footbridge dilemma or the trolley dilemma, in which one can save the five other people by turning the trolley onto a side track, killing one person instead. In these two dilemmas, the consequences are identical but the nature of the action is different. In the footbridge case, the harm is causally necessary to achieve the goal (a means to an end), while the harm is incidental (a side effect) in the trolley dilemma. These dilemmas also differ in whether the agent applies "personal force" to the victim (Greene et al., 2009), essentially the difference between directly pushing the victim or harming the victim in a more indirect, mechanically mediated way, such as hitting a switch (see also Royzman & Baron, 2002; Cushman et al., 2006; and Moore et al., 2008). As predicted, people responding to the footbridge dilemma reported more vividly imaging the person to be sacrificed, as compared to the five to be saved. We saw no such effect for the trolley case, and this difference in who gets visualized partially mediated the relationship between dilemma and judgment. In summary, it seems that we say "no" to pushing the man off the footbridge (at least partly), because we tend to visualize this violent event more than other morally consequential events, and because we tend to respond emotionally to that visualization. Convergent evidence comes from Conway and Gawronski (2013), who show that presenting visual displays of the potential victims in such dilemmas selectively enhances deontological inclinations.

VISUAL VERSUS VERBAL THINKING AND PRIMARY VERSUS SECONDARY EMOTIONS

Many researchers distinguish between *primary emotions* (e.g., anger and happiness) and *secondary emotions* (e.g., shame and pride). Primary emotions are thought of as being discrete and evolutionarily conserved, as relatively independent of cultural influence, as requiring less conceptual cognition, as having relatively short typical duration, and as evoking universally recognized facial expressions (Demoulin & Teixeira, 2010, Ekman, Friesen, & Ellsworth, 1972). Secondary emotions, in contrast, are thought of as being uniquely human (Gaunt, Leyens, & Demoulin, 2002; Leyens et al., 2001), as involving complex conceptual cognition, as having relatively long typical durations, and as being less readily observable (Demoulin et al., 2004). Some theorists have characterized secondary emotions as "self-conscious" (Tracy, Robins, & Tangney, 2007) or "moral" emotions (Haidt, 2003).

To summarize the previous points in a rough (and somewhat contentious) way, the primary emotions are thought to be more "primitive." One can say with more precision and confidence that vision is more primitive than language: Our ancestors have been seeing for hundreds of millions of years, whereas language is a relatively recent evolutionary development. If vision and primary emotion are both more primitive, operating in tandem for many millions of years, one might suppose further that there are more direct connections between visual processing and primary emotion. Likewise, one might suppose that secondary emotions are more dependent on language. Here we wish to be clear: We are by no means denying that visual thinking can cause secondary emotion. Nor are we claiming that verbal thinking cannot cause primary emotion. Our more modest hypothesis is that there may yet be a tighter relationship between visual thinking and primary emotion on the one hand, and between verbal thinking and secondary emotion on the other.

Preliminary data support this hypothesis. In one experiment (Amit, Chakroff, & Greene, in preparation), we had participants think about times when they experienced either primary or secondary emotions. At the same time, participants performed a 2-back visual or verbal working memory task, similar to the one used in the interference experiment described earlier. We found that performance on the visual task was worse when people recalled experiencing a primary emotion and that performance on the verbal task was worse when people recalled experiencing a secondary emotion. This pattern of interference is consistent with the idea that visual thinking preferentially supports the experience of primary emotion, while verbal thinking preferentially supports the experience of secondary emotions.[3]

If these preliminary data hold, they may have interesting implications for our understanding of emotion particularly and of complex, multimodal cognition more generally. First, they would provide further evidence for the controversial distinction between primary and secondary emotions. Second, the tendency to think more visually than verbally, and vice versa, may explain variation among emotional responses across individuals and situations. For example, some clinical disorders, such as phobia of spiders (which are concrete targets), seem to be more closely related to primary emotions, whereas others, such as generalized anxiety disorder (which has no specific, concrete target), seem to be more closely related to secondary emotions. If there is a preferential connection between visual cognition and primary emotions, or a preferential connection between verbal cognition and secondary emotions, understanding these connections may prove useful in understanding the causes of these disorders and possible avenues for treatment. Finally, one might wonder about the connection between visual processing and deontological judgment in light of the previous discussion of primary versus secondary emotions. This discussion suggests that deontological judgments may be preferentially supported by one or more primary emotions. However, it is not clear which primary emotion or emotions would be involved. Fear? Disgust? Or perhaps such judgments are driven by emotions that are in some ways like primary emotions but less well understood. This is an interesting avenue for future research.

CONCLUDING THOUGHTS

Dual-process theories are both powerful and pervasive, making sense of a wide range of phenomena in social judgment and decision making. In particular, the dual-process framework has deepened our understanding of moral psychology and provided a bridge between moral psychology and cognitive neuroscience. But this framework leaves open many questions, including the causes and representational nature of the automatic and controlled processes that (typically) put the "dual" in dual process. Here, we have attempted to integrate several widely used cognitive distinctions: deontological versus utilitarian, concrete versus abstract, proximal versus distal, visual versus verbal, and primary versus secondary. Construal level theory (Trope & Liberman, 2010) connects the abstract–concrete distinction to the proximal–distal distinction. Research by Amit (Amit, Algom, & Trope, 2009; Amit, Wakslak, & Trope, 2013) connects these two distinctions to the visual–verbal distinction. Research we have done together (Amit & Greene, 2012) connects the visual–verbal distinction to the deontological–utilitarian distinction, a connection suggested in at least two distinct ways: (1) Deontological judgments and visual representations both tend to be more emotional (perhaps specifically primary emotions); (2) deontological judgments are focused on means rather than ends, suggesting a low level of construal, which is associated with psychological proximity, which is associated with visual representation. Our research (Amit et al., in preparation) also (tentatively) connects the visual–verbal distinction to the distinction between primary and secondary emotions. As noted earlier, some or all of the distinctions may have analogs in the domain of neural mechanisms (e.g., default network vs. other large-scale networks) and evolutionary history (ancient widespread adaptations vs. recent and uniquely human adaptations).

Thus, we have in this chapter attempted to connect many dots. We acknowledge that the connections we have drawn do not yet form a clear picture, but we nevertheless strongly suspect that these connections are not random. If forced to identify a central node in this conceptual network, we would put our finger on the abstract–concrete distinction: Over evolutionary time, our brains evolved the capacity for increasingly abstract representation. In the moral domain, this enables us to judge actions by their consequences ("How many lives were saved?"), which may vary dramatically from context to context, rather than by observable features of the acts themselves ("Does it involve intentional pushing?"). Abstraction allows us to think about things that are far away in space and in time (next year's trip to London), glossing over unknown or irrelevant details (the outbound flight number). Likewise, abstraction allows us to set and pursue high-level goals (visiting London), independent of the specific concrete means that we may use to achieve them (taking Flight 228 to Heathrow). Abstraction allows us to represent things as good or bad, not merely because of their immediate value ("Tasty food makes me feel happy") but because of the value they take on in their social contexts ("Providing food for others makes me feel pride"). And words enable us to represent abstract concepts that can be represented imperfectly, or perhaps not at all, with visual (or otherwise sensory) representations. In light of the previous discussion, one might think that there is a deep connection between our capacity for abstraction and our capacity for dual-process cognition, and perhaps that is true. However, we suspect that there is no simple mapping here. In particular, some automatic processing seems to involve representations that are very abstract, such as the mathematical intuitions of mathematicians or, more prosaically, the use of abstract social categories to make dispositional attributions (Nussbaum, Trope, & Liberman, 2003). Thus, many puzzles remain concerning the relationships among abstract versus concrete thinking, visual versus verbal thinking, and the two sides of dual-process cognition. We hope that this discussion has provided some useful clues.

NOTES

1. Exceptions include abstract art.
2. Exceptions include onomatopoeia.
3. We emphasize that these data are preliminary. We had also predicted that the visual memory task would decrease intensity ratings for the recalled primary emotion and that the verbal task would decrease intensity ratings for the recalled secondary emotion. Neither of these predictions held. We are in the process of attempting to replicate the results described here to understand why some of our predicted results have held but others have not.

REFERENCES

Amit, E., Algom, D., & Trope, Y. (2009). Distance-dependent processing of pictures and words. *Journal of Experimental Psychology: General, 138*, 400–415.

Amit, E., Algom, D., Trope, Y., & Liberman, N. (2008). "Thou shalt not make unto thee any graven image": The distance-dependence of representation. In K. D. Markman, W. M. P. Klein, & J. A. Suhr (Eds.), *The handbook of imagination and mental simulation* (pp. 53–68). New York: Psychology Press.

Amit, E., Chakroff, A., & Greene, J. D. (in preparation). *Primary and secondary emotions rely on visual and verbal processing.*

Amit, E., & Greene, J. D. (2012). You see, the ends don't justify the means: Visual imagery and moral judgment. *Psychological Science, 23*(8), 861–868.

Amit, E., Rim, S., Halbeisen, G., Algom, D., & Trope, Y. (in preparation). *Distance-dependent memory for pictures and words.*

Amit, E., Wakslak, C., & Trope, Y. (2013). The use of visual and verbal means of communication across psychological distance. *Personality and Social Psychology Bulletin, 39*(1), 43–56.

Bartels, D. (2008). Principled moral sentiment and the flexibility of moral judgment and decision making. *Cognition*, 108, 381–417.

Bartels, D. M., & Pizarro, D. A. (2011). The mismeasure of morals: Antisocial personality traits predict utilitarian responses to moral dilemmas. *Cognition, 121*(1), 154–161.

Buckner, R. L., Andrews-Hanna, J. R., & Schacter, D. L. (2008). The brain's default network. *Annals of the New York Academy of Sciences, 1124*(1), 1–38.

Cacioppo, J. T., & Petty, R. E. (1982). The need for cognition. *Journal of Personality and Social Psychology, 42*(1), 116–131.

Chaiken, S., & Trope, Y. (Eds.). (1999). *Dual-process theories in social psychology.* New York: Guilford Press.

Chib, V. S., Rangel, A., Shimojo, S., & O'Doherty, J. P. (2009). Evidence for a common representation of decision values for dissimilar goods in human ventromedial prefrontal cortex. *Journal of Neuroscience, 29*(39), 12315–12320.

Ciaramelli, E., Muccioli, M., Ladavas, E., & di Pellegrino, G. (2007). Selective deficit in personal moral judgment following damage to ventromedial prefrontal cortex. *Social Cognitive and Affective Neuroscience, 2*, 84–92.

Conway, P., & Gawronski, B. (2013). Deontological and utilitarian inclinations in moral decision making: A process dissociation approach. *Journal of Personality and Social Psychology, 104*(2), 216–235.

Crockett, M. J., Clark, L., Hauser, M. D., & Robbins, T. W. (2010). Reply to Harris and Chan: Moral judgment is more than rational deliberation. *Proceedings of the National Academy of Sciences USA, 107*(50), 184.

Cushman, F., Gray, K., Gaffey, A., & Mendes, W. B. (2012). Simulating murder: The aversion to harmful action. *Emotion, 12*(1), 2–7.

Cushman, F. A., & Greene, J. D. (2012). Finding faults: How moral dilemmas reveal cognitive structure. *Social Neuroscience, 7*(3), 269–279.

Cushman, F. A., Young, L., & Hauser, M. D. (2006). The role of reasoning and intuition in moral judgments: Testing three principles of harm. *Psychological Science, 17*(12), 1082–1089.

De Houwer, J., & Hermans, D. (1994). Differences in the affective processing of words and pictures. *Cognition and Emotion, 8*, 1–20.

DeLoache, J. S., Pierroutsakos, S. L., & Uttal, D. H. (2003). The origins of pictorial competence. *Current Directions in Psychological Science, 12*, 114–118.

DeLoache, J. S., Pierroutsakos, S. L., Uttal, D. H., Rosengren, K. S., & Gottlieb, A. (1998). Grasping the nature of pictures. *Psychological Science, 9*, 205–210.

Demoulin, S., Leyens, J. P., Paladino, M. P., Rodriguez-Torres, R., Rodriguez-Perez, A., & Dovidio, J. (2004). Dimensions of "uniquely" and "non-uniquely" human emotions. *Cognition and Emotion, 18*(1), 71–96.

Demoulin, S., & Teixeira, C. P. (2010). Social categorization in interpersonal negotiation:

How social structural factors shape negotiations. *Group Processes and Intergroup Relations, 13*(6), 765–777.

Ekman, P., Friesen, W. V., & Ellsworth, P. (1972). *Emotion in the human face: Guidelines for research and an integration of findings*. Oxford, UK: Pergamon Press.

Evans, J. S. B. (2008). Dual-processing accounts of reasoning, judgment, and social cognition. *Annual Review of Psychology, 59*, 255–278.

Gaunt, R., Leyens, J. P., & Demoulin, S. (2002). Intergroup relations and the attribution of emotions: Control over memory for secondary emotions associated with the ingroup and outgroup. *Journal of Experimental Social Psychology, 38*(5), 508–514.

Glaser, W. R. (1992). Picture naming. *Cognition, 42*, 61–105.

Goodman, N. (1976). *Languages of art: An approach to a theory of symbols*. Cambridge, MA: Hackett.

Greene, J. D. (2007). The secret joke of Kant's soul. In W. Sinnott-Armstrong (Ed.), *Moral psychology: Vol. 3. The neuroscience of morality: emotion, disease, and development* (pp. 59–66). Cambridge, MA: MIT Press.

Greene, J. D., Cushman, F. A., Stewart, L. E., Lowenberg, K., Nystrom, L. E., & Cohen, J. D. (2009). Pushing moral buttons: The interaction between personal force and intention in moral judgment. *Cognition, 111*(3), 364–371.

Greene, J. D., Morelli, S. A., Lowenberg, K., Nystrom, L. E., & Cohen, J. D. (2008). Cognitive load selectively interferes with utilitarian moral judgment. *Cognition, 107*, 1144–1154.

Greene, J. D., Nystrom, L. E., Engell, A. D., Darley, J. M., & Cohen, J. D. (2004). The neural bases of cognitive conflict and control in moral judgment. *Neuron, 44*, 389–400.

Greene, J. D., Sommerville, R. B., Nystrom, L. E., Darley, J. M., & Cohen, J. D. (2001). An fMRI investigation of emotional engagement in moral judgment. *Science, 293*, 2105–2108.

Gusnard, D. A., & Raichle, M. E. (2001). Searching for a baseline: Functional imaging and the resting human brain. *Nature Reviews Neuroscience, 2*(10), 685–694.

Haidt, J. (2003). The moral emotions. In R. J. Davidson, K. R. Scherer, & H. H. Goldsmith (Eds.), *Handbook of affective sciences* (pp. 852–870). New York: Oxford University Press.

Hauser, M. D. (2006). The liver and the moral organ. *Social Cognitive and Affective Neuroscience, 1*(3), 214–220.

Holmes, E. A., & Mathews, A. (2005). Mental imagery and emotion: A special relationship? *Emotion, 5*, 489–497.

Holmes, E. A., Mathews, A., Dalgleish, T., & Mackintosh, B. (2006). Positive interpretation training: Effects of mental imagery versus verbal training on positive mood. *Behavior Therapy, 37*(3), 237–247.

Holmes, E. A., Mathews, A., Mackintosh, B., & Dalgleish, T. (2008). The causal effect of mental imagery on emotion assessed using picture–word cues. *Emotion, 8*, 395–409.

Jacoby, L. L. (1991). A process dissociation framework: Separating automatic from intentional uses of memory. *Journal of Memory and Language, 30*(5), 513–541.

Kahneman, D. (2003). A perspective on judgment and choice: Mapping bounded rationality. *American Psychology, 58*, 697–720.

Kahneman, D. (2011). *Thinking fast and slow*. New York: Farrar, Straus & Giroux.

Kensinger, E. A., & Schacter, D. L. (2006). Processing emotional pictures and words: Effects of valence and arousal. *Cognitive, Affective, and Behavioral Neuroscience, 6*, 110–126.

Kirchner, W. K. (1958). Age differences in short-term retention of rapidly changing information. *Journal of Experimental Psychology, 55*, 352–358.

Knutson, B., Taylor, J., Kaufman, M., Peterson, R., & Glover, G. (2005). Distributed neural representation of expected value. *Journal of Neuroscience, 25*(19), 4806–4812.

Koenigs, M., Young, L., Adolphs, R., Tranel, D., Cushman, F., Hauser, M., et al. (2007). Damage to the prefrontal cortex increases utilitarian moral judgments. *Nature, 446*, 908–911.

Koven, N. S. (2011). Specificity of meta-emotion effects on moral decision-making. *Emotion, 11*(5), 1255–1261.

Kraemer, D. J., Rosenberg, L. M., & Thompson-Schill, S. L. (2009). The neural correlates of visual and verbal cognitive styles. *Journal of Neuroscience, 29*(12), 3792–3798.

Leyens, J. P., Rodriguez-Perez, A., Rodriguez-Torres, R., Gaunt, R., Paladino, M. P., Vaes, J., et al. (2001). Psychological essentialism and the differential attribution of uniquely human emotions to ingroups and outgroups. *European Journal of Social Psychology, 31*(4), 395–411.

Liberman, N., & Trope, Y. (2008). The psychology of transcending the here and now. *Science, 322*, 1201–1205.

Lieberman, M. D., Gaunt, R., Gilbert, D. T., & Trope, Y. (2002). Reflection and reflexion: A social cognitive neuroscience approach to attributional interference. In M. P. Zanna (Ed.), *Advances in experimental social psychology* (pp. 199–249). San Diego: Academic Press.

Loewenstein, G. (1996). Out of control: Visceral influences on behavior. *Organizational Behavior and Human Decision Processes, 65*(3), 272–292.

Mendez, M. F., Anderson, E., & Shapira, J. S. (2005). An investigation of moral judgment in frontotemporal dementia. *Cognitive and Behavioral Neurology, 18*, 193–197.

Metcalfe, J., & Mischel, W. (1999). A hot/cool-system analysis of delay of gratification: Dynamics of willpower. *Psychological Review, 106*, 3–19.

Mikhail, J. (2000). *Rawls' linguistic analogy: A study of the "generative grammar" model of moral theory described by John Rawls in* A Theory of Justice. Unpublished doctoral dissertation, Cornell University, Ithaca, NY.

Mikhail, J. (2011). *Elements of moral cognition: Rawls' linguistic analogy and the cognitive science of moral and legal judgment.* Cambridge, UK: Cambridge University Press.

Miller, E. K., & Cohen, J. D. (2001). An integrative theory of prefrontal cortex function. *Annual Review of Neuroscience, 24*(1), 167–202.

Mobbs, D., Petrovic, P., Marchant, J. L., Hassabis, D., Weiskopf, N., Seymour, B., et al. (2007). When fear is near: Threat imminence elicits prefrontal-periaqueductal gray shifts in humans. *Science, 317*(5841), 1079–1083.

Moore, A., Clark, B., & Kane, M. (2008). Who shalt not kill?: Individual differences in working memory capacity, executive control, and moral judgment. *Psychological Science, 19*(6), 549–557.

Moretto, G., Ladavas, E., Mattioli, F., & di Pellegrino, G. (2010). A psychophysiological investigation of moral judgment after ventromedial prefrontal damage. *Journal of Cognitive Neuroscience, 22*, 1888–1899.

Navarrete, C. D., McDonald, M. M., Mott, M. L., & Asher, B. (2012). Virtual morality: Emotion and action in a simulated three-dimensional "trolley problem." *Emotion, 12*(2), 364–370.

Nussbaum, S., Trope, Y., & Liberman, N. (2003). Creeping dispositionism: The temporal dynamics of behavior prediction. *Journal of Personality and Social Psychology, 84*(3), 485–497.

Paivio, A. (1986). *Mental representations.* New York: Oxford University Press.

Paxton, J. M., Bruni, T., & Greene, J. D. (2013). Are "counter-intuitive" deontological judgments really counter-intuitive?: An empirical reply to Kahane et al. (2012). *Social Cognitive and Affective Neuroscience, 102.*

Paxton, J. M., Ungar, L., & Greene, J. D. (2011). Reflection and reasoning in moral judgment. *Cognitive Science, 36*(1), 163–177.

Perkins, A. M., Leonard, A. M., Weaver, K., Dalton, J. A., Mehta, M. A., Kumari, V., et al. (2012). A dose of ruthlessness: Interpersonal moral judgment is hardened by the anti-anxiety drug lorazepam. *Journal of Experimental Psychology: General, 142*(3), 612–620.

Petrinovich, L., O'Neill, P., & Jorgensen, M. (1993). An empirical study of moral intuitions: Toward and evolutionary ethics. *Journal of Personality and Social Psychology, 64*(3), 467–478.

Royzman, E. B., & Baron, J. (2002). The preference for indirect harm. *Social Justice Research, 15*, 165–184.

Schaich Borg, J., Hynes, C., Van Horn, J., Grafton, S., & Sinnott-Armstrong, W. (2006). Consequences, action, and intention as factors in moral judgments: An fMRI investigation. *Journal of Cognitive Neuroscience,18*(5), 803–817.

Shenhav, A., & Greene, J. D. (2010). Moral judgments recruit domain-general valuation mechanisms to integrate representations of probability and magnitude. *Neuron, 67*, 667–677.

Shiffrin, R. M. & Schneider, W. (1977). Controlled and automatic human information processing: Perceptual learning, automatic attending, and a general theory. *Psychological Review, 84*(2), 127–190.

Sloman, S. A. (1996). The empirical case for two systems of reasoning. *Psychological Bulletin, 119*, 3–22.

Stanovich, K. E., & West, R. F. (2000). Individual differences in reasoning: Implications for the rationality debate. *Behavioral and Brain Sciences, 23*, 645–665.

Stenberg, G. (2006). Conceptual and perceptual factors in the picture superiority effect. *European Journal of Cognitive Psychology, 18*, 813–847.

Strohminger, N., Lewis, R. L., & Meyer, D. E. (2011). Divergent effects of different positive emotions on moral judgment. *Cognition, 119*(2), 295–300.

Suter, R. S., & Hertwig, R. (2011). Time and moral judgment. *Cognition, 119*(3), 454–458.

Tangney, J. P., & Fischer, K. W. (1995). *Self-conscious emotions: The psychology of shame, guilt, embarrassment, and pride.* New York: Guilford Press.

Thomas, B. C., Croft, K. E., & Tranel, D.(2011). Harming kin to save strangers: Further evidence for abnormally utilitarian moral judgments after ventromedial prefrontal damage. *Journal of Cognitive Neuroscience, 23*(9), 2186–2196.

Thomson, J. (1985). The trolley problem. *Yale Law Journal, 94*, 1395–1415.

Tracy, J. L., Robins, R. W., & Tangney, J. P. (Eds.). (2007). *The self-conscious emotions: Theory and research.* New York: Guilford Press.

Trémolière, B., Neys, W. D., & Bonnefon, J. F. (2012). Mortality salience and morality: Thinking about death makes people less utilitarian. *Cognition, 124*(3), 379–384.

Trope, Y., & Liberman, N. (2010). Construal level theory of psychological distance. *Psychological Review, 117*, 440–463.

Valdesolo, P., & DeSteno, D. (2006). Manipulations of emotional context shape moral judgment. *Psychological Science, 17*(6), 476–477.

Vallacher, R., & Wegner, D. M. (1985). *A theory of action identification.* Hillsdale, NJ: Erlbaum.

CHAPTER 24

Prolonged Thought

Proposing Type 3 Processing

Ap Dijksterhuis, Madelijn Strick, Maarten W. Bos, and Loran F. Nordgren

> Our clear concepts are like islands which arise above the ocean of obscure ones . . . yet it is not easy to conceive that a thing can think and not be conscious that it thinks.
>
> —GOTTFRIED WILHELM LEIBNIZ[1]

The Latin verb for "to think" is *cogitare*—a contraction from co and agito—and it literally means "to shake together" or "to move together." Thinking, in other words, is a process in which different pieces of information—sometimes lots of them—are combined and transformed into a useful product such as an idea, an estimate, a decision, or a solution to a problem.

Thought processes can vary with respect to several parameters. People can think quickly or slowly, associatively or logically, and, at least according to Leibniz, consciously or unconsciously. Most theories that describe and explain thought processes assume that there are two different systems, or processes (Kahneman, 2003; Stanovich & West, 2000). The first system or process is the intuitive system, whereas the second produces reasoning.

In some publications, researchers have used a terminology of systems, whereby System 1 is the intuitive system and System 2 is the rational system (Kahneman, 2003; Stanovich & West, 2000). However, it has been argued that it may be more accurate to avoid the term *system*, because it suggests brain systems, which is, according to Stanovich, West, and Toplak (2011, p. 104), "a stronger assumption than most people wish to make." Hence, it may be more apt to refer to Type 1 and Type 2 processing (see also Evans, 2008; Stanovich, 2004). We concur with this analysis and use the labels Type 1 and Type 2 processing as well.

The two types of processing differ in various respects. *Type 1 processing* is usually defined as fast, automatic, effortless and associative, whereas *Type 2 processing* is slower, controlled, effortful, and governed by rules. Examples of Type 1 processing are quick estimates or judgments that we make on the basis of heuristics, such as the affect heuristic (Slovic, Finucane, Peters, & MacGregor, 2002) or the availability heuristic (Tversky & Kahneman, 1973). Examples of Type 2 processing are the deliberative efforts in which we engage when we do arithmetic or make a pros and cons list, as Benjamin Franklin advised us to do long ago; or before we purchase a new house, a new laptop, or a new lawnmower.

Thought processes precede, among other things, judgments and decisions, creative ideas, and solutions to problems that we face. In our view, a lot of real-life thought processes are perfectly well captured and explained by Type 1 processing or Type 2 processing (or, as happens often, a combined effort of the two). However, we argue that there are phenomena that do not seem to fit this taxonomy. These phenomena have one thing in common: They seem to be characterized by prolonged periods of thought.

PROLONGED THOUGHT

Recently, one of the authors of this chapter (A. Dijksterhuis) asked students in an introductory psychology class how long it had taken them to choose the destination of their last summer holiday. The median was 2 weeks. Subsequently, students were asked to reflect on how long it had taken them to choose their major. The answers varied wildly, and ranged from 3 minutes to 3 years, with a median of 4 months (see Dijksterhuis, van Dijk, Driessen, & Scheffers, 2013). Indeed, whereas we make the vast majority of our decisions in seconds, minutes, or at least within an hour, most of us are able to recall at least a few instances in which we made decisions that took days, or weeks, or even longer. The decision to take a new job is a good example of a decision that happens over an extended period of time.

Other examples of prolonged thought processes can be found in the domain of creativity. Anecdotes abound of scientists who are immersed in a topic for a long time before they are, often seemingly suddenly, struck by a solution that presents itself to consciousness (a "Eureka experience"; see, e.g., Ghiselin, 1952). Indeed, scientific discoveries are often the result of a similar series of psychological stages. First, people gather all the necessary information and ponder on things consciously. Subsequently, a period follows during which people put the problem aside and are not really consciously engaged in it, and finally, an answer is found. As the British scientist C. Lloyd Morgan put it long ago, when you want to solve a scientific problem "saturate yourself through and through with your subject with all that bears, or may bear upon it, and wait" (Koestler, 1964, p. 145). The intermediate process during which people are primarily dealing with the problem on an unconscious level has often been called *incubation* (Wallas, 1926) but also *unconscious thought* (Andreasen, 2005; Dijksterhuis & Nordgren, 2006), or, a long time ago, *unconscious rumination* (Schopenhauer, 1851/1970).

We also rely on such unconscious thought or incubation processes during the process of writing. When you promise yourself to start writing the next morning or when a writing session ends without satisfactory subjective closure, such as when a subsection you intended to write is not finished because you were called to a meeting unexpectedly, thoughts about the paper or chapter you are writing may intrude into consciousness. The author Norman Mailer put it this way (cited by Bargh, 2011, p. 638):

> Over the years, I've found one rule. It is the only one I give on those occasions when I talk about writing. It's a simple rule. If you tell yourself you are going to be at your desk tomorrow, you are by that declaration asking your unconscious to prepare the material. You are, in effect, contracting to pick up such valuables at a given time. Count on me, you are saying to a few forces below: I will be there to write. . . . On the other hand, you can sometimes say to yourself, "I'm not going to work tomorrow" and the unconscious may even by now be close enough in accord not to flood your mind with brilliant and all-too-perishable material. That is also important. Because in the course of going out and having the lively day and night you're entitled to, you don't want to keep having ideas about the book you're on.

Other intrusions in consciousness that may point to periods of prolonged unconscious thought are what we may call "nagging doubts" (Jordan, Logel, Spencer, Zanna, & Whitfield, 2009). You may be close to making a decision (or worse, you may have made a decision already), such as a hiring decision, or the purchase of a new car, and you are plagued with a recurrent, vague, and difficult-to-verbalize feeling that there is something not quite right. The person you are about to hire is very well qualified, but something makes you feel uneasy around him. The car seems fine enough, but some aspect of the salesperson's behavior makes you distrust her. Such feelings are presumably also the consequence of prolonged thought, or thought-like, activity.

In summary, creativity, problem solving and decision making can take time. While we solve problems or make decisions that require a lot of time we are, obviously, not continuously aware of the problem or decision. Instead, when for a couple of weeks one contemplates a job offer from a different university, the decision itself intrudes on consciousness sporadically, because most of the time consciousness is occupied with different matters.

An important question is what happens in between the moments you deal with a problem consciously. Although one may argue that people simply do nothing between these periods of conscious engagement, we believe that, at least under certain conditions, people continue to process or "think" about their decisions unconsciously. If we are right and unconscious thought does occur, it begs the question: How should we categorize unconscious thought in a dual-systems framework? It clearly is not Type 2 processing, but unconscious thought does not share many Type 1 processing properties either. Thus, beyond offering prescriptions for how one ought to make decisions, the notion of unconscious thought represents an interesting puzzle for the many two-modes-of-thought theories. Below, we review evidence for unconscious thought processes.

ACTIVE UNCONSCIOUS THOUGHT, OR MERELY DISTRACTION?

Before we delve into the scientific evidence for unconscious thought, it may be fruitful to define thought more carefully. As said, we define *thought* according to the original Latin definition: "to shake together" or "to move together." As we said in our opening paragraph, *thinking* is a process in which different pieces of information are (re) organized into a useful product such as an idea, an estimate, a decision, or a solution. According to this definition, thought represents more than, for instance, mere changes in accessibility due to priming. It is an integrative process.[2]

Whether people can really think unconsciously or not is a very old question. Plotinus proposed the idea around the year 250, and since then many other important thinkers have done the same. In the 17th century, the idea became much more controversial. Some, such as Leibniz, thought that the fact that people can think unconsciously was obvious; others, such as Locke, thought this was ridiculous (Whyte, 1962). More recently, the question has been of central importance in the scientific literature on incubation processes (Poincaré, 1913; Wallas, 1926). Research has shown (see Sio & Ormerod, 2009, for a recent review) that a period of incubation can help creativity. Relative to people who have to come up with a solution to a problem immediately, people who put the problem aside for a while to let it "incubate" sometimes reach better or more creative solutions. However, such demonstrations do not yet show that during incubation, actual unconscious thought took place. It is possible to argue that during a period of incubation no thought takes place at all and that people merely benefit from a period of distraction, because it allows them to return to a problem later on with a "fresh look" (see also Dijksterhuis, 2004).

Indeed, Schooler and Melcher (1995) have reviewed research in which a period of distraction can lead to change in a "mental set." In such cases, the role of the unconscious is passive and there is no reason to assume unconscious thought. People often approach a problem with wrong ideas, wrong heuristics, and/or wrong information. After a period of distraction, such inaccurate approaches become less accessible or are forgotten altogether. The effects of distraction on a change of mental set can be strong (e.g., when one tries to solve a chess problem and initially gets truly fixed in thinking along a wrong path) or relatively subtle (e.g., when distraction merely attenuates the biasing influence of primacy or recency effects). Although we fully agree that putting a problem aside for a while allows for a fresh, unbiased new start, we propose that under at least some conditions active unconscious thought takes place during periods of incubation. Let us look at some findings that suggest unconscious thought effects take place.

Participants in an experiment by Betsch, Plessner, Schwieren, and Gütig (2001) looked at advertisements shown on a computer screen. They were told that their memory for the ads would be probed later on; hence, they were asked to pay close attention. While the ads were shown, the numerical increases and decreases of five hypothetical shares were shown on the bottom of the screen. In total, participants saw 75 pieces of information. Afterwards, participants were first asked a few very concrete questions about the five shares, such as the shares' average money returns. As it turned out, the participants were clueless. However, when they were merely asked to give their attitudes, they seemed to know the best and worst shares. That is, they had developed a "gut feeling" toward the shares, indicating that they had—unconsciously—processed and integrated the information.

Evidence for unconscious thought processes in the domain of creativity comes from experiments by Bowers, Regehr, Balthazard, and Parker (1990). Their participants were asked to guess target words, while from time to time they were given a hint, such as an associated word. After each hint, participants were asked to guess. When people solve such problems, it "feels" as if they suddenly know the answer. And indeed, the answer suddenly pops up in consciousness ("man" . . . "glue" . . . "star" . . . of course, they mean "super"!). However, the experimenters closely looked at people's successive guesses and determined that the process is not quite as sudden if seen from the perspective of the unconscious. Successive guesses converged, and participants unconsciously seemed to be "closing in" on the correct answer quite a while before the answer became accessible to consciousness.

Other researchers later built on the seminal work by Bowers and colleagues (1990). In research on the tip-of-the-tongue (TOT) phenomenon, Yaniv and Meyer (1987) offered participants definitions of rare words that they could not recall but felt they knew. In a *lexical decision task*—a task that measures the accessibility of words and concepts—the target TOT words were highly accessible. That is, although the words were inaccessible to consciousness, the unconscious had found and activated them. Zhong, Dijksterhuis and Galinsky (2008) used a paradigm comparable to that used by Bowers and colleagues. Their participants were presented with Remote Associates Test (RAT; Mednick, 1962) items. RAT items comprise three words that are all related to a fourth, target word that participants need to produce. RAT items can be both easy (*state, large, Houston*) and difficult (*forward, flush, razor*). In one of the experiments, Zhong and colleagues presented very difficult RAT items to participants. After a period of distraction, participants were asked for their answers. Participants solved some but not others, and subsequently completed a lexical decision task with the answers to the RAT items. As it turned out, even for items participants could not solve, the answers were highly accessible. This means that during the few minutes of distraction, participants unconsciously searched their memories for the correct answers.

Another way to show that people can actively think during distraction is by looking at how the representation or organization of information changes while people are distracted. In an experiment that was part of a series on unconscious thought and decision making (Dijksterhuis, 2004, Experiment 5: see also Bos, Dijksterhuis, & van Baaren, 2008), participants were asked to form an impression of a fictitious person named Jeroen, who was described by 18 different sentences; each sentence was pretested to load on one of three trait categories (intelligence, extroversion, and liberal). Participants either recalled as many sentences as they could immediately, or after a period of distraction (the experiment contained more experimental conditions, but we stick to what is relevant now). The results showed that the recall results of the people who were distracted had a greater degree of organization—the information was clustered around the three trait concepts—than the protocols of the control participants. During distraction, a process had taken place that is reminiscent of the classic definition of thinking: The information had been shaken together.

Finally, yet another way to demonstrate unconscious thought is to compare people who are distracted while they are motivated to solve a problem or make a decision with people who are distracted exactly the same way but who do not have the goal to think. Bos et al. (2008) asked participants to choose between four hypothetical cars. Both groups were given a distraction task after reading information about the cars. Members of one group of participants were told that, after this task, they would be asked some questions about the cars. Members of the other group were instead told that they would not have to work on the decision problem anymore, and that they would not be asked anything about the cars later on. In other words, one group had the goal to process the decision information further, whereas the other group had no such goal. Results showed that the former group made better decisions than the latter. That is, merely distracting people does not help; people need a goal before they engage in active unconscious thought. Zhong et al. (2008) made the same distinction between people who were merely distracted and people who were given the goal unconsciously to think, and found that only the latter group showed evidence of a memory search for answers to the RAT items while they were distracted.

In summary, there is evidence for psychological processes we can easily categorize as real thought processes that are, at the same time, taking place unconsciously. One may note that the processes described in this section fail to resemble perfectly the real-life processes discussed in the section "Prolonged Thought." A few minutes of distraction is not the same as an incubation period of days or even weeks. The problem is that prolonged thought effects are very difficult to study with the standard methodology of social cognition or cognitive psychology. Experimental psychologists like to observe psychological processes closely as they unfold, and one simply cannot house participants in the laboratory in order to spend a couple of weeks on an important decision (although we can study the beneficial effects of a night of sleep, as we shall see later on).

However, the empirical findings described here do show one thing that is vital for our understanding of prolonged thought processes: Thought processes can continue, even while we are not consciously aware of these thought processes. In fact, it seems that we can think unconsciously while we do something completely different consciously.

In our view, the findings we have just discussed cannot be explained by Type 1 or Type 2 processing, and most likely also not by a combination of Type 1 and Type 2 processing. It seems that incubation or unconscious thought often follows activity of Type 2 processing—such as when a scientist first reads about a problem or discusses a problem with colleagues, and later engages in incubation—but the process itself is quite different.

Perhaps, then, it is useful to propose Type 3 processing. In what follows, we give some clues regarding its characteristics. Importantly, we concede that significant parts of the second half of this chapter are speculative. Our main goal is to encourage thinking about how we may theoretically accommodate processes that we labeled earlier as prolonged thought processes. Our goal is not to specify a concrete theory.

By the way, the answers to the two RAT items presented earlier are *Texas* and *straight,* respectively.

TYPE 3 PROCESSING

> The giant computer that is our unconscious silently crunches all the data it can from the experiences we've had, the people we've met, the lessons we've learned, the books we've read, the movies we've seen, and so on, and it forms an opinion.
>
> —MALCOLM GLADWELL

Guy Claxton (1997), an educational scientist, presented a model on thought processes in which he differentiated among three modes of thought: The first mode is very fast and deals with problems that require immediate action. This mode works effortlessly and automatically. The second mode, which Claxton calls D mode (with the D coming from deliberation), is what most people would associate with normal thought. It is slower than the first system and, indeed, closely resembles System 2 in Kahneman's (2003) taxonomy. D mode has various characteristics. It is more interested in finding answers than in examining the questions; it is precise; it values conscious, articulate understanding; it is purposeful and effortful rather than playful; and it relies on language.

Importantly, there is a third mode that, according to Claxton (1997) "proceeds slower still. It is often less purposeful and clear-cut, more playful, leisurely, and dreamy. In this mode we are ruminating or mulling things over; being contemplative or meditative" (p. 2). It deals with problems that cannot be solved by simply applying logic. This mode, as described by Claxton, forms the backbone of our view of Type 3 processing. In addition, in specifying Type 3 processing, we also partly rely on unconscious thought theory (UTT), a theory that we published earlier (Dijksterhuis & Nordgren, 2006).

What are the characteristics of Type 3 processing? This list potentially is almost endless, but in this chapter we would like to discuss five aspects of Type 3 processing that we think are important and at the same time insightful in distinguishing Type 3 processing from Type 1 and Type 2 processing. Type 3 processing, in our view, is (1) largely unconscious, (2) very slow, (3) abstract and exploratory, (4) goal-dependent, and (5) and largely, but not completely, effortless (see Table 24.1, for a schematic overview). We now turn to each aspect individually.

First of all, Type 3 processing works largely, but not completely, unconsciously. It is important to realize that we do not fully equate Type 3 processing with unconscious thought as we defined it earlier (Dijksterhuis, 2004; Dijksterhuis & Nordgren, 2006). Most Type 3 processing is unconscious thought, but Type 3 processing is also characterized by conscious intermezzi. There seem to be at least two kinds of conscious "intrusions" that result from Type 3 processing.

The first kinds of intrusions occur in the face of problems. Research on unconscious goal pursuit (see, e.g., Bargh & Chartrand, 1999; Bargh, Gollwitzer, Lee-Chai, Barndollar, & Trötschel, 2001; Custers & Aarts, 2005; Dijksterhuis & Aarts, 2010) shows that although people often pursue goals unconsciously, they become consciously aware of their goals when progress toward achieving the goal becomes problematic. For instance, when people are surreptitiously primed with the goal to achieve and are then given very difficult RAT items to solve, they become consciously aware of their achievement goal more often than do people who were not primed with the goal, or people who were primed with achievement but solved easy RAT items (e.g., Bongers, Dijksterhuis, & Spears, 2010). It is likely that Type 3 processing is also characterized by such intrusions. While thinking unconsciously about a certain problem, in the face of an obstacle, people again become temporarily consciously aware of this problem.

The second kinds of intrusions occur when one finds an answer to a question, or a solution to a problem or some important subaspect of a problem. When working on an article, it sometimes occurs to the person that while doing something completely different—daydreaming during a commute, for instance—a thought suddenly intrudes into consciousness: The person knows what the title for the article should be and quickly looks for a pen and a piece of paper to scribble things down before he or she forgets the thought. A well-known intrusion is the "Eureka experience," the wonderful moment when the answer to a complex creative problem suddenly comes to mind.

In summary, we can experience conscious intrusions when goal progress is problematic or when we clearly make progress. These two kinds of conscious intrusions are not only relevant to understanding the way Type 3 processing works, but they are also helpful in distinguishing Type 3 processing from unconscious thought. We defined *unconscious thought* as cognitive and/or affective task-relevant processes that take place outside conscious awareness (see Dijksterhuis, 2004; Dijksterhuis & Nordgren, 2006). However, although we maintain that Type 3 processing takes place outside of conscious awareness most of the time, these conscious intrusions make clear that Type 3 processing consists of more than unconscious thought.

While distinguishing unconscious thought from Type 3 processing it is also good to note

TABLE 24.1. Main Characteristics of the Three Types of Processing

Type 1 processing	Type 2 processing	Type 3 processing
Unconscious	Conscious	Largely unconscious
Fast	Slow	Very slow
Associative	Logical, rule-based	Abstract and exploratory
Automatic	Goal-directed	Goal-dependent
Effortless	Effortful	Largely effortless

that most of our own and others' research on unconscious thought has focused on a paradigm in which unconscious thought was studied by distracting participants for a few minutes (Dijksterhuis, 2004; see Strick et al., 2011, for a recent meta-analysis). In our view, research with this paradigm has been useful, because it has shown (1) that unconscious thought truly exists, in that people can think while they are distracted (for the most important articles, see Bos, Dijksterhuis, & van Baaren, 2008; Strick, Dijksterhuis, & van Baaren, 2010), and (2) that a period of unconscious thought can improve decisions (especially relative to no thought). However, apart from the fact that the results obtained with this paradigm have been shown to be unstable, the paradigm does lack ecological validity when one wants to investigate decisions that take days, weeks, or longer.

A second characteristic of Type 3 processing is that it is very slow. In most taxonomies, Type 1 processing is seen as fast, whereas Type 2 processing is seen as slow, but according to the taxonomy we propose, Type 3 processing is even slower than Type 2 processing. The most beautiful processes in which Type 3 processing is involved (in combination with Type 2 processing; more on that later) are the scientific discoveries made after scientists have been occupied with a problem for months or even years. George Spencer Brown (Claxton, 1997, page 58; see also Dijksterhuis, 2004), who described the way Sir Isaac Newton worked, once famously said, "To arrive at the simplest truth, as Newton knew and practiced, requires years of contemplation. Not activity. Not reasoning. Not calculating. Not busy behavior of any kind. Not reading. Not talking. Not making an effort. Not thinking. Simply bearing in mind what it is that one needs to know."

In addition, Type 3 processing is abstract and exploratory. These characteristics come from UTT research (Dijksterhuis & Nordgren, 2006). Type 3 processing is able to handle large amounts of information and has an automatic tendency to extract the gist of incoming information, and to organize, or cluster, incoming information based on its gist (see, e.g., Bos et al., 2008; Dijksterhuis, 2004; Reyna & Brainerd, 1995). In addition, Type 3 processing polarizes and weights information (Bos, Dijksterhuis, & van Baaren, 2011), and over time renders important information even more important and accessible, at the same time making unimportant information less important and accessible. Furthermore, Type 3 processing is exploratory in that it forms links or associations between previously unassociated information. Unlike Type 2 processing that works in a logical, analytic, and convergent way, Type 3 processing is largely divergent.

Importantly, Type 3 processing is goal-dependent. In the past 15 years, social psychology has witnessed a surge in research on unconscious goal pursuit, and we see Type 3 processing as a form of unconscious goal pursuit. Simply put, Type 3 processing only works when one—either consciously or unconsciously—wants it to work. The earlier quotation by Norman Mailer describes an eloquent example in this regard. In fact, it is very well possible—though this awaits testing—that the strength of a goal determines how hard Type 3 processing works to tackle a problem.

The previously discussed experiment by Bos et al. (2008) is highly relevant here. Participants processed information about four cars before they were distracted, and only the group of participants given the goal to choose between the cars before being distracted made sound decisions. In the same article, these authors also report an experiment in which participants read information about two decision problems simultaneously. They were presented with information about three cars and three roommates. They then engaged in a distraction task that lasted for a few minutes, but before they did this, some participants were told they had to choose among the cars, whereas others were told they had to choose among the roommates. After the distracting task, participants were asked to make both decisions, and as it turned out, their goals had influenced their decisions. Participants who were asked to decide among the cars indeed made better decisions on the car problem than participants who were asked to decide among the roommates, whereas the latter group was better able to choose among the roommates.

Finally, Type 3 processing requires more effort than Type 1 processing but much less than Type 2 processing. Goals guide attention, in the sense that we pay much more attention to goal-relevant stimuli or goal-relevant processes than to matters that are goal-irrelevant. Hence, and despite the fact that Type 3 processing works largely unconsciously, Type 3 processing does require resources. Again, the literature on unconscious goal pursuit is helpful here. Even goals that are pursued wholly unconsciously do take up some working memory capacity (Hassin, Bargh, Engell, & McCulloch, 2009; see also Hassin, 2011). Also, recent evidence shows that working memory is involved in thought that is not directly task-relevant, such as mind wandering (Levinson, Smallwood, & Davidson, 2012). The idea that Type 3 processing requires some effort is also supported by the finding that incubation produces better results when the distracter task is not too taxing—that is, not taking up too many resources (Sio & Ormerod, 2009). Furthermore, a recent study on unconscious thought showed that easier distraction tasks produce greater unconscious thought results than do difficult ones (McMahon, Sparrow, Chatman, & Riddle, 2011).

Given these proposed characteristics, it should generally be easy to distinguish Type 3 processing from Type 2 processing and Type 1 processing. Type 2 processing is conscious, needs full attention, and is relatively short-lived, whereas Type 3 processing is mostly unconscious (though they do sometimes need temporary conscious guidance), requires limited effort, and can take very long. Likewise, Type 1 processing is very fast and automatic, whereas Type 3 processing is slow and goal-dependent.

It may be useful also to discuss briefly the relation between Type 3 processing and intuition. We define *intuition* as a gut feeling based on unconscious information processing (see also Dijksterhuis & Nordgren, 2006), and as such, an intuition can be the consequence of both Type 3 and Type 1 processing. For example, a gut feeling based on a few seconds of interaction with a car salesperson that tells one that he should not be trusted is the consequence of Type 1 processing, whereas the nagging but vague feeling that there is something just not quite right with the car company one went to a week ago is the consequence of Type 3 processing.

It is perhaps in the domain of expert intuition that the boundaries between Type 1 and Type 3 processing become complicated. In Malcolm Gladwell's (2005) famous example of the fake (?) Kouros bought by the Getty Museum, some experts quickly saw that there was something wrong. There are different ways to look at this. One can say that Type 1 processing led to these experts' fast assessments. Another way is to say that the very brief period of unconscious thought really is truncated Type 3 processing that proceeds very fast because the thought process was aided by an enormous knowledge base. Yet another way to look at the process is to assume that the first assessment was based on Type 1 processing, but that it elicited Type 3 processing afterwards (this was not described by Gladwell, but no doubt the experts kept on mulling over the authenticity of the Kouros for a while). Future thinking and research may shed more light on the distinction between Type 1 processing and Type 3 processing.

COOPERATION OF TYPE 2 PROCESSING AND TYPE 3 PROCESSING

A taxonomy of different types of processing may lead to the idea that people use only one type to solve a given problem or make a decision. However, it feels as if, intuitively at least, most important decisions and most creative ideas spring from a cooperation between Type 2 processing and Type 3 processing. Hence, in order to understand better how people make important decisions in their daily lives, we should explore how Type 3 processing and Type 2 processing collaborate. It seems that there are at least a few ways in which this cooperation can take place.

First, sometimes an intrusion into consciousness by Type 3 processing, caused by lack of progress (see earlier discussion), leads to more than just fleeting moments of awareness of the problem one is trying to solve. When unconsciously mulling over the choice for one of three apartments for a number of days, one may find the need to make a pros and cons list of the financial aspects (price of apartments, initial investments that need to be made [the old kitchen in one of the apartments needs to be replaced!], various monthly costs, differences in costs of commute, etc.). In other words, conscious intrusions of Type 3 processing may lead to

Type 2 processing. Such Type 2 processing interventions may occur when new information is encountered.

Type 2 processing and Type 3 processing can also work on different aspects of the same decision problem, because each has its own strengths and weaknesses. Type 2 processing can follow strict rules, whereas Type 3 processing may be much better at integrating large amounts of information (Dijksterhuis & Nordgren, 2006). In a recent experiment, Nordgren, Bos, and Dijksterhuis (2011) had participants choose between 12 different apartments. Some apartments were generally more desirable than others, and whereas some violated certain rules (the monthly rent was too high), others did not. Participants who thought consciously were particularly good at choosing rule-abiding options, whereas participants who thought unconsciously were better able to determine which apartments were most desirable. However, participants who first thought consciously and subsequently thought unconsciously, made the best decisions: They chose apartments that were desirable and rule-abiding at the same time. Again, we do not equate unconscious thought with Type 3 processing (nor do we equate conscious thought with Type 2 processing), but this may point at a division of labor that is intuitively compelling. When we think about a decision among alternatives (think about a hiring decision or the choice for a house), we first use Type 2 processing to reject a few alternatives, then apply Type 3 processing to choose between the two or three best ones (and perhaps end with a return to Type 2 processing to make some final checks, such as when we read a contract before we sign it).

Another hypothesis is that the use of Type 3 processing is, for many problems we face, a default option. It may be the case that Type 2 processing only kicks in when Type 3 processing is not able to solve the problem. Some people never use lists of pros and cons or seem to engage in elaborate, logical, conscious decision strategies for important personal decisions, such as the choice of a place to live, or the choice between one's current job and a job offer. There may be many reasons for this, but one reason could be that these people simply do not need to do this because their Type 3 processing takes care of their choices.

An intriguing and somewhat strange example of the fact that Type 2 processing is needed when Type 3 processing does not fully deal with something comes from the domain of creativity. Once, while the famous poet Housman took a walk, he suddenly "wrote" a poem. Housman did not have to do anything; the poem just presented itself to consciousness, at least so the story goes (Ghiselin, 1952). In other words, the poem intruded into consciousness ready made by Type 3 processing. All Housman had to do was record it, as if he were listening to someone else recite the poem. Housman immediately knew that the poem was supposed to have four verses. Now, unfortunately, his unconscious, his Type 3 processing, only presented three such verses, then stopped. The fourth verse Housman had to work hard for, and it had to be constructed, consciously, step-by-step, by Type 2 processing.

Finally, another hypothesis we would like to propose is that there are decisions, or problems that, because of their inherent characteristics, fit one of the systems better than the others (see also Dijksterhuis & Nordgren, 2006). For instance, decisions that need to be dealt with instantaneously require Type 1 processing; decisions that require logical, analytical thought require Type 2 processing; and complicated decisions that do not necessarily require logic but do involve multiple "vague" and difficult-to-verbalize pieces of information require Type 3 processing. Not many people think it is very sane to make pros and cons list for various potential romantic partners—relationships seems to need Type 3 processing, not Type 2 processing—but when buying a new laptop, it seems ignorant not to engage in at least some conscious deliberation (in this case, Type 2 processing) about the specific characteristics one wants.

The idea of fit between decisions (or problems in general) and the different systems also implies that one can apply a system when one should not, and that this can lead to suboptimal decisions. Indeed, this has been shown in various experiments by Wilson and colleagues. If one uses Type 2 processing for decisions that really need to be taken care of by Type 1 or Type 3 processing, decisions actually suffer (Wilson & Schooler, 1991; Wilson et al., 1993; see also

Dijksterhuis & Aarts, 2010; Levine, Halberstadt, & Goldstone, 1996). Likewise, Payne, Samper, Bettman, and Luce (2008) showed that when people are forced to use Type 2 processing for a longer period than they normally would, their decision outcomes become worse.

TYPE 3 PROCESSING AND SLEEP

I learned not to think about anything that I was writing from the time I stopped writing until I started again the next day. That way my subconscious would be working on it.

—ERNEST HEMINGWAY

One of the most famous poems ever written—*Kubla Kahn: Or, a Vision in a Dream* by Samuel Taylor Coleridge—was revealed to the author in a dream. In 1865, Friedrich August Kekulé awoke from a strange dream in which a snake had been forming a circle while biting its own tail. The story goes that the dream made Kekulé realize the structure of benzene, something the scientific community had been working on for quite a while. People, so it seems, can think up remarkable things while they sleep. What is the empirical evidence for thought-like processes that occur while we sleep?

Wagner, Gais, Haider, Verleger, and Born (2004) showed that sleep more than doubled the likelihood of acquiring insight into a hidden rule. Participants completed a task in which they had to solve problems involving number sequences. These sequences could be solved in a slow, stepwise fashion, but they could also be completed much faster with a hidden, abstract rule. Participants practiced for a while, and this initial training session was followed by 8 hours of nighttime sleep, nighttime wakefulness, or daytime wakefulness. Of the people who slept before they resumed the task, almost 60% had discovered the rule, as opposed to only 23% of the people who had not slept (see also Stickgold & Walker, 2004). Recently, Cai, Mednick, Harrison, Kanady, and Mednick (2009) showed that improved creativity after sleep is at least partly caused by the fact that during rapid eye movement (REM) sleep, unassociated information is integrated.

Sleep also facilitates memory, and it does so in various ways. Perhaps the most well-known finding (or more precisely, set of related findings) is that sleep fosters memory consolidation. Concretely, at night, memories can become more stable, and they can also be enhanced, making them more effective (see Stickgold & Walker, 2007, for a review). In addition, sleep also helps the integration of newly learned information. In a fascinating experiment, Ellenbogen, Hu, Payne, Titone, and Walker (2007) presented to experimental participants information about the relations between various stimuli (of the sort of $A > B$, $B > C$, $C > D$, etc.). Immediately after the experiment, participants understood the close relations (e.g., $A > B$), but only after hours of engaging in other work did they understand the moderately remote ones ($A > C$). Finally, participants needed a good night's sleep in order to grasp the most abstract and remote relations ($A > E$).

The beneficial effects of sleep on memory can be even further enhanced by reactivating recently learned information during sleep. Rasch, Büchel, Gais and Born (2007) coupled an odor with information during a learning task that participants performed in the evening. After associations between the odor and the information were formed, participants slept. For some participants, the associated odor was again presented during sleep, and indeed, these participants showed better memory in the morning than control participants who were presented only with a control odor. Ritter, Strick, Bos, van Baaren, and Dijksterhuis (2012) replicated this finding in the domain of creativity. Participants in their experiment were asked, in the evening, to come up with ideas for a problem that required a creative solution. For some participants, this problem was coupled with the presence of an odor. During the night some participants had to put a scent diffuser next to their beds with the same odor; others, a scent diffuser with a different odor; and still others were not given a scent diffuser. The participants who were presented with the same odor during the night produced more creative ideas the next morning than participants in the other two groups, presumably because their goal to be creative remained active during the night.

The current state of affairs in the literature on cognitive processes that take place during sleep is somewhat unclear (see Stickgold & Walker, 2007, for a review), but it is clear that sleep can contribute to creativity and problem solving, and that sleep can therefore help—or it may even play a vital role—during the prolonged thought processes that we like to lump together under the umbrella of Type 3 processing.

TYPE 3 PROCESSING: WHERE AND HOW?

In sketching out the appearance of Type 3 processing, a final question to be answered is whether there are indications as to which brain processes might be involved. One of the implicit messages of the previous section is that Type 3 processing (like Type 1 and Type 2 processing, but probably moreso) comprises many different subprocesses (see also Dijksterhuis & Nordgren, 2006); hence, isolating a single brain area to explain all Type 3 processing seems unrealistic at the outset.

However, one tempting hypothesis that warrants further exploration is that Type 3 processing at least partly relies on the default network (e.g., Buckner, Andrews-Hanna, & Schacter, 2008). The default network comprises various related subsystems that integrate self-relevant information. Concretely, the medial temporal lobe offers information from past experience on which mental simulations are based, whereas the medial prefrontal subsystem fosters the flexible use of this information in the actual construction of these simulations (e.g., Buckner et al., 2008). Especially the fact that the default network is involved in processes that are both future-oriented and clearly self-relevant points to a relation with Type 3 processing. After all, Type 3 processing—that is, prolonged thought processes—seems to be involved mostly with (creative) problems that we are highly motivated to solve, and very important decisions we are facing. The idea of a relation between Type 3 processing and the default network is also consistent with the finding that default network activity increases when (conscious) cognitive control activity decreases. After all, unconscious thought also works better when people perform a relatively relaxing distracter task rather than a taxing one (McMahon et al., 2011; Sio & Ormerod, 2009). In addition, a possible relation between Type 3 processing and the default network is consistent with the finding that activation of the default network is correlated with mind wandering (Mason et al., 2007) and with the first evidence that creative incubation (Type 3 processing, in current terminology) is facilitated by mind wandering (Baird et al., 2012).

Finally, recent research shows that the default network is related to unconscious processes in general (Vincent et al., 2007; Yang, Weng, Zang, Xu, & Xu, 2010) and to creativity. For instance, activity in the default network facilitates the associations between object features (Bar, 2007), and this is crucial for creativity. Moreover, there is initial evidence that creativity correlates with structural differences in grey matter volume of the default network (Kühn, Ritter, Müller, Brass, Van Baaren, & Dijksterhuis, in review).

The relation between Type 3 processing and the default network could be an interesting topic for further study and theorizing. However, we again point out that Type 3 processing should not be associated with just a single area or network. As alluded to earlier, Type 3 processing is goal-dependent, and goals, even unconscious ones, do require some working memory guidance (Hassin et al., 2009). This shows that the default network is not solely responsible for all Type 3 processing.

CONCLUDING REMARKS

We have proposed Type 3 processing in order to better understand prolonged thought processes in which people engage when they solve creative problems or make decisions. We sketched possible outlines of Type 3 processing, only some of which were based on empirical evidence. Some aspects were merely based on anecdotes or on introspection, yet others were derived from—as science goes—a combination of the authors' own Type 2 processing and Type 3 processing.

However, we hope this chapter encourages thinking about how we may explain and understand processes of prolonged thought, and that it offers fruitful hints for further empirical research. In our view, there are various questions on which it may be interesting to shed further light. How effortless is Type 3 processing? And how slow is Type 3 processing? Can experts in a certain domain speed up Type 3 processing processes because of their large database of relevant knowledge? Is Type 3 processing, the way we have described it, indeed a default process that we often rely on, and is Type 2 processing the system that kicks in when Type 3 processing cannot solve a problem? Or is the relation between Type 2 processing and Type 3 processing quite different? And perhaps the most fundamental question: Is it indeed useful to propose Type 3 processing, or is it possible after all to accommodate prolonged thought in our existing dual-process framework, perhaps by adding some nuts and bolts to Type 1 processing and/or Type 2 processing?

ACKNOWLEDGMENTS

This chapter was supported by an NWO Vici grant (No. 453-05-004) awarded to Ap Dijksterhuis.

NOTES

1. Cited in Whyte (1962, p. 93).
2. One may note that the definition of *thought* in the Oxford dictionary also allows thought to be unconscious. *Thinking* is defined as "directing one's mind towards someone or something; use one's mind actively to form connected ideas." Furthermore, the process of thought is defined as "careful consideration or attention." Sometimes, attention is equated with consciousness, but attention—the resources we spend on a problem—is not the same as consciousness. Theoretically, attention and consciousness should be seen as orthogonal, though correlated in real life, as we are often consciously aware of things to which we pay a lot of attention (for more on this important distinction, see Dehaene, Changeux, Naccache, Sackur, & Sergent, 2006; Dijksterhuis & Aarts, 2010; Koch & Tsuchiya, 2006; Lamme, 2003).

REFERENCES

Andreasen, N. C. (2005). *The creative brain*. New York: Plume.

Baird, B., Smallwood, J., Mrazek, M. D., Kam, J., Franklin M. S., & Schooler, J. W. (2012). Inspired by distraction: Mind-wandering facilitates creative incubation. *Psychological Science, 23*(10), 1117–1122.

Bar, M. (2007). The proactive brain: Using analogies and associations to generate predictions. *Trends in Cognitive Sciences, 11*, 280–289.

Bargh, J. A. (2011). Unconscious thought theory and its discontents: A critique of the critiques. *Social Cognition, 29*, 629–647.

Bargh, J. A., & Chartrand, T. L. (1999). The unbearable automaticity of being. *American Psychologist, 54*, 462–479.

Bargh, J. A., Gollwitzer, P. M., Lee-Chai, A. Y., Barndollar, K., & Trötschel, R. (2001). Bypassing the will: Automatic and controlled self-regulation. *Journal of Personality and Social Psychology, 81*, 1014–1027.

Betsch, T., Plessner, H., Schwieren, C., & Gütig, R. (2001). I like it but I don't know why: A value-account approach to implicit attitude formation. *Personality and Social Psychology Bulletin, 27*, 242–253.

Bongers, K. C. A., Dijksterhuis, A., & Spears, R. (2010). On the role of consciousness in goal pursuit. *Social Cognition, 28*, 262–272.

Bos, M. W., Dijksterhuis, A., & van Baaren, R. B. (2008). On the goal-dependency of unconscious thought. *Journal of Experimental Psychology, 44*, 1114–1120.

Bos, M. W., Dijksterhuis, A., & van Baaren, R. B. (2011). The benefits of "sleeping on things": Unconscious thought leads to automatic weighting. *Journal of Consumer Psychology, 21*, 4–8.

Bowers, K. S., Regehr, G., Balthazard, C., & Parker, K. (1990). Intuition in the context of discovery. *Cognitive Psychology, 22*, 72–110.

Buckner, R. L., Andrews-Hanna, J. R., Schacter, D. L. (2008). The brain's default network: Anatomy, Function, and relevance to disease. *Annals of the New York Academy of Sciences, 1124*, 1–38.

Cai, J. D., Mednick, S. A., Harrison, E. M., Kanady, J. C., & Mednick, S. C. (2009). REM, not incubation, improves creativity by priming associative networks. *Proceedings of the National Academy of Science, 106*, 10130–10134.

Claxton, G. (1997). *Hare brain, tortoise mind: How intelligence increases when you think less.* New York: HarperCollins.

Custers, R., & Aarts, H. (2005). Positive affect as implicit motivator: On the nonconscious operation of behavioral goals. *Journal of Personality and Social Psychology, 89*(2), 129–142.

Dehaene, S., Changeux, J., Naccache, L., Sackur, J., & Sergent, C. (2006). Conscious, preconscious, and subliminal processing: A testable taxonomy. *Trends in Cognitive Sciences, 10,* 204–211.

Dijksterhuis, A. (2004). Think different: The merits of unconscious thought in preference development and decision making. *Journal of Personality and Social Psychology, 87,* 586–598.

Dijksterhuis, A., & Nordgren, L. F. (2006). A theory of unconscious thought. *Perspectives on Psychological Science, 1,* 95–109.

Dijksterhuis, A., van Dijk, J., Driessen, M., & Scheffers, M. (2013). *On how people make decisions in real life: Distinguishing Systems 1, 2 and 3.*

Ellenbogen, J. M., Hu, P. T., Payne, J. D., Titone, D., & Walker, M. P. (2007). Human relational memory requires time and sleep. *Proceedings of the National Academy of Sciences, 104,* 7723–7728.

Evans, J. St. B. T. (2008). Dual-processing accounts of reasoning, judgment and social cognition. *Annual Review of Psychology, 59,* 255–278.

Ghiselin, B. (1952). *The creative process.* New York: New American Library.

Gladwell, M. (2005). *Blink: The power of thinking without thinking.* New York: Little, Brown.

Hassin, R. R. (2011). Consciousness might still be in business, but not in this business. *Consciousness and Cognition, 20,* 299–300.

Hassin, R. R., Bargh, J. A., Engell, A. D., & McCulloch, K. C. (2009). Implicit working memory. *Consciousness and Cognition, 18,* 665–678.

Hemingway, E. (1964). *A moveable feast.* London: Arrow Books.

Jordan, C. H., Logel, C., Spencer, S. J., Zanna, M. P., & Whitfield, M. L. (2009). The heterogeneity of self-esteem: Exploring the interplay between implicit and explicit self-esteem. In R. E. Petty, R. H. Fazio, & P. Briñol (Eds.), *Attitudes: Insights from the new implicit measures* (pp. 251–284). New York: Psychology Press.

Kahneman, D. (2003). A perspective on judgment and choice. Mapping bounded rationality. *American Psychologist, 58,* 697–720.

Koch, C., & Tsuchiya, N. (2006). Attention and consciousness: Two distinct brain processes. *Trends in Cognitive Sciences, 11,* 16–22.

Koestler, A. (1964). *The act of creation.* London: Penguin.

Kühn, S., Ritter, S. M., Müller, B. C. N., Brass, M., van Baaren, R. B., & Dijksterhuis, A. (under review). *The importance of unconscious processes in creativity—a structural MRI Study.*

Lamme, V. A. F. (2003). Why visual attention and awareness are different. *Trends in Cognitive Sciences, 7,* 12–18.

Levine, G. M., Halberstadt, J. B., & Goldstone, R. L. (1996). Reasoning and the weighing of attributes in attitude judgments. *Journal of Personality and Social Psychology, 70,* 230–240.

Levinson, D. B., Smallwood, J., & Davidson, R. J. (2012). The persistence of thought: Evidence for a role of working memory in the maintenance in task-unrelated thinking. *Psychological Science, 23,* 375–380.

Mason, M. F., Norton, M. I., Van Horn, J. D., Wegner, D. M., Grafton, S. T. & Macrae, C. N. (2007). Wandering minds: The default network and stimulus-independent thought. *Science, 315,* 393–395.

McMahon, K., Sparrow, B., Chatman, L., & Riddle, T. (2011). Driven to distraction: The impact of distracter type on unconscious decision making. *Social Cognition, 29,* 683–698.

Mednick, S. A. (1962). The associative basis of the creative process. *Psychological Review, 69,* 220–232.

Nordgren, L. F., Bos, M. W., & Dijksterhuis, A. (2011). The best of both worlds: Integrating conscious and unconscious thought best solves complex decisions. *Journal of Experimental Social Psychology, 47,* 509–511.

Payne, J., Samper, A., Bettman, J. R., & Luce, M. F. (2008). Boundary conditions on unconscious thought in complex decision making. *Psychological Science, 19,* 1118–1123.

Poincaré, H. (1913). *The foundations of science.* Lancaster, PA: Science Press.

Rasch, B., Büchel, C., Gais, S., & Born, J. (2007). Odor-cues during slow-wave sleep prompt declarative memory consolidation. *Science, 315,* 1426–1429.

Reyna, V. F., & Brainerd, C. J. (1995). Fuzzy-trace theory: An interim synthesis. *Learning and Individual Differences*, 7, 1–75.

Ritter, S. M., Strick, M., Bos, M. W., van Baaren, R. B., & Dijksterhuis, A. (2012). Good morning creativity: Task reactivation during sleep enhances beneficial effects of sleep on creative performance. *Journal of Sleep Research*, *21*(6), 643–647.

Schooler, J. W., & Melcher, J. (1995). The ineffability of insight. In S. M. Smith, T. B. Ward, & R. A. Finke (Eds.), *The creative cognition approach* (pp. 97–134). Cambridge, MA: MIT Press.

Schopenhauer, A. (1970). *Essays and aphorisms*. London: Penguin. (Original work published 1851)

Sio, U. N., & Ormerod, T. C. (2009). Does incubation enhance problem-solving? A meta-analytic review. *Psychological Bulletin, 135*, 94–120.

Slovic, P., Finucane, M., Peters, E., & MacGregor, D. G. (2002). The affect heuristic. In T. Gilovich, D. Griffin, & D. Kahneman (Eds.), *Heuristics and biases* (pp. 397–420). New York: Cambridge University Press.

Stanovich, K. E. (2004). *The robots' rebellion: Finding meaning in the age of Darwin*. Chicago: University of Chicago Press.

Stanovich, K. E., & West, R. F. (2000). Individual differences in reasoning: Implications for the rationality debate. *Behavioral and Brain Sciences, 23*, 645–665.

Stanovich, K. E., West, R. F., Toplak, M. E. (2011). The complexity of developmental predictions from dual process models. *Developmental Review, 31*, 103–118.

Stickgold, R., & Walker, M. (2004). To sleep, perchance to gain creative insight? *Trends in Cognitive Sciences, 8*, 191–192.

Stickgold, R., & Walker, M. P. (2007). Sleep-dependent memory consolidation and reconsolidation. *Sleep Medicine, 8*, 331–343.

Strick, M., Dijksterhuis, A., Bos, M. W., Sjoerdsma, A., van Baaren, R. B., & Nordgren, L. F. (2011). A meta-analysis on unconscious thought effects. *Social Cognition, 29*, 738–763.

Strick, M., Dijksterhuis, A., & van Baaren, R. B. (2010). Unconscious-thought effects take place off-line, not on-line. *Psychological Science, 21*, 484–488.

Tversky, A., & Kahneman, D. (1973). Availability: A heuristic for judging frequency and probability. *Cognitive Psychology, 5*, 207–232.

Vincent, J. L., Patel, G. H., Fox, M. D., Snyder, A. Z., Baker, J. T., Van Essen, D. C., et al. (2007). Intrinsic functional architecture in the anaesthetized monkey brain. *Nature, 447*, 83–85.

Wagner, U., Gais, S., Haider, H., Verleger, R., & Born, J. (2004). Sleep inspires insight. *Nature, 427*, 352–355.

Wallas, G. (1926). *The art of thought*. New York: Harcourt Brace.

Whyte, L. L. (1962). *The unconscious before Freud*. Garden City, NY: Anchor Books.

Wilson, T. D., Lisle, D., Schooler, J. W., Hodges, S. D., Klaaren, K. J., & LaFleur, S. J. (1993). Introspecting about reasons can reduce post-choice satisfaction. *Personality and Social Psychology Bulletin, 19*, 331–339.

Wilson, T. D., & Schooler, J. W. (1991). Thinking too much: Introspection can reduce the quality of preferences and decisions. *Journal of Personality and Social Psychology, 60*, 181–192.

Yang, J., Weng, X., Zang, Y., Xu, M., & Xu, X. (2010). Sustained activity within the default mode network during an implicit memory task. *Cortex, 46*, 354–366.

Yaniv, I., & Meyer, D. E. (1987). Activation and metacognition of inaccessible stored information: Potential bases for incubation effects in problem-solving. *Journal of Experimental Psychology: Learning, Memory and Cognition, 13*, 187–205.

Zhong, C. B., Dijksterhuis, A., & Galinsky, A. (2008). The merits of unconscious thought in creativity. *Psychological Science, 19*, 912–918.

PART VII

HABITS, GOALS, AND MOTIVATION

CHAPTER 25

Habits in Dual-Process Models

Wendy Wood, Jennifer S. Labrecque, Pei-Ying Lin, and Dennis Rünger

Habits structure much of people's everyday activities. Habits for eating are some of the most striking. People consume about 91% of the food on their plates regardless of whether they are eating from a large or a small plate of food. Specifically, when given large plates, people served themselves and ate about half again more food as when given small plates (Wansink & Cheney, 2005). Thus, plate-cleaning habits persist despite the amount of food involved. People also develop habits to eat certain types of food. People with habits to eat popcorn at the movies consume approximately the same amount regardless of whether it is fresh and tasty or stale and spongy. Specifically, when popcorn was stale, habitual eaters at the cinema reported disliking it, but they consumed just as much as when it was fresh (Neal, Wood, Wu, & Kurlander, 2011). Thus, popcorn eating habits persist despite the palatability of the food. What propels people to eat habitually in this way, with minimal regard for the amount consumed or the way it tastes?

The answer to this question comes from an understanding of the nature of habits. Eating, like much of human behavior, can be repeated so that it becomes habitual. *Habits* are dispositions to give a response in a particular context. As people pursue goals in daily life, they experience myriad covariations between their actions (e.g., eating) and cues in the performance context (e.g., food on a plate, popcorn in a bag). Habit learning occurs when people repeat the same behavior in a specific context, so that associations between the behavior and the contextual cues can be formed. Once a habit is firmly established, perceiving relevant cues—the food on one's plate and the popcorn in the bag at the cinema—is sufficient to trigger the associated behavior.

In this chapter, we first develop a process-based account of habitual responding (see Wood & Neal, 2007, 2009), then consider the role of habits in dual-process theories. The remainder of the chapter focuses on the factors that promote or impair habitual control of action in relation to other action control mechanisms.

PROCESSES OF HABIT AUTOMATICITY

Following William James's (1890) notion of ideomotor action, we assume that a memory representation of the habitual response intervenes between cue perception and habit performance (see Figure 25.1). Due to the frequent repetition of the response, this representation is likely to be highly accessible in the sense of being strong, stable, and distinct. In addition, the frequent pairings of the context and the response produce a par-

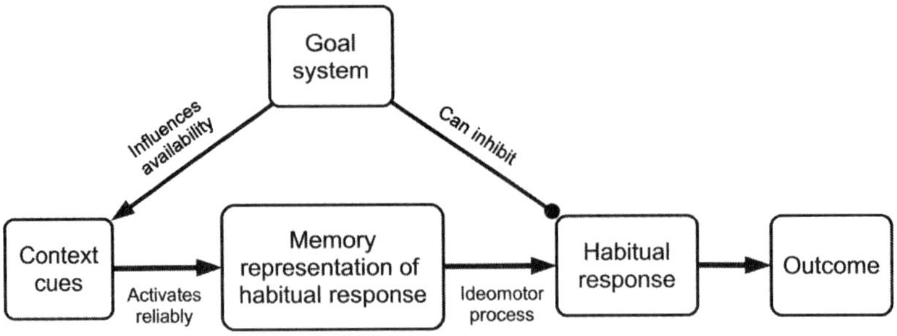

FIGURE 25.1. Processes by which habits are automatically triggered in memory by contexts, then integrated with goals to guide responding.

ticularly strong associative link between the memory representation of the context cues and that of the response. As a result, whenever an individual perceives the relevant cues, the habit representation is strongly and reliably activated.

Habitual responses have a high probability of being executed when their triggering conditions are met. One reason is the simple strength of habit representations in memory—they likely exceed the activation level of alternative actions. Contributing to this effect, alternative responses may decrease in accessibility as people repeatedly retrieve a particular response from memory (McCulloch, Aarts, Fujita, & Bargh, 2008; see retrieval-induced forgetting: Anderson, 2003). Also contributing to habit performance, people may misattribute externally cued representations to their own natural response to the situation, that is, to their internal preferences and desires (Loersch & Payne, 2011). With this misattribution, habitual responses can seem to be promoted by goals and intentions (see the section "Experience of Habits"). Nonetheless, as responses become more habitual, they come more directly under the control of the stimulus context and thereby lose sensitivity to the value of the consequences of that response.

The context cues that activate habits range from simple elements of the environment that covary with a response—including physical locations, other people, internal states, and preceding actions in a sequence—to complex conjunctions involving, for example, the standard place to meet a friend for lunch. The cueing process may proceed as envisioned in models of routine action, in which each response in a sequence is triggered by the current internal state given the response sequence, in conjunction with perceptions of the state of the environment (Botvinick & Plaut, 2004). Thus, when making coffee habitually, people may have learned that adding cream and the perception of the lighter color together cue the next response of adding sugar. In this view, habit learning amplifies aspects of context cues that were in the past informative for action selection. Thus, performance is tied not solely to a specific cue in a specific time and place (one's own coffee cup) but to other, similar context cues that share important features (other cups). Habit performance thereby can be triggered by a class of cues that might vary in irrelevant features.

Rewards for habit performance may be important initially to promote learning of context–response associations, but these consequences of responding become relatively unimportant once habits have developed (Neal, Wood, & Quinn, 2006). Thus, people with the relevant habits eat stale popcorn in the cinema despite its taste and eat most of the food on their plates regardless of whether they are still hungry. The stimulus-cued nature of habits yields this insensitivity to outcomes of the response.

The term *habit* is sometimes used interchangeably with automaticity. In contrast with this view, we argue that habits are characterized by a specific subset of the features that are commonly used to diagnose automaticity (De Houwer, Teige-Mocigemba, Spruyt, & Moors, 2009). Broadly speaking, habits are triggered by a relatively rigid form of context cueing that integrates with but is not flexibly responsive to people's goals and intentions. Habitual responses are initiated automatically in the sense that they are stimulus-driven, require only minimal or sporadic conscious monitoring and are therefore largely autonomous, and they do not depend on a goal for performance.

Despite these features of automaticity, habit responses are largely controllable. As illustrated in Figure 25.1, people do not necessarily act on a habit representation once it is brought to mind in a given context. Given an explicit goal that is incompatible with a habit, people can alter their responses in several ways (see Quinn, Pascoe, Wood, & Neal, 2010). Much like a dieter deciding to eat only half of the food on his or her plate, people can make decisions to inhibit an unwanted response. Also, when people are aware of the link between contextual cues and an unwanted habit, they can deliberately avoid habit triggers. Thus, dieters can decide not to walk by a favorite donut shop, and if they are aware of the tendency for cues to generalize on important dimensions, they should probably decide not to go to other restaurants filled with the sight and smell of donuts.

HABITS IN DUAL INFORMATION-PROCESSING SYSTEMS

In dual-process models, habit performance is mediated by a fast, automatic, unconscious processing system that reflects associations learned through experience. This automatic system typically is contrasted with slow, deliberative, conscious processing that requires access to a working memory system of limited capacity (Evans, 2008). A variety of dual-process models have been proposed, each providing a broad distinction between two partially independent processing systems, and each offering slightly different interpretations of automatic and deliberative processes (see Evans, 2008). The heterogeneous types of fast, automatic learning and retrieval capacities considered in these models are grouped under general labels such as *System 1* (Kahneman, 2003), the *impulsive system* (Strack & Deutsch, 2004), and the *reflexive system* (Lieberman, Gaunt, Gilbert, & Trope, 2002). This type of system includes habits, other features of automaticity, and low-effort processes such as relying on heuristic judgment rules.

It is surprising that few dual-process models identify habits as a distinct mechanism of action control. Habit also is largely absent from social psychology more generally. For example, the chapter on automaticity in Fiske, Gilbert, and Lindzey's (2009) *Handbook of Social Psychology* does not, according to the volume index, make even one mention of habit. Similarly, few textbooks in social psychology currently recognize habits, although this may change given the popular resurgence of interest (e.g., Duhigg, 2012).

Historically, habits were a central principle in William James's (1890) understanding of the mind. In the ensuing years, habits became linked with mechanistic approaches to learning, serving as a cornerstone of early learning models (Hull, 1934; Skinner, 1953). Subsequently, Squire and Zola-Morgan's (1991) classic model of memory systems differentiated skills and habits from other types of nondeclarative (implicit) processes, including priming, simple classical conditioning, and nonassociative learning. Building on these insights, Evans's (2008) review of dual-process models identified habits as one of three distinct types of low effort, automatic process. Recently, habits have become an important component of many neural models of memory systems (see the section "Habits in Neural Models of Memory"), and a number of theoretical analyses have outlined how habit mechanisms integrate with other aspects of action control (e.g., Wood & Neal, 2007; Yin & Knowlton, 2006).

By outlining the processes of habit automaticity, this chapter moves beyond global automatic versus controlled distinctions to the understanding of action control. We argue that habits involve characteristic neural mechanisms and cognitive representations, and that these characteristics are evident in particular patterns of response. In the next section, we explain how the neural mechanisms associated with habit memory subserve this automatic responding.

HABITS IN NEURAL MODELS OF MEMORY

Evidence of the neural substrates of habit performance comes from diverse research conducted on human and nonhuman primates, as well as rodents. Although it might seem that, in humans, habit memory is degraded or dependent on deliberative, higher cortical functions, research with selectively brain-damaged patients and with normal participants on a variety of tasks reveals that this learning mechanism is in fact well developed (Bayley, Frascino, & Squire, 2005). A common theme across these various research literatures is that repeated action and the formation of habits is accompanied by dynamic shifts in neural activity, especially in corticobasal ganglia circuits (Graybiel, 2008; Yin & Knowlton, 2006). The functional neuroanatomy of the corticobasal ganglia system underlies many of the characteristic features of habit automaticity, especially the cueing of responses by contexts with minimal responsiveness to goals.

As people repeat a response so as to form a habit, two corticobasal ganglia loops are particularly important (Graybiel, 2008; Yin & Knowlton, 2006). The first, the *associative loop*, supports working memory functions and goal-directed actions. This loop links the prefrontal cortex and associated areas with the caudate nucleus and the anterior portion of the putamen. The second, the *sensorimotor loop*, is thought to support the formation of inflexible stimulus–response associations that underlie automatic, habitual behaviors. This loop links the somatosensory and motor cortex with the medial and posterior portions of the putamen. The formation of habits and development of stimulus-cued responding are thought to involve a shift in behavioral control from the associative corticobasal ganglia loop to the sensorimotor loop (Graybiel, 2008; Yin & Knowlton, 2006).[1]

Evidence of the relative involvement of these two cortical–subcortical loops in the development of stimulus-driven responding comes from research on simple sequential motor tasks. In a 3-month study, monkeys practiced different sequences in a button-pressing task, with some new and some standard, habitual sequences (Miyachi, Hikosaka, Miyashita, Kárádi, & Rand, 1997). When the monkeys' associative striatum was temporarily inactivated (via muscimol injection), they were less able to perform the newly learned sequences but still able to enact the habitual ones. In contrast, inactivation of the sensorimotor striatum selectively disrupted performance of habits. Comparable shifts emerged in a monthlong study in which people practiced a sequence of finger movements (Lehéricy et al., 2005). With training, neural activation decreased in the associative loop systems linked with goal-directed actions (i.e., premotor and prefrontal cortical areas, anterior cingulate cortex, associative territories of the basal ganglia), whereas activation increased in the sensorimotor regions of the basal ganglia.

From a functional perspective, then, the goal-independence of habits is linked to the architecture of the basal ganglia, in particular the lack of reward-based modulation of neural activity in the sensorimotor loop. Evidence of this link comes from Tricomi, Balleine, and O'Doherty's (2009) research on habit formation in a button-press learning task. Participants received either chips or candy as a reward for pressing a button when one of two target images was presented. After extensive practice and habits had formed, participants continued to press the buttons to the target images regardless of whether they had just eaten their fill of the associated food reward. Importantly, the sensorimotor striatum was linked to this absence of reward modulation. Across this extensive training, participants showed increased neural activity in relevant sensorimotor territories of the basal ganglia.

Other features of habits, such as inflexible performance, also can be traced to particular neural substrates. Inflexibility arises in part from the unitization or *chunking* of action sequences over time. A *chunk* is an integrated memory representation that can be selected as a whole and executed with minimal attentional involvement. Research on the neural substrates of chunking has identified neural markers for the start and endpoints of action sequences, presumably at the start and end of the learned progression of responses, and minimal neural responding in the middle, suggesting an integrated sequence representation (Fujii & Graybiel, 2003).

Given the current research, it is tempting to conclude that the sensorimotor loop is responsible for the long-term retention of habits. This conclusion is challenged, however, by some evidence that habit performance, after especially extended learning, continues despite deactivation of the sensorimotor striatum (e.g., Desmurget &

Turner, 2010). With such extensive training, control of habitual behaviors may be further consolidated in transfer to extrastriatal areas, including the cortex. A neurocomputational model of automaticity in perceptual categorization by Ashby, Ennis, and Spiering (2007) offers an elegant account of this hypothesized transfer of control. The model assumes two pathways connecting sensory association areas with the premotor cortex—a slow reentrant corticobasal ganglia loop and a fast, direct corticocortical projection. Early performance is governed by goal-directed learning in the basal ganglia circuit. As training progresses, the appropriate corticocortical synapses are strengthened via Hebbian learning, and control is gradually transferred from the basal ganglia loop to the exclusively cortical network. This neural progression in learning was demonstrated in a procedural category learning task in which performance depended primarily on cortical areas once it became thoroughly automatic (Waldschmidt & Ashby, 2011). It may be, then, that the basal ganglia are not involved in the long-term storage of habitual behaviors. Their primary function in the development of automaticity could consist of training the direct corticocortical pathway.

In general, habits gradually develop as goal-responsive neural systems relinquish control to the sensorimotor system, and perhaps ultimately to cortical systems that control habits. Given that many everyday behaviors draw on multiple memory systems, their performance probably involves a combination of habit and other types of learning. Thus, the neural systems subserving habits are integrated with a variety of other substrates involved in action control. This interaction is enabled by neural architecture in which the sensorimotor striatal system associated with habit performance is embedded in broader corticobasal ganglia circuits that facilitate both stimulus-driven, habitual responding and more flexible, goal-oriented actions (Yin & Knowlton, 2006). Given interactions among these neural systems, habits interface with other action control systems to guide responding.

In the next section, we discuss the features of automaticity that comprise habit responding. We then address the multiple ways that habits integrate with other action control mechanisms.

HABITS ARE DIRECTLY BROUGHT TO MIND BY CONTEXT CUES

Evidence of Habit Automaticity

To test the cognitive associations that underlie habits, Neal, Wood, Labrecque, and Lally (2012, Study 1) assessed how quickly habitual runners detected the words *running* and *jogging* when presented in a lexical decision task. Before each detection trial, runners were subliminally primed with their personal (1) running locations (e.g., forest, gym) they usually frequented, or (2) goals (e.g., weight, relax) that motivated them to run. After subliminal exposure to their locations, runners with stronger habits were faster to detect running-related words. This suggests that their habitual behaviors were mentally linked with the contexts in which they performed that action. Also, suggesting that habits do not require goals, subliminal exposure to running goals did not activate thoughts of running for strongly habitual runners. Instead, a curvilinear association emerged between habits and goals. Specifically, for runners who were still developing habits, goals seemed motivating and therefore activated thoughts of running. Strongly habitual runners, however, relied on context–response associations rather than goals to activate running responses.

Additional evidence that habits are triggered directly by context cues comes from a study of sports fans. Reasoning that fans who frequently go to sports stadiums have acquired a habit of speaking loudly, Neal et al. (2012, Study 2) primed some participants with pictures of the stadiums they habitually visited. Control participants were primed instead with pictures of kitchens. The loudness of participants' speech was assessed from their verbal responses to a search task. Participants with stronger habits to visit sports stadiums spoke more loudly after being primed with pictures of stadiums but not kitchens. Furthermore, indicating that this direct context–response tie did not depend on a motivating goal, participants with strong habits spoke loudly regardless of whether they had a goal to visit the stadium. Across these two studies, then, cognitive representations of a habitual response, as well as performance of the response, were activated directly by context cues, without relying on a supporting goal.

Habits and Other Automatic Processes

Habit associations between contexts and responses have different features from the automaticity commonly studied by social psychologists. Automaticity in social psychology typically involves activation of concepts or goals. Even research on behavioral priming tests how activating a general construct in memory influences behavioral responses.

Concept priming occurs when activation of traits or other categories (e.g., elderly) brings to mind associated beliefs, plans, and schemas, and these in turn influence a variety of responses (e.g., cognitive wisdom, physical feebleness). These effects occur because priming a concept (1) activates a rich, complex array of associated constructs in memory (Wheeler & DeMaree, 2009) that may (2) bias interpretation of a variety of situational factors to provide answers to primary current concerns (Loersch & Payne, 2011). In contrast, *habit automaticity* involves the cueing of a particular learned response or sequence of responses.

Variability in response also typifies goal priming, in which environmental cues activate a particular need, along with a potential variety of responses to meet that need. For example, the goal of going shopping may activate associated behaviors (for Europeans, traveling by bicycle) that are a means of attaining that goal. Yet because of goal *equifinality*—or substitutability in the behavioral means to a goal—any one goal can activate a variety of behaviors (e.g., driving a car, walking). Even strongly desired goals that stably characterize people's motives yield a strategic orientation and not necessarily repetition of any behavioral means. Also, activated goals are moderated in their influence by a variety of factors. For example, people's explicit goals can moderate the influence of implicit goals, such as implementation intentions (Sheeran, Webb, & Gollwitzer, 2005). Thus, unlike habits, automated goal pursuit does not necessarily promote repetition of particular responses to particular cues.

In summary, habits produce a characteristic pattern of responding that differs from other types of automated processes. The repetition of habit responses can be contrasted with the variability of responses that results from automatic activation of concepts and goals.

HABITS INTERFACE WITH OTHER TYPES OF ACTION CONTROL

Habits arise from context–response learning that is acquired slowly with experience. The slow time course of such learning is likely functional, because it insulates habit dispositions against short-term changes in behavior that might be generated as people respond to current goals or enact nonhabitual responses. Only with extended repetition in stable contexts are behavior patterns likely to be represented in habit learning. By reflecting the recurring features of people's past experiences, the habit learning system shields existing knowledge against potential disruption from being overwritten or unduly distorted by new experiences.

Features of Habits Structure Action Control

These conservative features of habits provide a framework that organizes the interface between habits and other action control systems. Because habits are represented in slow-learning neural and cognitive systems that directly link contexts and responses, habit dispositions do not merge flexibly with other guides to action. Although learning of habits initially may be guided by goal pursuit, the unique nature of habit learning is suggested by double-dissociation studies of the neural systems underlying performance of habit-related versus other types of tasks (e.g., Knowlton, Mangels, & Squire, 1996). Specifically, amnesic patients with medial temporal lobe damage who could not easily memorize rules nonetheless performed normally on tasks that involved habit learning. In contrast, patients with Parkinson's disease and neostriatal impairment were challenged to learn habit associations through repetition despite having intact capacities for other learning processes.

Habits also represent a separable source of memory in *process dissociation* studies using a cued-recall paradigm (Yonelinas & Jacoby, 2012). In completing this task, participants rely on habits developed through repeated practice or on conscious recollection of the correct response. Dissociations have been documented in the factors that influence these types of performance: Amnesics with selective hippocampal damage, older adults, and people who are distracted or under time pressure during performance tend to perform the task by relying on habit-type knowledge, whereas younger people and those without distractions or time pressure rely more on conscious recall (Yonelinas & Jacoby, 2012).

Dissociations in neural mechanisms and in the factors that influence performance provide elegant ways to demonstrate separable habitual, automatic versus more deliberative, controlled systems. However, we suspect that these kinds of dissociations emerge primarily with particular tasks and with particular moderating factors. In daily life, it is more likely that habits interact in a variety of ways with other memory systems in guiding responding.

Habits Cooperate with Other Systems

Habit learning and other forms of action control often interact cooperatively in the sense that both systems provide compatible guides to responding. Illustrating this cooperation, some actions that initially are goal-directed (e.g., a new exercise regimen) become habitual over time. In this sense, habits can be a vestige of past goal pursuit.

Perhaps because many everyday habits originate in goal pursuit, habitual actions often correspond with what people intend to do. Habits may blindly carry out the work of the goal that initially prompted people to respond repeatedly and therefore to develop the habit. In support, Ouellette and Wood's (1998) meta-analysis across 33 studies revealed that, for a variety of everyday behaviors, habit strength (as reflected in frequency of past performance) was positively correlated with favorability of behavioral intentions (r = .43, p < .01). For these behaviors, performance could reflect habit systems or other forms of action control, including explicit or implicit goal pursuit.

Habits Conflict with Other Systems

Habits also interact with other forms of action control when they conflict with people's goals. By definition, unwanted or bad habits counter current goals. Also, people sometimes slip and inadvertently perform habits when they intend to perform another response (Reason, 1992). We have argued that "good" and "bad" habits are guided by common psychological mechanisms—they differ primarily in terms of consistency with current goals (Neal, Wood, & Drolet-Rossi, 2013). However, we suspect that people are especially aware of their bad or unwanted habits because of the challenges they experience when trying to control or change them. Attempts to change unwanted lifestyle habits such as overeating, overspending, and addictive responses drain large amounts of people's time, energy, and money.

CONDITIONS PROMOTING AND IMPAIRING HABITUAL RESPONDING

Research on habit mechanisms tends to capitalize on instances in which habitual response tendencies (e.g., to eat most of the food on one's plate) are not in line with other forms of action control (e.g., the belief that eating less is healthy). Research has used this contrast strategy to isolate habits from other mechanisms guiding behavior. Then, to the extent that people are acting habitually, they are countering their deliberate intentions. To more directly pit habits against deliberate control of action, research in this tradition also evaluates moderators (e.g., habit strength, willpower) that are likely to alter the strength of habit cues or decrease deliberative reasoning. By testing for these kinds of moderators, habit research conforms to the basic structure of other work on dual-process models (Evans, 2008), while providing insight into the nature of stimulus-driven automaticity.

Habit Strength

Behavior prediction research with everyday behaviors highlights the moderating role of habit strength. In a typical study, researchers evaluate whether habits or explicit behavioral intentions are better predictors of future behavior. The basic finding is that, regardless of people's intentions, strong habits tend to predominate for riding bicycles, voting in national elections, drinking milk, eating snack food, watching TV, exercising, and purchasing fast food (Aldrich, Montgomery, & Wood, 2011; de Bruijn, Kremers, Singh, van den Putte, & van Mechelen, 2009; Danner, Aarts, & De Vries, 2008; Ji & Wood, 2007; see meta-analysis in Ouellette & Wood, 1998). Thus, people tend to repeat strongly habitual actions even given conflicting input from intentional systems.

Additional evidence that strong habits typically predominate over intentions comes from a meta-analysis of 47 studies of persuasive appeals and other interventions designed to change behavior (Webb & Sheeran, 2006). These intervention studies significantly changed people's intentions, and the question was whether they would change actual behavior. Suggesting that strong habits maintained, behaviors that people could repeat into habits (e.g., seat belt use) changed only minimally following changed intentions, whereas behaviors not conducive to habit formation (e.g., course enrollment) changed to correspond with the new intentions. Thus, people continued to repeat habits despite having adopted conflicting intentions.

Experimental evidence that strong habits persist despite conflicting goals comes from Neal et al.'s (2011) research on popcorn eating, mentioned at the beginning of the chapter. Moviegoers with strong cinema–popcorn habits ate comparable amounts of stale and fresh popcorn, despite reporting that they disliked it when stale. Thus, when in the cinema, moviegoers acted on strong habits even when these habits countered their evaluations.

People tend to act on habitual dispositions upon perception of associated cues because, as we argued at the beginning of this chapter, the cues are strongly associated with clear, distinct action representations in memory. In addition, not acting habitually can require effort, given that people have to inhibit the salient response tendency and make a decision to perform another response or no response (Quinn et al., 2010). As we explain below, deliberative forms of action control can be derailed by limited reasoning ability, absentmindedness, stress, and fluctuations in willpower. As a result, these factors can increase reliance on habits.

Limited Reasoning Ability

When their reasoning skills at a task are not very sophisticated, people may instead rely on simpler, habitual processes. This moderation of habits by skills was demonstrated in a study in which participants learned to navigate a route through a maze (Marchette, Bakker, & Shelton, 2011). Some participants spontaneously developed a response-learning, habit strategy (e.g., first turn left, then turn right), whereas others used a more flexible, cognitive mapping strategy of orienting toward the goal. The habitual, response-learning strategy was especially marked among participants with poor *deliberative skills,* defined as low scores on a test of spatial perspective taking. At the neural level, a habitual, response-learning strategy was subserved by activation in the bilateral caudate nucleus, whereas relying on the flexible mapping strategy was subserved by the hippocampus. At the behavioral level, participants using a habit strategy tended to repeat the specific response pattern they had learned even on trials in which shortcuts appeared that provided a faster route. In contrast, participants with better mapping skills were more likely to take advantage of available shortcuts. In short, behavioral and neural data indicated greater reliance on habits among participants with poor spatial reasoning skills.

Absentmindedness and Distraction

Habit performance also might be heightened when people are temporarily distracted and therefore unable to deliberate about how to act. Evidence comes from research on *action slips*, or instances in which people find themselves performing an unintended action (Norman, 1981). People tend to slip in this way when they are in settings in which they might typically perform a habit. In such settings, they may respond to habit triggers even when intending to engage in another action. A standard example is finding oneself on a weekend driving the route to work when actually intending to drive to the store. In Reason's (1979) experience-sampling studies of everyday behaviors, such *habit intrusions* or *capture errors* comprised up to 40% of all action slips. In evidence that amount of thought moderates habit performance, people were particularly likely to fall prey to such intrusions when they were distracted and thinking about something other than what they were doing (Reason, 1979, 1992).

Habit intrusions may be relatively common in daily life. They impede attempts to change behavior, as people fall back on old habits despite their best intentions to adopt a healthier lifestyle (Danner, Aarts, Papies, & de Vries, 2011). Habit intrusions even contribute to the challenges of introducing new products into the consumer market. New products may fail to gain traction when consumers cannot kick old habits. Fully 25% of the instances in which consumers failed to use a new product were due to habit interference (Labrecque, Wood, Neal, & Harrington, in preparation). In these instances, product use failures were not due to people disliking a product or having difficulty using it. Instead, consumers suffered *product slips* and simply forgot to use the products and reverted back to past habits. As with action slips in general, participants were especially likely to suffer product slips when they were not thinking about what they were doing and were therfore susceptible to habit triggers.

Stress

The experience of stress, or psychological strain, also can promote habit performance, because stress limits deliberative capacity. That is, stress is associated with restricted attention, heightened arousal, and corresponding reliance on more routinized behavioral responses. Demonstrating the moderating role of stress on habit performance, Schwabe and Wolf (2009) trained participants in an instrumental task to respond to different fractal images for a food treat. Some participants had earlier undergone a cold-pressor task that heightened their stress levels. When stress was raised in this way, participants increased their habitual responses to the fractals regardless of their desire for the food treat. That is, stress increased participants' habitual responses even when they had already satiated on the relevant food. Thus, stress seemed to limit participants' ability to deliberate about what response they wished to give.

Willpower

Variations in willpower also affect habit performance by influencing the capacity to act on intentions. When willpower is low, people may fall back on performing habits, because they have limited ability to inhibit the activated response in mind or to decide to engage in an intended action (Hagger, Wood, Stiff, & Chatzisarantis, 2010). In line with this idea, participants who had lowered willpower because they first performed a demanding task were less able to modify their habitual levels of self-disclosure to fit situational demands (Vohs, Baumeister, & Ciarocco, 2005). Thus, after willpower was lowered in this way, low-disclosure participants acted in a habitual, reticent way regardless of social demands to share information about themselves. Similarly, in a 3-week field study of habitual social drinkers, participants consumed more alcohol on days when they experienced more self-control demands and were therefore more depleted (Muraven, Collins, Shiffman, & Paty, 2005).

Given that habit automaticity does not require a supporting goal, lowered self-control can promote reliance on habits that are congruent or incongruent with goals. Although people may have different reasons for countering good, goal-congruent or bad, goal-incongruent habits, the underlying habit cueing mechanism is the same in both instances. People may decide to counter good habits for reasons such as conforming to the preferences of others and trying something new, whereas decisions to counter bad habits are typically to achieve a long-term goal. Demonstrating that lack of self-control boosts habit performance, Neal et al.'s (2013) participants with lowered willpower made more habitual choices when presented with healthful or unhealthful food options. Additional evidence comes from a study that experimentally trained good and bad eating habits (Lin, Wood, & Monterosso, in preparation). Good habits to avoid chocolates were trained by having participants push away a joystick in response to photos of eating chocolates, and bad habits to approach chocolates were trained by having participants pull a joystick toward themselves in response to the photos. Some participants then had willpower depleted by performing a demanding self-control task, and finally all participants ate as many chocolates as they desired in the guise of a consumer study. When depleted, approach-trained participants ate more chocolates, whereas avoidance-trained ones showed a trend to eat less. Thus, much as with naturally occurring habits, depleted participants fell back on their experimentally formed habitual responses.

In summary, the relative influence of habits and more deliberative guides to action depends on a variety of moderating factors. In research designs that pit habitual responses against other forms of action control, habits predominate when they are stronger rather than weaker, and when circumstances limit people's ability to deliberate about their actions. Specifically, habits are promoted by circumstances that are distracting, heighten stress, reduce reasoning ability, and lower willpower, presumably because of people's lowered capacity to inhibit cued, habitual responses and to make decisions to do something else (or nothing at all). Also, the increase in arousal linked to stress, and perhaps to other factors limiting deliberation, likely promotes performance of dominant, habitual responses. Although habit performance appears robust given these limitations on deliberative ability, we explain in the next section that habit performance is sensitive to shifts in context cues.

HABIT PERFORMANCE DEPENDS ON RECURRING CONTEXTS

Habit performance can be disrupted by experimental manipulations of cues, as well as by naturally occurring changes in life circumstances (Rothman, Sheeran, & Wood, 2009). These context changes break the automatic cueing of habit and promote responsiveness to intentions and newly acquired information (Verplanken & Wood, 2006). Building on the insight that controlling cues provides a way of controlling habits, researchers suggest that smokers may improve their chances of quitting by removing items from their home or workplace that remind them of smoking (Prochaska & DiClemente, 1983). Eating habits also can be modified through changes in the structure of eating environments (van't Riet, Sijtsema, Dagevos, & De Bruijn, 2011). Tendencies to eat mindlessly or habitually are less likely to be triggered when food is out of reach, out of sight, and available in small portions or serving amounts (e.g., Wansink & Cheney, 2005). Thus, behavior change experts recommend that people take control of their local performance environments in order to control unwanted habits (van't Riet et al., 2011).

Experimental evidence that changes in context cues disrupt habit performance comes from Neal et al.'s (2011) popcorn-eating study mentioned previously. When at the cinema, participants with strong habits continued to eat fresh or stale popcorn, but habits were not cued in this way when participants were in a darkened conference room watching music videos. In this novel environment without strong habit associations, participants ate what they liked, and consumed more fresh than stale popcorn.

Along with experimental demonstrations, a growing literature addressing *habit discontinuity* illustrates how naturally occurring context changes disrupt habit cueing and enable people to act on their intentions. In one study, college students transferring to a new university reported 1 month before and 1 month after the transfer on their habits to exercise, read the newspaper, and watch TV (Wood, Tam, & Guerrero Witt, 2005). Students maintained their habits at the new campus when performance contexts were similar across the transfer (e.g., exercising at the gym in their apartment complex). However, when the context changed significantly, strong habits were disrupted. Without cues to habitual responding, students were guided by their current intentions so that, for example, they exercised only if they intended to do so. For students without habits, the similarity between pre- and post-transfer contexts had little effect on performance, and instead behavior was guided by intentions in both contexts. In other discontinuity research, moving to a new location disrupted car driving habits and increased use of public transit among new residents with strong environmental values (Verplanken, Walker, Davis, & Jurasek, 2008). This change in context provided the window of opportunity for new residents to adopt travel options in line with their values.

In summary, changes in performance contexts appear to disrupt habits but not other guides to action. Given the rigid structure of habits, a change in context can remove triggers to performance and lead to a collapse in habit performance (Bayley et al., 2005). In the absence of a ready habitual response, people are likely to respond in the new context based on their current motives and beliefs. In general, the moderator research we have reviewed suggests that factors influencing habit performance are relatively separable from the factors influencing more deliberative forms of action control.

EXPERIENCE OF HABITS

People are only occasionally aware of the influence of their habits within broader mechanisms of action control. As we noted earlier, people are likely most aware of habits that conflict with their current goals and intentions. It is not uncommon to hear people try to account for habit performance with comments such as "I can't help it, it's just a habit." Thus, habits inconsistent with current goals may be acknowledged as relatively autonomous guides to action.

More commonly, habits are consistent with goals (Ouellette & Wood, 1998); thus, people experience coherence in the forces guiding their behavior. Adding to this coherence, people may make inferences about their habits that highlight the consistency with goals. When people do not have direct access to the cognitions and motives guiding action, they draw inferences about such states by observing their behavior and external cues (Neal et al., 2012). Despite this limited insight, people may reason, "I do this often, so I must like to do it." Such reasoning is similar to situated inferences in which interpretation of experiences is influenced by current mental contents (Loersch & Payne, 2011), but in the case of habits, these interpretations often occur following behavior performance and therefore have limited impact on actual responding.

Inferences that goals motivate habit performance could be correct in a historical sense, because people might accurately remember the goals that initially guided habit formation. After all, people are most likely to repeat and thereby form habits for behaviors that attain desired goals or avoid undesired ones. In addition, people might generally be disposed to form positive evaluations of habits given the ease with which they are performed. Consumers often have a rational preference to stick with habitual products and actions over novel, more difficult ones (Labrecque et al., in preparation). Such preferences also might emerge from the positive affect generated by processing fluency that signals familiarity over uncertainty and success at processing and understanding. This positive affect could generalize to current activities (Reber, Schwarz, & Winkielman, 2004), yielding affective responses supporting habit performance.

The goals and cognitions that people use to account for repeated behaviors become largely epiphenomena as habits form and responses come to be cued directly by features of the performance context. Such inferences can make habits seem compatible with intentions. For example, inferences about the reasons for habitually listening to the radio while driving (e.g., liking music) could mask the fact that listening is actually cued as part of the driving experience. Suggesting that such inferences mask dissociations between habits and current intentions, participants in behavior prediction research were more certain of their intentions to perform strong than weak habits, despite the fact that their intentions to perform strong habits did not predict future behavior (Ji & Wood, 2007). That is, individuals behaved according to their strong habits, whether or not they intended to do so. Additional evidence comes from Neal et al.'s (2012) study of goal inferences made by habitual and nonhabitual runners. More habitual runners more strongly believed and rapidly inferred that their running was influenced by their goals, despite the fact that goals did not activate their thoughts of running. Thus, inferences that align cognitions and motives with habits can promote a sense of volition for habitual responding (Labrecque et al., in preparation).

In daily life, people often may not attend to or try to explain habitual responses. Even when performing a novel, implicit learning task, participants did not seem to be aware of repeating the same sequence of actions (Rünger & Frensch, 2008). However, participants were more likely to seek out explicit, reportable knowledge about their regular response patterns when they experienced an unexpected but systematic disruption in the task. It may be, then, that people generally do not attend to repeated behaviors or associated cues until some disturbance or unexpected event prompts them to make inferences about the nature of habit performance.

In summary, people may become aware of the influence of habits, especially unwanted habits. More commonly, people may not explain habit performance, or they may attribute it to corresponding motivations and cognitions that provide a volitional purpose behind the response.

CONCLUSION

In this chapter, we have argued that habit automaticity is stimulus-driven and largely autonomous, especially in that it is not dependent on goals. Understanding these distinctive features of habits in comparison with other types of action control is important given the prevalence of habits in daily life. In experience-sampling diary research in which participants reported once per hour on what they were thinking, feeling, and doing, about 45% of the behaviors participants listed tended to be repeated in the same physical location almost every day and were therefore potentially habitual (Wood, Quinn, & Kashy, 2002). Although habits appear to be a cornerstone of everyday human learning and performance, dual-process models rarely include habits, and instead tend to focus on the multiple ways that concepts and goals can guide responding.

Much as in nonhuman animals, habit learning is a robust mechanism in humans that gradually develops as goal-responsive neural systems relinquish control to the sensorimotor–basal ganglia system, and perhaps ultimately to exclusively cortical systems. Although habits are rigidly represented in non-goal-directed memories, they interact in various ways with goal/concept automaticity and with more deliberative, thoughtful processes. In daily life, this interaction takes the form of strong habits predominating, in part because of the strength of the cueing mechanism and in part because of limitations that can naturally occur in deliberative processes. Lack of reasoning skills, inattention or distraction, stress, and limited willpower all boost habit performance. When deliberation is restricted in these ways, people are not easily able to inhibit a habitual response and make a choice to respond differently.

Understanding habits is important from the applied perspective of human health and welfare. It is increasingly becoming evident, for example, that much of the global burden of disease comes from everyday lifestyle behaviors of overeating, smoking, addiction, and social isolation. As Marteau, Hollands, and Fletcher (2012) argued in a recent article in *Science*, behavior change interventions that encourage people to deliberate about their behaviors are unlikely to be successful at addressing such lifestyle diseases. Instead, effective interventions need to recognize the automatic, habitual processes that promote such responses regardless of people's best intentions.

NOTE

1. Initial, goal-directed learning does not appear necessary to guide habit formation in all tasks. With repetition, people may form habits to perform complex tasks successfully even when they cannot reason deliberatively abouto how to reach the correct outcome (Bayley et al., 2005).

REFERENCES

Aldrich, J. H., Montgomery, J. M., & Wood, W. (2011). Turnout as habit. *Political Behavior, 33*, 535–563.

Anderson, M. C. (2003). Rethinking interference theory: Executive control and the mechanisms of forgetting. *Journal of Memory and Language, 49*, 415–445.

Ashby, F. G., Ennis, J. M., & Spiering, B. J. (2007). A neurobiological theory of automaticity in perceptual categorization. *Psychological Review, 114*, 632–656.

Bayley, P. J., Frascino, J. C., & Squire, L. R. (2005). Robust habit learning in the absence of awareness and independent of the medial temporal lobe. *Nature, 436*, 550–553.

Botvinick, M., & Plaut, D. C. (2004). Doing

without schema hierarchies: A recurrent connectionist approach to normal and impaired routine sequential action. *Psychological Review, 111*, 395–429.

Danner, U. N., Aarts, H., & de Vries, N. K. (2008). Habit vs. intention in the prediction of future behaviour: The role of frequency, context stability and mental accessibility of past behaviour. *British Journal of Social Psychology, 47*, 245–265.

Danner, U. N., Aarts, H., Papies, E. K., & de Vries, N. K. (2011). Paving the path for habit change: Cognitive shielding of intentions against habit intrusion. *British Journal of Health Psychology, 16*, 189–200.

de Bruijn, G. J., Kremers, S. P. J., Singh, A., van den Putte, B., & van Mechelen, W. (2009). Adult active transportation: Adding habit strength to the theory of planned behavior. *American Journal of Preventive Medicine, 36*, 189–194.

De Houwer, J., Teige-Mocigemba, S., Spruyt, A., & Moors, A. (2009). Implicit measures: A normative analysis and review. *Psychological Bulletin, 135*, 347–368.

Desmurget, M., & Turner, R. S. (2010). Motor sequences and the basal ganglia: Kinematics, not habits. *Journal of Neuroscience, 30*, 7685–7690.

Duhigg, C. (2012). *The power of habit: Why we do what we do in life and business*. New York: Random House.

Evans, J. S. B. (2008). Dual-processing accounts of reasoning, judgment, and social cognition. *Annual Review of Psychology, 59*, 255–278.

Fiske, S. T., Gilbert, D. T., & Lindzey, G. (2010). *Handbook of social psychology*. Hoboken, NJ: Wiley.

Fujii, N., & Graybiel, A. M. (2003). Representation of action sequence boundaries by macaque prefrontal cortical neurons. *Science, 301*, 1246–1249.

Graybiel, A. M. (2008). Habits, rituals, and the evaluative brain. *Annual Review of Neuroscience, 31*, 359–387.

Hagger, M. S., Wood, C., Stiff, C., & Chatzisarantis, N. L. D. (2010). Ego depletion and the strength model of self-control: A meta-analysis. *Psychological Bulletin, 136*, 495–525.

Hull, C. L. (1934). The concept of the habit-family hierarchy and maze learning. *Psychological Review, 41*, 33–54.

James, W. (1890). *Principles of psychology*. New York: Holt.

Ji, M., & Wood, W. (2007). Purchase and consumption habits: Not necessarily what you intend. *Journal of Consumer Psychology, 17*, 261–276.

Kahneman, D. (2003). A perspective on judgment and choice: Mapping bounded rationality. *American Psychologist, 58*, 697–720.

Knowlton, B. J., Mangels, J. A., & Squire, L. R. (1996). Neostriatal habit learning system in humans. *Science, 273*, 1399–1402.

Labrecque, J. S., Wood, W., Neal, D. T., Harrington, N. (in preparation). *Product slips: Habit cueing can be friend or foe to new product use.*

Lehéricy, S., Benali, H., van de Moortele, P.-F., Pélégrini-Issac, M., Waechter, T., Uğurbil, K., et al. (2005). Distinct basal ganglia territories are engaged in early and advanced motor sequence learning. *Proceedings of the National Academy of Sciences USA, 102*, 12566–12571.

Lieberman, M. D., Gaunt, R., Gilbert, D. T., & Trope, Y. (2002). Reflexion and reflection: A social cognitive neuroscience approach to attributional inference. In M. P. Zanna (Ed.), *Advances in experimental social psychology* (Vol. 34, pp. 199–249). New York: Academic Press.

Lin, P., Wood, W., & Monterosso, J. M. (in preparation). *The role of good habits in facilitating long-term benefits.*

Loersch, C., & Payne, B. K. (2011). The situated inference model: An integrative account of the effects of primes on perception, behavior, and motivation. *Perspectives on Psychological Science, 6*, 234–252.

Marchette, S. A., Bakker, A., & Shelton, A. L. (2011). Cognitive mappers to creatures of habit: Differential engagement of place and response learning mechanisms predicts human navigational behavior. *Journal of Neuroscience, 31*, 15264–15268.

Marteau, T. M., Hollands, G. J., & Fletcher, P. C. (2012). Changing human behavior to prevent disease: The importance of targeting automatic processes. *Science, 337*(6101), 1492–1495.

McCulloch, K. C., Aarts, H., Fujita, K., & Bargh, J. A. (2008). Inhibition in goal systems: A retrieval-induced forgetting account. *Journal of Experimental Social Psychology, 44*, 614–623.

Miyachi, S., Hikosaka, O., Miyashita, K., Kárádi, Z., & Rand, M. K. (1997). Differential roles of monkey striatum in learning of sequential hand movement. *Experimental Brain Research, 115*, 1–5.

Muraven, M., Collins, R. L., Shiffman, S., & Paty, J. A. (2005). Daily fluctuations in self-control demands and alcohol intake. *Psychology of Addictive Behaviors: Journal of the Society of Psychologists in Addictive Behaviors, 19*(2), 140–147.

Neal, D. T., Wood, W., & Drolet-Rossi, A. (2013). How do people adhere to goals when willpower is low? The profits (and pitfalls) of strong habits. *Journal of Personality and Social Psychology, 104*(6), 959–975.

Neal, D. T., Wood, W., Labrecque, J., & Lally, P. (2012). How do habits guide behavior?: Perceived and actual triggers of habits in daily life. *Journal of Experimental Social Psychology, 48*, 492–498.

Neal, D. T., Wood, W., & Quinn, J. M. (2006). Habits: A repeat performance. *Current Directions in Psychological Science, 15*, 198–202.

Neal, D. T., Wood, W., Wu, M., & Kurlander, D. (2011). The pull of the past: When do habits persist despite conflict with motives? *Personality and Social Psychology Bulletin, 37*(11), 1428–1437.

Norman, D. A. (1981). Categorization of action slips. *Psychological Review, 88*, 1–15.

Ouellette, J. A., & Wood, W. (1998). Habit and intention in everyday life: The multiple processes by which past behavior predicts future behavior. *Psychological Bulletin, 124*, 54–74.

Prochaska, J. O., & DiClemente, C. C. (1983). Stages and processes of self-change of smoking: Toward an integrative model of change. *Journal of Consulting and Clinical Psychology, 51*(3), 390–395.

Quinn, J. M., Pascoe, A. M., Wood, W., & Neal, D. T. (2010). Can't help yourself?: Monitor those bad habits. *Personality and Social Psychology Bulletin, 36*, 499–511.

Reason, J. T. (1979). Actions not as planned. In G. Underwood & R. Stevens (Eds.), *Aspects of consciousness* (pp. 67–89). London: Academic Press.

Reason, J. T. (1992). Cognitive underspecification: Its variety and consequences. In B. J. Baars (Ed.), *Experimental slips and human error: Exploring the architecture of volition* (pp. 71–91). New York: Plenum.

Reber, R., Schwarz, N., & Winkielman, P. (2004). Processing fluency and aesthetic pleasure: Is beauty in the perceiver's processing experience? *Personality and Social Psychology Review, 8*, 364–382.

Rothman, A. J., Sheeran, P., & Wood, W. (2009). Reflective and automatic processes in the initiation and maintenance of food choices. *Annals of Behavioral Medicine, 38*(1), 4–17.

Rünger, D., & Frensch, P. A. (2008). How incidental sequence learning creates reportable knowledge: The role of unexpected events. *Journal of Experimental Psychology: Learning, Memory, and Cognition, 34*, 1011–1026.

Schwabe, L., & Wolf, O. T. (2009). Stress prompts habit behavior in humans. *Journal of Neuroscience, 29*(22), 7191–7198.

Sheeran, P., Webb, T. L., & Gollwitzer, P. (2005). The interplay between goal intentions and implementation intentions. *Personality and Social Psychology Bulletin, 31*, 87–98.

Skinner, B. F. (1953). *Science and human behavior*. New York: Free Press.

Squire, L. R., & Zola-Morgan, S. (1991). The medial temporal lobe memory system. *Science, 253*, 1380–1386.

Strack, F., & Deutsch, R. (2004). Reflective and impulsive determinants of social behavior. *Personality and Social Psychology Review, 8*, 220–247.

Tricomi, E., Balleine, B. W., & O'Doherty, J. P. (2009). A specific role for posterior dorsolateral striatum in human habit learning. *European Journal of Neuroscience, 29*(11), 2225–2232.

van't Riet, J., Sijtsema, S. J., Dagevos, H., & De Bruijn, G.-J. (2011). The importance of habits in eating behaviour: An overview and recommendations for future research. *Appetite, 57*(3), 585–596.

Verplanken, B., Walker, I., Davis, A., & Jurasek, M. (2008). Context change and travel mode choice: Combining the habit discontinuity and self-activation hypotheses. *Journal of Environmental Psychology, 28*(2), 121–127.

Verplanken, B., & Wood, W. (2006). Interventions to break and create consumer habits. *Journal of Public Policy and Marketing, 25*, 90–103.

Vohs, K. D., Baumeister, R. F., & Ciarocco, N. J. (2005). Self-regulation and self-presentation: Regulatory resource depletion impairs impression management and effortful self-presentation depletes regulatory resources. *Journal of Personality and Social Psychology, 88*, 632–657.

Waldschmidt, J. G., & Ashby, F. G. (2011). Cortical and striatal contributions to automaticity in information–integration categorization. *NeuroImage*, *56*, 1791–1802.

Wansink, B., & Cheney, M. M. (2005). Super bowls: Serving bowl size and food consumption. *Journal of the American Medical Association, 293*, 1727–1728.

Webb, T. L., & Sheeran, P. (2006). Does changing behavioral intentions engender behavioral change?: A meta-analysis of the experimental evidence, *Psychological Bulletin, 132*, 249–268.

Wheeler, S. C., & DeMarree, K. G. (2009). Multiple mechanisms of prime-to-behavior effects. *Social and Personality Psychology Compass, 3/4*, 566–581.

Wood, W., & Neal, D. T. (2007). A new look at habits and the habit-goal interface. *Psychological Review, 114*, 843–863.

Wood, W., & Neal, D. T. (2009). The habitual consumer. *Journal of Consumer Psychology, 19*, 579–592.

Wood, W., Quinn, J. M., & Kashy, D. (2002). Habits in everyday life: Thought, emotion, and action. *Journal of Personality and Social Psychology, 83*, 1281–1297.

Wood, W., Tam, L., & Guerrero Witt, M. (2005). Changing circumstances, disrupting habits. *Journal of Personality and Social Psychology, 88*, 918–933.

Yin, H. H., & Knowlton, B. J. (2006). The role of the basal ganglia in habit formation. *Nature Reviews Neuroscience, 7*, 464–476.

Yonelinas, A. P., & Jacoby, L. L. (2012). The process-dissociation approach two decades later: Convergence, boundary conditions, and new directions. *Memory and Cognition, 40*, 663–668.

CHAPTER 26

Conscious and Unconscious Goal Pursuit

Similar Functions, Different Processes?

Ruud Custers and Henk Aarts

Much of human behavior is directed at the attainment of desired outcomes, or goals. These outcomes can refer not only to certain states (e.g., being rich) but also behaviors (e.g., going out). In general, psychological theories assume that realization of these goals relies on conscious processes. In essence, the process of setting or adopting a goal is regarded as a decision-making process, in which people choose whether or not to pursue a certain goal, mainly based on its expected value. Once a decision has been made and an intention to pursue the goal is formed, another decision has to be made when it comes to selecting the proper actions that will lead to goal attainment in the situation at hand. Finally, in order to adapt to changes in the environment, the cognitive and behavioral processes involved in the pursuit of goals have to be controlled to keep attention and behavior on its course. As such, pursuing a goal seems to be a conscious affair.

Despite the fact that the three crucial functions required for goal pursuit—setting or adopting goals based on their expected value, selecting the proper action patterns, and controlling goal pursuit—are sometimes even by definition assumed to rely on conscious processes, recent findings suggest that the pursuit of goals can also unfold outside of conscious awareness. In this chapter, we discuss a framework that may help us to understand how such unconscious goal pursuit can occur. In essence, we argue that the three crucial functions mentioned earlier can be fulfilled by processes that operate outside of conscious awareness. We discuss how these processes may be different from their conscious counterparts, painting, at least in part, a dual-process picture of goal pursuit. At the end of this chapter, we discuss some of the current challenges for research on the role of consciousness in goal pursuit, such as how conscious and unconscious processes may work together to produce goal pursuit.

EVIDENCE FOR UNCONSCIOUS GOAL PURSUIT

Over the last decade, a growing number of studies has yielded evidence supporting the idea that goals can be triggered and pursued without conscious awareness (for reviews of this field, see Aarts & Custers, 2012; Bargh, Gollwitzer, & Oettingen, 2010; Custers & Aarts, 2010). Using priming as a technique to activate mental representations of goals without participants being aware of its influence on behavior, Bargh and colleagues, for instance, exposed people to achievement goal-related words (or control words) in a puzzle task (Bargh, Gollwitzer, Lee-Chai, Barndollar, & Trötschel, 2001). Effects on performance were tested on a second puzzle task. It was found that people who were primed with words related to the goal of achievement behaved more in line with these goals (they performed better on the second puzzle task), and that their behavior showed properties that are indicative of motivation and pursuit, such as persistence. As participants claimed to be unaware of the influences on their goal pursuits, these findings are taken as evidence for the idea that goal pursuit was initiated, and operated, under the radar of conscious awareness.

This study shows that motivational, goal-directed behavior can be automatically put in place if the representation of the goal is directly primed by semantic materials. These initial findings revealing unconscious goal pursuit spurred a lot of interest in the domain of automaticity and social cognition. Several researchers from different laboratories have identified specific aspects in the social environment that trigger goals and subsequent actions and thus cause people automatically to pursue goals. Goal pursuit has been found to result from exposure to names of significant others (e.g., parents, spouse) whose goals have been recurrently acted on in the past (Fitzsimons & Bargh, 2003; Kraus & Chen, 2009; Shah, 2003), as well as social roles (e.g., motherhood, leader or boss) that people associate with specific goals (Guinote, 2007; Shidlovski & Hassin, 2011; Smith & Galinsky, 2010). Other studies have illustrated how the mere processing of physical or semantic features of members of the stereotyped group (e.g., nurses or black people) instigates goal pursuit (e.g., effortful helping, striving for social equality), adding social stereotypes to the list of social triggers of goal pursuit (Aarts, Chartrand, et al., 2005; Campbell & Mohr, 2011; Custers, Maas, Wildenbeest, & Aarts, 2008; Moskowitz, Salomon, & Taylor, 2000). People also engage in goal pursuit upon inferring goals from other people's behavioral patterns (Aarts, Gollwitzer, & Hassin, 2004; Ackerman, Goldstein, Shapiro, & Bargh, 2009; Dik & Aarts, 2007; Friedman, Deci, Elliot, Moller, & Aarts, 2009; Lebreton, Kawa, d'Arc, Daunizeau, & Pessiglione, 2012; Loersch, Aarts, Payne, & Jefferis, 2008), which indicates how the observation of others' actions can prepare and motivate goal-directed behavior outside of awareness in interpersonal contexts. Finally, objects (e.g., a briefcase) and odors (e.g., the scent of citrus) seem to trigger associated goals (achievement or cleaning) and their pursuit (e.g., de Lange, Debets, Ruitenburg, & Holland, 2012; Holland, Hendriks, & Aarts, 2005; Kay, Wheeler, Bargh, & Ross, 2004).

The substantial body of research on goal priming and unconscious goal pursuit suggests that goals can be activated outside of people's awareness in various ways and that these unconsciously activated goals affect people's behavior by calling on several functions that are necessary for goal pursuit. First of all, people seem to be able to assess the rewarding value of an unconsciously triggered goal, thereby increasing their effort and motivation to engage in goal pursuit. Second, goals give direction to people's behavior: Priming a goal prepares the relevant action patterns instrumental to attaining the goal in the situation at hand. Third, some of the results, such a persistence of behavior over time, or in the face of obstacles, suggest that behavior is not only instigated but also controlled during goal pursuit. The same goes for behaviors that seem adaptive in the particular situation at hand. Although this may sound counterintuitive, these conclusions are in line with recent research suggesting that executive functions can operate without awareness (Lau & Rosenthal, 2011; Suhler & Churchland, 2009).

Together, these findings suggest that the only difference between conscious and unconscious goal pursuit is the subjective awareness that accompanies goal pursuit. However, assuming that people are able to access and select goals, to assess their value, to prepare instrumental actions, and to control their goal pursuit without conscious awareness seems to violate the very definitions of these processes. In the following section we propose a framework for understanding unconscious goal pursuit that assumes conscious and unconscious goal pursuit—at least partly—are based on distinct processes that fulfill the same functions.

A FRAMEWORK FOR UNDERSTANDING UNCONSCIOUS GOAL PURSUIT

It seems to be a commonly shared fact now that human thinking and doing are driven by brain processes that are not open to introspection. Hence, we are often not conscious of the processes underlying our thoughts and behavior (Bargh & Morsella, 2008; Blackmore, 2004; Lau & Rosenthal, 2011; Nisbett & Wilson, 1977; Nørretranders, 1991). Accordingly, in recent years, theory and research on the understanding of human conduct have started to focus on the basic functions and processes by which people's thinking and doing is produced outside awareness to examine and understand how their thoughts and actions gain access to conscious awareness. This process-oriented approach to the "unconscious mind" has been fruitfully applied to research on perception, cognition, emotion, and motor movement (Banks, 2009), and it slowly moves into the study on human goal pursuit. Building on this development, our framework for unconscious goal pursuit addresses a set of key functions that is pivotal for the pursuit of goals and investigates how those functions can be implemented by processes that operate outside of conscious awareness.

First, we suggest that goals are mentally represented as outcomes of actions, and that these goal representations incorporate information about not only an outcome but also its reward value or desirability (Custers & Aarts, 2005a, 2010). We propose that activation of a goal representation is accompanied by a reward signal that can directly mobilize effort that is required for effective goal pursuit, without a conscious assessment of value. Second, we assume that action and outcome representations are closely linked, which prepares relevant action patterns upon the activation of the goal, without the need for conscious selection or decision making. In essence, these two process (i.e., selection of desirable outcomes to pursue and the selection of the action patterns that will produce them in the situation at hand) fulfill the same two functions that are fulfilled by deliberative processes in contemporary theories of goal pursuit. Third, based on recent evidence, we also argue that upon activation of a goal representation, goals recruit executive functions outside of awareness, enabling humans to deal with the inherently dynamic nature of their mental and physical world and thereby rendering unconscious goal pursuit adaptive (Lau & Rosenthal, 2011). As such, we argue, the core functions that are required for goal pursuit (i.e., assessing the reward value and mobilizing effort, preparation of relevant action patterns, and controlling the execution of goal pursuit) can operate outside of conscious awareness. Below we discuss these components of our framework for unconscious goal pursuit (see Figure 26.1) in more detail.

Unconscious Reward Processing

Determining the reward value of potential goals and selecting them accordingly is a basic function to be fulfilled by any organism that is said to pursue goals. Indeed, theories on animal behavior recognize that this process plays a crucial role in motivation and goal-directed action. Incentive theory (see, e.g., Berridge, 2001) proposes that organisms will work for stimuli or states that are associated with rewards. While early in life rewards are tightly associated with stimuli that have biological importance, such as water and food, learning processes can create associations with any mental representation. Incentive theory grew out of several remarkable effects obtained in research on operant conditioning, called "misbehaviors." One such behavior is auto-shaping

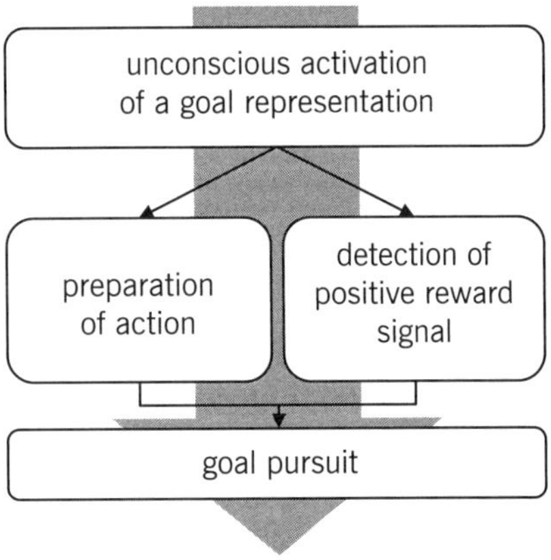

FIGURE 26.1. Framework for understanding unconscious goal pursuit. Based on Custers and Aarts (2010).

(Brown & Jenkins, 1968). For example, it has been observed that when presentation of food was repeatedly paired with a light signal, pigeons started vigorously to pick at the light bulb even though this behavior was not explicitly reinforced. This phenomenon has been explained by assuming that the reward associated with the food becomes linked to the light bulb, which therefore serves as an incentive for which the animal is motivated to work.

Neuroimaging research has discovered that rewarding properties of stimuli are processed by limbic structures, such as the nucleus accumbens and the ventral striatum (Schultz, 2006). These subcortical areas play a central role in determining the rewarding value of behaviors and outcomes, and are connected to corticofrontal areas that facilitate goal pursuit (Pessiglione et al., 2007). These reward centers in the brain respond not only to biologically relevant rewards (e.g., food and sexual stimuli) but also to learned rewards (e.g., money, status), or words (e.g., *good, nice*) associated with praise or rewards (Schultz, 2006). This demonstrates that such motivationally positive stimuli induce an internal reward signal, regardless of their shape or form (Shizgal, 1997).

Recent evidence suggests that reward information can increase motivation on a task, even when presented below the threshold of conscious awareness. In a recent study by Pessiglione and colleagues (2007), participants engaged in a task in which they could earn money by squeezing a hand grip. Before each trial, a picture of the maximal reward that could be earned—either a one pound or a one penny coin—was presented on the screen. It was found that even when this picture was presented subliminally participants invested more physical effort after a high-value reward cue, squeezing more forcefully than when they were exposed to a low-value reward cue. These effects appeared to be accompanied by activation in the limbic structures associated with reward processing and motivation (Bijleveld, Custers, & Aarts, 2009).

Because of these similar effects of conscious and unconscious reward cues, one could still argue that even though signal detection tests suggest otherwise, people may still have been aware of the primes to a certain extent, in which case, behavior may have been the result of conscious reflections on the reward after all. However, recently obtained diverging effects for conscious and unconscious reward cues render such an explanation unlikely.

In an experiment (Bijleveld, Custers, & Aarts, 2010), participants had to solve an arithmetic problem on each trial. They were told that the presented coins indicated the maximum reward that could be earned. They also learned that for accurate responses they would receive a percentage of this reward, but that this percentage would rapidly decrease with time. Hence, in order to obtain the highest percentage of the cued reward, they would have to be both fast and accurate. Results showed that on trials with subliminal reward cues, participants were faster on high-value than on low-value reward cues, while accuracy was equally high in both cases. For trials with consciously visible reward cues a different pattern emerged. Participants were slower on high- than on low-value reward trials, taking more time (hence, sacrificing a part of the reward) in order to be accurate and suggesting a more cautious mode of economic behavior (Rabin & Thaler, 2001). Thus, the results suggest that although both unconscious and conscious reward cues boosted the mental resources that people employed in the task, conscious reward cues on top of that led to strategic choices (see also Bijleveld, Custers, & Aarts, 2012a), in this case, to change speed–accuracy tradeoffs. Indeed, when the task was changed in a way that made such tradeoffs impossible, subliminal and supraliminal reward cues were found to increase speed to the same extent.

Together, these findings suggest that unconscious processing of reward value cues (a central feature of goal representations) boosts effort in a task through an initial rudimentary mechanism, and more so when demands on the body are higher (Bijleveld et al., 2012a). On top of these initial processes, participants engage in strategic analyses when reward cues can be consciously processed. Based on information about rewards and other aspects of the task, people may decide not to invest effort or change their tactics. As such, both conscious and unconscious reward cues motivate behavior, although conscious processes also affect behavior by means of decisions (Bijleveld, Custers, & Aarts, 2012b).

Unconscious Action Preparation

Pursuing a goal requires the selection of the appropriate action patterns that will lead to goal attainment. We argue, though, that these action patterns do not always have to be consciously selected. Research in various areas of psychology has demonstrated at several levels and in several ways that information about actions is stored as representations that contains two components: a representation of its observable effect or outcome (e.g., grasping the cup), as well as the action patterns or motor programs that contain information about the bodily movements that make it happen (Hommel, Muesseler, Aschersleben, & Prinz, 2001; Jeannerod, 1997). It is assumed that because execution of a certain motor program is usually followed by the perception of its effect, these two components become associated in memory, eventually sharing overlap and forming almost one representation. As a result, activating the representation of an action's effect or outcome can lead to the automatic preparation of the action patterns or motor programs that will produce it, even though the content of those programs is not always accessible to consciousness.

On the most basic level, mimicry provides evidence for such an overlap between outcome representations and action patterns. When it comes to actions such as lifting a finger or scratching one's arm, it is easy to think of the observable outcomes or consequences (the sight of a finger moving, the sound of the fingernail scratching one's arm). However, the actual motor programs that are executed (which muscles to contracts, which ones to relax) remain largely unknown to us. The only reason we know what to do is that the action patterns that make the outcome happen are associated with it. Hence, perceiving an action outcome, even in others, should to a certain extent activate and prepare the associated action patterns in ourselves; this effect is also known as the ideo-motor principle (e.g., James, 1890).

But outcomes do not have to be perceived directly to activate outcome representations. For instance, these representations can also be primed by objects that are associated with an action's effect. This corresponds with the notion that humans (and other organisms) perceive the world in terms of the action or outcomes it affords (Gibson, 1979). Perceiving a hammer, for instance, activates representations of outcomes related to functional properties of that object (e.g., grabbing, hitting) that prepare the associated action patterns. Zwaan and Taylor (2006) have described this activation of low-level action representation as *motor resonance*: the opportunities for action we perceive in the environment resonate in our motor system.

Such motor resonance has also been demonstrated for action outcomes that are not directly perceived but merely read about, thus causing (pre)motor activity by mere semantic processing. In a study by Pulvermüller (2005), participants read words meaning "lick," "pick," or "kick," which are related to tongue, hand, or foot moments, respectively. It was found that merely reading those words led to activation in not only the sensorimotor but also the premotor cortex, in the areas that are also activated when these actions are actually carried out by the corresponding body parts. Hence, it appears that regardless of whether activation of an outcome representation is caused by direct perception, associated stimuli, or communication, preparation of the associated action patterns follows.

On a more abstract level, things are not necessarily much different. It has been proposed that everyday goals are mentally represented in a network of associations that involve the desired outcome, the action patterns that produce it, and knowledge about situations in which these goals are pursued (Aarts & Dijksterhuis, 2000; Bargh, 1990; Kruglanski et al., 2002). As a result, activating a goal representation may activate the action patterns that lead to their attainment in a particular situation. This effect is the strongest when repeated pursuit of a goal via the same course of behavior has forged strong links between a goal representation and the representation of the behavior. For example, we do not have to deliberate about how to get to work in the morning, because the goal of going to work automatically activates the action pattern of using one's bike or car. In the same way, we do not have to consider all available bars when we go for a drink, since the goal of going for a drink may automatically activate the representation of walking to the bar we usually visit. Hence, although there may in reality be more than one means to a particular goal, the one that has proven itself in a particular situation in the past will be the representation that is most likely to be activated when a goal is primed.

Such automatic selection of habitual means or instrumental actions has been demonstrated in a number of studies and was first empirically demonstrated in the domain of travel mode choice behavior (e.g., Aarts & Dijksterhuis, 2000). Participants primed with certain travel goals (e.g., going to class) showed increased activation of certain means of traveling (e.g., biking). However, this effect only occurred in those students who habitually used the specific means (e.g., bicycle) to reach their travel goals. These findings have been replicated and extended to other goals. For instance, activating the goal to socialize has been found to increase consumption of alcohol as a habitual means (Danner, Aarts, & De Vries, 2008; Sheeran et al., 2005).

Unconscious Goal Pursuit as Function of Action Preparation and Reward Processing

So far, in the attempt to understand the human capacity for unconscious goal pursuit, reward value processing and preparation of action patterns have been treated separately. However, we argue that when a goal is primed, these two processes occur simultaneously. While the reward signal evoked by activation of the goal representation motivates pursuit of the goal, the activation of associated action patterns prepares one for the proper course of action.

The two processes have recently been demonstrated in an experiment (Aarts, Custers, & Marien, 2008) that employed a conditioning paradigm to manipulate the reward value of the goal that has been proven successfully to create goals in earlier research (Custers & Aarts, 2005a). Participants were given the task to squeeze a handgrip in response to a start sign, while the timing and physical effort of the behavior were measured. Prior to this task, words pertaining to the goal of physical exertion were subliminally presented (or not) together with a positive reward signal (e.g., positive words: *good, nice*) or not. It was found that subliminally priming the concept of exertion prepared participants for the squeezing behavior, causing them to start squeezing earlier (following a cue to squeeze), regardless of whether primes were presented together with positive words. However, only participants for whom the exertion was coactivated with a positive reward signal (i.e., positive words) showed more forceful and persistent squeezing. Moreover, self-reported motivation did not show any relation to the subliminal goal-priming manipulation. Hence, activating a goal representation gives behavior a head start by preparing the relevant actions, whereas the accompanying reward signal motivates behavior outside awareness.

Studies using the same manipulation have yielded similar results. Using cardiovascular measures to directly measure effort invested in a task, Capa, Cleeremans, Bustin, Bouquet, and Hansenne (2011; Capa, Cleeremans, Bustin, & Hansenne, 2011) primed words related to studying that were directly paired (or not) with positive words. They found that participants for whom studying was primed together with positive affect showed increased cardiovascular reactivity during a subsequent learning task, which is indicative of more effortful behavior and perseverance (Capa, Cleeremans, Bustin, Bouquet, et al., 2011). Further experimentation revealed that these effects were quite long-lasting, still showing up 25 minutes after the unconscious goal motivation treatment (see also Capa, Bouquet, Dreher, & Dufour, 2013).

Together, these studies show that primed goal representations prepare action, and particularly motivate behavior when they are associated with positive reward signals. As such, unconscious reward processing fulfills the function of selecting goals based on their expected value. Moreover, goals also activate the proper action representations, thus fulfilling the function of action selection. However, the persistence effects suggest that once a goal representation is activated, it remains active controlling behavior, thereby possibly rendering it more adaptive.

ADAPTIVITY OF UNCONSCIOUS GOAL PURSUIT

While it is known that activation of semantic items after priming decays in short-term memory quite rapidly, goal representations typically remain active over a longer period of time (Förster, Liberman, & Higgins, 2005). Increasing evidence suggests that goals that are activated unconsciously remain activated as well (Aarts, Custers, & Holland, 2007; Aarts, Custers, & Marien, 2009; Aarts, Custers, & Veltkamp, 2008; Bargh et al., 2001; Capa, Cleeremans, Bustin, Bouquet, et al., 2011; Capa, Cleeremans, Bustin, & Hansenne, 2011). For instance, in one study (Aarts et al., 2007), participants were either subliminally primed with the goal to socialize or not, and tested 2.5 minutes later for accessibility of the goal in a task measuring the speed of recognizing words related to the goal. Results showed that the representation of the goal remained accessible when participants were primed to attain the goal, but only when the goal represented an outcome they were motivated to attain. Similar persistent activation effects—even after 5 minutes of goal priming—have been obtained for behavioral measures (Aarts et al., 2004; Bargh et al., 2001).

Other studies have shown that unconsciously activated goals have the ability to inhibit interfering information (Aarts et al., 2007; Shah, Friedman, & Kruglanski, 2002) and to facilitate monitoring and feedback processing by preparing the instrumental actions that resolve discrepancies between the primed goal and the actual state of the world (Custers & Aarts, 2005b, 2007). These findings suggest that goal representations play an active role in controlling behavior by potentially rendering behavior adaptive and persistent by giving it direction.

A recent set of studies tested this hypothesis more directly (Marien, Custers, Hassin, & Aarts, 2012). Based on the notion that executive control processes are limited in capacity, their recruitment should incur costs on other tasks that rely on resources for executive control (Barrouillet, Bernardin, Portrat, Vergauwe, & Camos, 2007; Cocchini, Logie, Sala, MacPherson, & Baddeley, 2002). We examined the possibility that, if unconsciously activated goals actively control behavior, they make (at least partly) use of the same executive functions that are necessary for the control of conscious goal pursuit. In other words, when put in place, an unconscious goal "hijacks" the executive function for its own attainment, leaving less capacity for other processes.

One way to test this is first to activate a goal outside of awareness, then directly measure executive control performance on an unrelated task. Using a standard task for measuring the executive function (Smith & Jonides, 1999) we indeed found that priming goals such as socializing, or idiosyncratic goals, diminishes performance on a subsequent task that relies on executive control processes. This effect was demonstrated to be independent of task motivation, and it only occurred on the specific trials that required the executive function. Furthermore, the executive function was found to be similarly affected by unconscious and consciously activated goals (see also Masicampo & Baumeister, 2011, for conscious goal activation and executive control). Finally, an unconsciously activated goal occupied the executive function more strongly when the personal value of the goal was higher. These results suggest that unconscious goals recruit the executive functions required for their attainment, which may explain previous results indicating that subliminally primed goals cause people actively to maintain the goal, to inhibit interfering information, and to monitor and realize attainment by reacting to goal discrepancies.

DISCUSSION AND FUTURE DIRECTIONS

Process models of social behavior recognize two separate routes or systems to describe the nature of human behavior (Chaiken & Trope, 1999; Kahneman, 2011; Strack & Deutsch, 2004). In general, these dual-process models assume that social behavior results from more automatic (or unconscious) and controlled (conscious) processes, and assign distinctive functions and operations to these two systems. This framework and evidence we have discussed suggest that the control of human goal pursuit results from a set of key functions that can be fulfilled outside of conscious awareness. Moreover, our analysis suggests that conscious and unconscious goals may (partly) compete for the same resources to control behavior. How, then, does our framework deal with the distinction between unconscious and conscious processes in human goal pursuit?

Given the empirical evidence collected so far on this topic we are not in a position to formulate a firm answer to this question. However, one way to address this issue is to acknowledge and appreciate that our thinking, feeling, and doing originate from brain processes that are not open to our introspection; hence, in essence, *all* our behaviors start in the unconscious (Dennett, 2003; Libet, 1985; Nørretranders, 1991). Consciousness is called to the fore and may modulate the course of behavior when goals enter conscious awareness, and control is enforced when unconscious processes cannot deal with the task at hand (Baars & Franklin, 2003; Cleeremans, 2008; Jackendoff, 1987). In line with this argument, we suggest that the basic *functions* required for goal pursuit can be realized without conscious awareness, and that conscious goal pursuit likely builds on, and interacts with, the processes by which these functions are implemented for unconsciously activated goals. Because of this scaffolding relation and cross talk between the unconscious and consciousness, conscious and unconscious goal pursuit may diverge under certain circumstances. Clearly, this view of goal pursuit is rather speculative or at least premature. More importantly, it challenges the contemporary notion of dual-process models of behavior. We briefly discuss a few of these challenges below in the context of understanding and examining unconscious goal pursuit.

Controlled or Automatic?

Even though goal pursuit may be instigated and unfold outside of awareness, by definition and according to some of the evidence presented earlier, it is controlled. Because control is normally thought to result from conscious intentions, this raises the question that has already been eloquently addressed by Wegner (2005): "Who is the controller of controlled processes?" In this case, the answer would be "the goal itself." This conclusion corresponds with Bargh's (Bargh, Green, & Fitzsimons, 2008) notion of "the selfish goal," which holds that the reason goals occupy people's minds is for their own attainment. Such views call for a definition of controlled processes in terms of their functions (e.g., active maintenance, discrepancy detections) rather than their origin.

This does not mean that people do not experience control over their unconscious goal pursuits. Recent research has made clear that experiences of control or agency heavily rely on an inference process that arises when there is a match between the action–outcome representations activated in our minds and the outcomes we observe in the world (Aarts, Custers, & Wegner, 2005; Wegner & Wheatley, 1999). While such matches between previewed outcomes and actual outcomes naturally occur for successful conscious goal pursuits, they can also occur for unconscious goal pursuit. In fact, we have recently demonstrated that one of the key functions that promotes unconscious goal pursuit—that is, active maintenance of unconsciously activated desired outcome representations in mind—enhances experiences of agency when the outcome is attained (Aarts et al., 2009).

However, the fact that unconscious goal pursuit may in a sense be regarded as a controlled process does not mean that it is not automatic. Applying the four horsemen of automaticity (Bargh, 1994) to the influences that goal primes have on goal pursuit, these influences can be said to occur without awareness of the primes; they are therefore hard to control and appear not to be dependent on conscious intentions, other than perhaps the participant's intention to participate in the tasks offered. However, the remaining criterion of efficiency may not be met. We discuss this issue separately and examine more specifically how it relates to awareness.

Awareness and Efficiency

Whereas conscious processes are often characterized as effortful, unconscious (automatic) processes have been considered to be efficient and, to some extent, almost free, because the capacity of the unconscious has been assumed to be much larger than that of consciousness (Nørretranders, 1991). To investigate this relation between efficiency and awareness, we need to look at the different phases of the process of goal pursuit separately.

This relation may hold up for the first phases (i.e., the selection of goals and the proper instrumental actions). When a goal (and the reward value attached to it) is activated, there is no need for conscious deliberation about pros and cons of pursuing the goal, which may render this process more efficient than conscious goal setting. The same may be true for the selection of the specific actions by which the goal will be pursued. However, a different picture emerges when it comes to the control processes that operate during goal pursuit. As our studies on the hijacking of the executive function (Marien et al., 2012) indicate, unconsciously activated goals significantly tax the control capacity that is available for conscious goal pursuit (in the case of the study, performing the executive function task itself). Thus, conscious and unconscious goals may compete for the same resources, with unconscious goal pursuit being far from free in that respect.

As such, awareness and efficiency may be two aspects of goal pursuit that are quite unrelated. This finding is in line with the suggestion that full automaticity may be rare (e.g., Moors & De Houwer, 2006), and that each aspect of automaticity should be considered separately (Bargh, 1994). This independence may help to demystify the idea of unconscious goal pursuit: The control processes involved in goal pursuit require resources, regardless of whether goals are activated outside of awareness.

At this point, though, it is necessary to distinguish between different forms of awareness to understand the relation with efficiency. Although our priming manipulations (and those of others) to a reasonable extent warrant claims about unawareness of the source of goal activation, it is much harder to establish whether activated goals operate outside of awareness downstream. That is, even though people may not have been aware of the primes, activated goals may still reach conscious awareness. As a result, goal priming could affect behavior through conscious intentions and deliberations (see, e.g., Loersch & Payne, 2011), which may in turn affect behavior through conscious processes, or processes that are the result of conscious goals but operate outside of awareness (see, e.g., Balcetis & Dunning, 2010).

Some studies even suggest that the probability of unconsciously activated goals popping up in consciousness is more likely when goal pursuit is hampered (Bongers, Dijksterhuis, & Spears, 2010; Klinger, 1996; Martin & Tesser, 1996). Although this is often seen as an adaptive mechanism in which consciousness comes to the rescue if unconscious processes are not up to the job, the current take on unconscious goal pursuit suggests another explanation. Perhaps in those situations, unconscious goals take over so much of the executive function, thereby disrupting the ongoing tasks of consciousness, that they force it to focus on the issues with which the unconsciously activated goal is dealing. Such a shared-platform explanation would solve the mystery of how unconscious goals call consciousness to their rescue: They simply rob it of its resources, so the only content is the very goal that occupies the executive function. According to this perspective, awareness and efficiency may become less independent when goal pursuit requires a lot of executive function capacity.

It is worth noting that even though it is hard to rule out that people become conscious of primed goals or rewards, not all effects on pursuit described in this chapter are consistent with this possibility. In several of the discussed studies on unconscious reward processing, conscious and unconscious reward cues lead to different effects on motivation measures (Bijleveld et al., 2010; Zedelius, Veling, & Aarts, 2011). If the effect of unconscious reward cues were always mediated by conscious goals or intentions (e.g., "I think this is a high-reward trial, I'm gonna try harder"), one would expect the same effects (though perhaps of a different strength) in both conditions.

To conclude, whereas we have found that primed goals tax executive functions, it is hard to determine whether people may become aware of the primed goal along the way. However, dissociations between the effects of conscious and unconscious reward primes on motivation measures suggest that such mediation by conscious processes does not always occur.

Same or Different Platforms?

It appears that conscious and unconscious goal pursuit operate partly on the same and partly on different platforms. When it comes to the function of selecting goals based on expected value, unconscious processes rely on rudimentary brain structures that detect the reward value and recruit the effort necessary for goal pursuit accordingly. Because these same structures are also known to be involved in detecting the reward value of conscious stimuli (Shizgal, 1997), these processes may share the same platform. However, on top of that, conscious goal setting includes other information, relevant or irrelevant, that people may feel they should take into account, and may produce different results than unconscious selection of goals. As recent research on reward processing shows, being conscious of what is at stake may cause people to use different strategies, or it may distract them with thoughts about success or failure (Bijleveld et al., 2010; Zedelius et al., 2011). This can be true for consciously activated goals as well (Wegner, 2009).

When it comes to executive control, conscious and unconscious processes may largely operate on the same platform. Whereas decision-making processes can be replaced by perhaps cruder selection mechanisms to fulfill the goal and action selection functions, basic processes that are necessary for adaptive goal pursuit (e.g., active maintenance of goal representations, tuning of ongoing behavior) cannot. However, conscious processes may increase adaptivity in situations in which tuning of ongoing behavior is not enough and new strategies have to be formed and selected, possibly based on building new representations and retrieving information that has not been consulted for a while. In such situations, the capacity of consciousness for integrating information may prove beneficial, allowing new decisions to be made.

Such a role of consciousness has been proposed in recent models of action control that assume conscious awareness supports, and even results from, the broadcasting of available information over the whole brain (e.g., Baars, 2001; Dehaene & Naccache, 2001). This integrating role of consciousness may lie at the heart of the distinction between goal pursuit that arises from conscious versus unconscious sources: As long as specific brain mechanisms can take care of a task (e.g., determining reward value, preparing action patterns), goal pursuit can in principle emerge without conscious awareness. Hence, consciousness may not be required for any specific phase of goal pursuit (determining what we want, how to get it, or keeping behavior on course), but may instead be required for problem solving that requires communication between various brain areas, if those problems cannot be taken care of by specific mechanisms that operate on previously acquired knowledge.

CONCLUSION

In summary, even though goals may be activated outside conscious awareness, this does not mean that their pursuit relies on processes that are the same as those used by conscious goal pursuit. The functions they fulfill, though, are dictated by the very nature of goal pursuit and, of course, have to be supported by some processes. These processes may be different for conscious and unconscious goal pursuit when it comes to selecting goals and actions, although conscious goal pursuit may have simply extended these rudimentary processes with additional processes that involve deliberative decision making. Because of these additional processes, conscious and unconscious goal pursuit may diverge under certain circumstances.

Whereas unconscious selection of goals and actions has by now been fairly well studied, the real challenge lies in investigating the control processes that are instigated by unconscious goals. Because a certain level of adaptivity may already be built in into the selection processes of goals and actions in interaction with the environment, demonstrating processes that are exclusive to executive functions may require more than behavioral data (Lau & Passingham, 2007; Van Gaal & Lamme, 2012). Only by breaking down functions required for goal pursuit into processes that can be investigated separately will we be able to tell whether unconscious control of behavior is similar to conscious control.

REFERENCES

Aarts, H., Chartrand, T. L., Custers, R., Danner, U. N., Dik, G., Jefferis, V. E., et al. (2005). Social stereotypes and automatic goal pursuit. *Social Cognition*, *23*, 464–489.

Aarts, H., & Custers, R. (2012). Unconscious goal pursuit: Nonconscious goal regulation and motivation. In R. M. Ryan (Ed.), *Oxford handbook of motivation* (pp. 232–247). Oxford.

Aarts, H., Custers, R., & Holland, R. W. (2007). The nonconscious cessation of goal pursuit: When goals and negative affect are coactivated. *Journal of Personality and Social Psychology*, *92*, 165–178.

Aarts, H., Custers, R., & Marien, H. (2008). Preparing and motivating behavior outside of awareness. *Science*, *319*, 1639.

Aarts, H., Custers, R., & Marien, H. (2009). Priming and authorship ascription: When nonconscious goals turn into conscious experiences of self-agency. *Journal of Personality and Social Psychology*, *95*, 967–979.

Aarts, H., Custers, R., & Veltkamp, M. (2008). Goal priming and the affective–motivational route to nonconscious goal pursuit. *Social Cognition*, *26*, 555–577.

Aarts, H., Custers, R., & Wegner, D. M. (2005). On the inference of personal authorship: Enhancing experienced agency by priming effect information. *Consciousness and Cognition*, *14*, 439–458.

Aarts, H., & Dijksterhuis, A. (2000). Habits as knowledge structures: Automaticity in goal-directed behavior. *Journal of Personality and Social Psychology*, *78*, 53–63.

Aarts, H., Gollwitzer, P. M., & Hassin, R. R. (2004). Goal contagion: Perceiving is for pursuing. *Journal of Personality and Social Psychology*, *87*, 23–37.

Ackerman, J. M., Goldstein, N. J., Shapiro, J. R., & Bargh, J. A. (2009). You wear me out: The vicarious depletion of self-control. *Psychological Science*, *20*, 326–332.

Baars, B. J. (2001). *In the theater of consciousness: The workspace of the mind*. New York: Oxford University Press.

Baars, B. J., & Franklin, S. (2003). How conscious experience and working memory interact. *Trends in Cognitive Sciences*, *7*, 166–172.

Balcetis, E., & Dunning, D. (2010). Wishful seeing: More desired objects are seen as closer. *Psychological Science*, *21*, 147–152.

Banks, W. P. (Ed.). (2009). *Encyclopedia of consciousness* (1st ed.). Oxford, UK: Elsevier.

Bargh, J. A. (1990). Auto-motives: Preconscious determinants of social interaction. In E. T. Higgins & R. M. Sorrentino (Eds.), *Handbook of motivation and cognition* (pp. 93–130). New York: Guilford Press.

Bargh, J. A. (1994). The four horsemen of automaticity: Awareness, intention, efficiency, and control in social cognition. In R. S. Wyer, Jr. & T. K. Srull (Eds.), *Handbook of social cognition* (Vol. 2, pp. 1–40). Hillsdale, NJ: Erlbaum.

Bargh, J. A., Gollwitzer, P. M., Lee-Chai, A., Barndollar, K., & Trötschel, R. (2001). The automated will: Nonconscious activation and pursuit of behavioral goals. *Journal of Personality and Social Psychology*, *81*, 1014–1027.

Bargh, J. A., Gollwitzer, P. M., & Oettingen, G. (2010). Motivation. In S. T. Fiske, D. T. Gilbert, & G. Lindzey (Eds.), *Handbook of social psychology* (5th ed., pp. 268–316).

Bargh, J. A., Green, M., & Fitzsimons, G. M. (2008). The selfish goal: Unintended consequences of intended goal pursuits. *Social Cognition*, *26*, 534–554.

Bargh, J. A., & Morsella, E. (2008). The unconscious mind. *Perspectives on Psychological Science*, *3*, 73–79.

Barrouillet, P., Bernardin, S., Portrat, S., Vergauwe, E., & Camos, V. (2007). Time and cognitive load in working memory. *Journal of Experimental Psychology: Learning, Memory, and Cognition*, *33*, 570–585.

Berridge, K. C. (2001). Reward learning: Reinforcement, incentives, and expectations. In D. L. Medin (Ed.), *The psychology of learning and motivation: Advances in research and theory* (pp. 223–278). San Diego: Academic Press.

Bijleveld, E., Custers, R., & Aarts, H. (2009). The unconscious eye opener: Pupil dilation reveals strategic recruitment of resources upon presentation of subliminal reward cues. *Psychological Science*, *20*, 1313–1315.

Bijleveld, E., Custers, R., & Aarts, H. (2010). Unconscious reward cues increase invested effort, but do not change speed-accuracy tradeoffs. *Cognition*, *115*, 330–335.

Bijleveld, E., Custers, R., & Aarts, H. (2012a). Adaptive reward pursuit: How effort requirements affect unconscious reward responses and conscious reward decisions. *Journal of Experimental Psychology: General*, 728–742.

Bijleveld, E., Custers, R., & Aarts, H. (2012b). Human reward pursuit: From rudimentary to higher-level functions. *Current Directions in Psychological Science*, *21*, 194–199.

Blackmore, S. (2004). *Consciousness: An introduction*. New York: Oxford University Press.

Bongers, K. C. A., Dijksterhuis, A., & Spears, R. (2010). On the role of consciousness in goal pursuit. *Social Cognition*, *28*, 262–272.

Brown, P. L., & Jenkins, H. M. (1968). Autoshaping of the pigeon's key-peck. *Journal of the Experimental Analysis of Behavior*, *11*, 1–8.

Campbell, M. C., & Mohr, G. S. (2011). Seeing is eating: How and when activation of a negative stereotype increases stereotype-conducive behavior. *Journal of Consumer Research*, *38*, 431–444.

Capa, R. L., Bouquet, C. A., Dreher, J., & Dufour, A. (2013). Long-lasting effects of performance-contingent unconscious and conscious reward incentives during cued task-switching. *Cortex*, *49*(7), 1943–1954.

Capa, R. L., Cleeremans, A., Bustin, G. M., Bouquet, C. A., & Hansenne, M. (2011). Effects of subliminal priming on nonconscious goal pursuit and effort-related cardiovascular response. *Social Cognition*, *29*, 430–444.

Capa, R. L., Cleeremans, A., Bustin, G. M., & Hansenne, M. (2011). Long-lasting effect of subliminal processes on cardiovascular responses and performance. *International Journal of Psychophysiology*, *81*, 22–30.

Chaiken, S., & Trope, Y. (1999). *Dual-process theories in social psychology*. New York: Guilford Press.

Cleeremans, A. (2008). Consciousness: The radical plasticity thesis. In R. Banerjee & B. K. Chakrabarti (Eds.), *Models of brain and mind: Physical, computational and psychological approaches* (Vol. 168, pp. 19–33). Amsterdam: Elsevier.

Cocchini, G., Logie, R., Sala, S., MacPherson, S., & Baddeley, A. (2002). Concurrent performance of two memory tasks: Evidence for domain-specific working memory systems. *Memory and Cognition*, *30*, 1086–1095.

Custers, R., & Aarts, H. (2005a). Positive affect as implicit motivator: On the nonconscious operation of behavioral goals. *Journal of Personality and Social Psychology*, *89*, 129–142.

Custers, R., & Aarts, H. (2005b). Beyond priming effects: The role of positive affect and discrepancies in implicit processes of motivation and goal pursuit. In M. Hewstone & W. Stroebe (Eds.), *European review of social psychology* (pp. 257–300). Hove, UK: Psychology Press/Taylor & Francis.

Custers, R., & Aarts, H. (2007). Goal-discrepant situations prime goal-directed actions if goals are temporarily or chronically accessible. *Personality and Social Psychology Bulletin*, *33*, 623–633.

Custers, R., & Aarts, H. (2010). The unconscious will: How the pursuit of goals operates outside of conscious awareness. *Science*, *329*, 47–50.

Custers, R., Maas, M., Wildenbeest, M., & Aarts, H. (2008). Nonconscious goal pursuit and the surmounting of physical and social obstacles. *European Journal of Social Psychology*, *38*, 1013–1022.

Danner, U. N., Aarts, H., & De Vries, N. K. (2008). Habit vs. intention in the prediction of future behaviour: The role of frequency, context stability and mental accessibility of past behaviour. *British Journal of Social Psychology*, *47*, 245–265.

de Lange, M. A., Debets, L. W., Ruitenburg, K., & Holland, R. W. (2012). Making less of a mess: Scent exposure as a tool for behavioral change. *Social Influence*, *7*, 90–97.

Dehaene, S., & Naccache, L. (2001). Towards a cognitive neuroscience of consciousness: Basic evidence and a workspace framework. *Cognition*, *79*, 1–37.

Dennett, D. (2003). *Freedom evolves*. New York: Penguin.

Dik, G., & Aarts, H. (2007). Behavioral cues to others' motivation and goal pursuits: The perception of effort facilitates goal inference and contagion. *Journal of Experimental Social Psychology*, *43*, 727–737.

Fitzsimons, G. M., & Bargh, J. A. (2003). Thinking of you: Nonconscious pursuit of interpersonal goals associated with relationship partners. *Journal of Personality and Social Psychology*, *84*, 148–163.

Förster, J., Liberman, N., & Higgins, E. T. (2005). Accessibility from active and fulfilled goals. *Journal of Experimental Social Psychology*, *41*, 220–239.

Friedman, R., Deci, E. L., Elliot, A. J., Moller, A. C., & Aarts, H. (2009). Motivational synchronicity: Priming motivational orientations with observations of others' behaviors. *Motivation and Emotion*, *34*, 34–38.

Gibson, J. J. (1979). *The ecological approach to visual perception*. Boston: Houghton Mifflin.

Guinote, A. (2007). Power and goal pursuit. *Personality and Social Psychology Bulletin, 33*, 1076–1087.

Holland, R. W., Hendriks, M., & Aarts, H. (2005). Smells like clean spirit: Nonconscious effects of scent on cognition and behavior. *Psychological Science, 16*, 689–693.

Hommel, B., Muesseler, J., Aschersleben, G., & Prinz, W. (2001). The theory of event coding (TEC): A framework for perception and action planning. *Behavioral and Brain Sciences, 24*, 849–937.

Jackendoff, R. S. (1987). *Consciousness and the computational mind*. Cambridge, MA: MIT Press.

James, W. (1890). *Principles of psychology*. New York: Holt.

Jeannerod, M. (1997). *The cognitive neuroscience of action*. Oxford, UK: Blackwell.

Kahneman, D. (2011). *Thinking, fast and slow*. New York: Farrar, Straus & Giroux.

Kay, A. C., Wheeler, S. C., Bargh, J. A., & Ross, L. (2004). Material priming: The influence of mundane physical objects on situational construal and competitive behavioral choice. *Organizational Behavior and Human Decision Processes, 95*, 83–96.

Klinger, E. (1996). The contents of thoughts: Interference as the downside of adaptive normal mechanisms in thought flow. In I. G. Sarason, G. R. Pierce, & B. R. Sarason (Eds.), *Cognitive Interference: Theories, methods, and findings* (pp. 3–23). Mahwah, NJ: Erlbaum.

Kraus, M. W., & Chen, S. (2009). Striving to be known by significant others: Automatic activation of self-verification goals in relationship contexts. *Journal of Personality and Social Psychology, 97*, 58–73.

Kruglanski, A. W., Shah, J. Y., Fishbach, A., Friedman, R., Chun, W. Y., & Sleeth-Keppler, D. (2002). A theory of goal-systems. In M. P. Zanna (Ed.), *Advances in experimental social psychology* (Vol. 34, pp. 331–378). San Diego: Academic Press.

Lau, H. C., & Passingham, R. E. (2007). Unconscious activation of the cognitive control system in the human prefrontal cortex. *Journal of Neuroscience, 27*, 5805–5811.

Lau, H. C., & Rosenthal, D. (2011). Empirical support for higher-order theories of conscious awareness. *Trends in Cognitive Sciences, 15*, 365–373.

Lebreton, M., Kawa, S., d'Arc, B. F., Daunizeau, J., & Pessiglione, M. (2012). Your goal is mine: Unraveling mimetic desires in the human brain. *Journal of Neuroscience, 32*, 7146–7157.

Libet, B. (1985). Unconscious cerebral initiative and the role of conscious will in voluntary action. *Behavioral and Brain Sciences, 8*, 529–566.

Loersch, C., Aarts, H., Payne, K. B., & Jefferis, V. E. (2008). The influence of social groups on goal contagion. *Journal of Experimental Social Psychology, 44*, 1555–1558.

Loersch, C., & Payne, B. K. (2011). The situated inference model. *Perspectives on Psychological Science, 6*, 234–252.

Marien, H., Custers, R., Hassin, R. R., & Aarts, H. (2012). Unconscious goal activation and the hijacking of the executive function. *Journal of Personality and Social Psychology, 103*, 399–415.

Martin, L. L., & Tesser, A. (1996). Some ruminative thoughts. In *Ruminative thoughts* (pp. 1–47). Hillsdale, NJ: Erlbaum.

Masicampo, E. J., & Baumeister, R. F. (2011). Unfulfilled goals interfere with tasks that require executive functions. *Journal of Experimental Social Psychology, 47*, 300–311.

Moors, A., & De Houwer, J. (2006). Automaticity: A theoretical and conceptual analysis. *Psychological Bulletin, 132*, 297–326.

Moskowitz, G. B., Salomon, A. R., & Taylor, C. M. (2000). Preconsciously controlling stereotyping: Implicitly activated egalitarian goals prevent the activation of stereotypes. *Social Cognition, 18*, 151–177.

Nisbett, R. E., & Wilson, T. D. (1977). Telling more than we can know: Verbal reports on mental processes. *Psychological Review, 84*, 231–259.

Nørretranders, T. (1991). *The user illusion: Cutting consciousness down to size*. New York: Penguin.

Pessiglione, M., Schmidt, L., Draganski, B., Kalisch, R., Lau, H. C., Dolan, R. J., et al. (2007). How the brain translates money into force: A neuroimaging study of subliminal motivation. *Science, 316*, 904–906.

Pulvermüller, F. (2005). Brain mechanisms linking language and action. *Nature Reviews Neuroscience, 6*, 576–582.

Rabin, M., & Thaler, R. H. (2001). Anomalies: Risk aversion. *Journal of Economic Perspectives, 15*, 219–232.

Schultz, W. (2006). Behavioral theories and the neurophysiology of reward. *Annual Review of Psychology*, *57*, 87–115.

Shah, J. Y. (2003). Automatic for the people: How representations of significant others implicitly affect goal pursuit. *Journal of Personality and Social Psychology*, *84*, 661–681.

Shah, J. Y., Friedman, R., & Kruglanski, A. W. (2002). Forgetting all else: On the antecedents and consequences of goal shielding. *Journal of Personality and Social Psychology*, *83*, 1261–1280.

Sheeran, P., Aarts, H., Custers, R., Rivis, A., Webb, T., & Cooke, R. (2005). The goal-dependent automaticity of drinking habits. *British Journal of Social Psychology*, *44*, 47–63.

Shidlovski, D., & Hassin, R. R. (2011). When pooping babies become more appealing: The effects of nonconscious goal pursuit on experienced emotions. *Psychological Science*, *22*, 1381–1385.

Shizgal, P. (1997). Neural basis of utility estimation. *Current Opinion in Neurobiology*, *7*, 198–208.

Smith, E. E., & Jonides, J. (1999). Storage and executive processes in the frontal lobes. *Science*, *283*, 1657–1661.

Smith, P. K., & Galinsky, A. D. (2010). The nonconscious nature of power: Cues and consequences. *Social and Personality Psychology Compass*, *4*, 918–938.

Strack, F., & Deutsch, R. (2004). Reflective and impulsive determinants of social behavior. *Personality and Social Psychology Review*, *8*, 220–247.

Suhler, C. L., & Churchland, P. S. (2009). Control: Conscious and otherwise. *Trends in Cognitive Sciences*, *13*, 341–347.

Van Gaal, S., & Lamme, V. A. F. (2012). Unconscious high-level information processing: Implication for neurobiological theories of consciousness. *The Neuroscientist*, *18*, 287–301.

Wegner, D. M. (2005). Who is the controller of controlled processes? In R. R. Hassin, J. S. Uleman, & J. A. Bargh (Eds.), *The new unconsciousness* (pp. 1–36). New York: Oxford University Press.

Wegner, D. M. (2009). How to think, say, or do precisely the worst thing for any occasion. *Science*, *325*, 48–50.

Wegner, D. M., & Wheatley, T. (1999). Apparent mental causation: Sources of the experience of will. *American Psychologist*, *54*, 480–492.

Zedelius, C. M., Veling, H., & Aarts, H. (2011). Boosting or choking: How conscious and unconscious reward processing modulate the active maintenance of goal-relevant information. *Consciousness and Cognition*, *20*, 355–362.

Zwaan, R. A., & Taylor, L. J. (2006). Seeing, acting, understanding: Motor resonance in language comprehension. *Journal of Experimental Psychology: General*, *135*, 1–11.

CHAPTER 27

The Implicit Volition Model

The Unconscious Nature of Goal Pursuit

Gordon B. Moskowitz

The set of "dual-process models" that emerged from the 1970s through the 1990s revolutionized the way we think about the nature of consciousness and processing in the mind that is unconscious. These models reinvigorated research on motivation in order to better understand not merely what motivates behavior but what motivates the use of either systematic or heuristic thought processes, as well as the transition from one to the other during self-regulation. These models of a motivated social cognition typically described a default processing system that quickly makes sense of stimuli in a fashion that relies on the mere triggering of associations but one that can be modified by a separate system where one may alter these outputs through new processing, processing that would allow one to initiate operations that promote achieving some end. This regulation of responding to serve the intentions and goals of the individual is how *control* is defined. Despite the utility of these models, there are two issues that arise from research inspired by this dual-process approach that are the focus of analysis in this chapter

The first is that contrasting controlled processes with automatic processes suggests that there are some forms of social cognition that are goal-directed and motivated (controlled), and others that are not, that happen too quickly for control to be deployed (e.g., Fazio, 1990). I argue here that this distinction, while a useful metaphorical device, is likely a false dichotomy. It is true that most dual-process models have described these two types of processes in terms of a continuum in which the endpoints reflect absolute states, with most implicit processing reflecting some degree of control. Bargh (1990) distinguished between the purely automatic process and the goal-dependent automatic process, once again capturing the idea that much of social cognition that happens outside awareness may still be motivated. However, these distinctions do not go far enough. All cognition is social (in that it occurs within the norms, values, expectations, and shared beliefs of the environment and culture in which it occurs), and a defining aspect of social cognition is its goal-directedness. Even low-level implicit cognition, such as how and where to place attention selectively, what from among a complex stimulus array we perceive, how we categorize, and the experience of the passage of time are controlled by goals. It does not make sense, beyond the metaphorical level, to talk about controlled as opposed to other types of cognitive processing. Cognitive processing is a tool used to serve the needs of the organism, and, therefore, is controlled.

This is linked to the second issue I analyze in this chapter, that of consciousness and control. In the initial wave of dual-process models, the distinction between a motivated/goal-directed process and an automatic process made sense, because control was defined as borne of the conscious will and the explicit desire to attain an end. The defining features of an automatic process (aside from its inability to be controlled) were said to be its efficiency and ability to be triggered and run to completion without conscious intent or awareness. This implied that control had to be defined as requiring awareness, effort, and conscious intent. Control meant either (1) explicitly using processing to modify the outputs of an automatic process so that goals were better attained (e.g., Devine, 1989; Fiske & Neuberg, 1990; Gilbert, 1989; Strack, Schwarz, Bless, Kübler, & Wänke, 1993), or (2) consciously setting desired ends and engaging operations for the explicit purpose of delivering a desired state. In each case monitoring and feedback processes provide requisite information about progress toward the goal that allows the system to know whether to continue and at what pace (e.g., Carver & Scheier, 1981). In the intervening years, however, a growing line of research on unconscious goals has rendered the "automatic–controlled" distinction muddier. It is not merely that all cognition is controlled, but that this is possible because control need not be defined as conscious.

The conceptualization of control as not being synonymous with effort, inefficiency, and conscious contemplation of goals was first discussed in earnest in work on mindsets and the phases of goal pursuit (e.g., Gollwitzer, 1990), the theory of lay epistemics (Kruglanski, 1990), Bargh's (1990) auto-motive model, and my own research in graduate school on goal effects on implicit inference (Moskowitz, 1993; Uleman & Moskowitz, 1994) and priming effects (Thompson, Roman, Moskowitz, Chaiken, & Bargh, 1994). Yet it must be recognized that much of the classic theorizing on human goal pursuit (e.g., Lewin, 1936; Zeigarnik, 1927) and animal goal pursuit (Tolman, 1932) had long ago conceptualized goal pursuit as not requiring consciousness.[1] Other classic approaches between the 1930s and the implicit goal "revival" of the 1990s were merely agnostic on the issue, with models that focused on conscious goals, but that were amenable to the notion of unconscious goals, had one thought to introduce them (e.g., Atkinson, 1964; Carver & Scheier, 1981). Having consciousness does not mean humans lack the ability to process without it, and this key point took some time to be rediscovered when it comes to issues relating to control.

While synthesizing decades of research on implicit versus explicit cognition, dual-process models have fallen short in synthesizing research on implicit versus explicit volition. Even modern models have not fully integrated this conceptualization of control. For example, Payne (2006) proposed a process dissociation model to explain stereotype-based biases that persist in responding even when one intends to be unbiased. Payne argued that dual-process theories such as that introduced by Payne, Lambert, and Jacoby (2002) "attempt to explain when, how, and why behavior is driven by automatic versus intentionally controlled aspects of thought. . . . [We] have proposed a particular dual-process theory to account for both intentional control over decisions and the patterns of unintended bias seen in snap judgments" (p. 288). Payne posited that faces of black men trigger automatic associations (semantic and emotional) that dictate responding when controlled processing fails. A "weapons task" was used to examine whether control fails or succeeds (and what default processing occurs when it fails). In this task, faces of black or white men preceded an image of either a weapon or a tool, and participants needed to identify the object as a weapon or tool. Results showed that with ample time participants were accurate (but still faster to decide "weapon" when they had seen a black man's face). However, when pressured for time, participants could not implement control via the "required" effort, and control failed: Participants were more likely to report seeing a weapon when *any* image was preceded by a black face. Payne concluded that activation of weapons when participants saw black faces was automatic. Control is relegated to a conscious/effortful process in which the prevention of the expression of those stereotypes may occur. The bias even emerges when people are instructed not to stereotype, strengthening Payne's conclusion that activation of a stereotype is more efficient than control:

"In this and other studies, the weapon bias seems largely independent of intent. This is important because it means that the bias can coexist with conscious intentions to be fair and unbiased" (p. 288). While it is true that they can coexist, the implication that this makes the bias uncontrollable is not true.

A striking majority of modern dual-process accounts have yet to acknowledge the unconscious role of goals. For example, in the domain of prejudice, Mahzarin Banaji, a developer of the Implicit Association Test (IAT), noted on the television show *The Cycle* (February 14, 2013) how we can view the control of prejudice: "Some of us have used the power of our conscious minds to tell ourselves that information simply is not correct, whereas others have not. . . . And that's really the difference." The association of bias with a group cannot be controlled, according to this account, but behavior can under the appropriate conditions be predicated on awareness of the bias and the conscious motivation to rectify (overturn) the bias.

This failure to incorporate a role for implicit goals in control over implicit cognition, such as the activation of stereotypes or the implicit association of negative affect to a group, has implications not only for theory but also for how policymakers and practitioners approach the control of unwanted bias. For example, Devine, Forscher, Austin, and Cox (2012) developed a bias reduction training program for medical practitioners based on the following logic: "When they believe they have acted with bias, people who endorse values opposed to prejudice are motivated to inhibit the expression of implicit bias by seeking out information and putting effort into tasks they believe would help them break the prejudice habit" (p. 1268). The intervention draws from dual-process model notions of control, aimed at training people to develop new conscious responses when faced with awareness of a bad habit (implicit bias). Such a strategy based on effort can be effective, but fails to acknowledge the complementary role for goals that do not require effort.

An example of a model that has altered/modernized its conception of control is Sherman's (2006) quadruple-process model. This model identifies many types of automatic and controlled processes that can be summarized as falling within four general categories of processes—two classes of automatic and two classes of control processes. The first class of control is what Sherman called regulation, or *overturning bias* (OB), processes in which one is attempting to inhibit or overturn unwanted information that one has detected in one's response (e.g., the presence of a stereotype, or any unwanted thought). The second type of control is what Sherman called *discrimination* or *detection processes,* in which the person exerts consciousness and effort to analyze stimulus items in the service of a goal to get accurate information (to determine the quality of a persuasive message, the attributes of a person, etc.). Whether the role of consciousness and effort in control is necessary is challenged by Sherman's model. Though not the central purpose of that model, it has the flexibility to incorporate unconscious control by offering a processing model "that does not treat automaticity/control as the central or defining distinction among processes. Instead, the particular nature of the process is the key question (i.e., What does the process do?) and the automatic versus controlled nature of the process is only one important feature of the process" (p. 181). Calanchini and Sherman (2013) recently reiterated this stance:

> The operation of Detection [D] and Overcoming Bias [OB] demands a more nuanced portrayal of automaticity and control because D and OB possess features of both. For example, though it is clear that their operation can be disrupted, it also is clear that they are sufficiently efficient to influence responses during the performance of implicit tasks. This suggests two important points. First, researchers should resist the temptation to describe processes as either automatic or controlled. . . . Second, we need to broaden the range of processes that may be characterized as automatic.

However, a fully explicated account of how implicit volition is integrated into the model has yet to be developed. For all the emerging evidence supporting dissociating the four processes of the quadruple-process model (e.g., Calanchini & Sherman, 2013), none has yet focused on unconscious goals.

Most approaches to control fall squarely into what Sherman (2006) called an OB response, yet do not offer the flexibility of

Sherman's model for conceptualizing OB as an implicit process. And because they are contingent on conscious awareness of a biasing influence, they circumvent the possibility of unconscious control. While stages of the control process may be automated, they describe the enterprise of control as contingent upon the existence of (1) awareness of bias, (2) explicit motivation to counteract that bias, (3) the possession of a theory regarding how to counteract the bias accurately, (4) the ability (cognitive resources) to deploy a strategy to counteract the bias, and (5) lack of disruption from concomitant mental operations. Indeed, this set of contingencies describes not only how people may regulate the goal of being nonbiased but also a more general form of explicit self-regulation that can apply to the pursuit of any goal. This is why rather than use the term *overturning bias,* the implicit volition model (IVM) describes such control processes as *reactive control.*

Reactive control is initiated as a reaction to an existing state in which a shortcoming, or relative failure, in the pursuit of a desired end is detected (e.g., a goal not being met, a bias in one's responding). Importantly, the IVM further stipulates that these processing stages in reactive control that compensate for or counteract a failure or a shortcoming in attaining a desired goal do not need to be conscious. The bias or shortcoming can be implicitly triggered, as can the motivation to counteract the bias, as well as theories about the operations that need be initiated to achieve the goal and the operations themselves. Stating that the processes in reactive control need not be conscious does not in any way undermine the value of reactive approaches to control that are rooted in consciousness. It simply highlights that such approaches are limited, constrained by the assumption that control cannot be implicit. Reactive control is only complemented and extended by allowing for implicit goals.

The allowance for implicit goals does not merely extend how we understand reactive control. It also highlights a second set of control processes that can be contrasted to reactive control—*proactive control.* Rather than seeing control as a reaction to feedback, Sherman (2006) described "discrimination" or "detection" processes as a set of control processes that directs how stimulus information is analyzed when a goal has been adopted (e.g., a goal to get accurate information leading to closer attention to individuating information about a person). This reflects a classic goal-setting approach to control, in which goal pursuit is set in motion by the selection of a desired state (through deliberation among possible choices and evaluation of inputs, e.g., Carver & Scheier, 1981; Chaiken, Liberman, & Eagly, 1989; Gollwitzer, 1990) rather than as a counteractive response to negative feedback. The IVM refers to such processes as *proactive control,* or control that involves triggering a goal that then directs cognition and behavior in the service of goal attainment. Again, such control can be wholly implicit—one need not be aware of either the desired state or of the processes engaged to move toward goal attainment (the host of mental operations initiated relating to the implementation and strategies for pursuing the goal). For example, in the Stroop task we see a controlled process of naming a color interfered with by a so-called "automatic process" of reading words and inferring the meaning in those words. But the latter process is no less controlled than the former process. We simply fail to recognize the goal that directs the latter process. Though participants performing a Stroop task are explicitly asked to pursue the goal of naming colors, they also bring with them their habitual goal of distilling meaning from words This latter goal has receded into the background and operates implicitly, but this does not make its pursuit and influence any less controlled.

To illustrate the distinction between reactive and proactive control let us return to the example of an unwanted thought associated with a group, such as a prejudice or a stereotype. Models that focus on reactive control (1) assume that control occurs to compensate for bias, and that such bias is introduced by the typical operations of the mind that trigger stereotypes outside of awareness, without conscious intent, even among low-prejudice people, and (2) implicate awareness of bias as necessary to engage the counteractive steps deemed necessary for control. While this is a useful procedure for reducing bias, anything other than this reactive path to control will be ignored by a model positing that control over implicit stereotypes and prejudices must be more effortful than the implicit processes that trigger them (and such assumptions define most dual process models). This discounts the viability of proactive control, because the processes that give rise to stereotyping and prejudice would be beyond the reach of such control, leaving only modification of these outputs of automatic processing as a viable control strategy.

The IVM proposes that not only is the reactive approach not limited to conscious control attempts, but also that the implication of implicit control opens the door to proactive control of these biases. There is no reason to assume that to prevent stereotyped responses is more effortful than the processes that trigger them. For example, when goals are accessible that are antithetical with stereotyping they proactively initiate implicit processes associated with those goals that promote goal attainment. This includes processes that dictate how the person is categorized and whether stereotypes are activated or inhibited (Moskowitz, Gollwitzer, Wasel, & Schaal, 1999; Moskowitz & Li, 2011). The cognitive processes triggered in response to any given target vary from situation to situation as one's goals in the situation dictate. And one's goals need not dictate stereotypes being retrieved from memory, despite the ease with which this may occur when pursuing some types of goals. A thought experiment, though extreme, illustrates the point. Imagine a white American injured in a terrorist attack, who is bloodied and worrying about amputation, when a black man emerges from the crowd and says, "Relax, I'm a doctor. I can help you." Will cultural stereotypes of black people be activated? A model of implicit, proactive control argues that they will not, because one's goals lead not to the recruitment of those associations but to associations related to a different category (doctor), inhibiting interfering associations and inferences. From this perspective, proactive stereotype control is more than preventing a stereotype's activation. Such activation is itself serving a goal (e.g., to understand what a person is like and likely to do, to make predictions, to feel power, to enable feelings of ingroup superiority, etc.). It is just that the goal is not visible.

There is no need to describe either proactive or reactive control as limited to consciousness, or to describe one as more automatic than the other (though many people find reactive control more intuitively obvious as a conscious reaction). The implicit operation of these forms of control may even provide a more efficient way to achieve a goal (e.g., not stereotyping) than explicitly pursuing the goal (e.g., when explicitly trying not to stereotype leads one ultimately to rely on stereotypes more). As Bargh and Huang (2009) argued, consciousness in goal pursuit captures only a small piece of *what* the goal system controls and *how* it exerts control. Much of what we think of as automatic is controllable, and much of what we think of as controlled is regulated outside conscious awareness in a manner that once would have been called "automatic" (Bargh, 1990; Custers & Aarts, 2010; Gollwitzer & Moskowitz, 1996; Kruglanski et al., 2002).

VOLITION NEEDS NO INFERENCES: THE 13 POSTULATES OF THE IMPLICIT VOLITION MODEL

The Sovereignty of the Implicit Goal System

Definitions of control as requiring awareness, consciousness, and effort are so prevalent that it led Wegner and Bargh (1998, p. 453) to state: "the term 'unconscious control' doesn't seem right at all." My purpose in this chapter is to extend the definition of control; to highlight that the automatic–controlled dichotomy is limited because control may lack the features of consciousness, effort, and awareness. It may be habitual, triggered through associations, in the way that automatic processes are typically defined. Ostrom (1984) famously declared the sovereignty of social cognition, heralding the arrival of a distinct field of inquiry that laid waste to the need to distinguish between social and nonsocial cognition. While undeniable that social and nonsocial objects have different properties (e.g., a rock cannot be motivated to cause harm, nor does it change across situations) that lead us to think about them differently, our thoughts regarding each are, nonetheless, social in nature. Ostrom (p. 3) proclaimed that "all knowledge is social knowledge, and all social knowledge derives from action on the environment." Ostrom's reasoning is extended here in a way that I hope does not alter his meaning: Action on the environment is always in the service of the goals of the organism within that environment.

That is, what makes cognition social is not merely that the content of one's processing may be people, but that the stimulus—whether person or object—must be acted and reacted toward, and that this reaction occurs in the service of the goals of the person in relation to that stimulus within a social environment (its norms, culture, opportunities, threats) at that point in time. What makes social cognition sovereign is the social nature of all cognition, and what makes it social is the motivated nature of *all* cognition—any commerce with the environment introduces needs, motives, values, and goals that are the guiding force of any response. Cognition is a tool servicing the needs, intentions, and goals of the organism accessible at that moment; it occurs in the context of the goals of the organism in that setting.

This point has its opponents. For example, Bargh (1989, 1990) has argued for classifying social cognition into its goal-dependent and goal-independent forms. Bargh provides examples of *preconscious* automaticity and *postconscious* automaticity, which are meant to reflect the types of processing that are independent of goals (indeed, the only events on which such processing is said to be contingent is the presence of a triggering stimulus and the allocation of attentional resources, so that these stimuli can be detected and processed by the sensory apparatus). The primary examples provided are those of social construct activation and evaluation extraction. Yet research on implicit goals has led to a reframing of such phenomena. Construct accessibility is now discussed as being motivated and understood only in a goal system (Eitam & Higgins, 2010). Implicitly associating affect with categories is also now conceived to be a controlled phenomenon (e.g., Dasgupta & Greenwald, 2001; Glaser & Knowles, 2008) and as occurring because automatic attitude activation helps organisms pursue survival goals by providing fast feedback, allowing them to avoid that which is harmful and approach that which is beneficial (e.g., Chen & Bargh, 1999; Eder & Rothermund, 2008). And even the allocation of attention is controlled (e.g., Moskowitz, 2002).

These developments have led some to argue that much of conscious control is an epiphenomenon, something experienced to deliver a feeling of agency (e.g., van der Weiden, Aarts, & Ruys, in press; Wegner & Wheatley, 1999). Huang and Bargh (in press) even argued that consciousness is an exaptation of the unconscious. Drawing from the animal literature, they conclude that our evolutionarily earlier ancestors, who lack consciousness in goal pursuit, provide an illustration that the development of conscious goals occurs after the development of unconscious goals. They argue that most models have it backwards, and unconscious goal pursuit is the evolutionarily older, dominant, and more common form of goal pursuit, with consciousness in goal pursuit built upon—a scaffold to—older processing structures.

However, I do not posit that the existence of an implicit volition system that directs all cognitive processing renders consciousness as being uninvolved in control, or epiphenomenal. Instead, I posit that implicit goals have their genesis in the conscious intentions and experiences of the individual. While it is true that consciousness can be epiphenomenal, the IVM is not contingent on a belief that this is typically the case, or that unconscious goals are more primary due to processes of evolution that favor them. Rather, the IVM argues that goal-directed responding becomes automated over the course of one's lifetime, through learning, deliberation, evaluation, and other forms of conscious processing. The needs of the organism specify what goals to pursue, under which circumstances, and the specific means to achieve those ends. Over time, the choices made to promote needs satisfaction that associate goals and contexts and means become routine and automatically engaged, as consciousness recedes from being necessary for goal-directed responding. The role of consciousness is often felt through its impact on establishing associations formed between cues, environments, people, means of responding, and goals.

It was a watershed moment for psychological science when Bargh (1990) reintroduced these ideas in the "auto-motive" model and amended existing models of human goal pursuit by highlighting the question that had been ignored: Why assume that one's goals in any moment arise from one's conscious selection of them? The IVM develops these ideas by removing consciousness as the point of focal interest in control and instead focusing on the processes through which control is implemented in both its reactive and proactive forms.

Postulate 1: Goals in Humans Are Derived from Needs, Motives, and Values

A *goal* is a desired end state one has not yet attained but is committed (to varying degrees, as a function of its value and ones efficacy) to approach or to avoid, with a focus toward attaining the desired end in the future. The "end" can range from the concrete ("Do not think about white bears") to the abstract ("Maintain a rosy outlook"), and the semantic meaning associated with the end state (what it means to be "rosy") can change with the context. The most dominant source of goals is needs (e.g., Deci & Ryan, 1991; McClelland, 1985).[2] *Needs* were once defined as biological states of the organism required to sustain life, but are now accepted to include psychological states that are essential for well-being and for survival in the social world. A need specifies classes of *incentives*, which comprise a broad set of environmental opportunities for action that can bring about desired outcomes (a product of needs and the context). *Motives* are broad classes of desires or preferred states that emerge from needs, a "tendency to desire or be fearful of a specific type of positive or negative experience in a particular life domain" (Elliot & Niesta, 2009, p. 61). They develop early in life through an infant's experience with incentives and become cognitively elaborated over time. Motives provide the direction and energy for action by linking desired end states within a broad domain to incentives and the means to pursue those incentives. Goals are lower level yet within this hierarchy, and "are viewed as the carriers or servants of higher-order motivational propensities [that are] . . . usually insufficiently precise to regulate behavior effectively in that no specific standard or guideline for behavior is provided" (Elliot & Niesta, p. 65).

Research throughout the 20th century informs us that that those actions that are more instrumental for attaining a goal are specified by opportunities for acquiring the incentives in the context, and by one's efficacy at pursuing those opportunities (e.g., Bandura, 1989; Lewin, 1936; Wicklund & Gollwitzer, 1982). This suggests that the specific goal selected at any moment is tied to (1) its desirability (value), which is specified by the goal's association to the person's respective need, and (2) beliefs about how the goal can be realized and whether it is feasible to expect goal attainment.

Postulate 2: Goals Are Cognitively Represented

Tolman (1932) posited that when, via experience, external cues in the environment come to satisfy a given need of an animal, this leads that organism to form an association between the need state and those environmental cues. The cues come to have value to the animal in terms of satisfying a goal. This association among goals, values, stimuli, and contexts was said to be "represented" (stored in memory) in the mind of the perceiving organism so that it would be triggered when the organism entered the appropriate context, initiating the relevant behavior that can deliver the value the stimulus affords. Humans also develop goal representations through associative experience. Bargh (1990, p. 100) stated:

> Goals and intents are represented in the mind in the same fashion as are social constructs, stereotypes, and schemas . . . goals and intents, and the procedures . . . and plans . . . associated with them, may become directly and automatically linked in memory with representations of environmental features to which they are frequently and consistently associated.

Kruglanski (1996) elaborated on this concept of goal representations by further positing them to have a hierarchical organization, in which desired end states are superordinate and processing routines and actions–behavior routes (means) are low-order components of the representation. This allows the representation to be marked by equifinality, in which many means are linked to one higher-order goal (e.g., Kruglanski, Pierro, & Sheveland, 2011). It can also be marked by multifinality (e.g., Kruglanski et al., 2013) in which several high-order ends are attained by the same means (killing two birds with one stone).

A state of multifinality suggests one way that people select an action from among the many means they might enact (given a state of equifinality); they select that which has value for multiple goals, which proffers compounded value. Evidence for a goal representation with such a multifinal configuration is provided by showing that the value assigned to multifinal means declines when a subset of the goals served by the means is deactivated and means lose their compounded value (e.g., Chun, Kruglanski, Friedman, & Sleeth-Keppler, 2011). Evidence for goal representations is also provided by the transfer of affect from superordinate to lower-order elements of a representation (e.g., energizing means with the motivational properties of the goal). Ferguson and Bargh (2004) showed that the implicit evaluation of its means is more positive when a goal is held more strongly (see also, Fishbach, Shah, & Kruglanski, 2004).

Postulate 3: Goal Representations Link Ends to Multiple Means and Implicit Processing Routines

Goal representations include not only an end state, but associations to relevant means for attaining the desired end. As an example, Cacioppo, Priester, and Berntson (1993; see also Chen & Bargh, 1999; Friedman & Förster, 2002) had participants enact means associated with approach and avoidance goals. Arm flexion (pulling the arm toward oneself) or extension (pushing it away from oneself) was enacted during a word evaluation task. They found that neutral words were evaluated more positively during flexion and negatively during extension. This could only occur if means (flexion) were associated with a goal (approach) and its affect, and this affect then transferred to the neutral object. Shah and Kruglanski (2003) illustrated that merely thinking about means, not enacting them, triggers goals associated with those means, while Aarts and Dijksterhuis (2000) showed that thinking about a goal activates its means.

Cognitive processing routines that prepare one for action are also part of a goal's representation, so the organism is tuned to detect stimuli relevant to the goal and is preconsciously processing relevant information. Gollwitzer (1990) made this point by focusing on *mindsets* associated with distinct phases of goal pursuit. For example, deliberative and implemental mindsets function when goals are being selected versus pursued. They affect thought production, recall of task-relevant information, analysis of desirability-related information, inferences based on feasibility-related information, and attention.

Processing styles are associated not only with broad phases of goal pursuit but also specific goal contents. Balcetis and Dunning (2006) have shown that early stages of visual processing are shaped by motives. Eye movements governing the perception of an ambiguous stimulus array were directed by preferences, so that a desired interpretation emerged as a result of implicit perceptual processing. Balcetis, Dunning, and Granot (2012) further showed that during binocular rivalry (where ambiguity is created by exposing each eye to different images), desires determined which of two images was experienced. This extends research of Bruner and colleagues (e.g., Bruner & Goodman, 1947; Postman, Bruner, & McGinnies, 1948) showing that values and needs control the thresholds at which stimuli are perceived.

Many goal representations have been shown to have associated cognitive processing routines that facilitate goal attainment. Examples include the following: A goal of thought suppression has associated implicit monitoring processes that provide feedback regarding the absence–presence in the mind of the unwanted thought (e.g., Galinsky & Moskowitz, 2007; Macrae, Bodenhausen, Milne, & Jetten, 1994; Wegner, 1994). A goal of being egalitarian toward members of a group leads to inhibition of stereotypes associated with that group (e.g., Moskowitz et al., 1999; Moskowitz & Li, 2011) and selective attention to cues related to the group (Moskowitz, Li, Ignarri, & Stone, 2011; Moskowitz, 2002). A goal of being creative leads to retrieval of remotely associated knowledge (Ward, Finke, & Smith, 1995). A goal of approaching gains leads to focusing concern on aspirations and accomplishments, and the strategic inclination to *approach matches* to desired end states, while a goal of avoiding risk leads to focusing concern on protection/safety and the strategic inclination to *avoid mismatches* to desired goals (Higgins, 2009).

Postulate 4: Goal Representations Specify Not Merely Means and Ends, but Value

Like vectors, goal representations are marked by not only a direction in which one is striving but also valence that marks the affect associated with attaining the end and its pursuit. The representation captures *anticipatory desire,* a sense that reaching the end state will have positive consequences. Most models of goal pursuit implicate the *value* of the goal state as a determining force for commitment to a goal and whether a goal is transformed into behavior (e.g., Ferguson, 2007), such that even infusing affect (outside consciousness) to neutral semantic knowledge transforms it to a goal (e.g., Custers, 2009; Custers & Aarts, 2005). And decreasing positive affect associated with a desired end state reduces the motivation to pursue it (e.g., Aarts, Custers, & Holland, 2007; Winkielman, Berridge, & Willbarger, 2005).

Postulate 5: Goal Representations Are Marked by Tension States Arising from Discrepancies

A *goal* is a desired end state toward which one is *striving.* Semantic knowledge of the end state is not sufficient to label a representation as a goal, nor is valuing the end state. Striving must also be represented, which is to say that feedback regarding progress toward the end state must indicate a shortcoming or *discrepancy* between the valued endpoint and one's current state (Lewin, 1936, 1951)—the desired end is not yet attained. When monitoring–feedback reveal such a discrepancy, an aversive tension arises that is similar to the *drive* associated with a physiological need. Lewin posited that goal discrepancies also produce a tension that must be reduced, providing motivational force that persists until that tension is satisfied. One is impelled to respond in goal-directed ways to eliminate the tension.

This principle was reintroduced into modern theorizing about goals by Wicklund and Gollwitzer (1982). They posit that when shortcomings with respect to a goal pursuit are encountered (discrepancy), one experiences self-definitional *incompleteness* (tension). Tension will be greatest when an individual is committed to a goal domain, when it is self-defining. One manner in which people compensate for the sense of incompleteness surrounding a challenged identity is by attempting to acquire alternative symbols of success in the domain or new symbols suggesting that one possesses positive qualities linked to the goal.

In order to know when the discrepancy has been reduced and the tension addressed, to know whether to cease or to continue responding, the processing system is engaged in monitoring processes. Monitoring of a goal pursuit provides two types of feedback regarding the discrepancy that informs the system's "decisions" (e.g., Jostmann & Koole, 2009). The first type of feedback is amount of progress toward a goal (Liberman & Dar, 2009). The second type is rate of progress toward the goal that informs the individual regarding matters of pace (Carver & Scheier, 1998). Together, these steps of monitoring, feedback, and operations aimed at discrepancy reduction comprise a negative feedback loop (Carver & Scheier, 1981; Miller et al., 1960) or closed-loop control system (Powers, 1973) that persists until the negative state has dissipated and the discrepancy is eliminated (Martin & Tesser, 2009).

Postulate 6: Goal Activation–Selection and Goal Pursuit–Implementation Need Not Be Conscious

There is nothing in Postulates 1–5 that needs to specify a role for consciousness in any given goal pursuit. The goal, and its ends, means, cognitive operations, affect, and discrepancies, by virtue of being mentally represented, can be selected and pursed in a given moment without requiring consciousness, just as with any other mental representation. Rather, what is specified in these postulates is a distinction being drawn between processes involved in the setting, selection, triggering, creating, and accessibility of a goal versus processes involved in the implementation, pursuing, monitoring, and attainment of a goal. This parallels the more general case of mental representation activation, in which a distinction is drawn between a construct's activation and its application (where the activated construct guides responding; e.g., Devine, 1989; Gilbert, 1989; Strack et al., 1993). Each can proceed without consciousness.

Goal activation can be called unconscious if it meets one of two criteria: (1) The stimulus activating the goal is not consciously detected (e.g., subliminal presentation) or (2) one's state of goal activation is not consciously noticed, even if at some point either the goal-relevant stimuli or the goal itself had been consciously detected. Chartrand and Bargh (1996) illustrated these criteria in two seminal experiments. In the first, goals were primed by subliminal exposure to goal-relevant words; in the second, by conscious exposure to the words as part of a "scrambled sentence task" (a set of words in jumbled order had to be arranged in a fashion that produced a coherent sentence). In each case the unconscious triggering of the goal yielded the same mental operations as when the goal in question had been consciously introduced.

Goal pursuit can be implicit when the processes serving the goal (1) are not consciously initiated or detected, or (2) they are consciously initiated but the connection between the response and the goal is not detected. Examples of the former, in which people engage in responses without knowing, are revealed using a host of tasks, such as eye tracking (e.g., Balcetis & Dunning, 2006), mouse trajectories (e.g., Freeman, Dale, & Farmer, 2011; Packer, Miners, Ungson, and Okten (in preparation), and reaction time measures (e.g., facilitating response times to a goal-relevant target when it is the focus of attention, and reducing response times to a focal target when it is not) are used to reveal selective attention (e.g., Custers & Aarts, 2007; Gollwitzer, 1993; Moskowitz, 2002; Shah, 2003). For example, Trawalter, Todd, Baird, and Richeson (2008) showed that white participants who had avoidance goals related to black people (due to feelings of threat) selectively directed attention towards black faces, even though the faces were presented for only 30 milliseconds, too brief a time to direct attention consciously to a face.[3]

Four general categories of goal pursuits emerge when crossing the dimension of presence versus absence of consciousness with the dimension of goal activation–setting versus goal pursuit–implementation. The first category is the consciously primed goal that has conscious operations (which has been the target of much of the history of research on goals). The second is the unconsciously primed goal that has unconscious operations (e.g., in the Stroop task in which goals to distill meaning lead to the reading of words to be the dominant response rather than color-naming). The third is the consciously primed goal with unconscious operations (e.g., when conscious attempts at thought suppression yield implicit monitoring processes). The fourth category is unconsciously primed goals with conscious operations (e.g., when conscious flexion is influenced by implicit approach goals). Of course, any given goal pursuit can have a mixture of conscious and unconscious operations, as well as any operation being able to serve multiple conscious and unconscious goals that are activated simultaneously.

Postulate 7: Goal Representations Vary in Their State of Accessibility (and Can Be Primed)

As stipulated in Postulate 6, because goals are representations, conscious deliberation about what goal to pursue is not necessary. A goal can be passively primed (attain a state of readiness by being accessible in working memory) either through internal mental operations or external cues associated with the goal (features of the environment) that serve to trigger the goal. Bargh (1990, p. 100) stated:

> The mechanism proposed here by which the social environment may control judgments, decisions, and behavior is the formation of direct and automatic mental links between representations of motives and goals in memory (and consequently the goals and plans associated with them) and the representations of the social situations in which those motives have been frequently pursued in the past. The result of this automatic associative link is that the motive–goal–plan structure becomes activated whenever the relevant triggering situational features are present in the environment.

Goal priming, as a subtype of construct priming more generally, is governed by the principles of activation and inhibition that apply to other representations, such as stereotypes, categories, and attitudes. The probability that goal representations are "activated directly by environmental information is a joint function of their applicability to the information and their accessibility in memory" (Bargh, p. 100).[4] To review illustrations of goal priming the literature is next divided according to ways goals are primed.

The Unconscious Triggering of a Goal by an Undetected Stimulus

Goals are unconsciously primed by subliminal exposure to words linked to the goal (e.g., Chartrand & Bargh, 1996), but this is not the only way. Since significant others are associated with specific goals, subliminal exposure to those significant others can prime the goal (e.g., Fitzsimons & Bargh, 2003; Shah, 2003). And not all implicit primes are in the external environment. It is possible to prime a goal from one's mental activity. For example, observing others' behavior leads one to infer the goals of those others, often without awareness that inferences have been made and, implicitly priming that goal (Aarts, Gollwitzer, & Hassin, 2004).

The Unconscious Triggering of a Goal by Consciously Detected Stimuli

Similar to the scrambled sentence task of Chartrand and Bargh (1996), Bargh, Gollwitzer, Lee-Chai, Barndollar, and Trötschel (2001) triggered a goal in participants unconsciously by having them work consciously on word search puzzles containing goal-relevant words. Aarts and Dijksterhuis (2003) used a picture of an environment to increase accessibility of goals associated with that environment. Williams and Bargh (2008) showed that physical sensations associated with an object trigger goals with which those sensations are metaphorically linked. Kay, Wheeler, Bargh, and Ross (2004) showed that goals may be primed by objects in the room. And people with whom we interact trigger goals linked with those people (e.g., Moskowitz et al., 2011; Richeson & Shelton, 2007; Trawalter et al., 2008).

Consciously Selected Goals That Implicitly Retain Accessibility

A goal consciously selected at one point in time can retain its accessibility in later contexts in which the individual lacks awareness that the goal is now accessible. This can be illustrated when one believes that he or she has disengaged from a goal. This type of priming is seen in the research of Dijksterhuis, Bos, Nordgren, and Van Barren (2006), in which problem-solving goals were consciously relinquished prior to resolving the problem. Goal accessibility was shown to linger by participants continuing to work on the problem unconsciously. Research on *implementation intentions* (specifying if–then plans that link cues to responses) is another example (e.g., Gollwitzer, 1993; Parks-Stamm & Gollwitzer, 2009). Consciousness is needed to form an intention but not to trigger a plan. The mere presence of a cue specified by the plan implicitly initiates the response.

Goals That Attain Heightened Accessibility from Discrepancy Detection

Discrepancies can be primed (e.g., Custers & Aarts, 2007) as well as consciously detected (either by external agents giving feedback or by one's monitoring processes). Even if consciously detected, the discrepancy can ultimately recede into the unconscious if responses are made at a later point in time, when one is not aware of its lingering accessibility. This occurs not only when a response is temporally distanced from discrepancy detection but also when the response bears no surface resemblance to the goal and does not seem relevant to it (e.g., Koole, Smeets, van Knippenberg, & Dijksterhuis, 1999; Gollwitzer, Wicklund, & Hilton, 1982; Monteith, Ashburn-Nardo, Voils, & Czopp, 2002; Moskowitz, 2002).

Chronic Goals

Bargh (1990) provided an extensive review of goals that, through consistent and habitual pursuit, acquire a chronic state of heightened accessibility that persists across a variety of contexts. These goals are associated with individuals' long-standing interests and are highly relevant to their most cherished values and motives (e.g., Moskowitz, 1993, 2002; Moskowitz et al., 1999).

Consciously Selected Goals That Explicitly Retain Accessibility

This category of goal priming occurs when one's goals attain heightened accessibility by being consciously selected, with conscious focus on the goal and its relevance to one's behavior both being maintained throughout goal pursuit.

Postulate 8: Goals Are Regulated by Compensatory Responses That Include Implicit Cognition

Wegner and Pennebaker (1993) provide a framework in which *control of mind* is combined under the same umbrella as *control of behavior.* Just as a goal discrepancy triggers tension and goal-relevant behavioral responses, so too does it trigger goal-relevant mental operations. Cognition initiated in self-regulation, whether in the form of reactive or proactive control, is compensatory in that it exists to counteract the tension arising from a discrepancy between a current and a desired state. Automating such responses facilitates goal attainment by providing greater efficiency for initiation and regulation of a goal pursuit. It allows for (1) heightened readiness to attend to, detect, and respond to stimuli; (2) the retrieval and inhibition of semantic knowledge; and (3) activation of compatible and inhibition of incompatible goals (a horizontal communication among goals called *goal shielding*; Shah, Friedman, & Kruglanski, 2002).

Three examples illustrate the compensatory nature of even extremely low-level cognitive functioning. First, Van Bavel, Packer, and Cunningham (2011) examined a variant of "own-race bias." Rather than study preferential recall for members of one's *racial* group, they examined biased processing of people with whom one shared a *randomly* assigned group membership. They proposed that motivation to process members of one's own (nonracial) group preferentially would be reflected by implicit modulation at even low-level stages of face processing. Since facial recognition processes originate within 100–200 milliseconds of stimulus onset in an area of the fusiform gyrus called the fusiform face area (FFA), they used functional magnetic resonance imaging (fMRI) to assess how FFA activity was impacted by faces made motivationally relevant through participants' assignment to a randomly determined ingroup. The results showed greater FFA activity for these goal-relevant faces. The goal of preferential processing of ingroup members triggered compensatory control processes of face perception in the FFA.

Examples of *goal shielding* provide a second illustration of the implicit nature of compensatory cognition. Shah (2003) primed two goals: a consciously set analytic reasoning goal and an unconsciously primed creativity goal (via subliminal presentation of a picture of a significant other who valued the participant's creativity). For some participants, the conscious and unconscious goals were compatible; for others, the goals were irrelevant to each other. After being primed, participants performed a reasoning task. Goal shielding is observed in the form of response facilitation when the two goals are compatible. Priming with a compatible goal (creativity) initiated implicit operations that pulled the participant's attention toward and promoted reasoning goals. Aarts et al. (2007) illustrated goal shielding among incompatible goals in which we see inhibition rather than facilitation. Inhibitory processes ward off distractions and keep progress to a focal goal on track. Finally, goal shielding has also been shown to be a compensatory process when the obstacles to a goal serve to trigger heightened commitment to and accessibility of that goal. For example, Fishbach, Friedman, and Kruglanski (2003) had participants perform a task that exposed them to words related to a temptation (e.g., cake) to one of their goals (e.g., diet). This was followed by a task that assessed the ease of thinking about the goal compared to control items. After the temptation, thoughts of the goal were more prevalent. Temptation triggers a functional response when encountered: Relevant goals and means are brought to mind to counteract the temptation, what Fishbach et al. called *counteractive control.* This allows a temptation, ironically, to serve as a cue to avoid distractions and obstacles, and enhances staying on track in goal pursuit.

Finally, the direction of attention to goal-relevant stimuli illustrates yet a third implicit compensatory cognitive operation. Moskowitz (2002) gave participants the explicit goal of identifying the direction (up or down) in which a target item moved, while ignoring a distracting second target that moved in a different direction (left to right). Half of the participants also held an implicit egalitarian goal. Importantly, the targets in this task were actually words that moved too quickly to be identified as such, words that sometimes were relevant to egalitarian goals. The results showed that attention was distracted toward targets that were to be ignored, but only if one had an egalitarian goal, and only if the target was a goal-relevant word. Moskowitz et al. (2011) conceptually replicated this point using people as the goal-relevant targets. Participants were shown an array of four images of men and asked to identify (via a button press) which of them was wearing a bow tie. The correct response was always a white man in a bow tie, yet the array at times contained an image of a black man as one of the three nonfocal items. Participants once again showed displaced attention at speeds too fast for conscious control, but only if two conditions were met: (1) The array had to contain a black man's face, and (2) the participant had to have been primed previously with a goal of being egalitarian to black men.

Postulate 9: Goal Attainment Reduces Goal Accessibility

Once a goal is attained, the means and incentives that serve that goal are divested of their motivational force. This does not mean that the end state no longer has value. It merely means that striving to attain that state, enacting means to approach the value linked to the state, is not of use at that time and in that context. A goal requires both a discrepancy between a current state and an end state, and value being attached to that end state. If one values a state but there is no discrepancy between one's current state and that desired state, one does not have a goal. This is why one will *persist* at responding *until* a discrepancy is reduced and tension is alleviated (see Martin & Tesser, 2009). Evidence for this "persistence until" logic is provided by showing that so long as a discrepancy exists, one displays classic characteristics of motivated behavior, such as persistence in the face of obstacles and resumption of a disrupted task. But these characteristics are not seen when feedback signaling significant progress toward the goal is provided by the system's monitoring processes (e.g., Cesario, Plaks, & Higgins, 2006; Förster, Liberman, & Higgins, 2005; Koole et al., 1999; Liberman & Förster, 2000).

For example, Moskowitz et al. (2011, discussed earlier) found that the attention of white participants who held egalitarian goals was distracted to faces of black men. However, they also found that this act of compensatory cognition only persisted as long as the goal was not yet attained. When people who held egalitarian goals next wrote essays about success at being egalitarian, their attention was no longer diverted from the focal task. The essay afforded them a chance to compensate for their failure at being egalitarian, thus bringing implicit compensatory control (selective attention) to a halt. Moskowitz and Li (2011) also illustrated this principle, but using stereotype inhibition as the compensatory response that is halted.

Postulate 10: Goals Are Nested Within Goal Systems That Allow for Rotation among Goals

Kruglanski et al. (2002) described goals as embedded in a system of many horizontally linked goals that impact one another, with systemwide coordination among compatible and opposing forces. Goal systems therefore raise issues of how to determine what goal to select in any moment, and which, from among many possible means, to select to pursue that goal. Goals linked in a system can promote one another, and movement toward one can facilitate standing on another, but they can compete as well, and movement toward one goal may require inhibiting another. Which goal is selected in a given moment, when people rotate from one goal to another, and when one disengages from a goal comprises a complex set of issues that is beyond the scope of a complete review here. However, factors that are important to these issues are strength of commitment to the goal, opportunities that afford one a means to attain the goal, and the instrumental value those means possess. These can vary from moment to moment.

For example the value of the goal is impacted by one's history of goal pursuit within the context. Baumeister, Vohs, and Tice (2007) argued that successful goal regulation has a positively reinforcing impact on the value associated with the goal, increasing its desirability and strengthening its affective component, increasing the likelihood that the goal will again be set as the desired criterion. Commitment to a goal is impacted by a variety of factors, one of which is the number of equifinal means associated with the goal. Kruglanski et al. (2011) showed that while having many means linked to a goal decreases the commitment to any given means, it increases commitment to the goal (impacting subjective probability, the expectancy, that the goal can be achieved). Brehm and Self (1989) describe commitment as being determined by factors such as the strength of the need that yielded the goal and the incentive value of the task.

Finally, because goals are hierarchically linked to superordinate goals, motives, and needs, it is possible that pursuit of one goal within the system can contradict or conflict with a superordinate goal. The goal of feeling comforted may lead one to eat a cupcake despite this conflicting with a long term and superordinate goal of being healthy and eating well. As opportunities afford one chances to pursue a goal, and as the value of a goal waxes and wanes, we may see behavior that appears inconsistent. But apparent inconsistency may merely reflect rotation among goals as contexts and opportunities dictate.

Postulate 11: Goal Pursuit Is Limited by Resources

Goals are in competition for shared but limited resources (e.g., Vohs, Kaikati, Kerkhof, & Schmeichel, 2009). Any goal pursuit depletes this resource to a degree and can result in the resource pool being usurped. This results in a state called *ego depletion,* marked by a temporary loss of self-control. Ego depletion is not limited to the domain responsible for depletion; it represents general loss of ability to engage in executive functioning (e.g., Richeson & Trawalter, 2005; Schmeichel & Baumeister, 2004) and control (e.g., Vohs, Baumeister, & Ciarocco, 2005). Because ego depletion is a temporary state, regulatory ability returns after rest or other interventions. These resources can be bolstered with training. Gailliot, Plant, Butz, and Baumeister (2007) showed that practice at regulation makes one resistant to ego depletion. The biological basis for depletion and replenishing of the resource pool is not yet well understood (e.g., Molden et al., 2012).

Postulate 12: Implicit Control Involves Both Facilitation and Inhibition

The IVM incorporates the logic of goal shielding—that pursuit of a goal involves processes that not only facilitate attainment of a desired end, but also inhibit goals, temptations, and means that would serve as obstacles to attainment of that end. This makes possible an assortment of control strategies that previously had not been deemed possible according to dual-process theories. In a view of control that is largely conscious and reactive, the role of control is to overcome or counteract the effects of an implicit cognitive process that has been brought to one's awareness as a potential source of bias. The conscious efforts at correction that ensue represent an important method to regulate behavior and cognition. But this approach blinds us to seeing goals as more than mere conscious tools to deploy after we become aware of a problem to be counteracted. Control, if *proactive,* can prevent an unwanted (biasing) response from ever being produced. Implicit forms of proactive control initiate not only goal-relevant processing that circumvents the triggering of the unwanted response but also cognitive activity that inhibits undesired outputs. Concrete examples of such processes are seen in research on stereotype control.

In my own laboratory (e.g., Galinsky & Moskowitz, 2000, 2007; Moskowitz et al., 1999, 2011; Moskowitz, Salomon, & Taylor, 2000; Moskowitz & Li, 2011; Moskowitz & Stone, 2012; Sassenberg & Moskowitz, 2005), we have found behavioral evidence for the interplay of facilitative and inhibitory processes in proactive stereotype control, both with chronic goals and goals primed in the situation. While it is well established that stereotypes are associated with groups, and that thinking about the group often activates such stereotypes outside awareness (e.g., Devine, 1989), this is not an obstacle to proactive control. Indeed, it is argued that such efficient and effortless activation of stereotypes is itself a form of proactive control. Some goals, such as "sense making," are compatible with stereotype activation—the stereotyping is in the service of the goal. Thus, the prevalence of implicit stereotype activation is seen here as a reflection of the prevalence of goals that recruit stereotypes as part of goal operations. However, because stereotype *activation* is controlled by the self-regulatory system—it is a cognitive tool recruited for a reason—it is argued that one has the power quickly and efficiently *not to activate stereotypes* by exercising the same control system. Encountering a member of a stereotyped group who is relevant to one's goal will not lead to stereotype activation if that goal is incompatible with stereotyping. Rather, it will lead to heightened goal activation, to facilitated processing of goal relevant stimuli (such as tuning attention to goal-relevant stimuli; Moskowitz, 2002; Moskowitz et al., 2011; Trawalter et al., 2008); and to goal-shielding processes of stereotype inhibition. For example, an egalitarian goal is incompatible with stereotyping. Just as other goals recruit stereotypes as part of their operations of goal pursuit, egalitarian goals recruit compensatory cognitive operations that inhibit stereotypes due to their incompatibility with the goal.

Implicit but motivated *inhibition* of stereotypes when one is exposed to a stereotyped group was first illustrated by Moskowitz et al. (1999). Men with (and without) chronic egalitarian goals were recruited for an experiment. They were primed with faces (Experiment 3) and names (Experiment 4) of men and women, then asked to respond to words either related to the female stereotype or not. Participants without chronic egalitarian goals had stereotypes activated (facilitated responding to stereotypical words following female faces). But men with chronic egalitarian goals instead inhibited stereotypes of women (slower reaction times to stereotypical words following female faces). Moskowitz and Li (2011) extended this finding of implicit inhibition by shifting the stereotyped group to black men, and shifting the source of the goal from being chronically held to being manipulated. White subjects *without* a chronic egalitarian goal were brought to the laboratory. Half were primed with a goal to be egalitarian to black men. The results revealed a similar pattern of stereotype inhibition, this time for people with temporarily induced egalitarian goals—seeing a black man slowed responses to stereotype-relevant words (but not to control words). But stereotype activation occurred among people without primed egalitarian goals.

Such lack of stereotype activation is not merely a failure at control (e.g., poor regulation of a goal to stereotype), or an indication of nothing happening when a target is encountered. It is a goal-directed set of processes, including inhibition, being initiated that service the goal of being egalitarian. This is illustrated in several experiments in a variety of ways. First, using the "persistence until" logic reviewed earlier, stereotype inhibition ceases to occur if participants are given the opportunity to write an essay affirming their egalitarian goal prior to the reaction time task (e.g., Moskowitz & Li, 2011; Moskowitz & Stone, 2012). This indicates a motivated process being shut down rather than the lack of processing, or failure at an alternative goal pursuit. Moskowitz et al. (2000, see also Moskowitz & Stone, 2012) further showed that encountering goal-relevant people not only leads to inhibitory processes but also facilitates processing of goal-compatible stimuli and leads to heightened accessibility of the goal itself.

There is now evidence for proactive control of stereotypes across many laboratories. Mendoza, Gollwitzer, and Amodio (2010) had participants form implementation intentions not to stereotype. They found that implicitly triggering these plans later using environmental cues led to control over stereotype activation (as well as improved conscious control). Similarly, Devine, Plant, Amodio, Harmon-Jones, and Vance (2002) showed that people motivated to control prejudice for internal reasons do not respond as quickly as other individuals to negative words after being primed with black faces.

Cunningham, Van Bavel, Arbuckle, Packer, and Waggoner (2012) argue that even rapid responses to the race of a face are controlled by goals, such that race may be deemed irrelevant for processing. Instead, low-level processing is directed by the goals currently triggered, and this can include proactively avoiding race for a more instrumental response. Cunningham et al. used electroencephalography (EEG) to examine control over processes in the first 100 milliseconds of face perception that lead to racial biases in social categorization. They noted that "although the relationship between specific brain regions and ERP [event-related potential] waves is not perfectly precise, very early ERP waves, such as the P100 and N170 appear to subserve early face processing" (p. 2). They examined whether approach goals attenuate biased processing of black faces by collecting EEG data as participants performed a task that presented them with faces of white and black men. Consistent with prior evidence of racial bias, they found that white faces were associated with a larger P100 than black faces. But they also found proactive control, in that this effect interacted with goals. An approach goal altered the influence of race during the first 100 milliseconds of perceptual processing.

Amodio and Devine (2010) reviewed further neuroscience evidence to support proactive control. They posited that the anterior cingulate cortex (ACC) brain region monitors for conflicts between intended and automatic responses, thus representing a low-level, if not initial, step in control. Conflict is low when black targets are paired with stereotypical items; thus, ACC activity should be low. However, pairing black targets with nonstereotypical target items should lead to high ACC activity, indicating that control mechanisms are being recruited early, without conscious deliberation or awareness.

Postulate 13: Implicit Processes of Goal Pursuit Need Not Be the Same as Conscious Goal Pursuit

Implicit control in stereotyping revealed success at inhibiting "automatic" processes. Contrast this with findings from research on stereotype suppression (e.g., Wegner, 1994) and avoiding race bias (e.g., Payne, Lambert, & Jacoby, 2002), in which explicit goal pursuit led to control failures. Payne et al. demonstrated that explicit control is limited by resource demands, whereas Wegner (1994) found a more debilitating effect—ironically, stereotype activation increases with the explicit goal of suppressing stereotypes. A similar contrast emerges from work on creativity. Asking people to adopt a goal of having a creative solution to a problem leads to strikingly uncreative responses tethered to old examples that resemble plagiarism more than novelty. Priming creativity outside of consciousness produces the desired increase in creativity (e.g., Sassenberg & Moskowitz, 2005). Examining decision making, Dijksterhuis et al. (2006) revealed that providing ample time for conscious responding reduces the quality of the decisions reached relative to pursuing the goal of making an accurate decision when limited to implicit processing (under load).

However, some examinations have illustrated that implicit and explicit goal pursuit yield similar results following similar processes. Chartrand and Bargh (1996) found that an unconsciously primed goal to form an impression followed the same processing stages as when one consciously adopts the goal of impression formation. And Pessiglione et al. (2007) found that on a hand-grip task in which promise of a reward (money to be won on a given trial) was presented subliminally, the increase in effort was the same as when promise of reward was presented consciously, and the same region of brain activity moderated effort on the task.

Given that they share the same mechanisms of control (operations, monitoring, feedback, tension reduction, etc.), and many illustrations demonstrating that unconscious and conscious control follow identical processing steps, why do some studies demonstrate an apparent inconsistency—conscious goal pursuit fails, whereas implicit goal pursuit succeeds? In some cases, conscious processing can alter the meaning of the goal, because deliberation can recruit interpretive biases that yield changes to how the goal is framed or understood. The meaning of the goal "be a good student" can change when defined in terms of a standard set by one's beliefs about personal ability versus a standard set by what one ought to be to bring pride to others. Furthermore, conscious goals invoke *metacognition*—thoughts about the goal pursuit. This is especially likely when, for example, with the weapons task and stereotype suppression, the task itself invokes theories about how one is biased (that may or not be accurate) and what one needs to do to prevent/overturn bias (if it is perceived to have occurred). When a person is made aware of bias, the control process is not merely derailed by what may be incorrect theories of how control ought to be executed, but by processing limitations and restrictions in cognitive capacity. Even with an accurate theory, conscious execution of the steps may be rendered incomplete or inexact if one lacks ability to perform the work required, such as when resources for control are limited or responding is at a fast pace. Implicit control circumvents these pitfalls to control. Consciousness may at times be an obstacle to a goal better pursued implicitly; it can lead one astray by focusing one's attention on irrelevant information or causing one to rationalize an inappropriate response.

CONCLUSION

Dual-process models too often limit control to that which is conscious and effortful. Despite the counterintuitive feel of it, control can be, and often is, implicit. And unlike conceptions of the role of the unconscious in responding that have highlighted it as a source of error and bias (e.g., heuristic use in decision making), unconscious goals are an efficient and functional source for much human responding, perhaps guiding all cognition. It is just as likely that consciousness in control can introduce as much error and bias as can lack of consciousness. This suggests that consciousness is not a distinguishing factor in control: All cognition is controlled, often implicitly, and conscious control can have the same operations and outcomes as unconscious control. Conscious control need not mean a qualitatively different type of processing than implicit control. Nor need it suggest primacy of one form of control over the other. As Sherman (2006) stated: "Rather than treating automatic and controlled processes as separate categories of processes it would be more useful to treat automaticity and control as features of processes" (p. 181).

Implicit control suggests that the associations activated and inhibited when encountering a stimulus of any type are not independent of ones goals. One can respond to the same target in many ways as a function of the context, the opportunities for action within that context, and the goals of the individual relating to that target at that time in that context. For example, if one has the goal of cooperating with others, it may be that in a given context, the opportunity to pursue that goal is best afforded by a preference for people who share one's racial identity, which could promote stereotyping of outgroups. However, it may be that shared racial identity does not afford one the best opportunity to achieve the goal, and categorizing based on race would not occur and stereotypes would not be triggered. Alternatively, one could have a goal that does promote categorizing people into racial groups but discourages stereotype activation as the dominant association to the group (as illustrated by Moskowitz et al., 2011).

Stereotyping, like many unwanted responses, can be controlled not merely by reactively changing how we respond when our implicit goals encourage stereotyping. It can be controlled by changing one's goal and proactively initiating processes that never yield stereotype activation. Augmenting the well-elaborated power of conscious control is what many goal researchers now believe to be the more omnipresent form of control—unconscious goals that implicitly direct social cognition.

NOTES

1. Tolman (1932, p. 134) warned, regarding goal pursuits in animals, that "the reader will perhaps need constantly to remind himself that the use of the terms perception, mnemonization and memory implies nothing as to consciousness." It can be argued that the notion of unconscious goals and operations of goal pursuit got lost in the cognitive revolution when models of goal pursuit shifted from animal to human participants, with consciousness as the distinguishing factor elevating human above animal goal pursuits. With that shift came fervor for examining rationality and conscious choice as central to control.
2. Other sources of goals are theories (theories about the nature of ability; e.g., Grant & Dweck, 2003) and fantasies about future hopes (especially by contrasting those fantasies against a standard set by negative aspects of current reality; e.g., Oettingen, 2000).

3. Since conscious control is possible only after 600 milliseconds elapse once one encounters a stimulus (e.g., Fazio, 1990), responses made within this period occur without the benefit of conscious control. Thus, flashing a cue that triggers a goal can indicate an implicit goal if the cue and the goal-directed response occur within this period prior to consciousness.
4. However, there are also unique features of goal priming that make it distinct from other types of accessibility. First, accessibility strength and its impact on responding depend on the motivational value of a goal and instrumentality of opportunities in the environment (e.g., Eitam & Higgins, 2010). Second, with semantic knowledge, the accessibility strength decreases as time passes from the time of construct activation. The passage of time impacts goal accessibility differently. Goal representations contain a discrepancy, the state of which is being monitored and fed back through the system. Such operations keep the goal construct reactivated as time passes and increase accessibility strength, so that its ability to impact subsequent responding increases as time passes; the goal looms larger (e.g., Bargh et al., 2001; Curtis & D'Esposito, 2003; Förster, Liberman, & Friedman, 2007; Liberman & Förster, 2000).

REFERENCES

Aarts, H., Custers, R., & Holland, R. W. (2007). The nonconscious cessation of goal pursuit: When goals and negative affect are coactivated. *Journal of Personality and Social Psychology, 92*, 165–178.

Aarts, H., & Dijksterhuis, A. (2000). Habits as knowledge structures: Automaticity in goal-directed behavior. *Journal of Personality and Social Psychology, 78*(1), 53–63.

Aarts, H., & Dijksterhuis, A. (2003). The silence of the library: Environment, situational norm, and social behavior. *Journal of Personality and Social Psychology, 84*, 18–28.

Aarts, H., Gollwitzer, P. M., & Hassin, R. R. (2004). Goal contagion: Perceiving is for pursuing. *Journal of Personality and Social Psychology, 87*(1), 23–37.

Amodio, D. M., & Devine, P. G. (2010). Regulating behavior in the social world: Control in the context of intergroup bias. In R. R. Hassin, K. N. Ochsner, & Y. Trope (Eds.), *Self control in society, mind and brain* (pp. 49–75). New York: Oxford University Press.

Atkinson, J. W. (1964). *An introduction to motivation.* Princeton, NJ: Van Nostrand.

Balcetis, E., & Dunning, D. (2006). See what you want to see: Motivational influences on perception. *Journal of Personality and Social Psychology, 91*, 612–625.

Balcetis, E., Dunning, D., & Granot, Y. (2012). Subjective value determines initial dominance in binocular rivalry. *Journal of Experimental Social Psychology, 48*, 122–129.

Bandura, A. (1989). Perceived self-efficacy in the exercise of personal agency. *The Psychologist: Bulletin of the British Psychological Society, 2*, 411–424.

Bargh, J. A. (1989). Conditional automaticity: Varieties of automatic influence in social perception and cognition. In J. S. Uleman, & J. A. Bargh (Eds.), *Unintended thought* (pp. 3–51). New York: Guilford Press.

Bargh, J. A. (1990). Auto-motives: Preconscious determinants of social interaction. In E. T. Higgins & R. M. Sorrentino (Eds.), *Handbook of motivation and cognition: Foundations of social behavior* (Vol. 2, pp. 93–130). New York: Guilford Press.

Bargh, J. A., Gollwitzer, P. M., Lee-Chai, A., Barndollar, K., & Trötschel, R. (2001). The automated will: Nonconscious activation and pursuit of behavioral goals. *Journal of Personality and Social Psychology, 81*, 1014–1027.

Bargh, J. A., & Huang, J. Y. (2009). The selfish goal. In G. B. Moskowitz & H. Grant (Eds.), *The psychology of goals* (pp. 127–150). New York: Guilford Press.

Baumeister, R. F., Vohs, K. D., & Tice, D. M. (2007). The strength model of self-control. *Current Directions in Psychological Science, 16*(6), 351–355.

Brehm, J. W., & Self, E. A. (1989). The intensity of motivation. *Annual Review of Psychology, 40*, 109–131.

Bruner, J. S., & Goodman, C. D. (1947). Value and need as organizing factors in perception. *Journal of Abnormal Social Psychology, 42*, 33–44.

Cacioppo, J. T., Priester, J. R., & Berntson, G. G. (1993). Rudimentary determinants of attitudes: II. Arm flexion and extension have different effects on attitudes. *Journal of Personality and Social Psychology, 65*, 5–17.

Calanchini, J., & Sherman, J. W. (2013). Implicit

attitudes reflect associative, non-associative, and non-attitudinal processes. *Social and Personality Psychology Compass, 7*(9), 654–667.

Carver, C. S., & Scheier, M. F. (1981). *Attention and self-regulation: A control theory approach to human behavior.* New York: Springer.

Carver, C. S., & Scheier, M. F. (1998). *On the self-regulation of behavior.* New York: Cambridge University Press.

Cesario, J., Plaks, J. E., & Higgins, E. T. (2006). Automatic social behavior as motivated preparation to interact. *Journal of Personality and Social Psychology, 90,* 893–910.

Chaiken, S., Liberman, A., & Eagly, A. H. (1989). Heuristic and systematic information processing within and beyond the persuasion context. In J. S. Uleman & J. A. Bargh (Eds.), *Unintended thought* (pp. 212–252). New York: Guilford Press.

Chartrand, T. L., & Bargh, J. A. (1996). Automatic activation of impression formation and memorization goals: Nonconscious goal priming reproduces effects of explicit task instructions. *Journal of Personality and Social Psychology, 71*(3), 464–478.

Chen, M., & Bargh, J. A. (1999). Consequences of automatic evaluation: Immediate behavioral predispositions to approach or avoid the stimulus. *Personality and Social Psychology Bulletin, 25,* 215–224.

Chun, W. Y., Kruglanski, A. W., Friedman, R., & Sleeth-Keppler, D. (2011). Multifinality in unconscious choice. *Journal of Personality and Social Psychology, 101,* 1124–1137.

Cunningham, W. A., Van Bavel, J. J., Arbuckle, N. L., Packer, D. J., & Waggoner, A. S. (2012). Rapid social perception is flexible: Approach and avoidance motivational states shape P100 responses to other-race faces. *Frontiers in Human Neuroscience, 6,* 1–7.

Curtis, C. E., & D'Esposito, M. (2003). Persistent activity in the prefrontal cortex during working memory. *Trends in Cognitive Science, 7*(9), 415–423.

Custers, R. (2009). The role of affect in goal representations. In G. B. Moskowitz, & H. Grant (Eds.), *The psychology of goals* (pp. 179–202). New York: Guilford Press.

Custers, R., & Aarts, H. (2005). Positive affect as implicit motivator: On the nonconscious operation of behavioral goals. *Journal of Personality and Social Psychology, 89,* 129–142.

Custers, R., & Aarts, H. (2007). Goal-discrepant situations prime goal-directed actions if goals are temporarily or chronically accessible. *Personality and Social Psychology Bulletin, 33,* 623–633.

Custers, R., & Aarts, H. (2010). The unconscious will: How the pursuit of goals operates outside of conscious awareness. *Science, 329,* 47–50.

Dasgupta, N., & Greenwald, A. G. (2001). On the malleability of automatic attitudes: Combating automatic prejudice with images of admired and disliked individuals. *Journal of Personality and Social Psychology, 81,* 800–814.

Deci, E. L., & Ryan, R. M. (1991). A motivational approach to self. In R. Dienstbier (Ed.), *Nebraska Symposium on Motivation* (Vol. 38, pp. 237–288). Lincoln: University of Nebraska Press.

Devine, P. G. (1989). Stereotypes and prejudice: Their automatic and controlled components. *Journal of Personality and Social Psychology, 56,* 5–18.

Devine, P. G., Forscher, P. S., Austin, A. J., & Cox, W. T. L. (2012). Long-term reduction in implicit race bias: A prejudice habit-breaking intervention. *Journal of Experimental Social Psychology, 48,* 1267–1278

Devine, P. G., Plant, E. A., Amodio, D. M., Harmon-Jones, E., & Vance, S. L. (2002). The regulations of explicit and implicit race bias: The role of motivations to respond without prejudice. *Journal of Personality and Social Psychology, 82*(5), 835–848.

Dijksterhuis, A., Bos, M., Nordgren, L., & Van Baaren, R. B. (2006). On making the right choice: The deliberation-without-attention effect. *Science, 311,* 1005–1007.

Eder, A., & Rothermund, K. (2008). When do motor behaviors (mis)match affective stimuli?: An evaluative coding view of approach avoidance reactions. *Journal of Experimental Psychology: General, 137,* 262–281.

Eitam, B., & Higgins, E. T. (2010). Motivation in mental accessibility: Relevance of a representation (ROAR) as a new framework. *Social and Personality Psychology Compass, 3,* 1–17.

Elliot, A. J., & Niesta, D. (2009). Goals in the context of the hierarchical model of approach–avoidance motivation. In G. B. Moskowitz & H. Grant (Eds.), *The psychology of goals* (pp. 56–76). New York: Guilford Press.

Fazio, R. H. (1990). A practical guide of the use of response latency in social psychological review. In C. Hendrick & M. S. Clark (Eds.), *Research methods in personality and social psychology* (pp. 74–97). Newbury Park, CA: Sage.

Ferguson, M. J. (2007). On the automatic evaluation of end-states. *Journal of Personality and Social Psychology, 92*, 596–611.

Ferguson, M. J., & Bargh, J. A. (2004). Liking is for doing: The effects of goal pursuit on automatic evaluations. *Journal of Personality and Social Psychology, 87*(5), 557–572.

Fishbach, A., Friedman, R., & Kruglanski, A. W. (2003). Leading us not into temptation: Momentary allurements elicit overriding goal activation. *Journal of Personality and Social Psychology, 84*(2), 296–309.

Fishbach, A., Shah, J. Y., & Kruglanski, A. W. (2004). Emotional transfer in goal systems. *Journal of Experimental Social Psychology, 40*(6), 723–738.

Fiske, S. T., & Neuberg, S. L. (1990). A continuum of impression formation, from category-based to individuating processes: Influences of information and motivation on attention and interpretation. In M. P. Zanna (Ed.), *Advances in experimental social psychology* (Vol. 23, pp. 1–74). New York: Academic Press.

Fitzsimons, G. M., & Bargh, J. A. (2003). Thinking of you: Nonconscious pursuit of interpersonal goals associated with relationship partners. *Journal of Personality and Social Psychology, 84*(1), 148–163.

Förster, J., Liberman, N., & Friedman, R. S. (2007). Seven principles of goal activation: A systematic approach to distinguishing goal priming from priming of non-goal constructs. *Personality and Social Psychology Review, 11*, 211–233.

Förster, J., Liberman, N., & Higgins, E. T. (2005). Accessibility from active and fulfilled goals. *Journal of Experimental Social Psychology, 41*(3), 220–239.

Freeman, J. B., Dale, R., & Farmer, T. A. (2011). Hand in motion reveals mind in motion. *Frontiers in Psychology, 2*, 59.

Friedman, R. S., & Förster, J. (2002). The influence of approach and avoidance motor actions on creative cognition. *Journal of Experimental Social Psychology, 38*, 41–55.

Gailliot, M. T., Plant, E. A., Butz, D. A., & Baumeister, R. F. (2007). Increasing self-regulatory strength can reduce the depleting effect of suppressing stereotypes. *Personality and Social Psychology Bulletin, 33*, 281–294.

Galinsky, A. D., & Moskowitz, G. B. (2000). Perspective taking: Decreasing stereotype expression, accessibility, and in-group favoritism. *Journal of Personality and Social Psychology, 78*, 708–724.

Galinsky, A. D., & Moskowitz, G. B. (2007). Further ironies of suppression: Stereotype *and* counter-stereotype accessibility. *Journal of Experimental Social Psychology, 42*, 833–841.

Gilbert, D. T. 1989. Thinking lightly about others: Automatic components of the social inference process. In J. S. Uleman & J. A. Bargh (Eds.), *Unintended thought* (pp. 189–211). New York: Guilford Press.

Glaser, J., & Knowles, E. D. (2008). Implicit motivation to control prejudice. *Journal of Experimental Social Psychology, 44*, 164–172.

Gollwitzer, P. M. (1990). Action phases and mind-sets. In E. T. Higgins & R. M. Sorrentino (Eds.), *Handbook of motivation and cognition* (Vol. 2, pp. 53–92). New York: Guilford Press.

Gollwitzer, P. M. (1993). Goal achievement: The role of intentions. In W. Stroebe & M. Hewstone (Eds.), *European review of social psychology* (Vol. 4, pp. 141–185). Chichester, UK: Wiley.

Gollwitzer, P. M., & Moskowitz, G. B. (1996). Goal effects on action and cognition. In E. T. Higgins & A. Kruglanski (Eds.), *Social psychology: Handbook of basic principles* (pp. 361–399). New York: Guilford Press.

Gollwitzer, P. M., Wicklund, R. A., & Hilton, J. L. (1982). Admission of failure and symbolic self-completion: Extending Lewinian theory. *Journal of Personality and Social Psychology, 43*, 358–371.

Grant, H., & Dweck, C. S. (2003). Clarifying achievement goals and their impact. *Journal of Personality and Social Psychology, 85*, 541–553.

Higgins, E. T. (2009). Regulatory fit in the goal-pursuit process. In G. B. Moskowitz & H. Grant (Eds.), *The psychology of goals* (pp. 505–534). New York: Guilford Press.

Huang, J. Y., & Bargh, J. A. (in press). The selfish goal: Autonomously operating motivational structures as the proximal cause of human judgment and behavior. [Target Article] *Behavioral and Brain Sciences*.

Jostmann, N. B., & Koole, S. L. (2009). When persistence is futile: A functional analysis of action orientation and goal disengagement. In G. B. Moskowitz & H. Grant (Eds.), *The psychology of goals*. (pp. 337–361). New York: The Guilford Press.

Kay, A. C., Wheeler, C. S., Bargh, J. A., & Ross, L. D. (2004). Material priming: The influence of mundane physical objects on situational construal and competitive behavioral choice. *Organizational Behavior and Human Decision Processes, 95,* 83–96.

Koole, S. L., Smeets, K., van Knippenberg, A., & Dijksterhuis, A. (1999). The cessation of rumination through self-affirmation. *Journal of Personality and Social Psychology, 77,* 111–125.

Kruglanski, A. W. (1990). Motivations for judging and knowing: Implications for causal attribution. In E. T. Higgins & R. M. Sorrentino (Eds.), *Handbook of motivation and cognition* (Vol. 2, pp. 333–368). New York: Guilford Press.

Kruglanski, A. W. (1996). Goals as knowledge structures. In P. M. Gollwitzer & J. A. Bargh (Eds.), *The psychology of action* (pp. 599–618). New York: Guilford Press.

Kruglanski, A. W., Kopetz, C., Belanger, J. J., Chun, W. Y., Orehek, E., & Fishbach, A. (2013). Features of multifinality. *Personality and Social Psychology Review, 17,* 22–39.

Kruglanski, A. W., Pierro, A., & Sheveland, A. (2011). How many roads lead to Rome?: Equifinality set-size and commitment to goals and means. *European Journal of Social Psychology, 41,* 344–352.

Kruglanski, A. W., Shah, J., Fishbach, A., Friedman, R., Chun, W., Sleeth-Keppler, D., et al. (2002). A theory of goal systems. In M. P. Zanna (Ed.), *Advances in experimental social psychology* (Vol. 34, pp. 331–378). New York: Academic Press.

Lewin, K. (1936). *Principles of topological psychology.* New York: McGraw-Hill.

Lewin, K. (1951). *Field theory in social science: Selected theoretical papers.* New York: Harper & Row.

Liberman, N., & Dar, R. (2009). Normal and pathological consequences of encountering difficulties in monitoring progress toward goals. In G. B. Moskowitz & H. Grant (Eds.), *The psychology of goals* (pp. 277–303). New York: Guilford Press.

Liberman, N., & Förster, J. (2000). Expression after suppression: A motivational explanation of postsuppressional rebound. *Journal of Personality and Social Psychology, 79,* 190–203.

Macrae, C. N., Bodenhausen, G. V., Milne, A. B., & Jetten, J. (1994). Out of mind but back in sight: Stereotypes on the rebound. *Journal of Personality and Social Psychology, 67,* 808–817.

Martin, L. L., & Tesser, A. (2009). Five markers of motivated behavior. In G. B. Moskowitz and H. Grant (Eds.), *The psychology of goals* (pp. 257–276). New York: Guilford Press.

McClelland, D. C. (1985). *Human motivation.* Glenview, IL: Scott, Foresman.

Mendoza, S. A., Gollwitzer, P. M., & Amodio, D. M. (2010). Reducing the expression of implicit stereotypes: Reflexive control through implementation intentions. *Personality and Social Psychology Bulletin, 36,* 512–523.

Miller, G. A., Galanter, E., & Pribram, K. H. (1960). *Plans and the structure of behavior.* New York: Holt, Rinehart & Winston.

Molden, D. C., Hui, C. M., Scholer, A. A., Meier, B. P. Noreen, E. E., D'Agostino, P. R., & Martin, V. (2012). Motivational versus metabolic effects of carbohydrates on self-control. *Psychological Science, 23*(10), 1137–1144.

Monteith, M. J., Ashburn-Nardo, L., Voils, C. I., & Czopp, A. M. (2002). Putting the brakes on prejudice: On the development and operation of cues for control. *Journal of Personality and Social Psychology, 83,* 1029–1050.

Moskowitz, G. B. (1993). Individual differences in social categorization: The effects of personal need for structure on spontaneous trait inferences. *Journal of Personality and Social Psychology,* 65, 132–142.

Moskowitz, G. B. (2002). Preconscious effects of temporary goals on attention. *Journal of Experimental Social Psychology, 38,* 397–404.

Moskowitz, G. B., Gollwitzer, P. M., Wasel, W., & Schaal, B. (1999). Preconscious control of stereotype activation through chronic egalitarian goals. *Journal of Personality and Social Psychology, 77,* 167–184.

Moskowitz, G. B., & Li, P. (2011). Egalitarian goals trigger stereotype inhibition: A proactive form of stereotype control. *Journal of Experimental Social Psychology, 47*(1), 103–116.

Moskowitz, G. B., Li, P., Ignarri, C., & Stone, J. (2011). Compensatory cognition associated with egalitarian goals. *Journal of Experimental Social Psychology, 47*(2), 365–370.

Moskowitz, G. B., Salomon, A. R., & Taylor, C. M. (2000). Preconsciously controlling stereotyping: Implicitly activated egalitarian goals prevent the activation of stereotypes. *Social Cognition, 18,* 151–177.

Moskowitz, G. B., & Stone, J. (2012). The proactive control of stereotype activation: Implicit goals to *not* stereotype. *Journal of Psychology, 220*(3), 172–179.

Oettingen, G. (2000). Expectancy effects on behavior depend on self-regulatory thought. *Social Cognition, 18*, 101–129.

Ostrom, T. (1984). The sovereignty of social cognition. In R. S. Wyer, & T. K. Srull (Eds.), *Handbook of social cognition* (Vol. 1, pp. 1–38). Hilsdale, NJ: Erlbaum.

Packer, D. J., Miners, C. T. H., Ungson, N., & Okten, I. O. (in preparation). *Opportunities to influence group decisions decrease conformity in an Asch-like paradigm.*

Parks-Stamm, E. J., & Gollwitzer, P. M. (2009). Goal implementation: The benefits and costs of IF–THEN planning. In G. B. Moskowitz & H. Grant (Eds.), *The psychology of goals* (pp. 362–391). New York: Guilford Press.

Payne, B. K. (2006). Weapon bias: Split second decision and unintended stereotyping. *Current Directions in Psychological Science, 15*(6), 287–291.

Payne, B. K., Lambert, A. J., & Jacoby, L. L. (2002). Best laid plans: Effects of goals on accessibility bias and cognitive control in race based misperceptions of weapons. *Journal of Experimental Social Psychology, 38*, 384–396.

Pessiglione, M., Schmidt, L., Draganski, B., Kalisch, R., Lau, H., Dolan, R., et al. (2007). How the brain translates money into force: A neuroimaging study of subliminal motivation. *Science, 316*, 904–906.

Postman, L., Bruner, J. S., & McGinnies, E. (1948). Personal factors as selective factors in perception. *Journal of Abnormal and Social Psychology*, 43, 142–154.

Powers, W. T. (1973). *Behavior: The control of perception.* Chicago: Aldine.

Richeson, J. A., & Shelton, J. N. (2007). Negotiating interracial interactions: Costs, consequences, and possibilities. *Current Directions in Psychological Science, 16*, 316–320.

Richeson, J. A., & Trawalter, S. (2005). Why do interracial interactions impair executive function?: A resource depletion account. *Journal of Personality and Social Psychology, 88*, 934–947.

Sassenberg, K., & Moskowitz, G. B. (2005). Do not stereotype, think different!: Overcoming automatic stereotype activation by mindset priming. *Journal of Experimental Social Psychology, 41*(5), 317–413.

Schmeichel, B. J., & Baumeister, R. F. (2004). Self-regulatory strength. In R. F. Baumeister & K. D. Vohs (Eds.), *Handbook of self-regulation: Research, theory, and applications* (pp. 84–98). New York: Guilford Press.

Shah, J. (2003). Automatic for the people: How representations of significant others implicitly affect goal pursuit. *Journal of Personality and Social Psychology, 84*(4), 661–681.

Shah, J. Y., Friedman, R., & Kruglanski, A. W. (2002). Forgetting all else: On the antecedents and consequences of goal shielding. *Journal of Personality and Social Psychology, 83*, 1261–1280.

Shah, J. Y., & Kruglanski, A. W. (2003) When opportunity knocks: Bottom-up priming of goals by means and its effects on self-regulation. *Journal of Personality and Social Psychology, 84*(6), 1109–1122.

Sherman, J. W. (2006). On building a better process model: It's not only how many, but which ones and by which means? *Psychological Inquiry, 17*(3), 173–184.

Strack, F., Schwarz, N., Bless, H., Kübler, A., & Wänke, M. (1993). Awareness of the influence as a determinant of assimilation versus contrast. *European Journal of Social Psychology, 23*, 53–62.

Thompson, E. P., Roman, R. J., Moskowitz, G. B., Chaiken, S., & Bargh, J. A. (1994). Accuracy motivation attenuates covert priming effects: The systematic reprocessing of social information. *Journal of Personality and Social Psychology*, 66, 259–288.

Tolman, E. C. (1932). *Purposive behavior in animals and men.* Oxford, UK: Appleton-Century.

Trawalter, S., Todd, A. R., Baird, A. A., & Richeson, J. A. (2008). Attending to threat: Race-based patterns of selective attention. *Journal of Experimental Social Psychology 44*, 1322–1327.

Uleman, J. S., & Moskowitz, G. B. (1994). Unintended effects of goals on unintended inferences. *Journal of Personality and Social Psychology, 66*, 490–501.

Van Bavel, J. J., Packer, D. J., & Cunningham, W. A. (2011). Modulation of the fusiform face area following minimal exposure to motivationally relevant faces: Evidence of in-group enhancement (not out-group disregard). *Journal of Cognitive Neuroscience, 23*, 3343–3354.

van der Weiden, A., Aarts, H., & Ruys, K.

(in press). Inferring oneself as the cause of intended and unintended outcomes. *Social and Personality Psychology Compass*.

Vohs, K. D., Baumeister, R. F., & Ciarocco, N. J. (2005). Self-regulation and self-presentation: regulatory resource depletion impairs impression management and effortful self-presentation. *Journal of Personality and Social Psychology, 88*, 632–657.

Vohs, K. D., Kaikati, A. M., Kerkhof, P., & Schmeichel, B. J. (2009). Self-regulatory resource depletion: A model for understanding the limited nature of goal pursuit. In G. B. Moskowitz & H. Grant (Eds.), *The psychology of goals* (pp. 423–446). New York: Guilford Press.

Ward, T. B., Finke, R. A., & Smith, S. M. (1995). *Creativity and the mind: Discovering the genius within*. New York: Plenum.

Wegner, D. M. (1994). Ironic processes of mental control. *Psychological Review, 101*, 34–52.

Wegner, D. M., & Bargh, J. A. (1998). Control and automaticity in social life. In D. T. Gilbert, S. T. Fiske, & G. Lindzey (Eds.), *The handbook of social psychology* (4th ed., Vol. 1, pp. 446–496). Boston: McGraw-Hill.

Wegner, D. M., & Pennebaker, J. W. (1993). An introduction to mental control. In D. M. Wegner & J. W. Pennebaker (Eds.), *Handbook of mental control* (pp. 1–12). Englewood Cliffs, NJ: Prentice Hall.

Wegner, D. M., & Wheatley, T. (1999). Apparent mental causation: Sources of the experience of will. *American Psychologist, 54*(7), 480–492.

Wicklund, R. A., & Gollwitzer, P. M. (1982). *Symbolic self-completion*. Hillsdale, NJ: Erlbaum.

Williams, L. E., & Bargh, J. A. (2008). Experiencing physical warmth promotes interpersonal warmth. *Science, 322*, 606–607.

Winkielman, P., Berridge, K. C., & Wilbarger, J. L. (2005). Unconscious affective reactions to masked happy versus angry faces influence consumption behavior and judgments of value. *Personality and Social Psychology Bulletin, 31*(1), 121–135.

Zeigarnik, B. (1927). Das Behalten erledigter und unerledigter Handlungen [The retention of completed and uncompleted actions]. *Psychologische Forschung, 9*, 1–85.

CHAPTER 28

Promotion and Prevention:
How "0" Can Create Dual Motivational Forces

E. Tory Higgins

My personal "Story of 0" began when I moved from New York University to Columbia University in 1989. Because I moved to Columbia just after my first child was born, I did not think about what research I would be doing at Columbia until months after I had arrived there (in 1990). When I did think about it, I realized with a shock that I could no longer work on *self-discrepancy theory* as I had at NYU, because the research conditions at Columbia were completely different. There was a much larger subject pool at NYU than at Columbia, and at NYU all the students in the subject pool filled out a Battery booklet that included the Selves Questionnaire measuring individuals' self-discrepancies. Because there was no Battery at Columbia, my laboratory would have to run hundreds of participants just to obtain their self-discrepancies. Once we had done that, there would be no more subject hours to conduct the actual research. What was I to do?

It was while trying to find a solution to what to do about self-discrepancy theory that *regulatory focus theory* was born. I realized that I needed to find a way to test self-discrepancy theory without having to measure people's chronic self-discrepancies. But to make sense of this problem, I need to begin with some background about self-discrepancy theory, which was developed to answer a particular question: Why do people have such different emotional reactions to the same tragic event? More specifically, when people are emotionally overwhelmed by serious setbacks in their lives, such as the death of a child, the loss of a job, or the breakup of a marriage, why do some become depressed while others become anxious?

Self-discrepancy theory proposed that even when people have the same specific goals, they often vary in how they represent these goals. In self-discrepancy theory, the goals or standards that direct or guide our self-regulation are called *self-guides*. Some people represent their self-guides as hopes or aspirations, the kind of person they ideally want to be—*ideal* self-guides. Others represent their self-guides as duties or obligations, the kind of person they believe they ought to be—*ought* self-guides.

According to self-discrepancy theory (Higgins, 1987), it is this difference between failing to meet our ideals and failing to meet our oughts that explains why we have different emotional reactions to the same negative life event. When a negative life event happens to us, it is represented as saying something about how we are doing. We compare our current, actual self to our self-guides: "Compared to the kind of person I want to be (e.g., going to a good college; having a good marriage), how am I doing?" When there is a discrepancy between our actual self and a self-guide—a *self-discrepancy*—we suffer. An actual self-discrepancy from an ideal self-guide makes us feel sad, disappointed, discouraged—dejection-related emotions that relate clinically to depression. An actual self-discrepancy from an ought self-guide makes us feel nervous, tense, and worried—agitation-related emotions that relate clinically to anxiety disorders. Thus, different kinds of emotional suffering depend on which type of self-guide is emphasized in our self-regulation—suffering dejection/depression when ideals are emphasized and agitation/anxiety when oughts are emphasized.

Depression and generalized anxiety disorder (or social phobia) occur when there is a severe discrepancy between individuals' actual selves and their chronically accessible ideal or ought self-guides, respectively. However, consistent with already well-known principles of accessibility (Higgins, 1989), either ideal self-guides or ought self-guides can be more accessible at any one time, and whichever is more accessible determines which emotional syndrome the person experiences. This means that momentary situations can determine which syndrome is experienced by priming either ideal or ought self-guides. For example, there was already evidence that either actual–ideal discrepancies or actual–ought discrepancies could be made temporarily more accessible by exposing individuals to words that related to either an ideal or an ought they possessed. When such priming was done in an experiment, participants whose actual–ideal discrepancy was activated suddenly felt sad and disappointed, and fell into a depression-related state of low activity (e.g., they talked slower). In contrast, participants whose actual–ought discrepancy was primed suddenly felt nervous and worried and fell into an anxiety-related state of high activity (e.g., they talked faster). These kinds of effects had been found with both clinical (Strauman, 1989) and nonclinical samples (Strauman & Higgins, 1987).

According to self-discrepancy theory, these different emotional syndromes are produced by the different psychological situations that people experience. When events are related to our ideal self-guides (i.e., to our hopes and aspirations), we experience success as the presence of a positive outcome (a gain), which is a happy experience, and we experience failure as the absence of positive outcomes (a non-gain), which is a sad experience. However, when events are related to our ought self-guides (i.e., our beliefs about our duties and obligations), we experience success as the absence of a negative outcome (a non-loss), which is a relaxing experience, and we experience failure as the presence of a negative outcome (a loss), which is an anxious experience (see Higgins & Tykocinski, 1992; Strauman, 1992).

Now that I have provided some basic background about self-discrepancy theory and what it predicts, I can return to the problem I faced in 1990 after just moving to Columbia. Self-discrepancy theory was developed to test predictions about distinct kinds of emotional suffering that people experience—dejection/depression-related versus agitation/anxiety-related—as a function of their actual selves being discrepant from either their chronic ideal self-guides or their ought self-guides. To test this theory, chronic self-discrepancies had to be measured. But I no longer had the resources to measure the chronic self-discrepancies of 200 or more individuals in the way that I had done at NYU. The question, then, was how could I continue to test self-discrepancy theory.

Although most of our previous research testing self-discrepancy theory had examined the distinct emotional vulnerabilities associated with different kinds of self-discrepancies, occasionally we took advantage of previous work on priming and accessibility to make either actual–ideal or actual–ought discrepancies temporarily more accessible by priming either ideal or ought self-guides, respectively. In one study by Higgins, Bond, Klein, and Strauman (1986), for example, selected participants were either high in *both* actual–ideal and actual–ought discrepancies or low in both, and when they arrived for the study they were asked to discuss either their own and their parents' hopes and aspirations for them (ideal priming) or their own and their parents' beliefs concerning their duties and obligations (ought priming). The study found that when participants possessed high ideal and ought discrepancies, ideal priming produced dejection-related emotions, whereas ought priming produced agitation-related emotions.

Originally we used priming in order to have more experimental control over our tests of self-discrepancy theory by activating momentarily either actual–ideal or actual–ought discrepancies. We still thought of self-discrepancy theory in strictly personality terms. Although we knew from research going on during the same period that temporary accessibility from situational priming could trump, at least for awhile, chronic accessibility from established individual differences (Bargh, Lombardi, & Higgins, 1988), self-discrepancy theory was still about chronic individual differences in stored self-discrepancies. For individuals high in both ideal and ought discrepancies, as in the Higgins et al. (1986) study, we simply used the priming to make one or the other discrepancy more active at the moment.

So there I was in 1990, realizing that I could not conduct studies at Columbia that required measuring participants' self-discrepancies as I had earlier. To me that meant I could no longer do research on self-discrepancy theory. What was I to do? One thought was to return full-time to priming and accessibility research, but I was not yet ready to abandon self-discrepancy theory. Thinking about priming and accessibility while wanting to continue working on ideals and oughts made me think about the relevance of my problem to a chapter I had written on how certain psychological principles could function as a "common language" for personality and social psychology (Higgins, 1990).

What was critical to the "common language" idea was the notion of there being a psychological state that could have multiple sources—either chronic or momentary, or both—yet the state functioned the same way regardless of its source. For example, accessibility was a state, and the source of that state could be chronic accessibility, priming, or both (Higgins, 1989, 1990). And the effects on judgment as a result of a stored construct having higher accessibility were the same regardless of the source of that state. Accessibility illustrated how a psychological variable could provide a *common language* for persons (chronic accessibility) and situations (priming), which addressed the classic "person–situation" issue in a new way. I had also thought that standards provided another common language for persons (personal standards) and situations (contextual standards) (Higgins, 1990). But I had *not* fully appreciated what the notion of a common language implied, nor had I thought about how accessibility and standards could be combined.

What then dawned on me was that self-discrepancy theory restricted the distinction between ideal and ought self-regulation to a personality difference. But this was an unnecessary restriction, because a discrepancy is a psychological state and, as such, it would vary not only chronically across persons but also momentarily across situations. At any moment, people could be in a state of ideal self-regulation success or ideal self-regulation failure, or in a state of ought self-regulation success or ought self-regulation failure. And while these different states could be associated with chronic discrepancies (or congruencies) between the actual self and ideal or ought self-guides, they could also be induced by momentary situations. From a broader perspective, the story was not just about chronic discrepancies (or congruencies) between the actual self and ideal or ought self-guides. Rather, the story was about *two different systems of self-regulation*.

From this broader, two-distinct-systems perspective, the emotional and motivational implications of individuals being in a *state* of ideal self-regulatory success or failure versus a *state* of ought self-regulatory success or failure could be studied *without any need to measure individuals' chronic self-discrepancies*. What mattered was to study the implications of two distinct systems of self-regulation, in which one or the other *system* could be activated through priming or other experimental manipulations. It was *not* necessary to measure chronic self-discrepancies in order to study the implications of ideal and ought self-regulation being two different kinds of self-regulation.

My problem was solved! And, in solving the problem, a new theory was born—what I later called *regulatory focus theory*. This new theory was concerned with distinct self-regulatory *states* that varied across both persons *and* situations. Unlike self-discrepancy theory, it was *not* a personality theory. Whereas ideal and ought self-guides varied chronically across persons in self-discrepancy theory, ideal and ought self-regulation in regulatory focus theory varied across momentary situations and across persons. And this difference mattered, because it inspired research that would not have been generated by self-discrepancy theory, such as effects on decision making and performance from situationally induced promotion versus prevention states (see Higgins, 1998). Nonetheless, it is important to appreciate the historical relation between regulatory focus theory and self-discrepancy theory, because they share one very important emphasis—distinguishing between different kinds of positive and negative psychological situations related to ideal (promotion) versus ought (prevention) self-regulatory success and failure. As we will see, regulatory focus theory recognized that these distinct psychological situations were motivational states that could be induced in momentary situations and had significant implications for individuals' preferences in how to make decisions and pursue goals.

DISTINCT POSITIVE AND NEGATIVE PSYCHOLOGICAL SITUATIONS AS A FUNCTION OF FOCUS

From the ancient Greeks to 17th- and 18th-century British philosophers, to 20th century psychologists (see Kahneman, Diener, & Schwarz, 1999), the hedonic principle that people are motivated to approach pleasure and avoid pain has dominated our understanding of people's motivation. It is the basic motivational assumption of theories across all areas of psychology, including theories of emotion in psychobiology (e.g., Gray, 1982), conditioning in animal learning (e.g., Mowrer, 1960; Thorndike, 1935), decision making in cognitive psychology (e.g., Edwards, 1955; Kahneman & Tversky, 1979), consistency in social psychology (e.g., Festinger, 1957; Heider, 1958), and achievement motivation in personality (e.g., Atkinson, 1964). Even in *Beyond the Pleasure Principle*, when Freud (1920/1950) assigned a motivational role to the ego's reality principle, he made it clear that the reality principle "at bottom also seeks pleasure although a delayed and diminished pleasure," (p. 365). Perhaps the clearest statement on the importance of hedonic experiences to motivation was given by Jeremy Bentham (1781/1988, p. 1): "Nature has placed mankind under the governance of two sovereign masters, *pain* and *pleasure*. It is for them alone to point out what we ought to do, as well as to determine what we shall do. On the one hand the standard of right and wrong, on the other the chain of causes and effects, are fastened to their throne."

Within this historical context, the contribution of self-discrepancy theory and regulatory focus theory has been to emphasize the significance of different ways to regulate pleasure and pain. It is not enough to know that people approach pleasure and avoid pain. It is critical to know *how* they do so. To illustrate, for Gray (1982) and Mowrer (1960), as well as Carver and Scheier (1981, 1990a, 1990b), the important motivational distinction was between the behavioral approach system (BAS) and the behavioral avoidance or behavioral inhibition system (BIS). Gray (1982) and Mowrer (1960) explicitly included both approaching reward (the presence of a positive outcome) and approaching safety (the absence of a negative outcome) as *equivalent* cases of approaching a desired end state. In contrast, self-discrepancy theory (Higgins, 1987) and regulatory focus theory (Higgins, 1997) explicitly distinguished between the promotion–ideal system versus the prevention–ought system as *two different ways of approaching desired end states*. Rather than the hedonic principle per se, it was the difference between the two ways of approaching desired end states, and the two different ways of avoiding undesired end states, that mattered motivationally, because it produced different psychological situations associated with success and failure.

The distinction between ideal and ought self-regulation in self-discrepancy theory was initially described in terms of differences in the psychological situations represented by discrepancies and congruencies involving ideal versus ought self-guides (see Higgins, 1989). Actual self-congruencies to hopes, wishes, or aspirations (ideals) represent the presence of positive outcomes, whereas discrepancies represent the absence of positive outcomes. Thus, the psychological situations involved in (promotion) ideal self-regulation are the presence or the absence of positive outcomes.

The hopes, wishes, and aspirations represented in (promotion) ideal self-guides function like maximal goals. In contrast, the duties, obligations, and responsibilities represented in (prevention) ought self-guides function more like minimal goals (see Brendl & Higgins, 1996). These are goals that a person must attain or standards that must be met. When strong enough, such as biblical commandments, oughts can even function like necessities. Discrepancies to such minimal goals represent the presence of negative outcomes, whereas congruencies represent the absence of negative outcomes. Thus, the psychological situations involved in (prevention) ought self-regulation are the absence or the presence of negative outcomes. This distinction between ideal and ought self-regulation suggests that sensitivity to events involving the presence or the absence of positive outcomes should be greater when (promotion) ideal concerns predominate, whereas sensitivity to events involving the absence or the presence of negative outcomes should be greater when (prevention) ought concerns predominate. Like Kelly's (1955) personal construct systems that scan back and forth across the perceptual field and pick up "blips of meaning" (p.145), such chronic sensitivities to distinct psychological situations should influence how stimulus information is processed and remembered. Higgins and Tykocinski (1992) tested this prediction for chronic self-discrepancies.

Undergraduate participants were selected on the basis of their self-discrepancy scores. Self-discrepancies are measured using the Selves Questionnaire (see Higgins et al., 1986), which asks respondents to list up to eight or 10 attributes each for a number of different self-states, including their actual self and their ideal and ought self-guides. It is a spontaneous, idiographic measure (see Moretti & Higgins, 1990). The procedure for calculating the magnitude of an actual–ideal or actual–ought self-discrepancy involves comparing the actual self-attributes to the attributes listed in an ideal self-guide or an ought self-guide, respectively, to determine which attributes in the actual self match or mismatch the attributes in that particular self-guide. The self-discrepancy score is basically the number of mismatches minus the number of matches (see Higgins et al., 1986).

Participants in Higgins and Tykocinski's (1992) study were identified who had either predominant actual–ideal discrepancies (i.e., higher actual–ideal than actual–ought discrepancies) or predominant actual–ought discrepancies (i.e., higher actual–ought than actual–ideal discrepancies). All participants read the same essay about the life of a target person, in which events reflecting the four different types of psychological situations occurred, such as:

1. "I found a $20 bill on the pavement of Canal Street near the paint store" (the presence of positive outcomes)
2. "I've been wanting to see this movie at the 8th Street theater for some time, so this evening I went there straight after school to find out that it's not showing anymore" (the absence of positive outcomes).
3. "I was stuck in the subway for 35 minutes with at least 15 sweating passengers breathing down my neck" (the presence of negative outcomes).
4. "This is usually my worst school day. Awful schedule, class after class with no break. But today is election day—no school!" (the absence of negative outcomes).

Ten minutes after reading the essay, participants were asked to reproduce the essay word-for-word. The study found, as predicted, that predominant actual–ideal discrepancy participants remembered target events representing the presence or the absence of positive outcomes better than did predominant actual–ought discrepancy participants, whereas predominant actual–ought discrepancy participants remembered target events representing the absence or the presence of negative outcomes better than did predominant actual–ideal discepancy participants. This pattern of findings was independent of participants' prestudy mood, poststudy mood, or change in mood.

Approach versus Avoidance Strategies for Self-Regulation

The results of the Higgins and Tykocinski (1992) study support the proposal that self-regulation in relation to (promotion) ideals versus (prevention) oughts involves dinstinct sensitivities to different kinds of psychological situations—the presence or the absence of positive outcomes for (promotion) ideal self-regulation and the absence or the presence of negative outcomes for (prevention) ought self-regulation. The results of subsequent studies by Higgins, Roney, Crowe, and Hymes (1994) also support this general proposal in a different way, and, in addition, indicate that (promotion) ideal and (prevention) ought self-regulation differ in their predilection for approach versus avoidance strategies. The Higgins and Tykocinski (1992) study was conducted while I was at NYU. The Higgins et al. (1994) studies, conducted after I arrived at Columbia, represent the transition point from self-discrepancy theory to regulatory focus theory. It was a transition point because the studies examined sensitivities to ideal versus ought discrepancies and congruencies, but they did so in terms of conceptualizing ideal and ought self-regulation as constituting distinct self-regulatory systems and examining the different strategic preferences of these two systems.

Self-regulation in relation to (promotion) ideals and (prevention) oughts involves approaching desired end states at the system level by reducing discrepancies between current states and desired end states. But within approaching desired states at the system level, either approach or avoidance strategies can be used. Specifically, individuals can increase the likelihood that they will attain (or maintain) a desired end state by either approaching matches to that end state or by avoiding mismatches to that end state. For example, a person who wants to get a good grade on a quiz (a desired end state) could either study hard at the library the day before the quiz (approaching a match to the desired end state) or turn down an invitation to go out drinking with friends the night before the quiz (avoiding a mismatch to the desired end state).

Higgins et al. (1994) hypothesized that self-regulation in relation to ideal self-guides (hopes and aspirations), because of its concern with positive outcomes (their presence or their absence), would prefer the strategy of approaching matches to these desired end states. In contrast, self-regulation in relation to ought self-guides (duties and obligations), because of its concern with negative outcomes (their absence or their presence), would prefer the strategy of avoiding mismatches to these desired end states. To test these hypotheses, one study asked undergraduates to report either on how their hopes have changed over time (activating ideal self-guides) or on how their sense of duty has changed over time (activating ought self-guides). To reveal strategic inclinations, this study used a free recall technique similar to that used in the Higgins and Tykocinski (1992) study. But notice that in this study individuals' concern with (promotion) ideal self-regulation versus (prevention) ought self-regulation was situationally induced rather than being associated with personality differences in chronic self-discrepancies. The participants read about several episodes that occurred over a few days in the life of another student. In each of the episodes in which the target was trying to experience a desired end state, the target used either the strategy of approaching a match to the desired end state or the strategy of avoiding a mismatch to the desired end state, as in the following examples:

1. "Because I wanted to be at school for the beginning of my 8:30 psychology class, which is usually excellent, I woke up early this morning" (approaching a match to a desired end state).
2. "I wanted to take a class in photography at the community center, so I didn't register for a class in Spanish that was scheduled at the same time" (avoiding a mismatch to a desired end state).

As predicted, the participants remembered episodes that exemplified approaching a match to a desired end state significantly better when ideal self-regulation was activated than when ought self-regulation was activated, whereas they remembered episodes that exemplified avoiding a mismatch to a desired end state significantly better when ought self-regulation was activated than when ideal self-regulation was activated.

It turned out that this difference in strategic preferences between (promotion) ideal self-regulation and (prevention) ought self-regulation was very important, because it related to regulatory focus differences in decision-making and problem-solving processes. Eventually the (promotion) ideal preference for approaching a match to a desired end state was understood to represent a broader preference for *eager* means of advancing in goal pursuit, and the (prevention) ought preference for avoiding a mismatch to a desired end state was understood to represent a broader preference for *vigilant* means of being careful in goal pursuit.

Reinterpreting "0" as a Function of Ideal versus Ought Goal Pursuit

Another transition point from self-discrepancy theory to regulatory focus theory occurred around the same time as the Higgins et al. (1994) research. Miguel Brendl and I began working on a chapter for Mark Zanna's *Advances in Experimental Social Psychology* series that addressed the question, "What makes events positive or negative?" (Brendl & Higgins, 1996). When we were just beginning this project, I remember Miguel coming into my office with an air of excitement and telling me about a critical factor for understanding the nature of valence. His insight was that the nature of valence depended on how neutrality was determined: *to understand valence, you needed to understand "0."* It was a great insight that set the agenda for our chapter, which was to identify different principles that determine valence by determining what "0" meant.

With respect to the development of regulatory focus theory, the most relevant principle for judging valence that we reviewed was *the principle of goal supportiveness,* which refers to the degree to which an event is judged to support or impede the satisfaction of a set goal, with goal support producing judgments of positive valence quality and goal impediment producing judgments of negative valence quality. This principle has a long history. Lewin, Dembo, Festinger, and Sears (1944), for example, assumed that a goal separates positively valenced events from negatively valenced events, or an area of success from an area of failure, with the former being approached and the latter being avoided. More recent theories of emotion also assume that reaching versus frustrating a goal (Roseman, 1984; Lazarus, 1993; Ortony, Clore, & Collins, 1988) is experienced positively versus negatively.

Brendl and Higgins (1996) considered what this meant for the difference between the (promotion) ideal system and the (prevention) ought system. (When the chapter was written, regulatory focus was called *outcome focus,* promotion focus was called *positive outcome focus,* and prevention focus was called *negative outcome focus.* At a conference I attended in 1995, Marilynn Brewer pointed out that these earlier labels were very confusing [or worse], and they were, thankfully, replaced with the currently used labels, but too late for the *Advances* chapter.) We proposed that given the nature of ideal and ought goals, *"0" was* ***not*** *neutral.* Moreover, *"0" had a* ***different*** *valence for ideal and ought goal pursuit.*

We made these proposals because of the nature of goal supportiveness for ideal and ought goal pursuit. For (promotion) ideal goal pursuit, successfully attaining a positive outcome supports the goal pursuit, because it represents the *presence of a positive outcome,* and as such it has positive valence. Not attaining a positive outcome impedes (promotion) ideal goal pursuit, because it represents the *absence of a positive outcome,* and as such has negative valence. This means that simply maintaining a status quo "0" is ***not*** *experienced as neutral* in the (promotion) ideal system of goal pursuit; instead, it has *negative* valence, because it fails to attain a positive outcome (fails to advance). In contrast, for (prevention) ought goal pursuit, maintaining a status quo "0" has *positive* valence, because it represents the *absence of a negative outcome.* Thus, once again, "0" is ***not*** *experienced as neutral.* But for (prevention) ought goal pursuit, "0" has positive valence rather than the negative valence it has for promotion ideal goal pursuit. What has negative valence for (prevention) ought goal pursuit is failing to maintain a status quo "0", which represents the *presence of a negative outcome.*

REGULATORY FOCUS THEORY AND THE MOTIVATIONAL FORCE OF "0"

After the Brendl and Higgins (1996) chapter, there were subsequent developments in regulatory focus theory regarding the distinct nature and role of "0" for promotion versus prevention self-regulatory concerns. In 1997, I wrote an *American Psychologist* article called "Beyond Pleasure and Pain," in which I formally presented regulatory focus theory for the first time. Beyond introducing the new terminology (e.g., *promotion focus, prevention focus*), there were other noteworthy changes from self-discrepancy theory.

Self-discrepancy theory was concerned with self-regulation in relation to self-guides, distinguishing between self-regulation in relation to hopes and aspirations (ideals) versus duties and obligations (oughts). Regulatory focus was concerned with distinguishing more broadly between two distinct systems of self-regulation concerned with either growth and nurturance (promotion concerns) or safety and security (prevention concerns). Ideal concerns were part of promotion concerns, but there were other, more general concerns, such as concerns with nurturing, accomplishing, and advancing. Ought concerns were part of prevention concerns, but there were other, more general concerns with protecting and maintaining safety and security. Promotion concerns with growth and advancement naturally mean wanting to move in a positive direction forward (i.e., to make progress) away from a status quo "0." Prevention concerns with maintaining safety and security naturally mean wanting to maintain a status quo "0" and stop moving in a negative direction away from a status quo "0."

Another change introduced in Higgins (1997) was to emphasize more generally the promotion focus preference for eager strategies of goal pursuit rather than just approaching matches to ideal self-guides, and the prevention focus preference for vigilant strategies of goal pursuit rather than just avoiding mismatches to ought self-guides.

Related to this change of emphasis was a switch from describing ideal goal pursuit as concerned with the presence or the absence of positive outcomes to describing promotion goal pursuit as concerned with ensuring gains and ensuring against non-gains, and a switch from describing ought goal pursuit as concerned with the absence or the presence of negative outcomes to describing prevention goal pursuit as concerned with ensuring non-losses and ensuring against losses.

This change was also important because it more naturally highlighted the fact that maintaining status quo "0" had negative valence for a promotion focus, because it was a non-gain, whereas it had positive valence for a prevention focus because it was a non-loss. Admittedly, I did not fully appreciate this advantage at the time. What I did appreciate at the time, which led to several new tests of regulatory focus predictions regarding the promotion state being more creative and open to change than the prevention state (e.g., Crowe & Higgins, 1997; Friedman & Forster, 2001; Liberman, Idson, Camacho, & Higgins, 1999), was that individuals in a promotion state wanted to ensure hits (ensure gains) and ensure against errors of omission (ensure against non-gains), whereas individuals in a prevention state wanted to ensure correct rejections (ensure non-losses) and ensure against errors of commission (ensure against losses), which, generally speaking, would make individuals in a promotion state more willing to take chances than those in a prevention state.

A little later an insightful paper by Roese, Hur, and Pennington (1999) appeared that was also relevant, in its own innovative way, to the idea that what is negative in a promotion state is having failed to take action and do something positive that would have gained something, whereas what is negative in a prevention state is taking action that fails to maintain a current satisfactory state and should have been stopped to avoid a loss. When people feel bad about their action choices they sometimes engage in counterfactual thinking, in which they consider what might have happened "if only" they had taken certain actions or decided not to take certain actions (see Kahneman & Miller, 1986). Roese et al. (1999) investigated whether regulatory focus alters people's use of counterfactuals.

Roese et al. (1999) proposed that promotion preferences for eager strategies are related to the formation of *additive* counterfactuals, in which one imagines how one might have taken an action—rather than one's actual inaction—that would have led to a gain (e.g., "If only I had acted, I wouldn't have missed that opportunity for advancement"). They also proposed that prevention preferences for vigilant strategies are related to the formation of *subtractive* counterfactuals, in which one imagines how one instead might have refrained from taking the action that led to a loss (e.g., "If I hadn't acted, I would have avoided that mistake"). They reasoned that simulating the correction of a past error of omission, which occurs with additive counterfactuals, would be more consistent with promotion eagerness than prevention vigilance, and that simulating the correction of a past error of commission, which occurs with subtractive counterfactuals, would be more consistent with prevention vigilance than promotion eagerness.

In one study testing these hypotheses, Roese et al. (1999) had participants read scenarios involving failure situations, with half of the scenarios involving promotion failure (e.g., failure to attain an accomplishment goal) and the other half involving prevention failure (e.g., failure to attain a safety goal). Participants then completed sentences that began with the counterfactual "If only . . ." stem. As predicted, participants were more likely to complete the sentence with additive counterfactuals for the promotion than for the prevention failure scenario, and were more likely to complete the sentence with subtractive counterfactuals when the scenario invoked prevention rather than promotion failure.

In another study Roese et al. (1999) integrated self-discrepancy theory and regulatory focus theory in a novel way. They first induced either dejection or agitation by having participants think of a negative event in the past year that made them feel, respectively, either dejected, disappointed, discouraged, and so forth, or agitated, nervous, worried, and so forth. Afterwards, the participants were asked to give examples of any "If only" thoughts they had after experiencing the negative event. As predicted, the dejection that is associated with discrepancies from ideals (i.e., promotion failure) activated additive counterfactuals, whereas the agitation that is associated with discrepancies from oughts (i.e., prevention failure) activated subtractive counterfactuals.

The Roese et al. (1999) studies demonstrate in another way how the motivational force of "0" is different for promotion and prevention. For promotion, inaction and maintaining the status quo "0" is not neutral, because it gives up the possibility of a gain. Such inaction is a negative non-gain and leads people to think about what action they might have taken instead to ensure a gain (additive counterfactual thinking). To use our current way of describing regulatory focus forces (e.g., Higgins, 2009), promotion-focused individuals' concern with gains versus non-gains makes them sensitive to the difference between the status quo or neutral state and a positive deviation from that state—the difference between "0" and "+1." For them, staying at "0" is a failure and what is needed, even in imagination, is movement away from "0" to "+1." For prevention, on the other hand, taking unnecessary action that loses, or risks losing, the satisfactory status quo is a failure, and what is needed, even in imagination, if loss does occur, is to stop that action and maintain or restore "0." This is because prevention-focused individuals' concern with non-losses versus losses makes them sensitive to the difference between the status quo or neutral state and a negative deviation from that state—the difference between "0" and "–1." Having taken an action that led to a loss leads them to think about how that action might have been stopped to ensure a non-loss (subtractive counterfactual thinking).

Recent research on prevention motivational forces by Scholer, Zou, Fujita, Stroessner, and Higgins (2010) has discovered just how strongly prevention-focused individuals want to maintain the safety of the status quo "0" and, if they find themselves in a condition of loss, undo the loss and restore "0." Using a "two study" paradigm, participants in the first study were paid to complete a battery of questionnaires and were then given a choice to leave or to invest their payment in a second, stock investment study. They were told that, in general, participants walked away with additional money in the stock investment study, but that there was a chance they could lose their money. Most participants decided to invest in the stock investment study.

After making their initial investment decision, participants tracked the performance of their stock over time. At the end of the first round, all participants learned that they had lost not only their original investment but additional money (manipulation checks confirmed that participants did indeed experience their situation as a *real loss*). At this point, participants were given a choice between investing in two stocks for the second round of the study, a risky stock and a conservative stock. The expected value of these stocks was equivalent, but the risky stock was riskier both in the objective sense that its variance was greater and in the subjective sense that participants rated the risky stock as riskier.

The study found that participants who were *more* prevention-focused were *more* likely to choose the riskier stock. But this was not the end of the story. In this first stock investment study, only the risky option had the potential of returning participants to their break-even point. Thus, to restore the status quo "0", it was *necessary* to choose the risky option. What matters to prevention-focused individuals is to be vigilant and maintain a non-loss. In this first study, a risky tactical option supported being vigilant and restoring a non-loss by returning to "0." A second study included a different pair of options; *both* the risky and the conservative options had the potential of returning participants to their break-even point, with the more conservative option being more likely to reach "0", but only "0", and the more risky option being less likely to reach "0" but having some potential to go well beyond "0."

Now the more prevention-focused individuals were *less* likely to choose the risky option, because what mattered was restoring a non-loss by returning to "0", and the conservative option was more likely to do that. Another study showed that when strong prevention-focused participants chose the riskier option—because it was the only way to return to "0"—they did not like that option; rather, they disliked it less (because they saw it as a necessity). What these studies demonstrate is prevention's strong motivational force for maintaining the status quo "0", a satisfactory non-loss. If it is not maintained and a loss occurs, prevention-focused individuals will do what is necessary to restore it, and just it. They are motivated by "0" non-loss rather than by gain "+1."

PROMOTION AND PREVENTION WORKING TOGETHER

I conclude this chapter by considering the relation between the motivational forces of promotion and prevention. Do they operate in isolation, do they conflict, or do they work together? Our research findings suggest that all three, in some sense, are possible. Promotion and prevention motivational forces are both available to every individual. But they can each vary in strength, such that both could be high; both could be low; or one could be high, while the other is low. When one is high and the other is low, then one predominates and is the main determinant of what happens motivationally. This is the sense in which promotion or prevention can operate in isolation.

There are also cases in which promotion and prevention motivational forces can be in conflict. This would occur in a situation where one choice option supports moving from "0" to "+1" but with the danger of losing "0" and ending at "–1", and the other choice option supports maintaining "0" and stopping "–1" but precludes any possibility of advancing to "+1." The promotional motivational force would strongly push for (i.e., prefer) the former option, whereas the prevention motivational force would strongly push for the latter option. This would clearly produce a conflict between the promotion and prevention motivational forces.

But there is the third possibility as well of the promotion and prevention motivational forces working together. Indeed, even when one might think that these forces would surely be in conflict, this need not be the case. One example is the "classic speed–accuracy conflict." As the expression suggests, this is usually treated as an inherent conflict. But as Förster, Higgins, and Bianco (2003) point out, this need not be the case. Yes, it is true that promotion prefers speed (more gains) and prevention prefers accuracy (less losses). But individuals who are high in both promotion and prevention are strongly motivated to be *both* fast and accurate, and are so compared to individuals who are low in both.

Another example is the signal detection "conflict" between having a bias to say, "Yes, I have seen this before"—a promotion focus bias not to miss any "hits" (ensure against an error of omission)—and having a bias to say, "No, I have not seen this before"—a prevention focus bias not to commit a mistake (ensure against an error of commission). This would seem to be an obvious conflict between saying "Yes" and saying "No." However, individuals high in both promotion and prevention will be strongly motivated to ensure against *both* kinds of errors, and this will produce a resultant high discriminability (i.e., high d′).

More generally, promotion and prevention can work together in a highly functional way by setting constraints on the downside of each motivational force when it becomes too predominant (for a fuller discussion, see Higgins, 2012). All strong psychological forces have costs as well as benefits—tradeoffs. Unconstrained, promotion forces can result in people being overeager, which can produce impulsive and unrealistic choices. Unconstrained, prevention forces can result in people being hypervigilant, which can produce obsessive and compulsive behaviors. When a person or a team has both strong promotion and strong prevention forces directing choices, there is the possibility to have the benefits from each motivational force, with less of the costs. In this way, promotion and prevention motivational forces can *work together* effectively.

In regulatory focus theory, the distinction between promotion and prevention systems refers to two different self-regulatory systems that have different motivational concerns—promotion concerns with making progress from a current state to a better state that is associated with survival from growth and mastery, and prevention concerns with maintaining a satisfactory state that is associated with survival from safety and security. This is a different distinction than the distinction between automatic and controlled processing that is found in many other dual-systems models, because promotion and prevention regulation can each function in either automatic or controlled forms. Nonetheless, the promotion versus prevention distinction does relate in some ways to another distinction that is found in some dual-systems models—the classic distinction between two manners of establishing reality, and, especially, the reality that relates to evaluating something (Epstein, 1991; Smith & DeCoster, 2000; Strack & Deutsch, 2004): (1) a manner that relies on spontaneous feelings about and associations to something (the "heart" or "gut") versus (2) a manner that relies on reflection and propositional reasoning (the "head").

The output evaluation in the former might be "I can't explain it, but my heart (gut) tells me that this is what I have to do," whereas in the latter it might be "I don't feel good about it, but I have concluded from the evidence that this is what I have to do." The "heart" manner of establishing reality is often described as using an unconscious, uncontrolled, and almost effortless process to produce the output (i.e., the reality), whereas the "head" manner of establishing reality uses a conscious, controlled, and effortful process. However, this binary distinction is probably too simple (see, e.g., Bargh, 1989; Kruglanski, Erbs, Pierro, Mannetti, & Chun, 2006), and certainly promotion regulation and prevention pregulation can each occur in the presence or the absence of consciousness (or awareness), intentionality, controllability, and effort, and in multiple combinations and levels of these features. What is worth noting here, however, is that when making evaluations, individuals in a promotion focus place greater weight on their *feelings* than on their *reasons*, whereas the opposite is true for individuals in a prevention focus (Pham & Avnet, 2004; Avnet & Higgins, 2006).

Does this regulatory focus difference in emphasizing "heart" versus "head" (sometimes called "intuitive" vs. "rational" or "analytical") produce conflicts between the promotion and prevention systems or, once again, can promotion "heart" and prevention "head" worth together effectively? Stating it this way raises a classic issue in the psychological *and* philosophical literature. I agree with those who argue that each way of establishing reality—"heart" and "head"—can have both benefits and costs under different conditions, and striking a balance between them is generally the best way to proceed. A dual-process model that provides an especially compelling version of the "heart" versus "head" distinction describes how they can work together effectively (see Strack & Deutsch, 2004). Given the promotion emphasis on feelings and the prevention emphasis on reasons, this kind of model illustrates another way that the promotion and prevention systems can work together as partners.

REFERENCES

Atkinson, J. W. (1964). *An introduction to motivation*. Princeton, N J: Van Nostrand.

Avnet, T., & Higgins, E. T. (2006). How regulatory fit impacts value in consumer choices and opinions. *Journal of Marketing Research, 43*, 1–10.

Bargh, J. A. (1989). Conditional automaticity: Varieties of automatic influence in social perception and cognition. In J. S. Uleman & J. A. Bargh (Eds.), *Unintended thought* (pp. 3–51). New York: Guilford Press.

Bargh, J. A., Lombardi, W. J., & Higgins, E. T. (1988). Automaticity of chronically accessible constructs in person x situation effects on person perception: It's just a matter of time. *Journal of Personality and Social Psychology, 55*, 599–605.

Bentham, J. (1988). *The principles of morals and legislation*. Amherst, NY: Prometheus Books. (Original work published 1781)

Brendl, C. M., & Higgins, E. T. (1996). Principles of judging valence: What makes events positive or negative? In M. P. Zanna (Ed.), *Advances in experimental social psychology* (Vol. 28, pp. 95–160). New York: Academic Press.

Carver, C. S., & Scheier, M. F. (1981). *Attention and self-regulation: A control-theory approach to human behavior*. New York: Springer-Verlag.

Carver, C. S., & Scheier, M. F. (1990a). Principles of self-regulation: Action and emotion. In E. T. Higgins & R. M. Sorrentino (Eds.), *Handbook of motivation and cognition: Foundations of social behvior, Volume 2* (pp. 3–52). New York: Guilford Press.

Carver, C. S., & Scheier, M. F. (1990b). Origins and functions of positive and negative affect: A control-process view. *Psychological Review, 97*, 19–35.

Crowe, E., & Higgins, E. T. (1997). Regulatory focus and strategic inclinations: Promotion and prevention in decision-making. *Organizational Behavior and Human Decision Processes, 69*, 117–132.

Edwards, W. (1955). The prediction of decisions among bets. *Journal of Experimental Psychology, 51*, 201–214.

Epstein, S. (1991). Cognitive-experiential self theory: Implications for developmental psychology. In M. R. Gunnar & L. A. Sroufe (Eds.), *Self processes and development: The Minnesota Symposia on Child Psychology* (Vol. 23, pp. 79–123). Hillsdale, NJ: Erlbaum.

Festinger, L. (1957). *A theory of cognitive dissonance*. Evanston, IL: Row, Peterson.

Förster, J., Higgins, E. T., & Bianco, A. T. (2003). Speed/accuracy decisions in task performance: Built-in trade-off or separate strategic concerns? *Organizational Behavior and Human Decision Processes, 90*, 148–164.

Freud, S. (1950). *Beyond the pleasure principle*. New York: Liveright. (Original work published 1920)

Friedman, R. S., & Forster, J. (2001). The effects of promotion and prevention cues on creativity. *Journal of Personality and Social Psychology, 81*, 1001–1013.

Gray, J. A. (1982). *The neuropsychology of anxiety: An enquiry into the functions of the septo-hippocampal system*. New York: Oxford University Press.

Heider, F. (1958). *The psychology of interpersonal relations*. New York: Wiley.

Higgins, E. T. (1987). Self-discrepancy: A theory relating self and affect. *Psychological Review, 94*, 319–340.

Higgins, E. T. (1989). Knowledge accessibility and activation: Subjectivity and suffering from unconscious sources. In J. S. Uleman & J. A. Bargh (Eds.), *Unintended thought: The limits of awareness, intention and control* (pp. 75–123). New York: Guilford Press.

Higgins, E. T. (1990). Personality, social psychology, and person–situation relations: Standards and knowledge activation as a common language. In L. A. Pervin (Ed.), *Handbook of personality* (pp. 301–338). New York: Guilford Press.

Higgins, E. T. (1991). Development of self-regulatory and self-evaluative processes: Costs, benefits, and tradeoffs. In M. R. Gunnar & L. A. Sroufe (Eds.), *Self processes and development: The Minnesota Symposia on Child Psychology* (Vol. 23, pp. 125–165). Hillsdale, NJ: Erlbaum.

Higgins, E. T. (1997). Beyond pleasure and pain. *American Psychologist, 52*, 1280–1300.

Higgins, E. T. (1998). Promotion and prevention: Regulatory focus as a motivational principle. In M. P. Zanna (Ed.), *Advances in experimental social psychology* (Vol. 30, pp. 1–46). New York: Academic Press.

Higgins, E. T. (2009). Regulatory fit in the goal-pursuit process. In G. B. Moskowitz & H. Grant (Eds.), *The psychology of goals*. New York: Guilford Press.

Higgins, E. T. (2012). *Beyond pleasure and pain: How motivation works*. New York: Oxford University Press.

Higgins, E. T., Bond, R. N., Klein, R., & Strauman, T. (1986). Self-discrepancies and emotional vulnerability: How magnitude, accessibility, and type of discrepancy influence affect. *Journal of Personality and Social Psychology, 51*, 5–15.

Higgins, E. T., Roney, C., Crowe, E., & Hymes, C. (1994). Ideal versus ought predilections for approach and avoidance: Distinct self-regulatory systems. *Journal of Personality and Social Psychology, 66*, 276–286.

Higgins, E. T., & Tykocinski, O. (1992). Self-discrepancies and biographical memory: Personality and cognition at the level of psychological situation. *Personality and Social Psychology Bulletin, 18*, 527–535.

Kahneman, D., Diener, E., & Schwarz, N. (Eds.). (1999). *Well-being: The foundations of hedonic psychology*. New York: Russell Sage Foundation.

Kahneman, D., & Miller, D. T. (1986). Norm theory: Comparing reality to its alternatives. *Psychological Review, 93*, 136–153.

Kahneman, D., & Tversky, A. (1979). Prospect theory: An analysis of decision under risk. *Econometrica, 47*, 263–291.

Kelly, G. A. (1955). *The psychology of personal constructs*. New York: W. W. Norton.

Kruglanski, A. W., Erbs, H.-P., Pierro, A., Mannetti, L., & Chun, W. Y. (2006). On parametric continuities in the world of binary either ors. *Psychological Inquiry, 17*, 153–165.

Lazarus, R. S. (1990). Theory-based stress measurement. *Psychological Inquiry, 1*, 3–13.

Lewin, K., Dembo, T., Festinger, L., & Sears, P. S. (1944). Level of aspiration. In J. McHunt (Ed.), *Personality and the behavior disorders* (Vol. 1, pp. 333–378). New York: Ronald Press.

Liberman, N., Idson, L. C., Camacho, C. J., & Higgins, E. T. (1999). Promotion and prevention choices between stability and change. *Journal of Personality and Social Psychology, 77*, 1135–1145.

Moretti, M. M., & Higgins, E. T. (1990). Relating self-discrepancy to self-esteem: The contribution of discrepancy beyond actual-self ratings. *Journal of Experimental Social Psychology, 26*, 108–123.

Mowrer, O. H. (1960). *Learning theory and behavior*. New York: Wiley.

Ortony, A., Clore, G. L., & Collins, A. (1988). *The cognitive structure of emotions*. New York: Cambridge University Press

Pham, M., & Avnet, T. (2004). Ideals and oughts and the reliance on affect versus substance in persuasion. *Journal of Consumer Research, 30*, 503–518.

Roese, N. J., Hur, T., & Pennington, G. L. (1999). Counterfactual thinking and regulatory focus: Implications for action versus inaction and sufficiency versus necessity. *Journal of Personality and Social Psychology, 77*, 1109–1120.

Roseman, I. J. (1984). Cognitive determinants of emotion: A structural theory. *Review of Personality and Social Psychology, 5*, 11–36.

Scholer, A. A., Zou, X., Fujita, K., Stroessner, S. J., & Higgins, E. T. (2010). When risk-seeking becomes a motivational necessity. *Journal of Personality and Social Psychology, 99*, 215–231.

Smith, E. R., & DeCoster, J. (2000). Dual-process models in social and cognitive psychology: Conceptual integration and links to underlying memory systems. *Personality and Social Psychology Review, 4*, 108–131.

Strack, F., & Deutsch, R. (2004). Reflective and impulsive determinants of social behavior. *Personality and Social Psychology Review, 8*, 220–247.

Strauman, T. J. (1989). Self-discrepancies in clinical depression and social phobia: Cognitive structures that underlie emotional disorders? *Journal of Abnormal Psychology, 98*, 14–22.

Strauman, T. J. (1992). Self-guides, autobiographical memory, and anxiety and dysphoria: Toward a cognitive model of vulnerability to emotional distress. *Journal of Abnormal Psychology, 101*, 87–95.

Strauman, T. J., & Higgins, E. T. (1987). Automatic activation of self-discrepancies and emotional syndromes: When cognitive structures influence affect. *Journal of Personality and Social Psychology, 53*, 1004–1014.

Thorndike, E. L. (1935). *The psychology of wants, interests, and attitudes*. New York: Appleton-Century-Crofts.

PART VIII

SELF-REGULATION AND CONTROL

CHAPTER 29

Beyond Control versus Automaticity

Psychological Processes Driving Postsuppressional Rebound

Jens Förster and Nira Liberman

When the first author was invited to job interviews some years ago, advisors told him not to present his research on embodiment but to talk about his work on social cognition. At this time, embodiment research was neither very popular nor clearly perceived as "social psychology"; thus, they thought it would only hurt his chances to get a job. The first author noticed that it was very difficult not to not think about embodiment especially during the interviews, when the committee members asked him about his research interests and future projects. It occurred to him that almost all his future projects were related to embodiment. Moreover, whenever he came back from job interviews, his mind was occupied with ideas on embodiment and he felt an urge to do more research on this topic even though it was not on his research agenda before he started interviewing. It felt as if suppression had placed forbidden thoughts foremost in his mind and created high motivation to dig deeper into taboo material.

This anecdote illustrates an effect of *postsuppressional rebound* (PSR)—the tendency of a suppressed construct to become even more accessible than it would be without suppression attempts. It also points to some implications for behavior, namely, increased motivation to engage in the forbidden activity.

CAN'T GET THAT BEAR OFF MY MIND

Wegner, Schneider, Carter, and White (1987) were the first to demonstrate consequences of suppression, including PSR in the laboratory. In their classic study, participants in one group (the suppression group) were asked to not to think of white bears for a period of 5 minutes and to ring a bell each time the thought of a white bear crossed their minds. A different group of participants (the expression group) performed the first phase without suppression instructions. Following this initial phase, participants were instructed to think of anything they wanted for another phase of 5 minutes; they could also think of white bears. They were asked to ring a bell each time a white bear came to mind. The results showed two effects: First, suppression in the first phase was difficult for participants—most of them thought of white bears despite instructions not to think of them. Second, thoughts of white bears rebounded after suppression in the second phase, when participants were allowed to think about white bears. Results showed that the rate of thoughts about white bears during the expression phase was higher for participants in the first phase who had to suppress thoughts than those who could think about everything, indicating PSR.

The studies by the Wegner group inspired researchers to examine PSR in a variety of domains. To give only a couple of examples, PSR was demonstrated by suppression of moods (Wegner, Erber, & Zanakos, 1993), by not allowing participants to use certain color-words while they were asked to describe paintings (Liberman & Förster, 2000), or upon suppression of thoughts about a film showing a fire in an office building (Davies & Clark, 1998). In the more social domain, PSRs were observed upon suppression of thoughts about one's own former romantic relationships (Wegner & Gold, 1995), and after suppression of stereotypes that enhanced the accessibility of the stereotype led to more stereotypical judgments and enhanced discrimination (Förster & Liberman, 2001; Liberman & Förster, 2000; Macrae, Bodenhausen, & Milne, 1998; Macrae, Bodenhausen, Milne, & Jetten, 1994; Monteith, Spicer, & Tooman, 1998; Wyer, Sherman, & Stroessner, 1998). Recently, it has been shown that suppression of aggressive thoughts rebounded in subsequent aggression, and that suppression of thirst rebounded in enhanced drinking (Denzler, Förster, Liberman, & Rozenman, 2010). Finally, while in most studies participants were asked to suppress thoughts, a few studies showed that suppression of behavior can have behavioral rebound effects as well. For example, the suppression of laughter rebounded in more laughing afterward (Denzler et al., 2010), and the suppression of scratching enhanced scratching (Reuven-Magril, Rosenman, Liberman, & Dar, 2009).

In order to explain PSR, Wegner (1994; Wegner & Wenzlaff, 1996) developed a dual-process account, the "ironic monitoring model of suppression." According to this model, suppressing a thought involves a *controlled search for distracters* (i.e., contents other than the one being suppressed), and *automatic monitoring for suppression failures*, or occurrences of the suppressed construct. More specifically, the automatic monitor "reviews potentially conscious material, noting items that imply failed control and increasing their activation. This increases the likelihood that the items will surface in consciousness so that the operating process can renew its work" (Wegner, 1994, p. 38). For example, when trying to suppress thoughts of a former lover, people try to think about other things (e.g., their work, their vacation) and at the same time monitor for occurrences of thoughts related to the former lover. This monitoring process notes suppression failures (e.g., "I thought of my last vacation. I remember this dinner with him on the beach. Oops, I should not have thought about this vacation!") and directs thoughts to a new subject upon detection of a failure (e.g., "Let's go to a new restaurant. They serve sushi. Oops, this was his favorite dish"). Although this process successfully pushes thoughts of the to-be suppressed construct out of consciousness, the ironic monitor remains sensitized to constructs related to it through the entire period of suppression and therefore makes it accessible. When the suppression period is over, the accessibility of the suppressed construct is manifested in faster and more frequent use of the construct.

Critically, the ironic monitor is said to increase *accessibility* of the suppressed construct during the act of thought suppression (Macrae, Bodenhausen, & Milne, 1998)—accessibility that decays slowly thereafter. Accessibility, in turn, increases the likelihood of correspondent behavior.

This reasoning is in line with both central models of semantic priming (for reviews, see Förster & Liberman, 2007; Higgins, 1996), and models of behavioral priming (e.g., Dijksterhuis & Bargh, 2001). In semantic priming, recent and frequent activation of a concept leads to high accessibility that then slowly decays over time. To illustrate, a semantic activation of the construct "doctor" usually enhances subsequent speed in lexical decisions of semantic associates, such as "nurse" (Neely, 1991). Decay of accessibility is a matter of time and intensity: The longer the time interval between the prime and the target, the less facilitation can be expected (i.e., *the recency principle*). Furthermore, the stronger the initial activation (or the more often the prime is presented) the more facilitation can be expected (i.e., *the frequency principle*).

The importance of the effects of accessibility for judgment and behavior made it highly relevant for central issues of social psychology. Thus, models of semantic priming suggest that accessible knowledge activated in an unrelated previous phase of the experiment (e.g., the concept of "hostility") influences further judgment (e.g., judging a person's ambiguous behavior as aggressive; Srull & Wyer, 1979). Moreover, current models suggest also that "perceptual inputs are translated automatically into corresponding behavioral outputs" (Dijksterhuis & Bargh, 2001, p. 1). As a result, increased accessibility of a concept (e.g., thinking about older adults) can trigger correspondent behavior (e.g., walking slowly down the hallway; Bargh, Chen, & Burrows, 1996). Most relevant to this chapter, according to the ironic monitoring model, suppressed thoughts are made highly accessible via the ironic monitor, increasing the likelihood of PSR on thinking, judgments, and behavior.

The ironic monitoring model is a prime example of a dual-process model, demonstrating the operation of automatic and controlled processes. We do not question the notion that PSR is produced by both controlled and automatic processes; rather, we believe that probably there is no complex human behavior that is *not* produced by both automatic *and* controlled processes (Förster & Jostmann, 2012). For one thing, the last decade of research on automaticity has shown that automatic processes are more dynamic than formerly assumed (see Dijksterhuis & Nordgren, 2006; Liberman & Förster, 2005). Moreover, critics warned that the focus on an automatic versus controlled distinction obstructs the view of processes that operate beyond it (Kruglanski & Thompson, 1999). In the domain of PSR this seems especially important, because the ironic monitoring model paints a rather pessimistic picture of means to prevent unwanted rebounds. In a nutshell, Wegner (2011) concluded with respect to successful suppression (and a reduced PSR) that "we can do this in large parts by escaping thought suppression itself" (p. 672). In other words, as soon as we start suppressing, we are deemed to fall prey to PSR. However, recent research conducted in a different theoretical framework has discovered strategies that successfully prevent PSR even when participants engage in suppression. We first describe the framework and the research it generated, then return to the more general question of its implications for the dual-process models.

YES YOU CAN: HOPE FOR FREEING THE BEARS

Recently, we (Liberman & Förster, 2000, 2005; Förster & Liberman, 2001, 2004a, 2004b) suggested another model, the motivational inference model (MIMO) of PSR. We first propose that people may infer from the difficulty they experience during suppression or from suppression failures that they are motivated to use the suppressed construct. For example, a person trying to not think about his former lover may find this difficult and thinks: "If it is so hard for me to get him out of my mind, then it must be because I really want to think of him." We propose that this attribution of difficulty to motivation enhances the motivation to think of the suppressed construct, thereby also enhancing its accessibility, which in turn eventually produces PSR. As we discuss shortly, these attribution processes can enhance and even eliminate rebound.

A second fundamental difference between the models is that whereas the ironic monitoring model is based on semantic priming, the MIMO, according to which people infer motivation, is based on goal priming (Förster & Liberman, 2006; Förster, Liberman, & Friedman, 2007). Accessibility of goals is more dynamic than semantic priming, and follows different activation and decay patterns. In the following we summarize evidence for the inference process involved in PSR, then report studies showing that goal priming plays a role in PSR.

MIMO has been described in detail in former articles (Förster & Liberman, 2001, 2004a, 2004b; Liberman & Förster, 2000, 2005); therefore, we only briefly summarize the basic assumptions, then describe findings that support MIMO and bear relevance to models of "dual processes."

INFERENCE MECHANISMS: IT'S NOT YOU! IT'S ALL ABOUT THE BEARS!

According to self-perception theory (Bem, 1972) and the overjustification framework (Nisbett & Valins, 1972; Pittman & Heller, 1987), motivation may be inferred from overt behavior. For example, classic research has shown that providing extrinsic rewards for engaging in an attractive activity may undermine intrinsic interest and subsequent engagement in that activity (Lepper, Greene, & Nisbett, 1973). Presumably, people who thought that they performed an activity for a reward inferred that they were not interested in the activity. Perhaps even more relevant to suppression, imposing an extrinsic restriction on an initially unattractive activity was shown to enhance subsequent intrinsic motivation to engage in it (Wilson & Lassiter, 1982). Again, attribution processes could have played a role, in that people who performed an activity despite a threat of being punished for it inferred that the activity must be attractive. Such findings illustrate that people attribute their engagement in the activity (or refraining from it) to extrinsic causes and discount (or augment) their intrinsic motivation.

MIMO suggests that subjective difficulty typically (but not always) experienced during suppression may be used as informational input in self-relevant inferences. The general importance of difficulty in inference processes has been repeatedly demonstrated by Norbert Schwarz and his colleagues (Schwarz et al., 1991; Wänke, Schwarz, & Bless, 1995; Winkielman, Schwarz, & Belli, 1998). In a typical study (Schwarz et al., 1991), participants are asked to remember either a large number or a small number of diagnostic behavioral events (e.g., either six or 12 incidents of assertive behavior they performed), then rate themselves on a relevant dimension (e.g., indicate how assertive they are). These studies repeatedly find that listing a large number of events (which is relatively difficult) reduced ratings on the corresponding dimension. To illustrate, people rated themselves as less assertive after listing 12 assertive behaviors than after listing six. Presumably, people inferred from the experienced difficulty of retrieving 12 assertive behaviors a lack of assertiveness on their part.

In support of the proposed underlying inferences, Schwarz and his colleagues (1991) have shown that these effects may be altered by a misattribution manipulation. Thus, when participants were led to believe that the music played in the experimental room inhibited recall of 12 (vs. six) events, they did not reduce their self-ratings on assertiveness after recalling many incidents of assertive behavior. Presumably, in this case, they attributed the difficulty of retrieval to an external source (the music) and did not think it was indicative of lack of assertiveness on their part.

Combining self-perception, overjustification, and feelings-as-information accounts, we suggest that people may use experienced difficulty to infer their own motivations (see also Liberman & Förster, 2006). How could motivational inferences produce PSR? For example, in the studies by Wegner et al. (1987; Wegner & Gold, 1995), participants experienced suppression failures or intrusions of the suppressed thought. Participants may lack the knowledge that most people experience a substantial number of such intrusions (i.e., that the task is objectively difficult). They may then conclude that the failures are informative of their own motivational state: "If thoughts of white bears keep popping into my mind despite my attempts to suppress them, and I seem to be incapable of avoiding these stupid thoughts, I really need to finish at least these few white bear thoughts to get them off my mind." We therefore suggest that suppressing a certain thought activates the goal to think the forbidden thought.

In more natural social situations, as with suppression of stereotypes or tempting thoughts, the assumed attribution of motivation is even more plausible than in the original example of white bears. People may think: "If it is so hard for me to suppress thoughts about food, then I must want to eat," or "If it is hard for me not to think of my former lover, then it must be the case that I really want to think of him or her." Of course, in many situations people may have strong motivations and be well aware of them before engaging in suppression. In fact, they often attempt suppression precisely because they have that motivation. For example, people may want to eat, and may like to entertain thoughts about eating. In these cases, suppression that is accompanied by inferences from suppression difficulty could intensify these motivations: "If I try to suppress thought about food but find myself thinking of it again and again, it must be the case that I am craving it even more than I thought." This process is reminiscent of the experiments that instructed kids not to play with an unattractive toy, which made them more likely to do so (Wilson & Lassiter, 1982). What is important from the perspective of the MIMO model is not whether the motivation existed beforehand, but that as a result of these attributions, the motivation was created or intensified, therefore also enhancing the accessibility of goal-related constructs. Note that in order to start such inference processes, suppression failures are not necessary—experienced *difficulty, in the absence of actual failures to suppress* may suffice. This is consistent with research showing that PSR can also occur after rather successful suppression attempts, such as when participants asked to write nonracist descriptions about minority members and successfully avoided any stereotypes in their writing, yet felt that they had to put much effort in this task.

In summary, we suggest that people infer from suppression failures and the perceived difficulty of the suppression process that they are compelled to think of the suppressed construct (i.e., they infer a motivation to use the suppressed construct). This motivation, in turn, enhances the accessibility of goal-related constructs (Bargh, 1997; Bruner, 1957; Higgins & King, 1981) and thereby produces PSR.

If this is true, one would assume that any factors that influence difficulty, such as practice, cognitive load, or intrinsic motivation to suppress, would also influence the size of PSR. We now discuss some examples that bear on that reasoning.

CLASSIC STRATEGIES FOR TAMING THE BEARS

Practice

Practice seems to reduce PSR. For example, Kelly and Kahn (1994) found that suppression of frequently occurring intrusive thoughts, unlike suppression of novel thoughts provided by the experimenter, did not produce rebound effects. The ironic monitoring account argues that the strenuous process of suppression may become more efficient (i.e., more automatic) with practice, and therefore requires fewer resources and shifts the balance toward more effective suppression (Monteith, Spicer, et al., 1998; Wegner, 1994). MIMO, on the other hand, suggests that practice simply makes suppression easier: In other words, according to MIMO, the critical component of practice is that it provides less room for inferences from difficulty, not that it makes suppression more automatic.

Load

Research has shown repeatedly that PSR is stronger when participants engage in thought suppression under cognitive load compared to a no-load condition (Wegner, 1992, 1994; Wegner et al., 1987). Ironic monitoring theory explains that cognitive load interferes with the controlled process of looking for distractors, but not with the automatic process of ironic monitoring (e.g., Wegner, 1994). As a result, the ironic monitor, which enhances accessibility of the suppressed construct, also enhances PSR. Another possibility, in line with MIMO, is that load makes suppression more difficult, and that people may interpret this difficulty as indicating a particularly strong motivation to engage in the suppressed activity.

Galinsky and Moskowitz (2007) added complexity to the general notion that load enhances PSR. They showed that suppression of stereotypes not only causes high accessibility of stereotypical concepts but also brings counterstereotypical information to mind (e.g., the construct "honest" became more accessible to U.S. students upon suppressing thoughts of African Americans). This, however, only occurred when participants were not under cognitive load. When under cognitive load, stereotypical concepts were more accessible than counterstereotypical ones. The ironic monitoring model may explain such results via the interruption of a conscious search for valuable distractors, which in the case of stereotypes could be counterstereotypes (suppression in this study was induced by asking participants to not use any stereotypes in their descriptions, which may have naturally led to a focus on the opposite, counterstereotypical constructs). According to MIMO, however, participants under cognitive load may have struggled with finding counterstereotypical descriptions and may at the same time have felt that unwanted stereotypes popped into their minds. This could have shifted the motivation from thinking about counterstereotypes toward stereotypical information.

While load is the major variable in dual-process research, within MIMO it is only one among many variables that make suppression difficult. Moreover, MIMO suggests also other factors that may enhance or reduce PSR, namely, factors that alter the attributions people make for the experienced difficulty rather than the experience of difficulty itself. MIMO predicts that if participants are led to attribute the experienced difficulty to an external factor (e.g., the extra task that produces load) rather than to their motivation to think of the suppressed construct, then the effect of load on rebound would be undermined. Ironic monitoring theory, on the other hand, predicts the same effect of load on rebound regardless of the attribution participants make for the experienced difficulty.

Internal Motivation

In a study on the suppression of stereotypes, Monteith, Spicer, et al. (1998) showed that PSR does not occur with low-prejudice people. They theorized that low-prejudice people possess an internal (as opposed to external) motivation to suppress stereotypes (Monteith, Sherman, & Devine, 1998). Along the same line, a study by Gordijn, Hindriks, Koomen, Dijksterhuis, and van Knippenberg (2004) suggests that participants with high levels of internal motivation to respond without prejudice required no additional cognitive resources to suppress stereotypes, nor did they experience PSR. The latter study may suggest that low-prejudice people may not experience difficulty during suppression; it is possible that they have proceduralized strategies that make suppression easy to them (Kelly & Kahn, 1994). Another possibility is that the inferences that normally activate the motivation to use the suppressed construct are weaker with intrinsically motivated suppression than with extrinsically motivated suppression. Possibly, people who are convinced that they are not racist at all may be less inclined to interpret difficulty of suppression as a desire to use or think about the suppressed construct. Perhaps due to preexisting beliefs, low-prejudice people may find it easier to attribute difficulty to external sources.

A study conducted by Natalie Wyer (2007; Experiment 1) shed light on the motivational processes involved in suppression. She measured both modern racism (McConahay, 1986) and the motivation to control prejudiced responses (Dunton & Fazio, 1997), and assessed PSR upon suppression of racial stereotypes. Her study demonstrated that, generally, participants with high motivation to control prejudice were better in suppressing stereotypes in the first, suppression phase than those with low motivation—presumably because participants who did not want to control prejudice in general simply did not comply with suppression instructions. The latter group also showed less pronounced PSR than the group that efficiently suppressed stereotypes. However, racism moderated this effect, in that high PSR was found especially in people who scored high both in motivation to control prejudice and in modern racism. One may conclude then that people who scored low in racism with a high motivation to control racism either did not find suppression difficult (e.g., because they had likely proceduralized it), or did not attribute experienced difficulty to motivation to use the suppressed construct (e.g., because they knew that they did not have this motivation). As a result, they did not show PSR. On the other hand, racist people with a high motivation to control racism might have experienced difficulty during the suppression task and noticed a strong discrepancy between their ideal (e.g., not being racist) and their actual behavior (i.e., having racist thoughts), which in the end could lead to the conclusion: "If I try to control stereotypes so hard but still stereotypes are popping up, I must be really compelled to think about stereotypes." This is exactly the condition for which MIMO predicts the strongest PSR. In the following, we report research that points more directly to the assumed attribution processes as proposed by MIMO.

TAMING BEARS BY ATTRIBUTIONS

A series of studies examined more directly the processes of motivational inference that underlie PSR by altering the meaning of experienced difficulty (Förster & Liberman, 2001). Our first studies used the white bear paradigm and added a misattribution paradigm from Yzerbyt, Schadron, Leyens, and Rocher (1994). More specifically, during the first phase, in which participants were asked to suppress thoughts of white bears, they listened to a recording of unintelligible speech, which was an extract from a novel read aloud and played backwards. We told some participants that the tape would make it easy for them to suppress thoughts of white bears, because it would subliminally introduce concepts that interfere with such thoughts ("suppression-easy condition"). In contrast, other participants were told that the tape would make it difficult for them to suppress thoughts of white bears, because it would subliminally introduce these thoughts ("suppression-difficult condition"). We reasoned that for participants in the suppression-easy condition the inference process would be something like, "If it is difficult for me to suppress the thought in spite of the purported helpful effect of the tape, it must be because I am really compelled to think of white bears." Participants in the suppression-difficult condition, on the other hand, would engage in a different inference process, something like, "It is difficult for me to suppress the thoughts, but it must be the effect of the tape and not something special about me." We also included a no-attribution group, in which no tape was played in the first phase, and a control group, in which no suppression was introduced in the first phase. Relative to the no-tape condition, we predicted more rebound in the suppression-easy condition and less in the suppression-difficult condition.

Results were consistent with this prediction of MIMO: Telling participants that the tape would make suppression difficult not only reduced PSR but also actually eliminated it. The number of white bear thoughts in this condition was lower than in the no-tape condition and did not differ from the control (no suppression) condition. Telling participants that the tape would make suppression easy, however, enhanced rebound as compared to the no-tape condition. Thus, the study demonstrated both reduction and enhancement of rebound relative to the baseline level of rebound obtained in the no-tape condition.

A look at the correlations between suppression failures (the number of white bear thoughts during the suppression phase) and rebound (the number of white bear thoughts during the expression phase) is also informative. If participants interpreted suppression failures as indicating either high or low motivation to use the suppressed construct, then MIMO should predict a higher correlation between the two measures in the suppression-easy condition than in the suppression-difficult condition. This is precisely what we found. Finally, the correlations in the control condition were positive, significant, and closer to the suppression-easy condition than to the suppression-difficult condition, as would be expected naturally if people interpret suppression failures as indicating a high motivation to think about the suppressed construct. In another study, we replicated these results with a more direct manipulation of attribution, in which we explicitly told participants that suppression failures reflect either high or low motivation.

These studies point to possibilities to reduce PSR. Could the model be used to reduce unwanted PSR, such as rebound after suppression of stereotypes or after suppression of unwanted behavior such as aggression and (over) eating? Could there be more practical, easily implemented manipulations along the lines of those in the MIMO? What would happen if we merely informed participants about the fact that suppression of thoughts is difficult for everybody? In a series of studies we predicted that this simple manipulation would eliminate rebound via inferences such as "If it is difficult for everybody to suppress, then the difficulty I experience does not reflect my own motivation to think about the thing I am trying to suppress (or to do the thing I am trying not to do)."

In one series of studies, we asked German participants to suppress or not to suppress stereotypes while writing a story about a foreign worker, a stereotype that contained associations with crime (Förster & Liberman, 2001). Participants in the "suppression-difficult" condition were told that recent research has shown that avoiding stereotype use is difficult, even for people who are not prejudiced. We hypothesized that participants in this condition would not attribute the difficulty they experienced during suppression to their motivation to use the stereotype and would therefore not exhibit PSR. After writing the story for 5 minutes, participants were stopped, and the dependent measures were handed out. In one study, we gave participants a word stem completion task, with stems that could be solved with stereotypical words or words unrelated to the stereotype. This study showed that suppression without instructions compared to no suppression led to PSR; however, the mere instruction that "suppression is difficult" eliminated PSR even when participants suppressed stereotypes in the first phase. Importantly, in most of the studies, the descriptions that participants wrote during the suppression phase did not differ between the suppression groups and the suppression-difficult group with respect to stereotypicality. Thus, overall, telling participants that a difficulty to suppress is normative did not relax suppression attempts and legitimize stereotyping.

These results and others that conceptually replicated the studies with a diversity of dependent measures supported a MIMO account: In all the experiments, providing an external attribution for the difficulty to suppress ("This is difficult for everybody") eliminated PSR.

Interestingly, this intervention was also shown to reduce PSR after suppression of behavior (Denzler, Förster, Liberman, & Rozenman, 2010). In fact, MIMO is especially relevant for behavioral PSR because of its direct relation to motivational inferences and the assumed process of goal activation rather than semantic activation.

In a recent test of the implications of MIMO for behavioral rebound, in the first stage of the experiment, participants took the perspective of a protagonist watching her lover make love with her best friend. After having read the story, participants were asked to write down what they had in mind. Participants in the no-suppression group did not receive any further instructions. Participants in the suppression group were asked to suppress aggressive thoughts. Participants in the external attribution condition were told, in addition, that it is usually difficult for everybody to suppress aggressive thoughts in this type of situation. Using a lexical decision task containing aggression-related and -unrelated words, we found higher accessibility of aggression-related words in the suppression group compared to the control group, reflecting PSR. However, as predicted by MIMO, PSR was eliminated when participants were told that suppression is usually difficult.

In addition, as a behavioral aggression measure, we applied a picture selection task in which participants are asked to select 10 pictures out of 30 for another person, whom they did not know. Some of the photographs presented aversive scenes, and aggression was measured as the mean score of aversiveness of the pictures selected (Mussweiler & Förster, 2000). Participants who suppressed aggressive thoughts chose more negative pictures than participants who did not engage in suppression. Importantly, those who suppressed aggressive thoughts but were informed that suppression is difficult did not show this behavioral form of PSR. They selected about the same number of negative pictures as the control group. Findings were conceptually replicated with suppression of drinking and suppression of laughter (Denzler et al., 2010), and with suppression of scratching while reading about itching events (e.g., ants; Reuven-Magril et al., 2009).

To sum up, studies conducted in the framework of MIMO found that providing participants with external attribution for experienced difficulty to suppress thoughts reduced rebound of thoughts and behavior. Similarly, giving reasons to believe that suppression is easy increased PSR, presumably because in that case participants attributed suppression difficulty to their own motivation to think about the forbidden thought. We think that the studies support MIMO assumptions that inferences about motivation affect PSR. Let us now turn to the second main assumption of MIMO, namely, that motivation-related accessibility underlies PSR.

GOAL-PRIMING MECHANISMS: LET'S JUST TALK ABOUT THAT BEAR!

The second theoretical assumption of MIMO is that because suppression produces or intensifies the motivation to use the suppressed construct, PSR is based on goal priming rather than semantic priming. Because this distinction has been widely applied in the past, we summarize it only briefly (for more detailed reviews, see Förster, Liberman, & Friedman, 2007, 2009; Förster & Liberman, 2007; Liberman & Förster, 2005).

Many theories propose that motivational states, such as needs, goals, intentions, and concerns, are characterized by enhanced accessibility of motivation-related constructs, accessibility that eventually supports goal pursuit (Bruner, 1957; Anderson, 1983; Higgins & King, 1981; Wyer & Srull, 1989; Goschke & Kuhl, 1993; Kuhl, 1983, 1987; Gollwitzer & Moskowitz, 1996). Accessibility from motivational sources seems to have several characteristics that distinguish between it and accessibility from semantic priming.

First, accessibility from motivation persists as long as the motivation is active, therefore typically undergoing slower decay than semantic priming effects, at least before the goal as fulfilled. For example, Goschke and Kuhl (1993) had participants rehearse a series of actions, then informed them that they would either perform the actions (a goal) or observe another person performing them (no goal). Using a recognition test, they found faster and more accurate responses to the actions in the goal condition than in the no-goal condition, even when rehearsal of the actions was not possible in the intervening time. In both groups, the stimuli were processed to a similar extent, with similar time elapsed between processing and the measurement of accessibility. Nevertheless, accessibility was higher in the goal group than in the no goal group. These results were interpreted as supporting the notion of more persistent accessibility when motivation is involved compared to a nonmotivational, semantic priming state. Other evidence for the persistence of accessibility until goal fulfillment comes from research on frustrated goals. It was theorized that unfulfilled goals underlie rumination and intrusive thoughts (Martin & Tesser, 1996). Such activation remains until the individual reaches the original goal, reaches a substitute goal, or disengages from the goal all together (Lewin, 1951; Martin & Tesser, 1996). Consequently, unfulfilled goals may maintain the accessibility of goal-related constructs over extended periods of months or even years. In stark contrast, semantic priming usually decays after as little as a few minutes (Higgins, 1996).

Furthermore, accessibility from motivational sources is inhibited upon fulfillment of the goal, which reduces the corresponding motivation (Förster, Liberman, & Higgins, 2005; Marsh, Hicks, & Bink, 1998; Lewin, 1951; Marsh, Hicks, & Bryan, 1999; Zeigarnik, 1927). To illustrate, Marsh et al. (1998, 1999) extended the paradigm of Goschke and Kuhl (1993), mentioned earlier, and used a lexical decision task to examine the accessibility of intended actions both before and after completion. Replicating the work of Goschke and Kuhl, Marsh et al. (1998, 1999) found that prior to completion, accessibility of intended actions was enhanced relative to unintended (i.e., to be observed) actions. More importantly, after performance, the accessibility of the completed action was inhibited and became lower than that of observed actions, a result that is suggestive of postfulfillment inhibition (see also Förster et al., 2005; Liberman, Förster, & Higgins, 2007).

The proposed activation–deactivation pattern of accessibility from motivational sources is consistent with a functional view of the motivation–cognition interface, because it is conducive to efficient self-regulation (Lewin, 1951). Heightened accessibility of goal-related constructs helps in detection of stimuli that are instrumental for efficient goal pursuit in the environment (see Ach, 1935; Kuhl, 1983; Gollwitzer, 1999). However, upon goal fulfillment, "clearing up" the mental system from such constructs could be highly instrumental, because the accessibility of goal-related constructs loses its functionality and could potentially interfere with other tasks an individual faces.

According to MIMO, goal-related accessibility is underlying PSR. Specifically, MIMO suggests that participants infer a motivation to use the suppressed construct while they suppress it, and that enhanced accessibility after suppression is related to motivation. Thus, MIMO predicts that the accessibility of the suppressed construct persists as long as the motivation is active and would be inhibited once the motivation is fulfilled (i.e., in the context of suppression, after participants do the suppressed activity). Our model therefore predicts inhibition of motivation-related accessibility after goal fulfillment or, in other words, after expression. The ironic monitoring model is unspecific with respect to what kind of accessibility is produced by suppression, although some studies specifically related it to semantic priming (Macrae et al., 1998; Wegner & Erber, 1992). Importantly, semantic priming models predict an increase in accessibility after expression because of the aforementioned "recency principle." To give an example, expressing a stereotype would, according to semantic priming, increase accessibility. However, if expressing a stereotype constitutes fulfillment of a goal that got activated as a result of attributional processes during suppression, then it should decrease accessibility of the suppressed and then expressed construct.

To test this prediction, we conducted a series of experiments (Liberman & Förster, 2000) in which participants either suppressed or did not suppress a construct, then, in the second stage, either expressed or did not express the same construct. We expected first to replicate PSR, showing that when no expression is introduced, accessibility would be higher after suppression than after no suppression (suppression–no expression: PSR high). Second, we predicted a classic priming effect for participants who did not suppress thoughts but only used them (no suppression–expression: semantic priming). The critical prediction concerned the way these two effects would combine. Specifically, if suppression produces accessibility by inducing motivation to express the forbidden construct, then expression after suppression should satisfy that motivation and instigate inhibition of related constructs (suppression–expression: no PSR). Therefore, it would result in lower accessibility than either suppression alone (a state in which an active goal continues to exist) or expression alone (a state in which accessibility due to semantic priming exists).

In a series of studies, participants were asked to describe a colorful Miró painting, so that another person would be able to imagine the picture without actually seeing it. Participants in the no-suppression condition received no further instructions, while participants in the suppression condition were told to avoid using any words related to color. After this first stage, half of the participants in each condition, assigned to the expression condition, were asked to describe a colorful Kandinsky painting, again, so that another person would be able to imagine the picture without seeing it. They were explicitly told to describe the picture by using many color words. The rest of the participants, assigned to the no-expression condition, did not describe a second picture and proceeded directly with the next stage, in which accessibility was measured. After completing the picture descriptions, all participants were introduced to a seemingly unrelated word stem completion task (including stems that could be solved with words related or unrelated to colors) measuring the accessibility of color words. Results showed that both suppressing and using color words (without suppression beforehand) enhanced the use of colors. More importantly, and as predicted, despite the fact that expression of color words obviously involved processing them, it reduced their accessibility when it *followed* suppression.

We also measured the experienced difficulty of writing the picture description and the motivation to use color words if participants had to describe another picture at the end of the study. The results showed that motivation to use colors was higher in the suppression, no-expression condition than in the other three conditions, which did not significantly differ from each other. This also means that introducing expression after suppression reduced the motivation to use colors. As a measure of difficulty, participants explicitly indicated how difficult it was to describe the picture. Central for our model especially were the relations among perceived difficulty, motivation, and accessibility of color words in the suppression, no-expression condition. Consistent with MIMO, the more difficult a person experienced the suppression task to be, the more accessible the suppressed construct. Most importantly, a mediational analysis showed that motivation mediated the effect of difficulty on the accessibility of color words in the suppression, no-expression condition: Thus, when participants had to describe the picture without using color words, they experienced difficulty and interpreted it as indicating a motivation to use color words. As a result, the accessibility and the motivation to use color words was enhanced.

Two additional studies examined our hypothesis with suppression of stereotypes. Here again, allowing participants to express stereotypes upon suppression eliminated PSR. Thus, across different content domains, introducing expression after suppression eliminated PSR, an effect that is consistent with our notion that the accessibility produced by suppression stems from a motivation to use the suppressed construct. Inasmuch the ironic monitoring model is based on semantic priming, such results cannot be explained by it.

More recent research shows other moderating variables of PSR that are consistent with this view of how goal fulfillment affects PSR (see Guinote, 2007). For example, Koole and van Knippenberg (2007) showed that self-affirmation after suppression of stereotypes eliminated PSR. More specifically, the authors asked participants to describe a bodybuilder and suppress stereotypes or to write a description, without further suppression instructions. After suppression they received fake positive (e.g., "You are very social") or neutral (e.g., "You are reasonably social") feedback on a personality questionnaire they had filled out before describing the bodybuilder. Afterwards a word stem completion measured accessibility of stereotypes related to bodybuilders. PSR was eliminated after self-affirmation.

The authors interpreted these results in line with MIMO, suggesting that a more general, global experience of goal completion suffices to eliminate PSR. Somewhat similarly, Martin and Tesser (1996) suggested that PSR is rumination about the failure to suppress. They presented results that indicated telling people they were good at suppression reduced PSR. It is possible that this positive feedback reduced the feeling that they had not completed the goal or perhaps eliminated unpleasant feelings, such as the feeling of difficulty to suppress.

It is important to note that Martin, Tesser, and Cornell (1996) suggested the operation of a slightly different goal as underlying PSR than the goal assumed by MIMO. Within MIMO, the goal to use the suppressed construct is driving PSR, whereas in a the model proposed by Martin et al., it is the goal to suppress that needs to be fulfilled in order to stop rumination processes. Experiencing success during suppression or accepting positive feedback on suppression attempts eliminates PSR, because it stops rumination about suppression failures. While MIMO can account for Martin et al.'s finding, it is difficult to explain our results by pure rumination based on failures to suppress. Future research should focus on these different motivations as possible precursors of PSR in order to deepen our understanding of PSR and the means to reduce it.

To summarize, studies conducted in the framework of MIMO provide evidence for the idea that suppression produces motivation-related accessibility. We think that this motivation is produced or enhanced by attributing the difficulty experienced during suppression or suppression failures to a motivation to perform the suppressed activity. Let us now consider this model and the research it generated within the broader context of dual-process models.

SUPPRESSION AS A DUAL PROCESS

We started this chapter by presenting Wegner's (1994) ironic monitoring model of suppression, according to which suppression involves controlled and automatic processes that work in opposition to each other.We then presented the MIMO, which is an attempt to replace this dual-process model with a single process of interpreting one's own experiences of suppression and the consequences of this inference process for goal-related accessibility. Our model is silent with respect to the question of whether this process is automatic or not. Indeed, our process is metacognitive in nature, in the sense that people interpret their own mental states. These inferences, like many other inferences, however, can be both conscious and unconscious (for an example of automatic trait inferences, see Willis & Todorov, 2006), efficient (due to extensive repetition and proceduralization, see Förster & Jostmann, 2012) or resource-consuming. They sometimes start without intention but at other times may be the product of an intended rumination about one's performance. Thus, examining separately the different criteria for automaticity (consciousness, efficiency, unintentionality; Bargh, 1994) leads to the conclusion that each criterion does not apply to all cases of

PSR, although PSR might, at times, satisfy each of them.

We think that suppression and PSR are flexible processes: The resources they take, their accessibility to awareness and intentionality, are not defining properties of these processes. Rather, the extent to which suppression and PSR are automatic is determined, as with many other cognitive, emotional, and behavioral processes, by their difficulty, by the other processes that run at the same time, as well as by the motivational, cognitive, and emotional state of the actor. We believe that the MIMO model contributes to the literature an attempt to replace a dual-process model with a model that is more akin to the unimodel view (Kruglanski & Thompson, 1999). Our single-process model assumes a process that is flexible, complex, and propositional (Mitchell, De Houwer, & Lovibond, 2009a, 2009b), yet may be performed efficiently and unconsciously.

Why is suppression so often difficult? Does it suggest that one's stream of thought runs automatically? Possibly. At times, our thoughts start unintentionally and proceed despite attempts to stop them. Trained in prospection, our mind paints for us future scenarios and counterfactual worlds that we did not ask it to produce. But suppression, we believe, is difficult for another reason, which is that it incorporates a paradox of negation—it is impossible to not think of a white bear without first representing that bear (Wegner et al., 2011).

CONCLUDING REMARKS

In this chapter, we have presented MIMO, a model that explains PSR as being the result of inferences about one's motivation. We have presented findings generated in the framework of this model that cannot be explained by Wegner's dual-system ironic monitoring account. Moreover, we do not think that a classic dual-process distinction applies to the processes we discovered. Whereas in the ironic monitoring model PSR naturally follows suppression and produces a vicious circle of activation, in MIMO it depends on inferences and goal activation that can be changed relatively easily. This is important, since recently PSR was introduced as a causal factor in a wide range of psychological disorders (Najmi & Wegner, 2008); therefore, it is also useful for practitioners to learn more about possible ways to alter PSR.

REFERENCES

Ach, N. (1935). Analyse des Willens. In E. Abderhalden (Ed.), *Handbuch der biologischen Arbeitsmethoden* [](Vol. VI). Berlin: Urban & Schwarzenberg [Analysis of will-acts. *Handbook of biological methods*].

Anderson, J. R. (1983). *The architecture of cognition.* Cambridge, MA: Harvard University Press. Harvard

Bargh, J. A. (1994). The four horsemen of automaticity: Awareness, intention, efficiency, and control in social cognition. In R. S. Wyer & T. K. Srull (Eds.), *Handbook of social cognition* (2 ed., pp. 1–40). Hilldale, NJ: Erlbaum.

Bargh, J. A. (1997). The automaticity of everyday life. In R. S. Wyer, Jr. & T. K. Srull (Eds.), *Handbook of social cognition* (Vol. 10, pp. 1–61). Hillsdale, NJ: Erlbaum.

Bargh, J. A., Chen, M., & Burrows, L. (1996). Automaticity of social behaviour: Direct effects of trait construct and stereotype activation on action. *Journal of Personality and Social Psychology, 71*, 230–244.

Bem, D. J. (1972). Self-perception theory. In L. Berkowitz (Ed.), *Advances in experimental social psychology* (Vol. 6, pp. 1–62). New York: Academic Press.

Bruner, J. S. (1957). Going beyond the information given. In H. E. Gruber, K. H. Hammond, & R. Jessor (Eds.), *Contemporary approaches to cognition* (pp. 41–69). Cambridge, MA: Harvard University Press.

Davies, M. I., & Clark, D. M. (1998). Thought suppression produces rebound effect with analogue post-traumatic intentions. *Behaviour Research and Therapy, 36*, 571–582.

Denzler, M., Förster, J., Liberman, N., & Rozenman, M. (2010). Aggressive, funny and thirsty: A motivational inference model (MIMO) approach to behavioral rebound. *Personality and Social Psychology Bulletin, 36*, 1385–1396.

Dijksterhuis, A., & Bargh, J. A. (2001). The perception–behavior expressway: Automatic effects of social perception on social behavior. In M. Zanna (Ed.), *Advances in experimental social psychology* (Vol. 33, pp. 1–40). San Diego: Academic Press.

Dijksterhuis, A., & Nordgren, L. F. (2006). A theory of unconscious thought. *Perspectives on Psychological Science, 1,* 95–109.

Dunton, B. C., & Fazio, R. H. (1997). An individual difference measure of motivation to control prejudiced reactions. *Personality and Social Psychology Bulletin, 23,* 316–326.

Förster, J., & Jostmann, N. (2012). What is automatic self-regulation? *Zeitschrift für Psychologie, 220*(3), 147–156.

Förster, J., & Liberman, N. (2001). The role of attribution of motivation in producing postsuppressional rebound. *Journal of Personality and Social Psychology, 81,* 377–390.

Förster, J., & Liberman, N. (2004a). A motivational model of post-suppressional rebound. *European Review of Social Psychology, 15,* 1–32.

Förster, J., & Liberman, N. (2004b). How motivational inferences influence post-suppressional rebound. In S. Shohov (Ed.), *Advances in psychology research* (Vol. 34, pp. 63–88). New York: Nova Science.

Förster, J., & Liberman, N. (2007). Knowledge activation. In E. T. Higgins & A. W. Kruglanski (Eds.), *Social psychology: Handbook of basic principles* (2nd ed.). New York: Guilford Press.

Förster, J., Liberman, N., & Friedman, R. (2007). Seven principles of goal activation: A systematic approach to distinguishing goal priming from priming of non-goal constructs. *Personality and Social Psychology Review, 11,* 211–233.

Förster, J., Liberman, N., & Friedman, R. (2009). What do we prime?: On distinguishing between semantic priming, procedural and goal priming. In E. Morsella , J. Bargh, & P. Gollwitzer (Eds.), *The Oxford handbook of human action* (pp. 173–193). New York: Oxford University Press.

Förster, J., Liberman, N., & Higgins, E. T. (2005). Accessibility from active and fulfilled goals. *Journal of Experimental Social Psychology, 41,* 220–239.

Galinsky, A. D., & Moskowitz, G. B. (2007). Further ironies of suppression: Stereotype and counter-stereotype accessibility. *Journal of Experimental Social Psychology, 42,* 833–841.

Gollwitzer, P. M. (1999). Implementation intentions: Strong effects of simple plans. *American Psychologist, 54,* 493–503

Gollwitzer, P. M., & Moskowitz, G. B. (1996). Goal effects on action and cognition. In E. T. Higgins & A. W. Kruglanski (Eds.), *Social psychology: Handbook of basic principles* (pp. 361–399). New York: Guilford Press.

Gordijn, E. H., Hindriks, I., Koomen, W., Dijksterhuis, A., & van Knippenberg, A. (2004). Consequences of stereotype suppression and internal suppression motivation: A self-regulation approach. *Personality and Social Psychology Bulletin, 30,* 212–224.

Goschke, T., & Kuhl, J. (1993). Representation of intentions: Persisting activation in memory. *Journal of Experimental Psychology: Learning, Memory, and Cognition, 19,* 1211–1226.

Guinote, A. (2007). Power and the suppression of unwanted thoughts: Does control over others decrease control over the self? *Journal of Experimental Social Psychology* 43, 433–440.

Higgins, E. T. (1996). Knowledge activation: Accessibility, applicability, and salience. In E. T. Higgins & A. W. Kruglanski (Eds.), *Social psychology: Handbook of basic principles* (pp. 133–169). New York: Guilford Press.

Higgins, E. T., & King, G. A. (1981). Accessibility of social constructs: Information-processing consequences of individual and contextual variability. In N. Cantor & J. Kihlstrom (Eds.), *Personality, cognition and social interaction* (pp. 69–122). Hillsdale, NJ: Erlbaum.

Kelly, A. E., & Kahn, J. H. (1994). Effects of suppression of personal intrusive thoughts. *Journal of Personality and Social Psychology, 66,* 998–1006.

Koole, S. L., & van Knippenberg, A. (2007). Controlling your mind without ironic consequences: Self affirmation eliminates rebound effects after thought suppression. *Journal of Experimental Social Psychology, 43*(4), 671–677.

Kruglanski, A. W., & Thompson, E. P. (1999). Persuasion by a single route: A view from the unimodel. *Psychological Inquiry, 10,* 83–110.

Kuhl, J. (1983). *Motivation, konflikt und handlungskontrolle* [Motivation, conflict and action]. New York: Springer.

Kuhl, J. (1987). Action control: The maintenance of motivational states. In F. Halisch & J. Kuhl (Eds.), *Motivation, intention, and volition* (pp. 279–291). New York: Springer.

Lepper, M. R., Greene, D., & Nisbett, R. E. (1973). Undermining children's intrinsic interest with extrinsic rewards: A test of the overjustification hypothesis. *Journal of Personality and Social Psychology, 28,* 129–137.

Lewin, K. (1951). *Field theory in social science.* New York: Harper.

Liberman, N., & Förster, J. (2000). Expression after suppression: A motivational explanation of post-suppressional rebound. *Journal of Personality and Social Psychology, 79,* 190–203.

Liberman, N., & Förster, J. (2005). Motivation and construct accessibility. In J. P. Forgas, K. D. Kipling, & S. M. Laham (Eds.), *Social motivation: Conscious and unconscious processes* (pp. 228–248). Cambridge, UK: Cambridge University Press.

Liberman, N., & Förster, J. (2006). Inferences from decision difficulty. *Journal of Experimental Social Psychology, 42,* 290–302.

Liberman, N., Förster, J., & Higgins, E. T. (2007). Completed vs. interruped priming: Reduced accessibility from post-fulfillment inhibition. *Journal of Experimental Social Psychology, 43,* 258–264.

Macrae, C. N., Bodenhausen, G. V., & Milne, A. B. (1998). Saying no to unwanted thoughts: Self-focus and the regulation of mental life. *Journal of Personality and Social Psychology, 72,* 578–589.

Macrae, C. N., Bodenhausen, G. V., Milne, A. B., & Jetten, J. (1994). Out of mind but back in sight: Stereotypes on the rebound. *Journal of Personality and Social Psychology, 67,* 808–817.

Marsh, R. L., Hicks, J. L., & Bink, M. L. (1998). Activation of completed, uncompleted and partially completed intentions. *Journal of Experimental Psychology: Learning, Memory, and Cognition, 24,* 350–361.

Marsh, R. L., Hicks, J. L., & Bryan, E. S. (1999). The activation of unrelated and canceled intentions. *Memory and Cognition, 27,* 320–327.

Martin, L. L., & Tesser, A. (1996). Some ruminative thoughts. In R. S. Wyer (Ed.), *Advances in social cognition* (Vol. 2, pp. 1–48). Hillsdale, NJ: Erlbaum.

Martin, L. L., Tesser, A., & Cornell, D. P. (1996). On the substitutability of self-protective mechanisms. In P. M. Gollwitzer & J. A. Bargh (Eds.), *The psychology of action: Linking cognition and motivation to behavior* (pp. 48–68). New York: Guilford Press.

McConahay, J. B. (1986). Modern racism, ambivalence, and the Modern Racism Scale. In J. F. Dovidio & S. L. Gaertner (Eds.), *Prejudice, discrimination and racism* (pp. 91–126). New York: Academic Press.

Mitchell, C. J., De Houwer, J., & Lovibond, P. F. (2009a). The propositional nature of human associative learning. *Behavioral and Brain Sciences, 32,* 183–198.

Mitchell, C. J., De Houwer, J., & Lovibond, P. F. (2009b). Link-based learning theory creates more problems than it solves. *Behavioral and Brain Sciences, 32,* 230–246.

Monteith, M. J., Sherman, J. W., & Devine, P. G. (1998). Suppression as a stereotype control strategy. *Personality and Social Psychology Review, 2,* 63–82.

Monteith, M. J., Spicer, C. V., & Tooman, J. D. (1998). Consequences of stereotype suppression: Stereotypes on and not on the rebound. *Journal of Experimental Social Psychology, 34,* 355–377.

Mussweiler, T., & Förster, J. (2000). The sex → aggression link: A perception–behavior dissociation. *Journal of Personality and Social Psychology, 79,* 507–520.

Najmi, S., & Wegner, D. M. (2008). Thought suppression and psychopathology. In A. Elliot (Ed.), *Handbook of approach and avoidance motivation* (pp. 447–459). Mahwah, NJ: Erlbaum.

Neely, J. H. (1991). Semantic priming effects in visual word recognition: A selective review of current findings and theories. In D. Besner & G. W. Humphreys, (Eds.), *Basic processes in reading: Visual word recognition* (pp. 264–336). Hillsdale, NJ: Erlbaum.

Nisbett, R. E., & Valins, S. (1972). Perceiving the causes of one's own behavior. In E. Jones, D. Kanouse, H. Kelly, R. Nisbett, S. Valins, & B. Weiner (Eds.), *Attribution: Perceiving the causes of behavior* (pp. 1–27). Morristown, NJ: General Learning.

Pittman, T. S. & Heller, J. F. (1987). Social motivation. *Annual Review of Psychology, 38,* 461–489.

Reuven-Magril, O., Rosenman, M., Liberman, N., & Dar, R. (2009). Manipulating metacognitive beliefs about the difficulty to suppress scratching: Implications for obsessive–compulsive disorder. *International Journal of Cognitive Therapy: Special Section: Metacognition, 2,* 143–151.

Schwarz, N., Bless, H., Strack, F., Klumpp, G., Rittenauer-Schatka, H., & Simons, A. (1991). Ease of retrieval as information: Another look at the availability heuristic. *Journal of Personality and Social Psychology, 61,* 195–202.

Srull, T. K., & Wyer, R. S. (1979). The role of category accessibility in the interpretation of information about persons: Some determinants and implications. *Journal of Personality and Social Psychology, 37,* 1660–1672.

Wänke, M., Schwarz, N., & Bless, H. (1995). The availability heuristic revisited: Experienced ease of retrieval in mundane frequency estimates. *Acta Psychologica, 89,* 83–90.

Wegner, D. M. (1992). You can't always think what you want: Problems in the suppression of unwanted thoughts. In M. Zanna (Ed.), *Advances in experimental social psychology* (Vol. 25, pp. 193–225). San Diego: Academic Press.

Wegner, D. M. (1994). Ironic processes of mental control. *Psychological Review, 101,* 34–52.

Wegner, D. M. (2011). Setting free the bears: Escape from thought suppression. *American Psychologist, 66,* 671–680.

Wegner, D. M., & Erber, R. (1992). The hyperaccessibility of suppressed thoughts. *Journal of Personality and Social Psychology, 63,* 903–912.

Wegner, D. M., Erber, R., & Zanakos, S. (1993). Ironic processes in the mental control of mood and mood related thought. *Journal of Personality and Social Psychology, 65,* 1093–1104.

Wegner, D. M., & Gold, D. G. (1995). Fanning old flames: Emotional and cognitive effects of suppressing thought of past relationship. *Journal of Personality and Social Psychology, 68,* 782–792.

Wegner, D. M., Schneider, D. J., Carter, S., & White, L. (1987). Paradoxical effects of thought suppression. *Journal of Personality and Social Psychology, 53,* 5–13.

Wegner, D. M., & Wenzlaff, R. M. (1996). Mental control. In E. T. Higgins & A. W. Kruglanski (Eds.), *Social psychology: Handbook of basic principles* (pp. 466–492). New York: Guilford Press.

Willis, J., & Todorov, A. (2006). First impressions: Making up your mind after a 100-ms exposure to a face. *Psychological Science, 17,* 592–598.

Wilson, T. D., & Lassiter, G. D. (1982). Increasing intrinsic interest with superfluous extrinsic constraints. *Journal of Personality and Social Psychology, 42,* 811–819.

Winkielman, P., Schwarz, N., & Belli, R. F. (1998). The role of ease of retrieval and attribution in memory judgments: Judging your memory as worse despite recalling more events. *Psychological Science, 9,* 124–126.

Wyer, N. A. (2007). Motivational influences on compliance with and consequences of instructions to suppress stereotypes. *Journal of Experimental Social Psychology, 43,* 417–424.

Wyer, N. A., Sherman, J. W., & Stroessner, S. J. (1998). The spontaneous suppression of racial stereotypes. *Social Cognition, 16,* 340–352.

Wyer, R. S., & Srull, T. K. (1989). *Memory and cognition in its social context.* Hillsdale, NJ: Erlbaum.

Yzerbyt, V. Y., Schadron, G., Leyens, J. P., & Rocher, S. (1994). Social judgeability: The impact of meta-informational cues on the use of stereotypes. *Journal of Personality and Social Psychology, 66,* 48–55.

Zeigarnik, B. (1927). Das Behalten erledigter und unerledigter Handlungen [The memory of completed and uncompleted tasks]. *Psychologische Forschung, 9,* 1–85.

CHAPTER 30

The Explicit and Implicit Ways of Overcoming Temptation

Ayelet Fishbach and Luxi Shen

The ability to exercise self-control and overcome temptation is the key to achieving many positive life outcomes, including academic and career success, good health, and strong social ties. Furthermore, the lack of self-control is associated with negative outcomes, including addiction, overspending, and crime (Baron, 2003; Baumeister & Tierney, 2011; Gottfredson & Hirschi, 1990; Loewenstein, 1996; Mischel, Cantor, & Feldman, 1996; Thaler & Shefrin, 1981). Indeed, the modern lifestyle of people in Western societies is a constant battle for self-control: People have the power and the skills to achieve positive life outcomes, but they often lack the ability to resist temptations that prevent these outcomes.

A *self-control dilemma* is an internal conflict between a high-order and often long-term goal and a low-order and often short-term temptation (Ainslie, 1992; Carver, 2005; de Ridder, Lensvelt-Mulders, Finkenauer, Stok, & Baumeister, 2012; Duckworth & Kern, 2011; Hoch & Loewenstein, 1991; Rachlin, 2000; Thaler, 1991). For example, a diner may want to keep in shape while enjoying a fatty dessert or a parent may hope to prevent future whining while also being willing to quiet a complaining child with candy. What marks a successful exercise of self-control, in turn, is the pursuit of high-order goals and overcoming temptation.

Traditionally, self-control researchers focused on the explicit processes of resisting temptation, suggesting that both the experience of a goal–temptation conflict and the response to the conflict require conscious awareness and effort (Mischel, Shoda, & Rodriguez, 1989; Muraven & Baumeister, 2000). A main conclusion from past research is that self-control is inherently dif?cult and bound to fail if overused. Although we agree that self-control can be a conscious and taxing process, we argue that it is not always. An implicit and nonconscious operation mode of self-control exists, and it enables a smooth pursuit of long-term interests (Alberts, Martijn, Greb, Merkelbach, & De Vries, 2007; Ferguson, 2008; Fishbach, Friedman, & Kruglanski, 2003; Fitzsimons & Bargh, 2004; Kroese, Adriaanse, Evers, & de Ridder, 2011; Wiers & Stacy, 2006). We further suggest that when people become aware they are exercising self-control, this awareness arises partially because the conflict they face is particularly difficult and therefore not resolved prior to the recruitment of conscious awareness. By definition, then, a self-control response that requires awareness is one that is elicited in reaction to a difficult-to-resolve conflict and will therefore be more likely to fail than an implicit self-control response that does not require awareness. Because self-control research mainly focuses on explicit processes (with notable exceptions), a general bias exists in this literature toward self-control failures.

In this chapter, we address the explicit and implicit processes of self-control. Specifically, we investigate the identification of and the response to a self-control conflict, and argue that each challenge—identifying and responding to a conflict—involves implicit processes that either accompany or substitute for explicit processes. We use the terms *explicit* and *implicit* to refer to the degree of conscious awareness involved in the self-control process. Although assuming that awareness varies by degree and represents a continuum is reasonable, for the sake of simplicity (and without compromising accuracy), we refer to two extreme situations: when the self-control process is completely under conscious awareness and when it is not.

Our analysis of self-control differs in an important aspect from other dual-process models of self-control (Bechara, Noel, & Crone, 2006; Fudenberg & Levine, 2006; Hofmann, Friese, & Strack, 2009; Metcalfe & Mischel, 1999; Strack & Deutsch, 2004): We focus on the similarities between the two modes, whereas other research addresses the differences. Other models distinguish between an implicit and associative process that promotes giving in to temptation and an explicit and rule-based (self-control) process that promotes goal adherence. We argue that explicit and implicit self-control modes operate in tandem and follow the same basic principles. Our model therefore echoes recent discoveries in attitude research. Traditional models of attitudinal control asserted that stereotyping is an automatic response that is overridden by controlled processes (Devine, 1989; Fazio, Sanbonmatsu, Powell, & Kardes, 1986). However, according to recent work, the implementation of control can become automatized to the same or to a similar extent as the initial activation of the attitude (Monteith, Ashburn-Nardo, Voils, & Czopp, 2002; Moskowitz, Gollwitzer, Wasel, & Schaal, 1999; Payne, 2001; Sherman et al., 2008). Similarly, we identify situations in which the corrective, self-control response is no less automatic than the direct activation of desire by the presence of temptation. Thus, in our model, both the direct response to temptation with desire and the self-control response that inhibits the desire involve implicit (as well as explicit) processes.

In what follows, we describe a two-stage model of exercising self-control that suggests self-control success requires that a person first identify a self-control conflict, then retrieve self-control operations designed to increase the motivational strength of the goal and decrease the motivational strength of temptation. We discuss the explicit and implicit processes in each of these stages.

A TWO-STAGE MODEL: IDENTIFICATION AND RESOLUTION

For successful self-control, individuals need to know when and how to exercise restraint (see Figure 30.1). With respect to "when," people implement self-control only if they have identified a self-control conflict. At times, the question of identification is trivial. Thus, the person who considers losing her temper in a meeting with her boss might easily recognize the long-term consequence of raising her voice at an employer. In addition, self-control researchers often provide their study participants with already identified self-control problems. For example, researchers asked children participants to delay the gratification of consuming a small candy now in favor of getting a large candy later (Mischel et al., 1989); they requested that adult participants inhibit thinking about a particular concept (e.g., "white bears"; Wegner, Schneider, Carter, & White, 1987) or inhibit various dominant responses (Muraven & Baumeister, 2000). However, at other times, identification is not trivial, because the cost of a single lack of restraint is negligible; for example, the cost of a single donut for a dieter's weight, a single cigarette for a smoker's health, and a single day off for a professional's career prospects is trivial. We coined the term *epsilon temptation* to describe situations in which the cost of a single indulgence, or unit consumption cost, is negligible, but that of extended consumption may prove serious. Such temptations are pervasive in modern life and pose the problem of conflict identification. We further

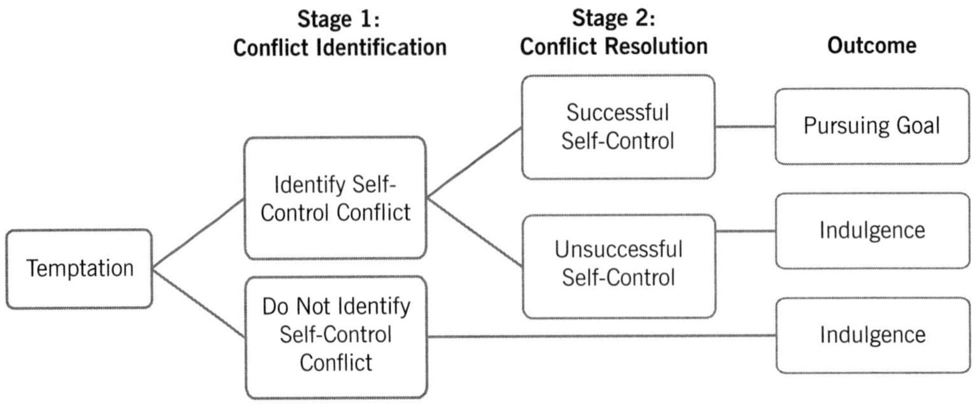

FIGURE 30.1. Two challenges of self-control: Identification and resolution. Data from Myrseth and Fishbach (2009).

argue the process of conflict identification is almost always of a nonconscious, implicit nature.

To the extent that a self-control conflict is identified upon presentation of temptation, the person is likely to exert self-control. Although identification processes can then be maintained or reactivated as part of resolving the conflict (e.g., when framing choice as a self-control problem promotes restraint), it is only to the extent that self-control conflict was identified in the first place that people exercise self-control. Our research on counteractive control theory describes the process by which individuals offset the influence of temptation on goal pursuit (Fishbach & Trope, 2005; Myrseth, Fishbach, & Trope, 2009; Sheldon & Fishbach, 2011; Trope & Fishbach, 2000; Zhang & Fishbach, 2010). According to this theory, self-control involves asymmetrical shifts in motivational strength: an increase in motivation to pursue a goal and a decrease in motivation to embrace temptation. Such asymmetrical shifts may be conscious or not. In what follows, we elaborate on the explicit and implicit operations of identifying conflict and responding to conflict with restraint.

CONFLICT IDENTIFICATION

Several factors contribute to conflict identification, mostly outside of conscious awareness, although once a conflict has been identified, people may be aware of it.

Width

Viewing an action opportunity in relation to future opportunities (i.e., a wide bracket) facilitates conflict identification, because doing so emphasizes the significant cost of aggregated temptation (Myrseth & Fishbach, 2009). Thus, the smoker who says, "One cigarette won't kill me," perceives the temptation in isolation, notes the trivial costs associated with smoking a single cigarette, and likely does not experience a conflict. The smoker who considers smoking this week or this month, however, may be more likely to perceive the cost of smoking for her long-term health, because she considers the impact of aggregated smoking. As an example of the effect of a wide frame, Read, Loewenstein, and Kalyanaraman (1999) found that when choosing several movies for several days simultaneously (i.e., a wide bracket), choosers selected more highbrow than lowbrow movies (e.g., *Schindler's List* vs. *My Cousin Vinny*) than when they chose sequentially, one day at a time (i.e., a narrow bracket). People apparently would like to watch highbrow movies but are tempted by lowbrow alternatives; therefore, planning their movie consumption for a period of time helps incorporate some highbrow movies.

Research on frame widths often assumes a conscious process of reasoning through the decision (Rachlin, 2000; Read, Loewenstein, & Rabin, 1999; Read, Loewenstein, & Kalyanaraman, 1999; Sussman & Alter, 2012; Wood & Neal, 2007). However, implicit and subtle cues also activate perception of a wide versus narrow bracket and promote conflict identification. In studies that illustrate this possibility, food choices suggesting predictable patterns of repetition promoted self-control more than one-time food choices. For example, Myrseth and Fishbach (2009) invited passersby to help themselves to an assortment of carrots and chocolates. In one condition, the food stand had a sign that read "April 12th Stand" (a narrow bracket), and in another condition, it read "Spring Food Stand" (a wide bracket). The narrow bracket led to greater consumption of chocolates (vs. carrots) than did the wide bracket.

Consistency

To activate perception of self-control conflict, an individual not only needs to consider a sequence of related choices, but should also see herself consistently making the same choice across these opportunities. If she perceives that she will exercise restraint on some opportunities and give in to temptations on others, the perception of a wide bracket would not promote restraint. A behavioral pattern that reflects consistency is titled "highlighting"—restraint promotes further effort to exercise restraint at the next opportunity. For example, a healthy entrée choice can encourage a person also to choose a healthy dessert. A behavioral pattern that reflects absence of consistency is titled "balancing"—restraint provides a psychological license to indulge. For example, a healthy entrée choice can justify an unhealthy dessert choice (Dhar & Simonson, 1999; Fishbach & Dhar, 2005; Fishbach, Dhar, & Zhang, 2006; Fishbach & Zhang, 2008; Koo & Fishbach, 2008).

Several situational cues activate a highlighting versus balancing choice dynamic and therefore influence conflict identification. For example, the presentation of goal and temptation options separately, in two separate displays, nonconsciously promotes identification of a self-control conflict and highlighting, whereas presenting these options together, in a single display, nonconsciously hinders conflict identification and promotes balancing. In one experimental demonstration, participants consumed more healthy carrots and fewer unhealthy chocolates when these items were served in separate bowls than when they were served together in one bowl (Fishbach & Zhang, 2008). This study further demonstrated that the choice of chocolates in the separate-bowls condition reflected the failure to identify a self-control dilemma: Individual differences in the strength of the weight-watching goal (i.e., how much the participant wanted to lose weight) predicted healthy over tempting choices only when the options were presented in separate bowls, but not when they were presented together in the same bowl. Physically presenting the temptation and goal options separately (vs. together) enabled psychological identification of the self-control conflict and the exercise of self-control.

At times, the perception of inconsistency across actions or choices (i.e., balancing) provides a psychological license to indulge or relax one's moral standards (Khan & Dhar, 2006; Mazar & Zhong, 2010; Monin & Miller, 2001). In these situations, people use past or future virtuous choices to justify giving in to temptation in the present. For example, people are more likely to choose a luxury over a utilitarian good after indicating their intent to engage in a charitable act (Khan & Dhar, 2006). Psychological licensing reflects a failure to see a particular choice or action as posing a self-control conflict, because a person assumes her behavior in the present is different than past or future behavior.

Ease of Monitoring

When monitoring indulgence is trivial, the individual can (consciously or not) take a mental note of relapses, which in turn eases conflict identification. In contrast, when monitoring is difficult, relapses go unnoticed and do not promote conflict identification. For example, when consuming cookies of irregular and uneven (vs. similar) shape, people often have difficulty monitoring consumption, because the unit for monitoring consumption—the number of cookies—is meaningless when the cookies are of different sizes. The result is that consumption of large quantities goes unnoticed (Carter & Fishbach, 2012). Indeed, Wansink and colleagues' research indicates that people rely on implicit cues such as "Eat one cookie," "Drink one cup," and "Do not fill up your plate twice" in monitoring consumption. Once these cues are missing or misleading, people fail to monitor indulgence and they increase consumption (Wansink, 2006; Wansink, Painter, & North, 2005; Kahn & Wansink, 2004). Similarly, research documented more deception in the form of exaggerated performance when participants completed a task in a dim (vs. well-lit) room, because monitoring the self in the dark was difficult (Zhong, Bohns, & Gino, 2010).

Diagnosticity

People are not only more likely to identify a self-control conflict when they are reminded of the consequences of their actions for their goals (as in wide brackets), but they are also sensitive to reminders of how their actions affect how they perceive themselves. People often choose their actions to signal valued traits and identities to the self (Bodner & Prelec, 2001). In turn, actions they deem to be more self-diagnostic are more likely to evoke self-control conflict.

A major cue that an action is diagnostic is how salient it is for the pursuer; therefore, people are more likely to identify a conflict and exercise self-control for their salient actions. To demonstrate this point, we explored self-control for actions presented as being at the beginning or end of a sequence (Touré-Tillery & Fishbach, 2012a). For many goals, a natural sequence of actions results in their completion, for example, when completing a series of assignments for class or a series of tasks at work. Similarly, for ongoing goals such as maintaining good health or financial responsibility, the perception often exists that some actions are at the beginning and end of a sequence (e.g., the beginning–end of the week), whereas other actions are in the middle. Actions at the beginning and end (vs. the middle) of goal sequences are more noticeable and memorable (Greene, 1986; Murdock, 1960); therefore, people perceived these actions to be more diagnostic of their own traits and abilities.

Thus, in one study, we documented people's adherence to the Jewish religious tradition of lighting the menorah candles on eight consecutive nights over the Hanukkah holiday. We found that people were more likely to light the candles on the first and last nights than on the nights in the middle of the sequence, and, as predicted, the more religious people were, the more likely they were to exhibit this U-shaped pattern in following religious tradition. Importantly, people further believed that lighting the menorah on the first and last nights (vs. the middle) is a better signal that a person follows religious traditions. Other studies explored adhering to standards or goals in privacy and documented similar patterns of greater self-control at the beginning and end (vs. the middle). For example, participants were less likely to engage in deceit at the beginning and end versus the middle of an experiment (Touré-Tillery & Fishbach, 2012a).

Perceptual salience also matters. For example, actions that make noise are more perceptually salient, better activate conflict identification, and evoke greater goal adherence than actions that do not make noise. And when people express their attitudes in color (vs. black) pens, those attitudes are more closely related to their long-term goals (Touré-Tillery & Fishbach, 2012b). In these studies, cues that an action is noticeable evoke identification of a self-control problem and greater adherence to important goals.

To summarize, cues that explicitly or implicitly remind people of a self-control conflict promote identification, which is the first step in exercising restraint. A failure to identify a conflict will result in self-control failure that is not accompanied by the exercise of restraint in the first place. We next move to the explicit and implicit self-control responses to conflict.

EXERCISING RESTRAINT

Self-control counteracts the influence of temptation on goal adherence. The presence of temptation directly decreases the likelihood of goal adherence; however, indirectly, temptation activates a self-control response, which increases the likelihood of goal adherence. When these two influences of temptation—the direct and indirect—cancel each other out, successful self-control ensues: The individual is no less likely to adhere to the goal when confronting temptation than not (Fishbach & Trope, 2005; Trope & Fishbach, 2000). For example, a college student who is invited to a party before an important exam faces a temptation not to study, which directly decreases her motivation to study. However, indirectly, an invitation to a party triggers the exercise of self-control, which increases her motivation to study. When these two influences of the invitation—the direct and the indirect—cancel each other out, the student successfully resolves the conflict by maintaining the motivation to study when invited to the party.

The strength of the self-control response increases proportionally with the strength of the anticipated temptation in order to diminish the impact of temptation on the individual's behavior. When people anticipate strong temptation, they increase their self-control responses, and their performance is better than when they do not anticipate temptation. For example, in the context of mixed-motive interactions (e.g., social dilemmas; Dawes, 1980; Messick & Brewer, 1983), people often recognize that the long-term benefits of cooperation outweigh the short-term payoffs of competition but nonetheless feel tempted to compete (Dewitte & De Cremer, 2001). People are then more likely to cooperate when they anticipate barriers to successful outcomes in advance than when they expect that doing well will be easy (Sheldon & Fishbach, 2011). In what follows, we address the explicit and implicit self-control responses to temptation, which enable restraint.

SELF-CONTROL OPERATIONS

Self-control involves asymmetrically shifting the motivational strengths of conflicting motivations. Goals are strengthened so they may override temptations. Temptations are weakened so they may be overridden by goals. These asymmetrical shifts in motivational strength may be achieved by modulating the situation or its mental representations. These shifts may further involve explicit or implicit operations (see Table 30.1).

Changing the Choice Situation

Self-control responses that operate on the choice situation enable people to resolve a self-control conflict in advance, before it occurs, by changing the situation so that it no longer presents a conflict.

Self-Imposed Penalties and Rewards

Self-imposed penalties and rewards change the actual value of giving in to temptation or pursuing a goal to decrease the incentive to deviate from the goal (Trope & Fishbach, 2000). Diet betting websites that let people write a personal contract with a set penalty

TABLE 30.1. Self-Control Strategies That Create Asymmetric Change in Motivational Strength of Goals versus Temptations

	Goals	Temptations
Changing the choice situation	Self-imposed rewards	Self-imposed penalties
	Precommitment to pursue	Precommitment to forgo
	Approach	Avoidance
Changing the psychological meaning of choice options	Bolster	Devalue
	Hot and concrete construal	Cool and abstract construal
	Setting high expectations	Setting low expectations
	Activate	Inhibit

for missing their weight-loss goal are one application of self-imposed penalties. A self-imposed reward is a complementary strategy by which people set rewards for meeting their goals. For example, in one study, participants chose to receive their payment on completing a painful procedure only after they finished it, as opposed to before, to maintain their incentive to complete the procedure (Trope & Fishbach, 2000). Whereas imposed penalties decrease motivation to give in to temptation, imposed rewards increase the motivation to adhere to the goal. These strategies require conscious planning and deliberation; hence, they are bound to fail when the person is preoccupied.

Precommitment

A precommitment strategy restricts the individual's options to pursue goal-consistent behavior (Ainslie, 1992; Ariely & Wertenbroch, 2002; Gourville & Soman, 1998; Meyvis, Oppenheimer, & Bennett, 2010; Schelling, 1984; Strotz, 1956; Thaler & Shefrin, 1981; Wertenbroch, 1998). For example, the grocery shopper who purchases a large quantity of produce and a small quantity of sweets precommits to eat healthily and abstain from unhealthy food until her next trip to the grocery store. The strategy of precommitment can require conscious planning, although once certain precommitments become a habit, this pattern of goal pursuit and forgoing temptation occurs without conscious awareness (Wood & Neal, 2007).

Implicit Approach and Avoidance Responses

People further engage in implicit processes that shape their choice situations: They approach goals and avoid temptations. For example, the dieter who asks a waiter to take away her half-finished dessert plate can be mindless of the self-control function of her behavior. People further implicitly pull themselves toward others who facilitate their goals, and move away from those who hinder these goals. For example, a hard-working student may look for the proximity of others who also work hard, and distance herself from those friends who like to party (Fitzsimons & Fishbach, 2010).

Our research has documented automatic dispositions to approach goals and avoid temptations by assessing the time people take to respond to goal- and temptation-related words by either pushing a joystick away or pulling it toward themselves (Fishbach & Shah, 2006). An approach orientation enables faster pulling of a lever, whereas an avoidance orientation enables faster pushing away of a lever (Chen & Bargh, 1999; Markman & Brendl, 2005; Solarz, 1960). Using goal and temptation words (e.g., *exercise* vs. *alcohol*), we found faster response to goal-related (vs. temptation-related) words when participants responded with pulling, and faster response to temptation-related (vs. goal-related) words when participants responded with pushing. In the academic context, implicit dispositions to approach academic words and avoid nonacademic words were associated with a higher grade point average; hence, implicit dispositions predicted important self-regulatory outcomes.

Changing the Psychological Meaning of Choice Options

In addition to altering the choice situation, people may alter their motivation to pursue goals and embrace temptation by changing the psychological meaning of these options.

Bolstering Goals, Devaluing Temptations

People bolster the value of goals by linking the attainment of these goals to their self-standards (Bandura, 1989) or by elaborating on what makes the goals positive (e.g., important, appealing, attractive, etc.; Beckmann & Kuhl, 1985; Fishbach, Shah, & Kruglanski, 2004; Kuhl, 1984). They may further devalue temptations by disassociating these motives from the self, or by ignoring aspects that make them value temptations positively (Zhang, Huang, & Broniarczyk, 2010). The availability of temptations should then affect judgments of their subjective value. When potential temptations are available, they evoke changes in evaluation.

Indeed, research on explicit valuation presented exercisers on their way out of the gym with a choice between health bars and chocolate bars (Myrseth et al., 2009). Almost everybody chose a health bar to take home with them, and the researchers examined how they evaluated their two available options. For those choosers who evaluated the food options before making a choice, the chocolates represented a tempting alternative to the health bar that was consistent with their long-term health goals. These choosers counteracted this temptation by dampening their positive evaluations of the chocolates relative to the health bars. In contrast, other choosers in this study evaluated the foods after making their choice. These people rated the health bars and chocolate bars as equally attractive.

Bolstering goals and devaluing temptations take place outside of conscious awareness, and people's lack of awareness secures the effectiveness of evaluative biases. Further research directly demonstrated the implicit manifestation of counteractive evaluations (Fishbach, Zhang, & Trope, 2010). For example, using an implicit evaluation task (Bargh, Chaiken, Govender, & Pratto, 1992; Fazio, Jackson, Dunton, & Williams, 1995), Fishbach et al. documented implicit positive evaluations of healthy foods and negative evaluations of unhealthy foods, after participants viewed food temptations they wanted to forgo (e.g., ice cream, fried chicken). Thus, people devalued unhealthy foods and bolstered healthy foods only after they considered the various foods that tempt them away from their goals. Notably, participants in this study were aware of the initial exposure to temptation and may have been conscious of the self-control conflict it evoked, but they were unaware of their self-control response.

Hot versus Cool Construal

Abstract thinking facilitates self-control because, in big-picture thinking, goals weigh more than temptation (Fujita & Han, 2009; Fujita, Trope, Liberman, & Levin-Sagi, 2006; Marguc, Förster, & Van Kleef, 2011). But beyond abstract thinking, the construal of the goal and temptation activities themselves matters. The mental representation of goals and temptations varies between "hot" and abstract on one extreme and "cool" and concrete on the other (Kross, Ayduk, & Mischel, 2005; Metcalfe & Mischel, 1999). Whether, for example, a person construes the goal of studying as "gaining knowledge" (abstract) or as "reading pages" (concrete) would then influence pursuit of this goal. An abstract construal of a temptation stimulus "cools it down." For example, in the classic delay-of-gratification paradigm, children were better able to resist the temptation of eating a single marshmallow in order to receive a larger reward later if they thought of the marshmallows as "white, puffy clouds" or "round, white moons" (a cool construal) than if they thought of the marshmallows as "sweet and chewy and soft" (a hot construal; Mischel & Baker, 1975). In addition, a concrete, hot construal of a goal makes people more likely to pursue it. For example, research on implementation intentions documented that forming concrete behavioral plans to study facilitates studying among students (Gollwitzer, 1999; Gollwitzer & Brandstätter, 1997). As with other strategies, the construal that promotes self-control is asymmetrical: To promote their long-term interests, people think concretely about goals and abstractly about temptation, and these construals likely involve implicit operations.

Setting Expectations

Counteractive optimism is a self-control strategy that involves setting optimistic expectations to increase engagement with the goal and decrease engagement with temptation (Zhang & Fishbach, 2010). When people expect an obstacle or a temptation to hinder their goal attainment, they set more optimistic expectations that are asymmetrical: They expect greater goal pursuit and less pursuit of temptation. For example, examinees predicted a faster turnover of a take-home exam when they expected it to be difficult (vs. easy) to complete. In another study, students planned to devote more time to studying if they first listed the amount of time they would spend on social activities that day. Furthermore, they planned to devote less time to social activities if they first listed the amount of time they would spend studying that day.

Research on counteractive optimism has documented a somewhat counterintuitive pattern: The greater the obstacle, the more optimistic people are in their goal adherence. We find this pattern using various measures of motivation, from speed of completion to likelihood of attainment and level of performance. Because optimistic predictions act as performance standards, they implicitly motivate people's investment in effort to achieve the self-imposed standard (Locke & Latham, 1990; Wright & Brehm, 1989).

Inhibiting Temptations, Activating Goals

Implicit counteractive control most clearly manifests itself in the inhibition of temptations and activation of goals (Fishbach et al., 2003). By activating constructs related to a goal in response to reminders of interfering temptations, individuals increase the relative mental availability of goal-consistent behaviors. Alternatively, by inhibiting temptation-related constructs in response to reminders of overriding goals, individuals decrease the relative mental availability of temptation-related behaviors. For example, in one study that used participants' stated goal–temptation pairs (e.g., *class–sleep, save–spend*), in a sequential priming paradigm, participants recognized goal-related words (*class*) more quickly after subliminal presentation of relevant temptation-related words (*sleep*) than after subliminal presentation of irrelevant temptation. Consistent with work on "goal shielding," (Shah, Friedman, & Kruglanski, 2002), we also found participants took longer to recognize temptation-related words (*sleep*) after subliminal presentation of relevant goals (*class*) than irrelevant goals. We take these patterns of activation to suggest that temptations (vs. control primes) activate goals, and goals (vs. control primes) inhibit temptations, although further investigation would be required to separate amount of inhibition from lack of activation empirically (see Sherman et al., 2008).

These patterns of activation minimally tax working memory, in that we find similar patterns of goal activation and temptation inhibition under cognitive load, that is, when one's working memory is preoccupied. Nonconscious processes are often assumed to operate in an effortless fashion; however, recent research has shown that two aspects of automaticity—consciousness and effort—are distinct, and certain mental processes can consume effort in the absence of conscious awareness (Dijksterhuis & Aarts, 2010; Marien, Custers, Hassin, & Aarts, 2012). Accordingly, although self-control operations take place largely outside awareness, the process of exercising self-control could be taxing (Muraven & Baumeister, 2000; Vohs & Heatherton, 2000). In contrast with nonconscious yet taxing self-control, the implicit responses of inhibiting temptations and activating goals require limited working memory resources (i.e., they sustain cognitive load; see also Fujita, 2011).

Other research suggests that implicit temptation inhibition and goal activation are employed more frequently by successful self-regulators than by unsuccessful ones. For example, successful dieters exhibit these patterns, but dieters who frequently fail do not (Papies, Stroebe, & Aarts, 2008). Interestingly, because successful dieters respond to food temptations with activation of dieting goals, some researchers have concluded that fatty food causes weight loss (e.g., Kroese, Evers, & de Ridder, 2009). However, we assume that the presence of temptation would activate sufficient self-control to cancel out the impact of temptation but not increase goal adherence beyond what one would expect in the absence of temptation. The presence of temptation will only facilitate goal pursuit if the positive impact of the self-control response is stronger than the negative, direct impact of the temptation.

In summary, self-control operations increase the motivational strength of the goal and decrease the motivational strength of the temptation, to promote goal adherence. The self-control response can take an explicit form whenever individuals deliberately and consciously implement self-control. However, more often, these responses take an implicit form whenever individuals engage in mental operations that resolve the self-control conflict outside of conscious awareness.

CONCLUDING REMARKS

Self-control is a two-stage process. To succeed at goal pursuit, individuals facing temptations must first identify the conflict between those temptations and their goals. Once they have identified the conflict, they then have the opportunity to draw on self-control strategies to promote goal pursuit. We have described the conditions for identifying a self-control conflict: Conflict identification is more likely when a person considers multiple opportunities to act (width), expects to make consistent choices at each opportunity (consistency), finds her behavior easy to monitor (ease of monitoring), and finds her action meaningful for making self-inferences beyond their impact on goal attainment (diagnosticity).

We further portray the process of self-control as a process of asymmetrical response to goals versus temptations, such that self-control operations either increase the motivational strength of goals or decrease that of temptations. As we have shown, in response to temptation, individuals engage in a variety of operations, some that involve conscious deliberation and others that are elicited spontaneously without awareness and deliberation, and, at times, with minimal attentional resources.

Our analysis of self-control behavior portrays a process that is different from other dual-process models of self-control (Bechara et al., 2006; Fudenberg & Levine, 2006; Hofmann et al., 2009; Metcalfe & Mischel, 1999; Strack & Deutsch, 2004) in a key aspect: We assume that there is a single process that can involve an explicit or implicit operation mode. Whereas some work has portrayed the self-control conflict as involving a discrepancy between explicit and implicit modes, with the implicit mode more aligned with temptation and the explicit mode more aligned with goals, we suggest that implicit processes are as likely as explicit processes to be in the service of goals. At times, implicit processes may even override an explicit tendency to give in to temptation. Thus, neither mode is more closely aligned with high-level interests.

Importantly, our model does not refer to situations in which the presence of temptations only activates the self-control response and there is no impulse for temptation any more (e.g., when a cigarette loses its appeal for the smoker). Rather, the temptation in our model (and studies) directly activates the desire, and it is only through the simultaneous activation of self-control operations that the attraction is canceled out and the temptation is inhibited. We therefore assume opposite (simultaneous) effects of temptation, such that it activates desire and self-control responses at the same time. Researchers, then, observe inhibition of temptation (rather than activation) whenever the net effect of self-control is stronger and it overrides the effect of desire or attraction.

As a final note, we suggest that individuals do not face temptation defenseless and vulnerable. Rather, individuals facing temptation have an arsenal of operations designed to identify the problem and promote long-term interests in response to a self-control conflict.

REFERENCES

Ainslie, G. (1992). *Picoeconomics: The strategic interaction of successive motivational states within the person.* Cambridge, UK: Cambridge University Press.

Alberts, H., Martijn, C., Greb, J., Merkelbach, H., & De Vries, N. (2007). Carrying on or giving in: The role of automatic processes in overcoming ego depletion. *British Journal of Social Psychology, 46*(2), 383–399.

Ariely, D., & Wertenbroch, K. (2002). Procrastination, deadlines, and performance: Self-control by precommitment. *Psychological Science, 13*(3), 219–224.

Bandura, A. (1989). Self-regulation of motivation and action through internal standards and goal systems. In L. A. Pervin (Ed.), *Goal concepts in personality and social psychology* (pp. 19–85). Hillsdale, NJ: Erlbaum.

Bargh, J. A., Chaiken, S., Govender, R., & Pratto, F. (1992). The generality of the automatic attitude activation effect. *Journal of Personality and Social Psychology, 62*(6), 893–912.

Baron, S. W. (2003). Self-control, social consequences, and criminal behavior: Street youth and the general theory of crime. *Journal of Research in Crime and Delinquency, 40*(4), 403–425.

Baumeister, R. F., & Tierney, J. (2011). *Willpower: Rediscovering the great human strength.* New York: Penguin Press.

Bechara, A., Noel, X., & Crone, E. A. (2006). Loss of willpower: Abnormal neural mechanisms of impulse control and decision making in addiction. In R. W. Wiers, & A. W. Stacy (Eds.), *Handbook of implicit cognition and addiction* (pp. 215–232). Thousand Oaks, CA: Sage.

Beckmann, J., & Kuhl, J. (1985). *Action control: From cognition to behavior.* Berlin: Springer-Verlag.

Bodner, R., & Prelec, D. (2001). Self-signaling and diagnostic utility in everyday decision making. In I. Brocas & J. Carillo (Eds.), *Collected essays in psychology and economics* (pp. 1–22). New York: Oxford University Press.

Carter, T. J., & Fishbach, A. (2012). *The role of self-deception in the exercise of self-control.* Working paper, University of Chicago.

Carver, C. S. (2005). Impulse and constraint: Perspectives from personality psychology, convergence with theory in other areas, and potential for integration. *Personality and Social Psychology Review, 9*(4), 312–333.

Chen, M., & Bargh, J. A. (1999). Consequences of automatic evaluation: Immediate behavioral predispositions to approach or avoid the stimulus. *Personality and Social Psychology Bulletin, 25*(2), 215–224.

Dawes, R. M. (1980). Social dilemmas. *Annual Review of Psychology, 31*, 169–193.

de Ridder, D., Lensvelt-Mulders, G., Finkenauer, C., Stok, F. M., & Baumeister, R. F. (2012). A meta-analysis of how trait self-control relates to a wide range of behaviors. *Personality and Social Psychology Review, 16*(1), 76–99.

Devine, P. G. (1989). Stereotypes and prejudice: Their automatic and controlled components. *Journal of Personality and Social Psychology, 56*(1), 5–18.

Dewitte, S., & De Cremer, D. (2001). Self-control and cooperation: Different concepts, similar decisions?: A question of the right perspective. *Journal of Psychology, 135*(2), 133–153.

Dhar, R., & Simonson, I. (1999). Making complementary choices in consumption episodes: Highlighting versus balancing. *Journal of Marketing Research, 36*(1), 29–44.

Dijksterhuis, A., & Aarts, H. (2010). Goals, attention, and (un)consciousness. *Annual Review of Psychology, 61*, 467–490.

Duckworth, A. L., & Kern, M. L. (2011). A meta-analysis of the convergent validity of self-control measures. *Journal of Research in Personality, 45*(3), 259–268.

Fazio, R. H., Jackson, J. R., Dunton, B. C., & Williams, C. J. (1995). Variability in automatic activation as an unobstrusive measure of racial attitudes: A bona fide pipeline? *Journal of Personality and Social Psychology, 69*(6), 1013–1027.

Fazio, R. H., Sanbonmatsu, D. M., Powell, M. C., & Kardes, F. R., (1986). On the automatic activation of attitudes, *Journal of Personality and Social Psychology, 50*, 229–238.

Ferguson, M. J. (2008). On becoming ready to pursue a goal you don't know you have: Effects of nonconscious goals on evaluative readiness. *Journal of Personality and Social Psychology, 95*(6), 1268–1294.

Fishbach, A., & Dhar, R. (2005). Goals as excuses or guides: The liberating effect of perceived goal progress on choice. *Journal of Consumer Research, 32*(3), 370–377.

Fishbach, A., Dhar, R., & Zhang, Y. (2006). Subgoals as substitutes or complements: The role of goal accessibility. *Journal of Personality and Social Psychology, 91*(2), 232–242.

Fishbach, A., Friedman, R., & Kruglanski, A. (2003). Leading us not unto temptation: Momentary allurements elicit automatic goal activation. *Journal of Personality and Social Psychology, 84*(2), 296–309.

Fishbach, A., & Shah, J. Y. (2006). Self-control in action: Implicit dispositions toward goals and away from temptations. *Journal of Personality and Social Psychology, 90*(5), 820–832.

Fishbach, A., Shah, J. Y., & Kruglanski, A. W. (2004). Emotional transfer in goal systems. *Journal of Experimental Social Psychology, 40*, 723–738.

Fishbach, A., & Trope, Y. (2005). The substitutability of external control and self-control in overcoming temptation. *Journal of Experimental Social Psychology, 41*, 256–270.

Fishbach, A., & Zhang, Y. (2008). Together or apart: When goals and temptations complement versus compete. *Journal of Personality and Social Psychology, 94*, 547–559.

Fishbach, A., Zhang, Y., & Trope, Y. (2010). Counteractive evaluation: Asymmetric shifts in the implicit value of conflicting motivations. *Journal of Experimental Social Psychology, 46*, 29–38.

Fitzsimons, G. M., & Bargh, J. A. (2004). Automatic self-regulation. In R. F. Baumeister & K. D. Vohs (Eds.), *Handbook of self-regulation: Research, theory, and applications* (pp. 151–170). New York: Guilford Press.

Fitzsimons, G. M., & Fishbach, A. (2010). Shifting closeness: Interpersonal effects of personal goal progress. *Journal of Personality and Social Psychology, 98*(4), 535–549.

Fudenberg, D., & Levine, D. K. (2006). A dual-self model of impulse control. *American Economic Review, 96*(5), 1449–1476.

Fujita, K. (2011). On conceptualizing self-control as more than the effortful inhibition of impulses. *Personality and Social Psychology Review, 15*(4), 352–366.

Fujita, K., & Han, H. A. (2009). Moving beyond deliberative control of impulses: The effect of construal levels on evaluative associations in self-control conflicts. *Psychological Science, 20*(7), 799–804.

Fujita, K., Trope, Y., Liberman, N., & Levin-Sagi, M. (2006). Construal levels and self-control. *Journal of Personality and Social Psychology, 90*(3), 351–367.

Gollwitzer, P. M. (1999). Implementation intentions: Strong effects of simple plans. *American Psychologist, 54*(7), 493–503.

Gollwitzer, P. M., & Brandstätter, V. (1997). Implementation intentions and effective goal pursuit. *Journal of Personality and Social Psychology, 73*(1), 186–199.

Gottfredson, M. R., & Hirschi, T. (1990). *A general theory of crime*. Stanford, CA: Stanford University Press.

Gourville, J., & Soman, D. (1998). Payment depreciation: The behavioral effects of temporally separating payments from consumption. *Journal of Consumer Research, 25*(2), 160–174.

Greene, R. L. (1986). Sources of recency effects in free-recall. *Psychological Bulletin, 99*(2), 221–228.

Hoch, S. J., & Loewenstein, G. F. (1991). Time-inconsistent preferences and consumer self-control. *Journal of Consumer Research, 17*, 492–507.

Hofmann, W., Friese, M., & Strack, F. (2009). Impulse and self-control from a dual-systems perspective. *Perspectives on Psychological Science, 4*, 162–176.

Kahn, B. E., & Wansink, B. (2004). The influence of assortment structure on perceived variety and consumption quantities. *Journal of Consumer Research, 30*(4), 519–533.

Khan, U., & Dhar, R. (2006). Licensing effect in consumer choice. *Journal of Marketing Research, 43*(2), 259–266.

Koo, M., & Fishbach, A. (2008). Dynamics of self-regulation: How (un)accomplished goal actions affect motivation. *Journal of Personality and Social Psychology, 94*(2), 183–195.

Kroese, F. M., Adriaanse, M. A., Evers, C., & de Ridder, D. T. (2011). "Instant success": Turning temptations into cues for goal-directed behavior. *Personality and Social Psychology Bulletin, 37*(10), 1389–1397.

Kroese, F. M., Evers, C., & de Ridder, D. T. D. (2009). How chocolate keeps you slim: The effect of food temptations weight watching goal importance, intentions, and eating behavior. *Appetite, 53*(3), 430–433.

Kross, E., Ayduk, O., & Mischel, W. (2005). When asking "why" does not hurt: Distinguishing rumination from reflective processing of negative emotions. *Psychological Science, 16*(9), 709–715.

Kuhl, J. (1984). Volitional aspects of achievement motivation and learned helplessness: Toward a comprehensive theory of action control. In B. A. Maher (Ed.), *Progress in experimental personality research* (Vol. 13, pp. 99–171). New York: Academic Press.

Locke, E. A., & Latham, G. P. (1990). *A theory of goal setting and task performance*. Upper Saddle River, NJ: Prentice Hall.

Loewenstein, G. (1996). Out of control: Visceral influences on behavior. *Organizational Behavior and Human Decision Processes, 65*(3), 272–292.

Marien, H., Custers, R., Hassin, R. R., & Aarts, H. (2012). Unconscious goal activation and the hijacking of the executive function. *Journal of Personality and Social Psychology, 103*(3), 399–415.

Marguc, J., Förster, J., & Van Kleef, G. A. (2011). Stepping back to see the big picture: When obstacles elicit global processing. *Journal of Personality and Social Psychology, 101*(5), 883–901.

Markman, A. B., & Brendl, C. (2005). Constraining theories of embodied cognition. *Psychological Science, 16*(1), 6–10.

Mazar, N., & Zhong, C. (2010). Do green products make us better people? *Psychological Science, 21*(4), 494–498.

Messick, D. M., & Brewer, M. B. (1983). Solving social dilemmas: A review. *Review of Personality and Social Psychology, 4*, 11–44.

Metcalfe, J., & Mischel, W. (1999). A hot/cool system analysis of delay of grati?cation: Dynamics of willpower. *Psychological Review, 106*(1), 3–19.

Meyvis, T., Oppenheimer, D. M., & Bennett, A. (2010). Pre-commitment to charity. In D. M. Oppenheimer & C. Y. Olivola (Eds.), *The science of giving: Experimental approaches to the study of charity* (pp. 35–48). New York: Taylor & Francis.

Mischel, W., & Baker, N. (1975). Cognitive appraisals and transformations in delay behavior. *Journal of Personality and Social Psychology, 31*(2), 254–261.

Mischel, W., Cantor, N., & Feldman, S. (1996). Principles of self-regulation: The nature of willpower and self-control. In E. T. Higgins & A. W. Kruglanski (Eds.), *Social psychology:*

Handbook of basic principles (pp 329–360). New York: Guilford Press.

Mischel, W., Shoda, Y., & Rodriguez, M. L. (1989). Delay of gratification in children. *Science, 244*(4907), 933–938.

Monin, B., & Miller, D. T. (2001). Moral credentials and the expression of prejudice. *Journal of Personality and Social Psychology, 81*(1), 33–43.

Monteith, M. J., Ashburn-Nardo, L., Voils, C. I., & Czopp, A. M. (2002). Putting the brakes on prejudice: On the development and operation of cues for control. *Journal of Personality and Social Psychology, 83*, 1029–1050.

Moskowitz, G. B., Gollwitzer, P. M., Wasel, W., & Schaal, B. (1999). Preconscious control of stereotype activation through chronic egalitarian goals. *Journal of Personality and Social Psychology, 77*, 167–184.

Muraven, M. R., & Baumeister, R. F. (2000). Self-regulation and depletion of limited resources: Does self-control resemble a muscle? *Psychological Bulletin, 126*, 247–259.

Murdock, B. B. (1960). The distinctiveness of stimuli. *Psychological Review, 67*(1), 16–31.

Myrseth, K. O. R., & Fishbach, A. (2009). Self-control: a function of knowing when and how to exercise restraint. *Current Directions in Psychological Science, 18*(4), 247–252.

Myrseth, K. O., & Fishbach, A., & Trope, Y. (2009). Counteractive self-control: When making temptation available makes temptation less tempting. *Psychological Science, 20*(2), 159–163.

Papies, E. K., Stroebe, W., & Aarts, H. (2008). The allure of forbidden food: On the role of attention in self-regulation. *Journal of Experimental Social Psychology, 44*(5), 1283–1292.

Payne, B. K. (2001). Prejudice and perception: The role of automatic and controlled processes in misperceiving a weapon. *Journal of Personality and Social Psychology, 81*, 181–192.

Rachlin, H. (2000). *The science of self-control.* Cambridge, MA: Harvard University Press.

Read, D., Loewenstein, G., & Kalyanaraman, S. (1999). Mixing virtue and vice: Combining the immediacy effect and the diversification heuristic. *Journal of Behavioral Decision Making, 12*(4), 257–273.

Read, D., Loewenstein, G., & Rabin, M. (1999). Choice bracketing. *Journal of Risk and Uncertainty, 19*(1–3), 171–197.

Schelling, T. C. (1984). Self-command in practice, in policy, and in a theory of rational choice. *American Economic Review, 74*(2), 1–11.

Shah, J. Y., Friedman, R., & Kruglanski, A. W. (2002). Forgetting all else: On the antecedents and consequences of goal shielding. *Journal of Personality and Social Psychology, 83*, 1261–1280.

Sheldon, O. J., & Fishbach, A. (2011). Resisting the temptation to compete: Self-control promotes cooperation in mixed-motive interactions. *Journal of Experimental Social Psychology, 47*(2), 403–410.

Sherman, J. W., Gawronski, B., Gonsalkorale, K., Hugenberg, K., Allen, T. J., & Groom, C. J. (2008). The self-regulation of automatic associations and behavioral impulses. *Psychological Review, 115*, 314–335.

Solarz, A. K. (1960). Latency of instrumental responses as a function of compatibility with the meaning of eliciting verbal signs. *Journal of Experimental Psychology, 59*(4), 239–245.

Strack, F., & Deutsch, R. (2004). Reflective and impulsive determinants of social behavior. *Personality and Social Psychology Review, 8*(3), 220–247.

Strotz, R. H. (1955–1956). Myopia and inconsistency in dynamic utility maximization. *Review of Economic Studies, 23*, 165–180.

Sussman, A. B., & Alter, A. L. (2012). The exception is the rule: Underestimating and overspending on exceptional expenses. *Journal of Consumer Research, 39*, 800–814.

Thaler, R. H. (1991). *Quasi rational economics.* New York: Russel Sage Foundation.

Thaler, R. H., & Shefrin, H. M. (1981). An economic theory of self-control. *Journal of Political Economy, 89*(2), 392–406.

Touré-Tillery, M., & Fishbach, A. (2012a). The end justifies the means, but only in the middle. *Journal of Experimental Psychology: General, 141*(3), 570–583.

Touré-Tillery, M., & Fishbach, A. (2012b). *Making an impact on the self: How colors and sounds promote adherence to prosocial goals.* Working paper, University of Chicago.

Trope, Y., & Fishbach, A. (2000). Counteractive self-control in overcoming temptation. *Journal of Personality and Social Psychology, 79*(4), 493–506.

Vohs, K. D., & Heatherton, T. F. (2000). Self-regulatory failure: A resource-depletion approach. *Psychological Science, 11*(3), 249–254

Wansink, B. (2006). *Mindless eating: Why we*

eat more than we think. New York: Bantam-Dell.

Wansink, B., Painter, J. E., & North, J. (2005). Bottomless bowls: Why visual cues of portion size may influence intake. *Obesity Research, 13*(1), 93–100.

Wegner, D. M., Schneider, D. J., Carter, S., & White, T. (1987). Paradoxical effects of thought suppression. *Journal of Personality and Social Psychology, 53*(1), 5–13.

Wertenbroch, K. (1998). Consumption self-control by rationing purchase quantities of virtue and vice. *Marketing Science, 17*(4), 317–337.

Wiers, R. W., & Stacy, A. W. (2006). Implicit cognition and addiction. *Current Directions in Psychological Science, 15*(6), 292–296.

Wood, W., & Neal, D. T. (2007). A new look at habits and the interface between habits and goals. *Psychological Review, 114*(4), 843–863.

Wright, R. A., & Brehm, J. W. (1989). Energization and goal attractiveness. In L. A. Pervin (Ed.), *Goal concepts in personality and social psychology* (pp. 169–210). Hillsdale, NJ: Erlbaum.

Zhang, Y., & Fishbach, A. (2010). Counteracting obstacles with optimistic predictions. *Journal of Experimental Psychology: General, 139*(1), 16–31.

Zhang, Y., Huang, S., & Broniarczyk, S. M. (2010). Counteractive construal in consumer goal pursuit. *Journal of Consumer Research, 37*(1), 129–142.

Zhong, C., Bohns, V., & Gino, F. (2010). Good lamps are the best police: Darkness increases dishonesty and self-interested behavior. *Psychological Science, 21*, 311–314.

CHAPTER 31

Breaking the Prejudice Habit

Automaticity and Control in the Context of a Long-Term Goal

Patrick S. Forscher and Patricia G. Devine

The past two decades have witnessed an explosion of work on automaticity and control. This work has led to the creation of so-called "dual-process theories," which argue that people's behavior can be driven by either relatively automatic or relatively controlled processes. By focusing on the various factors that influence the type of processes activated in any given situation, dual-process theories have productively advanced our understanding of behavior, both in general (Strack & Deutsch, 2004; Smith & DeCoster, 2000), and in specific domains, such as person perception (e.g., Fiske & Neuberg, 1990; Brewer, 1988), attributional inference (Gilbert, 1989), and persuasion (Chaiken, 1980; Petty & Cacioppo, 1986).

One dual-process theory that stands out as unique from the others is the prejudice habit model (Devine, 1989; Devine & Monteith, 1993), which differentiates itself from other dual-process theories in two primary ways. First, rather than describing a particular class of behavior, the prejudice habit model develops a theoretical analysis of a particular social problem, that of lingering discrimination despite increasingly positive beliefs about outgroups. Second, because it deals with a social problem, the prejudice habit model concerns itself not only with the interplay between automatic and controlled processes within a single moment, but also with how this interplay is guided and structured by a person's long-term goals. Because of these two characteristics, the prejudice habit model is less specific than other dual-process theories in its assumptions about both the precise means through which automatic processes influence behavior (e.g., the activation of stereotypes vs. the activation of evaluations) and the precise controlled processes that oppose the influence of the automatic processes (e.g., inhibition, suppression, correction, or other control mechanisms). Instead, the model trades theoretical specificity for the ability to ground automaticity and control within a broad societal and temporal context.

In what follows, we describe the problem that motivated the development of the prejudice habit model, namely, that even people who report beliefs and attitudes that are opposed to prejudice can act in discriminatory ways. We then review the prejudice habit model and how it uses the distinction between controlled and automatic processes to understand lingering group disparities. We end our discussion with a review of topics for further research and implications of the prejudice habit model for other dual-process theories.

AUTOMATICITY AND THE PREJUDICE PARADOX

To understand the prejudice habit model, one must first understand the paradox the model was developed to explain. The Civil Rights Movement gave birth to dramatic changes in laws and personal norms that, in combination, made overt discrimination illegal and socially taboo. In the wake of these legal and normative changes, national surveys have revealed both increasingly positive attitudes toward minorities and decreasing endorsement of minority stereotypes (Schuman, Steeh, Bobo, & Krysan, 1997; Devine & Elliot, 1995). Despite these improvements, minority group members continue to have more adverse outcomes than majority group members in domains ranging from education (Steele, 1997) to employment (Bertrand & Mulllainathan, 2004) to health and well-being (e.g., Williams, Neighbors, & Jackson, 2003).

The societal-level paradox has been accompanied by a personal-level paradox. When people perform tasks that unambiguously measure prejudice, such as self-report measures of racial attitudes, their responses, consistent with the national survey data, are generally positive and nonprejudiced. However, when many people perform tasks on which the nonprejudiced response is ambiguous, their responses subtly favor majority group members over minority group members (Crosby, Bromley, & Saxe, 1980). This pattern of results occurs even among people who report that they believe prejudice is wrong (Devine, 1989).

The contradiction that people who disavow prejudice can still act with bias has presented scholars with a difficult problem, both theoretically and practically. Theoretically, the contradiction has led to ambiguity in the interpretation of responses to tasks for which participants are able to monitor their behavior, such as self-report measures. Some theorists have gone so far as to conclude that self-report measures are irrevocably contaminated by strategic self-presentation concerns (Gaertner & Dovidio, 1986), and that the apparent improvement in people's self-reported attitudes masks underlying negative "true attitudes" (Crandall, Eshleman, & O'Brien, 2002; Crosby et al., 1980). This type of reasoning leads to the pessimistic conclusion that the normative changes wrought by civil rights legislation are illusory in the sense that they have not created genuine intentions to act without prejudice.

If responses on measures permitting conscious monitoring are taken to reflect nonprejudiced intentions, an open theoretical question remains about the psychological process(es) that are responsible for the disparity between overt and subtle indicators of bias. In order to operate despite people's intentions, these processes must satisfy at least some of the formal criteria for automaticity (i.e., operate below the threshold of awareness, become activated quickly and unintentionally, and be difficult to control; Bargh, 1994).

The available evidence suggests that the processes leading to unintentional bias are not perfectly automatic (see Devine, 2001; Devine & Monteith, 1999). However, the biases are acquired easily, often after as little as a single exposure to negative evaluative information (Olsson, Ebert, Banaji, & Phelps, 2005), and early, perhaps as young as age 6 (Baron & Banaji, 2006). Once acquired, the biases are also frequently activated due to the saturation of stereotypic information within the social environment (Gerbner, 1998). These biases then become overlearned to the point that, even if they are not perfectly automatic, they are activated as quickly as 300–600 milliseconds after cue onset (Bartholow, Dickter, & Sestir, 2006; Ito, Thompson, & Cacioppo, 2004). Likewise, on tasks that occur quickly enough to preclude deliberative responding, merely instructing people to avoid bias appears to do little to prevent biases from occurring, suggesting that the processes leading to bias are difficult to control (e.g., Kim, 2003).

Thus, the debate about whether the processes leading to unintentional bias are "truly" automatic is in some ways unimportant, at least from the perspective of people concerned about the consequences of these processes. What is important is that these processes bias people's behavior, and that these biased behaviors can have dramatic consequences for outgroup members, such as false recognition of Black faces in crime contexts (Eberhardt, Goff, Purdie, & Davies, 2004), poorer quality interactions with majority group members (Richeson & Shelton, 2003), and disparate allocation of health and economic resources (Green et al., 2007; Amodio & Devine, 2006). Furthermore, these biased behaviors are ones that, if the perpetrators were aware of them, most would find immoral and unacceptable. The existence of lingering bias that is to some extent automatic leaves open the practical problem of whether the biases can be eliminated, and if so, how. Some theorists have argued that no methods will effectively reduce subtle biases, and that subtle biases are inevitable due to the natural constraints of human cognition (see Billig, 1985; Bargh, 1999). The prejudice habit model challenges arguments about both the inevitability of prejudice and the interpretation of self-report measures as merely reflecting strategic self-presentation (Devine, 1989; Devine & Monteith, 1993). The model draws on dual-process theory logic to argue that, like unwanted habits, relatively automatic implicit stereotypes and evaluations can cause otherwise well-intentioned people to unwittingly perpetuate discrimination. However, rather than concluding that the existence of automatic bias inevitably leads people to discriminate against outgroups, the prejudice habit model argues that if people have sufficient personal motivation to overcome bias and awareness of their bias, they can exert effort by deploying controlled processes to "break the prejudice habit." Even if this effort is not sufficient to disrupt the automatic processes leading to discrimination within a single moment, the effort can lead to increased efficiency in the regulation of prejudice in future situations, thereby increasing the probability that people will bring behavior in line with intention in situations where they might once have failed.

The importance of the prejudice habit model stems from both theoretical and practical concerns. Theoretically, the model allows a more nuanced understanding of the apparent paradox of so-called "modern" forms of prejudice. Although many people have genuinely renounced prejudice, lingering stereotypic and evaluative associations can still cause people to fail to live up to their intentions in ambiguous or time-pressured situations, leading to negative outcomes for outgroup members. The model therefore highlights the internal struggle of a person attempting to overcome prejudice (Allport, 1954), and understands that person's actions in any given moment as only one snapshot of his or her overall self-regulatory process. Practically, the model outlines the necessary conditions for breaking the prejudice habit over both short and long timescales. By outlining these conditions, the habit model offers a practical potential road map for eliminating lingering disparities linked to automatic bias.

In the following sections, we outline the conditions that the prejudice habit model argues are necessary to overcome prejudice—personal motivation to rid oneself of automatic bias, awareness of the bias, and efforts in deploying controlled processes to reduce the bias. All of these components are discussed in the context of a regulatory process to achieve the long-term goal of prejudice reduction.

THE COMPONENTS OF CONTROL

The Internal Struggle: Personal Motivation to Respond without Prejudice

The personal motivation to reduce prejudice stems from a long-term goal to reduce one's bias. Thus, before people can develop a personal motivation to reduce bias, they must establish an identity that is opposed to prejudice and thereby adopt a long-term goal to reduce prejudice. On the basis of this logic, Devine and Monteith (1993) argued that the establishment of an egalitarian self-concept is a necessary precondition for personally motivated regulation of bias to occur.

Once a long-term goal to reduce prejudice has been adopted, this goal, and the motivation that stems from it, structures people's orientations to their environment, changing how they interpret the situations they encounter and their reactions to those situations. This change in how people interpret their environment has three primary consequences. First, it leads people to adopt situational intentions consistent with the long-term goal of overcoming bias. Second, it leads people to establish self-regulatory standards that are used to monitor and evaluate progress toward the long-term goal. Third, it heightens the affective consequences of acting in ways that are inconsistent with the long-term goal.

The first consequence, the adoption of situational intentions conducive to the elimination of prejudice, is a dynamic process that occurs after one has identified a situation as relevant to the regulation of prejudice (i.e., after the identification of a situation as relevant to one's long-term goals). The identification of a situation as goal-relevant generates a search for opportunities to behave in ways that are conducive to goal progress. Thus, in interracial interactions, for example, the personal motivation to respond without prejudice is linked to intentions to treat the interaction partner fairly (Plant & Devine, 2009; Plant, Devine, & Peruche, 2010). After a perceived self-regulatory failure, such as the rejection of a qualified job candidate on the basis of the candidate's sexual orientation (Monteith, 1993), personal motivation is linked to interest in and attention to materials perceived to be useful in eliminating subtle bias. By generating intentions to act in ways that are consistent with long-term goals, motivation orients a person to the situational affordances that further one's long-term goals.

The second change, the establishment of personally endorsed self-regulatory standards, allows people to monitor goal progress. Standards define the behaviors that are considered violations of a goal. Thus, through a comparison of standards to ongoing behavior, people can evaluate the extent to which their behavior is consistent with a given goal (Devine, Monteith, Zuwerink, & Elliot, 1991) and thereby draw conclusions about current progress towards that goal (Carver & Scheier, 1990). Greater personal motivation is related to stricter, better internalized, and more well-defined standards; thus, personal motivation indirectly determines the behaviors that are considered goal-relevant (Devine et al., 1991; Monteith, Devine, & Zuwerink, 1993).

The final change, heightening the affective consequences of behaving in goal-inconsistent ways, is interrelated with the establishment of standards to monitor goal progress. Once people establish well-defined standards to regulate bias, these standards engage an ongoing monitoring process that orients people's attention to violations of the standards. To the extent that people perceive the long-term goal of regulating bias as personally relevant, violations of the standards are interpreted as moral failures, generating guilt (Devine et al., 1991). Combined with the aforementioned intentions to eliminate prejudice, the guilt generated by violations of a person's standards motivates later efforts to bring behavior in line with that person's goals (Monteith, 1993; Monteith, Ashburn-Nardo, Voils, & Czopp, 2002; Amodio, Devine, & Harmon-Jones, 2007). Overall, personal motivation to respond without prejudice engages a dynamic self-regulatory process. When a situation is perceived to be relevant to the long-term goal of eliminating prejudice, motivation generates a situation-specific intention to act consistently with that goal. Motivation also leads people to adopt standards that allow people to monitor goal progress. Finally, motivation leads people to interpret behavior inconsistent with standards as moral failures, an interpretation that results in guilt and efforts to bring future behavior more in line with the standards.

The External Struggle: Being Motivated for Social Reasons

A personally endorsed goal is not the only reason people might be motivated to respond without prejudice. The establishment of norms and legislation that prohibit overt discrimination has created compelling external reasons to respond without prejudice.

The antidiscriminatory legislation was established at least in part under the hope that encouraging people to comply with this legislation would eventually lead to internal change in the form of personally endorsed intentions to respond without prejudice. Thus, an important question arising from the changes in legislation and norms is whether external motivation spurred these measures results in self-regulatory processes similar to those resulting from internal motivation. Answering this question would enable social scientists to evaluate the extent to which antidiscriminatory legislation was successful in creating internal change via external pressure.

To help address questions about the potentially different implications of internal (i.e., value and/or goal-driven) and external (i.e., social) motivations to respond without prejudice, Plant and Devine (1998) created separate measures of these motivations, namely, the Internal Motivation Scale (IMS) and the

External Motivation Scale (EMS). Interestingly, despite the hopes of activists and legislatures that external motivation would eventually lead to internal motivation, both Plant and Devine and subsequent researchers have consistently found that the internal and external scales are only mildly correlated, if at all (e.g., $r = -.15$; Plant & Devine, 1998; $r = -.05$ to $-.01$, Klonis, Plant, & Devine, 2005; $r = .14$, Ratcliff, Lassiter, Markman, & Snyder, 2006). This suggests that the two sources of motivation operate somewhat independently of each other. Subsequent research has found that external motivation also has very different self-regulatory implications than internal motivation.

First, in contrast to the intentions to eliminate prejudice that are associated with internal motivation, external motivation is associated with intentions serving the long-term goal of hiding prejudice from others (Plant & Devine, 2009). This subtle difference in intention can have dramatic consequences for behavior. Because externally motivated people are primarily concerned with how they appear to others, their behavior is strategic; if a given situation does not provide the proper affordances to hide prejudice from others, people who are primarily externally motivated do not attempt to regulate their prejudice. Thus, external motivation is associated with interest in and attention to materials perceived to prevent detectable (overt) forms of prejudice, but not necessarily undetectable (subtle) forms of prejudice (Plant & Devine, 2009). In interracial interactions, people who are externally motivated adopt intentions to hide their prejudice from their interaction partner. Unfortunately for people who are primarily externally motivated the intention to hide prejudice is not associated with strategies that create smooth interactions; thus, ironically, minority interaction partners perceive more prejudice from externally motivated people than from people who are not externally motivated (Plant et al., 2010). Overall, because internal and external motivations serve different long-term goals, people who are primarily internally and externally motivated are oriented to different kinds of situational affordances. These differences in orientation lead people who are primarily internally and externally motivated to adopt different intentions in the same situations and to attend to different aspects of these same situations.

Internal and external motivations to respond without prejudice also have different implications for the standards used to regulate prejudiced behavior. Whereas the standards of internally motivated people serve as a basis for determining whether their behavior is consistent with the long-term goal of eliminating bias, the standards of externally motivated people are functionally different, serving the long-term goal of hiding bias (Plant & Devine, 1998). Instead of using their own standards to regulate their behavior, people who are primarily externally motivated use what they perceive to be the standards of others, and they only use these standards in the presence of a perceived audience that is thought to disapprove of prejudice. Thus, while both internally and externally motivated people may regulate their prejudice in the presence of a perceived audience known to disapprove of prejudice, people who are primarily externally motivated relax their regulatory standards outside the presence of this perceived audience (Plant & Devine, 1998, 2001, 2009).

Finally, external motivation is related to different interpretations of violations of self-regulatory standards. Because people who are primarily externally motivated use the perceived standards of others to regulate their behavior, violations of the standards are interpreted as signals of imminent social sanctions, an interpretation which leads people who are primarily externally motivated to direct feelings of threat and anger at the perceived source of the social sanctions (Higgins, 1987; Plant & Devine, 1998). The implications of the threat and anger are that when social pressure to respond without prejudice is lifted, people who are primarily externally motivated experience backlash at the curtailment of their psychological freedom, attempting to restore this freedom by responding with greater prejudice than if pressure had not been applied in the first place (Plant & Devine, 2001). Though not tested to date, one provocative interpretation of this backlash is that at least some primarily externally motivated people come to view the expression of prejudice in spite of strong antidiscriminatory norms as good, moral, and consistent with their values. To the extent that the expression of prejudice comes to be viewed as a part of one's self-concept, this change in self-definition could lead to the development of a motivation to express prejudice.

Thus, accumulating evidence suggests that the changes in norms have not been uniformly successful in generating internally endorsed intentions to respond without prejudice. People who are strongly motivated to conform to these norms regulate themselves in a very different way from people who are motivated to respond without prejudice for internal reasons, experiencing an external struggle between norms and automatic bias rather than an internal struggle between values and automatic bias. The external struggle leads to differences in the intentions that guide self-regulatory efforts, the standards used to evaluate goal progress, and the interpretation of instances of goal failure. Overall, the external struggle may even lead to resentment and behavioral backlash, and, to the extent that people come to define their self-concepts by resisting social pressure through covert expressions of prejudice, perhaps even the development of a motivation to express prejudice.

The Role of Awareness in the Bias Reduction Process

Regardless of whether people are motivated to respond without prejudice for internal or external reasons, motivation seems to structure the intentions people adopt and the way they monitor and evaluate progress toward their goals. However, motivation by itself will not spur self-regulatory efforts unless people notice that they are succeeding or failing at their goals. This logic forms the basis of the awareness component of the prejudice habit model.

The prejudice habit model has generally distinguished between two types of awareness. The first type is *chronic* awareness, or the extent to which a person is chronically sensitive to one's level of bias (Devine & Monteith, 1993). The second type is *momentary* awareness, or the extent to which, within a given situation, one is aware of one's bias. Momentary awareness has been further subdivided into *prospective* awareness, or awareness that one has the potential to act with bias, and *retrospective* awareness, or awareness that one has already acted with bias (Monteith et al., 2002).

Both situational and chronic awareness are important to the regulation of prejudice. Chronic awareness generates a monitoring process that increases the likelihood that self-regulation will occur in any given situation (Monteith et al., 2002). However, this monitoring process must be triggered within a given situation for self-regulation to occur.[1] Thus, successful self-regulation occurs when people translate chronic awareness into situational awareness, resulting in the exertion of self-regulatory effort (Monteith & Mark, 2005).

Chronic awareness is closely linked to the standards that people have for regulating their bias. As people monitor the extent to which their actual responses differ from their standards, they develop a set of relatively enduring beliefs about the level of bias present in their ongoing behavior (Devine et al., 1991). Chronic awareness has thus been conceptualized as the extent to which a person's beliefs about the degree of bias in his or her behavior differs from his or her standards (Devine et al., 1991). The close linkage in the conceptualization of motivation and chronic awareness illustrates the theorized reciprocal relationships between motivation and chronic awareness. Because motivation generates standards to help evaluate and monitor goal progress, it also eventually generates beliefs about one's level of bias and, to the extent that these beliefs are accurate, chronic sensitivity to one's level of bias. To the extent that people believe that their actual level of bias differs from their standards, this discrepancy between beliefs and standards can also generate guilt and motivated tendencies to bring future behavior in line with the standards for that behavior. Thus, ongoing chronic awareness can eventually result in increased motivation, with all the downstream consequences resulting from that motivation.

Within a specific situation, awareness can be triggered either prior to a biased response (prospective awareness) or after a biased response has already occurred (retrospective awareness). Most of the research on awareness has focused on the consequences of retrospective awareness. As described in The Internal Struggle section, this work has revealed that retrospectively becoming aware of bias generates guilt, at least among people who are personally (i.e., internally) motivated to respond without bias (Devine et al., 1991). Although retrospective awareness has typically been portrayed as the product of a relatively effortful introspective process (e.g., see Monteith et al., 2002), attention can be recruited to bias-relevant errors very quickly and efficiently, particularly among people who are highly internally motivated to respond without bias (Amodio et al., 2008).[2]

Repeated retrospective awareness should also trigger increased chronic awareness, increasing overall sensitivity to future instances of bias. Monteith and her colleagues (2002) argue that the chronic awareness generated through retrospective reflection may be somewhat situation-specific; the guilt generated by the retrospective reflection becomes associated with the characteristics of that situation, which later become "cues for control" that help trigger future prospective awareness. Cues for control provide a warning that a person is at risk of acting in a biased way, recruiting attention to a given situation, so that the person can deploy controlled processes to inhibit stereotypic responses.

Bringing the Components Together: Effort

In many ways, the deployment of effort to exercise control over stereotypic responses is the culmination of the regulation of a person's biased responses. Although both motivation and awareness may be necessary for the successful regulation of bias, Devine and colleagues have argued forcefully that they are insufficient to produce enduring reductions in bias (e.g., Devine, Forscher, Austin, & Cox, 2012; Devine, 1989; Devine & Monteith, 1993). Indeed, they have argued that overcoming bias is likely to be a protracted process requiring considerable effort over time (Devine, 1989; Devine et al., 1991).

Accordingly, Devine and colleagues have found that, when people who are motivated to reduce their bias are made situationally aware of their bias, they feel guilty, and the guilt motivates efforts to reduce bias. For example, people who are made aware of their bias report more interest in and spend more time studying information that they believe will help to reduce their bias (Amodio et al., 2007; Monteith, 1993), and immediately after the guilt-evoking experience, these same people regulate their prejudice by attending to and slowing their responses and by putting effort into tasks that they believe will reduce their bias (Monteith, 1993; Monteith et al., 2002; Monteith, Mark, & Ashburn-Nardo, 2010).

In arguing that these experiences will be effective in reducing bias, theorists have made two assumptions. First, they have assumed that, to the extent that people exert effort intended to reduce their implicit bias immediately after a regulatory failure, they will be more efficient in regulating their bias in future situations. In effect, theorists have overlooked the question of whether effort exerted in one situation will actually be successful in reducing implicit bias in future situations by either decreasing the strength of future activation of bias or increasing the efficiency with which people deploy controlled processes. Second, theorists have assumed that people will know the proper strategies that, when deployed, will successfully reduce implicit bias. Effectively, participants have been left to their own devices to discover the strategies permitting successful regulation of bias.

Although little work has directly addressed the assumptions that effort will improve long-term self-regulatory attempts, some recent work has identified a promising set of strategies that may successfully help to regulate implicit bias. These strategies have typically been tested by simply asking participants to perform the strategy as part of an experimental task; thus, participants in these experiments were not regulating their prejudice but instead merely complying with the instructions of the experimenter. Despite the fact that the participants in these studies were not actively attempting to regulate their prejudice, many of these strategies, such as taking the perspective of stigmatized others (Galinsky & Moskowitz, 2000) and imagining counter-stereotypic examples (Blair, Ma, & Lenton, 2001; Dasgupta & Greenwald, 2001), lead to substantial reductions in implicit bias, at least for a short time (i.e., up to 24 hours). However, investigators have typically not tested whether the beneficial effects of these strategies on implicit bias endure beyond a single laboratory session. Additionally, the prejudice habit model, along with a few other dual-process theories in psychology (e.g., Smith & DeCoster, 2000; Strack & Deutsch, 2004), predicts that because the processes supporting automatic bias have developed through repeated activation from a lifetime of exposure to biasing information in the social environment (Devine, 1989), these processes are only likely to change in an enduring way after considerable time, effort, and/or intensity of experience. Thus, because one-shot interventions must counteract a large accretion of associative learning, they are unlikely to produce enduring change in automatic responses. Such change is likely only after the application of considerable goal-directed effort over time.

Devine and her colleagues (2012) recently attempted to address the aforementioned shortcomings by designing and testing longitudinally an intervention to produce enduring reductions in implicit bias. Because the goal of the intervention was to engage a complex self-regulatory process, and because of the difficulty of knowing a priori which components of the intervention would be necessary or sufficient to produce enduring reductions in implicit bias (Prochaska & Velicer, 1997), the intervention was intentionally multifaceted, containing components designed to engage awareness, motivation, and effort. All participants in the study first completed an implicit measure of bias and received feedback about their level of implicit bias. The completion of the implicit measure and the feedback served to make participants situationally aware of their bias. Participants who received the intervention then watched a 45-minute, narrated slide show. The slide show attempted to translate the situational awareness provided by the feedback into chronic awareness by educating participants about what implicit bias is, how it is measured, and its consequences for outgroup members. The slide show then described the situations in which implicit bias can lead to subtle discrimination.

To channel the motivation and awareness provided by the implicit bias education into effort that might have an impact on implicit bias, the slide show next described strategies culled from the literature that, were the participants to exert effort by practicing them in their everyday life, should lead to enduring reductions in implicit bias. These strategies were intentionally diverse, including stereotype replacement (Devine & Monteith, 1993), counter-stereotypic imaging (Blair et al., 2001), individuation (Brewer, 1988; Fiske & Neuberg, 1990), perspective taking (Galinsky & Moskowitz, 2000), and increasing opportunities for contact (Pettigrew, 1998). Devine and colleagues (2012) reasoned that presenting a wide variety of strategies would enable participants to select the strategies that best suited the participants' individual situations (Prochaska & Velicer, 1997). At 1 and 2 months following the randomized intervention, Devine and colleagues (2012) measured an array of variables related to the prejudice habit model, including motivation, chronic awareness, effort, and implicit bias.

The results of the study suggested that the intervention was successful. Participants who received the intervention experienced dramatic reductions in implicit bias that endured up to 2 months after the intervention. Participants who received the intervention also experienced increased chronic awareness and concern about discrimination, the last of which, Devine and colleagues (2012) argued, was a component of motivation. Moreover, the participants who were most concerned about discrimination after receiving the intervention experienced the greatest reductions in implicit bias, highlighting the importance of motivation in the regulation of subtle bias. Finally, Devine and colleagues also conducted a word-frequency analysis of free-response answers that participants gave to questionnaires about their strategy use. Importantly, the participants who used the greatest frequency of word stems relating to the implementation of the bias-reducing strategies (e.g., *implement**, *practice**, *appli**, *use**, *tri**) were the same participants who experienced the greatest reductions in implicit bias. This last finding underscores the importance of effort in the successful regulation of bias.

In developing an intervention that produces long-term reductions in implicit bias, increases in concern about discrimination, and increases in chronic awareness of one's bias, prejudice habit model researchers have come full circle. The theory was originally proposed to provide an understanding of the prejudice paradox that did not rely on arguments about the inevitability of prejudice or interpretations of all self-report measures as strategic self-presentation. Although the model proposed that implicit bias could be reduced in the long term given sufficient personal motivation, awareness, and effort, it was silent as to exactly how this process would unfold. Although many questions remain, we now have preliminary evidence supporting the original conceptualization that prejudice is a habit that can be broken.

UNANSWERED QUESTIONS AND RECOMMENDATIONS FOR FUTURE RESEARCH

Research on the prejudice habit model over the past two decades has been extremely productive. It has demonstrated the challenges faced by people experiencing the "internal struggle" to eliminate unwanted implicit bias. The research has also forcefully argued that although the process of overcoming bias may be arduous, people can harness controlled processes to overcome automatic biases given sufficient motivation, awareness, and effort. However, there are still many gaps in our understanding of how people overcome bias. In the following sections, we outline what we perceive to be the most pressing issues facing researchers using the habit framework. We organize our discussion according to the various components of the model. We finish our discussion with two methodological recommendations and a review of the model for other dual-process theories.

Developing an Understanding of Motivation's Development

Although we know that motivation shapes the way a person regulates bias, we have large gaps in our knowledge about how motivation develops, and how that development is affected by a person's long-term goals and values. Devine and Monteith (1993) argued that the motivation to respond without prejudice stems from values of equality, but to date we have little understanding of precisely how values of equality lead to a personal motivation to respond without prejudice. Because of the abstract nature of values, valuing equality does not guarantee that the value is seen as relevant to prejudice toward a particular group (see Maio, Hahn, Frost, & Cheung, 2009). Thus, the issue of how values of equality come to be seen as applicable to prejudice toward a particular group may be critical to understanding the relationship between values and motivation. Developing a more thorough understanding of the factors influencing the application of values to the regulation of prejudice might eventually enable us to develop interventions to change people's motivations.

Another important aspect of motivation that is currently not well understood is how internal and external motivations develop over time. On the basis of self-determination theory (Deci & Ryan, 2000), Devine, Plant, Amodio, Harmon-Jones, and Vance (2002) speculated that internal and external motivations follow a developmental trajectory whereby people first become motivated for external reasons, resulting in high levels of external motivation, then gradually internalize the external motivation, resulting in high levels of both internal and external motivation, and finally fully integrate the external motivation into their self-concepts, resulting in high internal motivation only (see also Crandall & Eshleman, 2003). Some evidence supports this argument; for example, compared to people who are motivated for both internal and external reasons, people who are motivated for only internal reasons have a preconscious sensitivity to bias-relevant errors (Amodio, Devine, & Harmon-Jones, 2008) and lower levels of implicit bias, as assessed by both the Implicit Association Test (Devine et al., 2002) and a startle eyeblink method (Amodio, Harmon-Jones, & Devine, 2003). This suggests that people who are motivated to respond without prejudice for only internal reasons are more efficient in their self-regulation than people who are both internally and externally motivated.

However, the evidence does not uniformly support a self-determination perspective on the development of internal and external motivations. For example, people who are primarily externally motivated have higher levels of explicit bias than people who are not motivated for either internal or external reasons (Devine et al., 2002; Plant & Devine, 1998), and they respond with higher levels of anger, threat, and other forms of backlash when pressured to comply with egalitarian norms (Plant & Devine, 2001). Although primarily externally motivated people do regulate their bias when doing so reduces the risk of receiving social sanctions, they appear to resent the external pressure to regulate their bias, and seem therefore to have internalized egalitarian norms to an even lesser extent than people who are neither internally nor externally motivated to respond without prejudice. Studying the developmental sequence of motivation will allow us to understand better the interplay between internal and external motivations, which will provide us with more tools for developing interventions to increase internal motivation.

Broadening Our Understanding of Awareness

Although researchers who study awareness have made a key distinction between momentary and chronic awareness, our knowledge of how chronic awareness becomes translated into momentary awareness (and how momentary awareness may lead to increased chronic awareness) is just emerging. Part of the reason for this lack of knowledge is methodological; neither chronic nor momentary awareness has typically been used as outcome variables in experimental studies, with the result that we have little knowledge of the factors that causally influence either variable (but see Devine et al., 2012). However, another potential reason for this lack of knowledge is that current researchers may have overlooked some of the complexities inherent in becoming aware of one's bias.

Developing awareness of one's bias, either momentary or chronic, requires the application of knowledge about bias to both a specific situation and to oneself. The specific content of this knowledge (i.e., a person's lay theory; Wilson & Brekke, 1994) may have dramatic implications for whether people develop chronic or momentary awareness in the first place. Without a lay theory of prejudice positing that discrimination can arise unintentionally, people who consciously renounce prejudice but still associate Black people with negative stereotypes will not notice unintentional forms of bias when this bias does arise, thus missing opportunities to engage in controlled processes to regulate their prejudice.

Lay theories of prejudice may also have important consequences for how people interpret biases that they do notice. For example, people who believe that biases arise from intentions may be more likely to make a dispositional attribution of prejudice when observing behavior that is believed to stem from prejudice or bias (Devine, Evett, & Vasquez-Suson, 1996). These dispositional attributions may have dramatic inter- and intrapersonal consequences; a dispositional inference of prejudice about another person may lead to avoidance of that person, while a dispositional inference of prejudice about oneself may lead to avoidance of intergroup interactions due to the assumption that self-regulation of prejudice is fruitless (for similar arguments, see Carr, Rattan, & Dweck, 2012).

Another way in which people's beliefs about bias may be important is in whether and how they calibrate their beliefs about their own bias to their actual level of bias. Accuracy in the beliefs people have about their bias is important, because these beliefs determine when and how much effort people deploy in correcting their behavior. Thus, having inaccurate beliefs may cause people to undercorrect their behavior in some situations and perhaps overcorrect in others. Accurately attuning beliefs to actual bias is not a trivial task; because discrimination can happen unintentionally and without awareness, merely reflecting about past experiences with bias is unlikely to give an accurate estimate of actual vulnerability to bias. The fact that beliefs about bias and actual levels of implicit bias are only modestly correlated ($r = .17$; Monteith, Voils, & Ashburn-Nardo, 2001) is consistent with the argument that most people's beliefs are not well-attuned with their actual levels of bias.

One final way in which general knowledge about bias might be important is in the application of general knowledge to a specific situation. Although, in some situations, there is a clear potential for discrimination and the nonprejudiced response is obvious, other situations are more ambiguous in these respects (Gaertner & Dovidio, 1986; see also Maio, 2010). Thus, whether people interpret a specific situation as relevant to the regulation of bias may be a key factor in triggering momentary awareness. One promising avenue for research on this component of awareness is investigating how knowledge of bias is represented in memory; to the extent that knowledge of bias is connected to specific types of situations (e.g., job interviews), encountering those situations should be more likely to trigger awareness of the potential for bias and subsequent self-regulatory efforts.

Effort: The Understudied Component

Although effort is an integral part the prejudice habit model, it is also the least studied. Only one published study to date has investigated effort as an outcome of a self-regulatory process (Devine et al., 2012), and that study lacks a direct, precise measure of effort. Consequently, the remaining questions about how effort plays into the self-regulatory process are numerous. For example, it is unclear precisely how much and what kinds of effort are required to produce changes in the various components of the prejudice habit model. Effort in monitoring one's thoughts could produce specialized increases in chronic awareness. In contrast, effort exerted in taking the perspective of outgroup members could produce specialized increases in motivation and concern about discrimination.

In a related question, we have little knowledge about the specific psychological processes that are affected by effort in reducing relatively automatic forms of bias. The prejudice habit model predicts that repeated deployment of effort should increase the efficiency of future control of one's bias; however, it is also possible that repeated deployment of effort directly reduces the activation of automatic biases. Forthcoming work suggests that the specific ways in which people overcome their bias (and maintain their bias at a low level) depend, at least in part, on the strategies people use to overcome their bias and the amount of effort they exert in the deployment of these strategies (Monteith & Lybarger, in preparation). Recently developed multinomial modeling techniques could help shed further light on the ways in which effort relates to the reduction of implicit bias (Payne, 2001; Conrey, Sherman, Gawronski, Hugenberg, & Groom, 2005).

Finally, it is unclear what factors determine whether effort exerted in one situation will translate into bias reductions in a different situation. Answering this question will be critical in understanding how effort creates long-term changes in outcomes related to implicit bias. Overall, investigations of effort are in their infancy, and these studies are some of the most exciting avenues for future research on the prejudice habit model.

Implications for Other Dual-Process Theories and Two Methodological Recommendations

As we noted at the beginning of this chapter, the main points of differentiation between the prejudice habit model and other dual-process models and the habit model's concern with a social problem and how, as a result, the prejudice habit model situates the interplay between automaticity and control within the context of the pursuit of a broader goal to treat people equally. This integration of dual-process theory logic into a broader self-regulatory framework is its main contribution to our understanding of dual-process theories generally.

However, to exploit the theoretical integration of a dual-process analysis with self-regulatory processes empirically, researchers should heed two methodological recommendations. First, researchers studying prejudice and implicit bias should broaden the range of outcome variables that they study. Perhaps because prejudice researchers have often had the metatheoretical goal of finding methods to reduce implicit bias, they have become preoccupied with using specific implicit measures of bias (e.g., the IAT) as their primary outcome measures. However, implicit bias is not a unitary construct, and as a result, any one implicit measure is unlikely to capture entirely the full range of psychological processes that lead to subtle discrimination (Amodio, 2009). Additionally, a preoccupation with implicit measures of bias for their own sake has contributed to a lack of theoretical clarity about the other psychological factors involved in the regulation and reduction of implicit bias, such as motivation, awareness, and effort. As shown by Devine et al. (2012), maintaining a full theoretical appreciation of these variables is critical to developing interventions that produce long-term change in subtle bias.

The second recommendation is closely related to the first. Because of its emphasis on the development and maintenance of long-term regulatory processes, the habit model has from its inception been a developmental model. It is therefore somewhat strange that until very recently researchers have not investigated the components of the model longitudinally. One-shot experiments do allow snapshot views of the regulatory process, but without longitudinal designs, we will not be able to appreciate properly people's regulatory struggles in the context of their long-term goals. A full investigation of the interplay of motivation, awareness, and effort in empowering people to control relatively automatic forms of bias demands the use of longitudinal designs.

Overall, the prejudice habit model has proved instrumental in advancing our knowledge of the process of reducing people's bias. It is our hope that it will continue to prove productive in incrementally advancing its original goal of decreasing lingering disparities and empowering people to bring their behavior in line with their intentions.

NOTES

1. It is possible that situational awareness need not be triggered in every situation for the regulation of bias to occur, at least in the sense that some people who successfully regulate their bias might not retrospectively report that they had any awareness of potential to act with bias. However, as we note later, the processes that lead to situational awareness can themselves become efficient to the point of being triggered preconsciously (Amodio, Devine, & Harmon-Jones, 2008), suggesting that the detection of bias need not necessarily coincide with a phenomenal state of awareness. Additionally, even if a phenomenal state of situational awareness is unnecessary for self-regulation in a given situation, the prejudice habit model predicts that chronic awareness is necessary for successful long-term self-regulation.
2. Note that the efficient preconscious recruitment of attention to prejudice-relevant errors only occurs for people who are both high in internal motivation and low in external motivation to respond without prejudice. Why the fast recruitment of attention occurs for this subgroup and no other is a question to which we return later in the chapter.

REFERENCES

Allport, G. W. (1954). *The nature of prejudice.* Cambridge, MA: Addison-Wesley.

Amodio, D. M. (2009). The social neuroscience of intergroup relations. *European Review of Social Psychology, 19*, 1–54.

Amodio, D. M., & Devine, P. G. (2006). Stereotyping and evaluation in implicit race bias: Evidence for independent constructs and unique effects on behavior. *Journal of Personality and Social Psychology, 91*, 652–661.

Amodio, D. M., Devine, P. G., & Harmon-Jones, E. (2007). A dynamic model of guilt: Implications for motivation and self-regulation in the context of prejudice. *Psychological Science, 18*, 524–530.

Amodio, D. M., Devine, P. G., & Harmon-Jones, E. (2008). Individual differences in the regulation of intergroup bias: The role of conflict monitoring and neural signals for control. *Journal of Personality and Social Psychology, 94*, 60–74.

Amodio, D. M., Harmon-Jones, E., & Devine, P. G. (2003). Individual differences in the activation and control of affective race bias as assessed by startle eyeblink response and self-report. *Journal of Personality and Social Psychology, 84*, 738–753.

Bargh, J. (1999). The cognitive monster: The case against the controllability of automatic stereotype effects. In S. Chaiken & Y. Trope (Eds.), *Dual-process theories in social psychology* (pp. 361–382). New York: Guilford Press.

Bargh, J. A. (1994). The four horsemen of automaticity: Awareness, intention, efficiency, and control in social cognition. In R. S. Wyer & T. K. Srull (Eds.), *Handbook of social cognition: Vol. 1. Basic processes* (2nd ed., pp. 1–40).). Hillsdale, NJ: Erlbaum.

Baron, A. S., & Banaji, M. R. (2006). The development of implicit attitudes. Evidence of race evaluations from ages 6 and 10 and adulthood. *Psychological Science, 17*, 53–58.

Bartholow, B. D., Dickter, C. L., & Sestir, M. A. (2006). Stereotype activation and control of race bias: Cognitive control of inhibition and its impairment by alcohol. *Journal of Personality and Social Psychology, 90*, 272–287.

Bertrand, M., & Mullainathan, S. (2004). Are Emily and Greg more employable than Lakisha and Jamal?: A field experiment on labor market discrimination. *American Economic Review, 94*, 991–1013.

Billig, M. (1985). Prejudice, categorization and particularization: From a perceptual to a rhetorical approach. *European Journal of Social Psychology, 15*, 79–103.

Blair, I. V., Ma, J. E., & Lenton, A. P. (2001). Imagining stereotypes away: The moderation of implicit stereotypes through mental imagery. *Journal of Personality and Social Psychology, 81*, 828–841.

Brewer, M. (1988). A dual-process model of impression formation. In T. Srull & R. Wyer (Eds.), *Advances in social cognition* (pp. 1–36). Hillsdale, NJ: Erlbaum.

Carr, P. B., Rattan, A., & Dweck, C. S. (2012). Implicit theories shape intergroup relations. In P. Devine & A. Plant (Eds.), *Advances in experimental social psychology* (Vol. 45, pp. 127–165). Amsterdam: Elsevier.

Carver, C. S., & Scheier, M. F. (1990). Origins and functions of positive and negative affect: A control-process view. *Psychological Review, 97*, 19–35.

Chaiken, S. (1980). Heuristic versus systematic information processing and the use of source versus message cues in persuasion. *Journal of Personality and Social Psychology, 39*, 752–766.

Conrey, F. R., Sherman, J. W., Gawronski, B., Hugenberg, K., & Groom, C. J. (2005). Separating multiple processes in implicit social cognition: The quad model of implicit task performance. *Journal of Personality and Social Psychology, 89*, 469–487.

Crandall, C. S., Eshleman, A., & O'Brien, L. (2002). Social norms and the expression and suppression of prejudice: The struggle for internalization. *Journal of Personality and Social Psychology, 82*, 359–378.

Crandall, C. S., & Eshleman, A. (2003). A justification-suppression model of the expression and experience of prejudice. *Psychological Bulletin, 129*, 414–446.

Crosby, F., Bromley, S., & Saxe, L. (1980). Recent unobtrusive studies of Black and White discrimination and prejudice: A literature review. *Psychological Bulletin, 87*, 546–563.

Dasgupta, N., & Greenwald, A. G. (2001). On the malleability of automatic attitudes: Combating automatic prejudice with images of admired and disliked individuals. *Journal of Personality and Social Psychology, 81*, 800–814.

Deci, E., & Ryan, R. (2000). The "what" and "why" of goal pursuits: Human needs and the self-determination of behavior. *Psychological Inquiry, 11*, 227–268.

Devine, P. G. (1989). Stereotypes and prejudice: Their automatic and controlled components. *Journal of Personality and Social Psychology, 56*, 5–18.

Devine, P. G. (2001). Implicit prejudice and stereotyping: How automatic are they?: Introduction to the special section. *Journal of Personality and Social Psychology, 81*, 757–759.

Devine, P. G., & Elliot, A. J. (1995). Are racial stereotypes really fading?: The Princeton trilogy revisited. *Personality and Social Psychology Bulletin, 21*, 1139–1150.

Devine, P. G., Evett, S. R., & Vasquez-Suson, K. A. (1996). Exploring the interpersonal dynamics of intergroup contact. In R. M. Sorrentino & E. T. Higgins (Eds.), *Handbook of motivation and cognition: Foundations of social behavior* (pp. 423–464). New York: Guilford Press.

Devine, P. G., Forscher, P. S., Austin, A. J., & Cox, W. T. L. (2012). Long-term reduction in implicit race bias: A prejudice habit-breaking intervention. *Journal of Experimental Social Psychology, 48*(6), 1267–1278.

Devine, P. G., & Monteith, M. J. (1993). The role of discrepancy-associated affect in prejudice reduction. In D. M. Mackie & D. L. Hamilton (Eds.), *Affect, cognition, and stereotyping: Interactive processes in group perception* (pp. 317–344). San Diego: Academic Press.

Devine, P. G., & Monteith, M. J. (1999). Automaticity and control in stereotyping. In S. Chaiken & Y. Trope (Eds.), *Dual-process theories in social psychology* (pp. 339–360). New York: Guilford Press.

Devine, P. G., Monteith, M. J., Zuwerink, J. R., & Elliot, A. J. (1991). Prejudice with and without compunction. *Journal of Personality and Social Psychology, 60*, 817–830.

Devine, P. G., Plant, E. A., Amodio, D. M., Harmon-Jones, E., & Vance, S. L. (2002). The regulation of explicit and implicit race bias: The role of motivations to respond without prejudice. *Journal of Personality and Social Psychology, 82*, 835–848.

Eberhardt, J. L., Goff, R. A., Purdie, V. J., & Davies, P. G. (2004). Seeing Black: Race, crime, and visual processing. *Journal of Personality and Social Psychology, 87*, 876–893.

Fiske, S. T., & Neuberg, S. L. (1990). A continuum of impression formation, from category-based to individuating processes: Influences of information and motivation on attention and interpretation. In M. P. Zanna (Ed.), *Advances in experimental social psychology* (Vol. 23, pp. 1–74). Amsterdam: Elsevier.

Gaertner, S., & Dovidio, J. F. (1986). The aversive form of racism. In J. F. Dovidio & S. Gaertner (Eds.), *Prejudice, discrimination, and racism* (pp. 61–89). Orlando, FL: Academic Press.

Galinsky, A. D., & Moskowitz, G. B. (2000). Perspective-taking: Decreasing stereotype expression, stereotype accessibility, and in-group favoritism. *Journal of Personality and Social Psychology*, *78*, 708–724.

Gerbner, G. (1998). Cultivation analysis: An overview. *Mass Communication and Society*, *1*, 175–194.

Gilbert, D. T. (1989). Thinking lightly about others: Automatic components of the social inference process. In J. S. Uleman & J. A. Bargh (Eds.), *Unintended thought* (pp. 189–211). New York: Guilford Press.

Green, A. R., Carney, D. R., Pallin, D. J., Ngo, L. H., Raymond, K. L., Iezzoni, L. I., et al. (2007). Implicit bias among physicians and its prediction of thrombolysis decisions for Black and White patients. *Journal of General Internal Medicine*, 22, 1231–1238.

Higgins, E. T. (1987). Self-discrepancy: A theory relating self and affect. *Psychological Review*, *94*, 319–340.

Ito, T. A., Thompson, E., & Cacioppo, J. T. (2004). Tracking the timecourse of social perception: The effects of racial cues on event-related brain potentials. *Personality and Social Psychology Bulletin*, *30*, 1267–1280.

Kim, D. (2003). Voluntary controllability of the Implicit Association Test (IAT). *Social Psychology Quarterly*, *66*, 83–96.

Klonis, S. C., Plant, E. A., & Devine, P. G. (2005). Internal and external motivation to respond without sexism. *Personality and Social Psychology Bulletin*, *31*, 1237–1249.

Maio, G. R. (2010). Mental representations of social values. In M. P. Zanna (Ed.), *Advances in experimental social psychology* (Vol. 42, pp. 1–43). Amsterdam: Elsevier.

Maio, G. R., Hahn, U., Frost, J., & Cheung, W. (2009). Applying the value of equality unequally: Effects of value instantiations that vary in typicality. *Journal of Personality and Social Psychology*, *97*, 598–614.

Monteith, M. J. (1993). Self-regulation of prejudiced responses: Implications for progress in prejudice-reduction efforts. *Journal of Personality and Social Psychology*, *65*, 469–485.

Monteith, M. J., Ashburn-Nardo, L., Voils, C. I., & Czopp, A. M. (2002). Putting the brakes on prejudice: On the development and operation of cues for control. *Journal of Personality and Social Psychology*, *83*, 1029–1050.

Monteith, M. J., Devine, P. G., & Zuwerink, J. R. (1993). Self-directed versus other-directed affect as a consequence of prejudice-related discrepancies. *Journal of Personality and Social Psychology*, *64*, 198–210.

Monteith, M. J., & Lybarger, J. E. (in preparation).

Monteith, M. J., & Mark, A. Y. (2005). Changing one's prejudiced ways: Awareness, affect, and self-regulation. *European Review of Social Psychology*, *16*, 113–154.

Monteith, M. J., Mark, A. Y., & Ashburn-Nardo, L. (2010). The self-regulation of prejudice: Toward understanding its lived character. *Group Processes and Intergroup Relations*, *13*, 183–200.

Monteith, M. J., Voils, C. I., & Ashburn-Nardo, L. (2001). Taking a look underground: Detecting, interpreting, and reacting to implicit racial biases. *Social Cognition*, *19*, 395–417.

Olsson, A., Ebert, J. P., Banaji, M. R., & Phelps, E. A. (2005). The role of social groups in the persistence of learned fear. *Science*, *309*, 785–787.

Payne, B. K. (2001). Prejudice and perception: the role of automatic and controlled processes in misperceiving a weapon. *Journal of Personality and Social Psychology*, *81*, 181–192.

Pettigrew, T. F. (1998). Integroup contact theory. *Annual Review of Psychology*, *49*, 65–85.

Petty, R. E., & Cacioppo, J. T. (1986). The elaboration likelihood model of persuasion. In L. Berkowitz (Ed.), *Advances in experimental social psychology* (Vol. 19, pp. 123–205). Orlando, FL: Academic Press.

Plant, E. A., & Devine, P. G. (1998). Internal and external motivation to respond without prejudice. *Journal of Personality and Social Psychology*, *75*, 811–832.

Plant, E. A., & Devine, P. G. (2001). Responses to other-imposed pro-Black pressure: Acceptance or backlash? *Journal of Experimental Social Psychology*, *37*, 486–501.

Plant, E. A., & Devine, P. G. (2009). The active control of prejudice: Unpacking the intentions guiding control efforts. *Journal of Personality and Social Psychology*, *96*, 640–652.

Plant, E. A., Devine, P. G., & Peruche, M. B.

(2010). Routes to positive interracial interactions: Approaching egalitarianism or avoiding prejudice. *Personality and Social Psychology Bulletin, 36*, 1135–1147.

Prochaska, J. O., & Velicer, W. F. (1997). The transtheoretical model of health behavior change. *American Journal of Health Promotion, 12*, 38–48.

Ratcliff, J. J., Lassiter, G. D., Markman, K. D., & Snyder, C. J. (2006). Gender differences in attitudes toward gay men and lesbians: The role of motivation to respond without prejudice. *Personality and Social Psychology Bulletin, 32*, 1325–1338.

Richeson, J. A., & Shelton, J. N. (2003). When prejudice does not pay: Effects of interracial contact on executive function. *Psychological Science, 14*, 287–290.

Schuman, H., Steeh, C., Bobo, L., & Krysan, M. (1997). *Racial attitudes in America: Trends and interpretations* (Rev. ed.). Cambridge, MA: Harvard University Press.

Smith, E. R., & DeCoster, J. (2000). Dual-process models in social and cognitive psychology: Conceptual integration and links to underlying memory systems. *Personality and Social Psychology Review, 4*, 108–131.

Steele, C. M. (1997). A threat in the air: How stereotypes shape intellectual identity and performance. *American Psychologist, 52*, 613–629.

Strack, F., & Deutsch, R. (2004). Reflective and impulsive determinants of social behavior. *Personality and Social Psychology Review, 8*, 220–247.

Williams, D. R., Neighbors, H. W., & Jackson, J. S. (2003). Racial/ethnic discrimination and health: Findings from community studies. *American Journal of Public Health, 93*, 200–208.

Wilson, T. D., & Brekke, N. (1994). Mental contamination and mental correction: Unwanted influences on judgments and evaluations. *Psychological Bulletin, 116*, 117–142.

CHAPTER 32

Emotion Generation and Emotion Regulation

Moving Beyond Traditional Dual-Process Accounts

Gal Sheppes and James J. Gross

From classical philosophers such as David Hume to early psychologists such as Sigmund Freud, the distinction between processes that generate emotion and those that regulate emotion has featured prominently. This distinction has also dominated modern emotion theory and research (e.g., Gross, 1998a, 2001; Gross & Thompson, 2007; Koole, 2009). However, an alternative view that describes emotion and regulation as inseparably bound up with one another has emerged in recent years (e.g., Campos, Frankel, & Camras, 2004; Kappas, 2011; Mesquita & Fridja, 2011; Thompson, 2011). Recently, we have attempted to reconcile these contrasting views by suggesting that different theoretical perspectives on emotion lead to preferences to make (or not make) such a distinction (Gross & Barrett, 2011; Gross, Sheppes, & Urry, 2011a), and we have tried to define when the distinction is useful and when it is not (Gross, Sheppes, & Urry, 2011b).

In this chapter, we revisit this debate from the standpoint of a dual-process perspective. To that end, we begin by clearly defining emotion generation and emotion regulation, and by describing considerations that justify their separation (Gross, Sheppes, & Urry, 2011a, 2011b). We then describe a dual-process model that uses a classic framework according to which emotion generation is executed via associative processes and emotion regulation via reflective processes (Gross & Thompson, 2007; Sheppes & Gross, 2011, 2012). Although this model is broadly consistent with prior experimental work in the field, we argue that emerging evidence challenges this classic categorization and suggests the value of making a further division within the emotion regulation concept that includes the operation of both associative and reflective processes (e.g., Berkman & Lieberman, 2009; Gyurak, Gross, & Etkin, 2011; Mauss, Bunge, & Gross, 2007).

DEFINITION OF TERMS

Emotions play a central part in our lives. The experience of fear may help us to be more vigilant when we walk in a dark alley at night, and surprise followed by happiness may facilitate our appreciation when we meet an acquaintance we did not expect to see. We can then experience sadness when the acquaintance shares with us his recent job loss experience or switch to experiencing anger or even genuine disgust (Chapman, Kim, Susskind, & Anderson, 2009) if we perceive the reason for the job termination to be fundamentally unfair. Though clearly central in our lives, emotions are invoked in unique circumstances and are not experienced all of the time. What are the unique circumstances in which emotions are called into being?

Emotion Generation

From an evolutionary perspective, emotions are induced to prepare the organism and to produce responses that will be advantageous to the organism or to its relations (Damasio, 1999). Specifically, emotions are generated when an organism attends to a certain situation that is given a valenced meaning, and this evaluation gives rise to a coordinated set of experiential, behavioral, and physiological responses (Gross, 1998a, 1998b, 2001, 2002). Going back to the previous example, if we attend to the features of the dark alley and appraise it as potentially dangerous, we experience fear, that involves behavioral (e.g., facial expressive behavior; Ekman, 1992) and physiological (e.g., increased sympathetic activation; Kreibig, 2010) responses.

In Figure 32.1, we present in schematic form the situation–attention–meaning–response sequence that constitutes an emotional response. We use a rather abstract definition here, which we call the "modal model" of emotion, because emotions form such a heterogeneous category, with different types, intensities, and durations, that it is difficult to make generalizations that apply to all cases. Despite fundamental differences between emotions, we wish to emphasize three common features for different emotional episodes.

First, emotions arise when a situation is construed as being relevant to one or more of an individual's personal strivings or active goals (Scherer, Schorr, & Johnstone, 2001). Some of these goals may be biologically based (e.g., avoiding physical harm). Others may be culturally derived (e.g., protecting familial dignity). Some of these goals may be social (e.g., helping an older adult cross the street). Others may be self-focused (e.g., wanting to meet one's own expectations). Because many goals are usually active at any one time, the most dominant goal dictates which, if any, emotion will be activated and to what degree. Whatever the details of the emotion-generating goals that are active at a particular point in time, and whatever the details of the situation the individual faces, it is ultimately the situational meaning in relation to a goal that gives rise to an emotion. As either the goal or the individual's construal of the situation changes, so will the emotion.

A second common feature is that emotions are multifaceted, embodied phenomena that involve loosely coupled changes in the domains of subjective experience, behavior, and peripheral physiology (Mauss, Levenson, McCarter, Wilhelm, & Gross, 2005). The experiential component of emotion, which is also defined as feeling, is a private state or an internal representation of the changes invoked by the emotional unfolding (Damasio, 1999). The behavioral component of emotion includes changes in activity in muscles of the face and body, and in what one says, as well as more general changes in basic motivational states, such as the likelihood of approaching or withdrawing from something in the environment (Frijda, 1986). The peripheral physiological component of emotion includes the autonomic and neuroendocrine responses that putatively provide metabolic support for anticipated and actual behavioral responses (Levenson, 1999).

A third common feature is that emotions play out in ways that are sensitive to the particular details of a given internal or external environment. This means that, under some circumstances, emotions can take full control (Frijda, 1986). For example, walking around the streets of Paris, a person's dominant goal may be sightseeing. But if a stranger pulls a knife and asks for all of the person's money, his or her dominant goal quickly becomes survival, and fear takes over. In this case, the emotion-related goal (survival) has overridden the non-emotion-related goal (sightseeing). However, emotions do not always trump other goal-driven

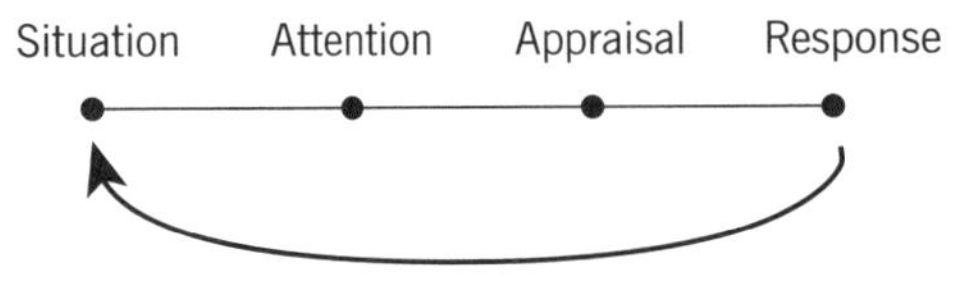

FIGURE 32.1. A schematic of the emotion generative process. From Gross and Thompson (2007). Copyright by The Guilford Press. Reprinted by permission.

processes (i.e., processes related to meeting active goals; e.g., sightseeing in the previous example that is unrelated to the emotion-generating goals). This means that emotions can be and often are adjusted to suit our needs in a given situation. It is this third common feature of emotion that permits us to regulate our emotions.

Emotion Regulation

Emotion regulation refers to the processes that influence which emotions we have, when we have them, and how we experience or express these emotions (Gross, 1998a). Recently, we highlighted that emotion regulation should be defined by the activation of a goal to modify the emotion generative process, and involves the motivated recruitment of one or more processes to influence emotion generation (Gross et al., 2011a). Whether we consult our own experiences or the empirical literature, it is clear that emotions may be regulated in many different ways (Gross, Richards, & John, 2006).

One important point of difference across emotion regulation episodes is whether the emotion regulatory goal is activated in the individual who is having (or is likely to have) an emotion episode or in someone else. An example of the first type of emotion regulation episode—which we refer to as *intrinsic emotion regulation*—is when someone tries not to think about something that is upsetting. An example of the second type of emotion regulation episode—which we refer to as *extrinsic emotion regulation*—is when a friend calms us down by putting an upsetting situation in perspective. While extrinsic emotion regulation remains important in adulthood, it is perhaps the most dominant form of emotion regulation in infancy where parents have a crucial role in helping infants to develop an ability to regulate their emotions (Macklem, 2008).

A second point of difference across emotion regulation episodes is whether the motivation to engage in emotion regulation is *hedonic* (the goal to feel less negative or more positive in the near-term) or *instrumental* (to achieve one's long-term goals) (Tamir, 2009). In some cases these two types of goals are congruent, for example, when a person tries to decrease fear and anxiety because it makes him or her jittery in the moment and at the same time can hurt his or her long-term health. At other times these goals can compete, for example, when one wants to avoid a certain dreaded situation in order to feel relief in the short run that in the long run perpetuates the situation.

Finally, emotions can be *down-regulated* when the goal is to decrease the magnitude or duration of a certain emotion response, or *up-regulated* when the goal is to increase the magnitude or duration of an emotional response. While the obvious examples of down-regulation involve decreasing negative emotions, and the obvious examples of up-regulation involve increasing positive emotions, there are many instances in which one's instrumental goals are to down-regulate positive emotions or up-regulate negative emotions (Tamir, 2009). For example, a person on a diet might try to reduce his or her joy when eating high- calorie food, or a person who wishes to avoid certain dangers might prefer to up-regulate his or her fear levels (Tamir & Ford, 2009). Though all of these types of emotion regulation are clearly important, we focus in this chapter on down-regulation of negative emotions, because it is one of the most common and important types of regulation.

Distinguishing Emotion Generation from Emotion Regulation

The difference between emotion generation and emotion regulation is a distinction between the processes that generate an emotion in a particular situation, and the processes that are engaged to modify these emotion generative processes.

Recently, we have argued that although both emotion generation and emotion regulation involve goals, a process is emotion regulatory if, and only if, it is instantiated in pursuit of a goal to influence an ongoing or future emotion (Gross et al., 2011a). Therefore, the target of an emotion regulation goal is always the emotion-generative process. This is in contrast to the goals that generate emotion, namely, those that are instantiated in pursuit of a particular outcome. Therefore, the target of an emotion generation goal can be either the internal or the external environment. As we explain below, it is often difficult to discern when a goal to regulate emotion has been activated, and emotion generation and emotion regulation often (but not always) co-occur. However, it is the targeting of an ongoing or future emotion generative process for change that constitutes emotion regulation.

In most everyday situations, the emotion trajectory that we observe is the result of a complex interplay between emotion generative and emotion regulatory processes. The challenge is to determine—for any given case—whether a goal to modify an emotion has been activated, leading to the recruitment of regulatory processes and (often) to the alteration of the emotion response trajectory. We find it useful to imagine a continuum of possibilities, ranging from cases where there are clear and compelling grounds for inferring that emotion regulation processes are operative to those in which there is little ground for thinking that emotion regulation processes are operative.

At one end of this continuum, there are clear signs that a stable, dominant emotion regulation goal has been activated, leading to the recruitment of regulatory processes and to the alteration of the emotion response trajectory. In these situations, it seems useful to postulate two separable factors that govern the way the individual is responding in that particular situation: emotion generation and emotion regulation. At the other end of the continuum, there is no clear indication that a stable, dominant emotion regulation goal has been activated or that the emotion response trajectory has been altered (e.g., the individual behaves in a way that is similar to his or her behavior when freely expressing a certain emotion). In this case, it seems most parsimonious to invoke only emotion generative (and not emotion regulatory) processes.

Perhaps most interesting are cases in which (1) there are clear indications that an emotion regulation goal has been activated, yet we cannot detect any change in the emotion trajectory, or (2) there is no clear sign that an emotion regulation goal has been activated, yet the emotion trajectory is altered. In the former case, we might invoke ineffective (or failed) emotion regulation. In the latter case, if there is no indication that an emotion regulation goal has been activated, and no evidence for the recruitment of emotion regulatory processes, the individual's response may best be explained more simply, in terms of emotion generative (and not emotion regulatory) processes. These "intermediate" cases may be more the norm than the exception as one moves away from controlled laboratory studies toward everyday social interactions, where most of our emotions play out, and where the interdigitation of emotion generation and emotion regulation may be most pronounced (Campos, Walle, Dahl, & Main, 2011).

Wherever we are on this hypothetical continuum, invoking emotion regulatory processes requires activation of an emotion regulatory goal, and in many cases results in an observed emotion trajectory that is different from the (hypothetical) emotion trajectory that would have unfolded in the absence of emotion regulation. This highlights the fact that statements about emotion regulation—like other psychological constructs—are inherently probabilistic.

A DUAL-PROCESS ACCOUNT OF EMOTION GENERATION AND EMOTION REGULATION

Distinctions between emotion generation and emotion regulation are important, but what is essential is defining the processes underlying each. Consider the process model of emotion regulation (for reviews, see Gross, 1998a, 2001, 2002; Gross & Thompson, 2007). According to this model, the analysis of emotion regulation processes involves considering which parts of the emotion generative process are primary targets of an active goal to influence emotion. To examine this dimension of variation, we take the emotion generation model depicted in Figure 32.1 as a starting point. Emotion regulatory acts are seen as having their primary impact on different stages of the emotion generative process (Gross, 2001). In Figure 32.2, we highlight five points in the emotion generative process at which individuals can regulate their emotions, corresponding to five families of emotion regulation processes: situation selection, situation modification, attentional deployment, cognitive change, and response modulation.

Situation selection refers to efforts individuals make to influence the situations they encounter, with a view toward increasing (or decreasing) the likelihood that certain

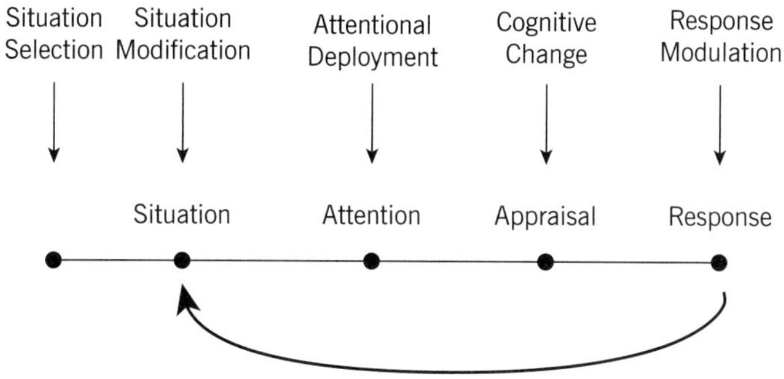

FIGURE 32.2. A process model of emotion regulation that highlights five families of emotion regulation strategies. From Gross and Thompson (2007). Copyright by The Guilford Press. Reprinted by permission.

emotions will arise. *Situation modification* refers to attempts to change the external features of a situation in a way that will alter one's emotional response to that situation. Moving from efforts to regulate the external features of an emotional situation to regulations efforts that influence internal representations (i.e., the "black box"), *attentional deployment* refers to directing attention in such a way that the emotion–response trajectory is altered. *Cognitive change* refers to altering a situation's meaning in a way that influences the emotions that situation will produce. Finally, *response modulation* refers to targeting the experiential, behavioral and/or physiological components of an activated emotion response for change.

Within this broad framework, of course, it is possible to drill down and analyze more specific processes of each of the strategies that make up each family of regulatory processes. For example, we recently considered in greater detail the underlying mechanisms involved in attentional deployment and cognitive change (Sheppes, 2014; Sheppes & Gross, 2011; Sheppes & Levin, 2013; Sheppes, Scheibe, Suri, & Gross, 2011; Sheppes et al., in press). According to our perspective, emotion regulatory strategies can modify the cognitive processing of emotional information at two major stages.

Incoming emotional information can be regulated at an early processing stage via a filtering mechanism that blocks it from capturing selective attention. Such early disengagement from cognitive processing of emotional information does not permit elaborative processing that may be important for fully evaluating the situation and preparing an adaptive response (Bradley, Codispoti, Cuthbert, & Lang, 2001; Wilson & Gilbert, 2008). However, early disengagement, before emotional information gathers force, can successfully modulate low and high emotional intensity information. A classic early disengagement regulation strategy is *distraction*, which involves disengaging from negative emotion by producing neutral thoughts, using an early filter that blocks emotional information before it is represented in working memory for further evaluative processing (see Figure 32.3a).

Incoming emotional information that passes the early filter can still be regulated at a late stage via a second filtering mechanism that operates at the semantic meaning level and determines the final output of the system. Engagement with emotional processing allows elaborated cognitive processing of emotional information, but because emotional information gathers force prior to its late modulation, it is less effective at modulating high-intensity emotional information. A classic late engagement strategy is *reappraisal*, which involves engaging with negative emotion by allowing emotional information to be represented in working memory and provided with elaborated meaning before it is reinterpreted via a late filter (see Figure 32.3b).

While the process model and its elaborations favor a separation between emotion generation processes and emotion regulation processes, an important ques-

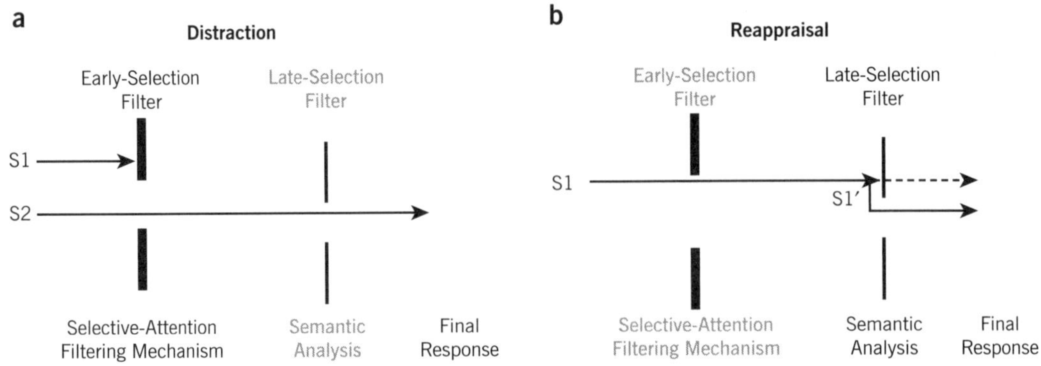

FIGURE 32.3. Illustrations of the underlying operation of distraction and reappraisal. The thickness of the lines representing the early-selection and late-selection filters reflects the ability of these filters to block emotional processing. In disengagement distraction, which is shown in Panel *a*, incoming emotional information (represented by the arrow for Stimulus 1, S1) is filtered out at an early attentional selection phase. A neutral stream of information (represented by arrow S2) that corresponds to the neutral thoughts produced in distraction and that is semantically independent from the original emotional information dominates the final response. In engagement reappraisal, which is shown in Panel *b*, incoming emotional information (represented by arrow S1) passes the early filter, is attended, undergoes semantic analysis, and is provided with elaborative meaning prior to modulation via a neutral reinterpretation (represented by arrow S1′), which is semantically dependent on the original emotional information. High-intensity emotional information (represented by the dashed arrow) passes through the late-selection filter and affects the final response. Adapted from Sheppes, Scheibe, Suri, and Gross (2011). Copyright by the Association for Psychological Science. Adapted with permission from Sage Publications, Inc.

tion is how best to capture the relationships between these two sets of processes. In neighboring fields such as that of self-regulation (which includes emotion regulation, as well as the regulation of thoughts, drives, beliefs, behaviors, and goals), classic dual-process accounts have been proposed (e.g., for reviews, see Hofmann, Friese, & Strack, 2009; Strack & Deutsch, 2004). For example, some models have highlighted that deliberate self-control is initiated when a conflict is identified between central goals and opposing associative temptations (e.g., Fujita & Carnevale, 2012; Myrseth & Fishbach, 2009). In these cases deliberate self-control is activated to resolve the conflict in accord with goal pursuit. Borrowing from these models, emotion generation has often been considered to involve an associative mode that involves lower-order mental operations that are achieved through relatively fast automatic and effortless processes, and emotion regulation has often been viewed as a reflective mode that involves higher-order mental operations that are achieved via relatively slow, deliberate, and effortful processes.

While the process model and its elaborations do not explicitly limit emotion generation to an associative mode and emotion regulation to a reflective mode, the most common interpretation of this model and related findings across multiple levels of analysis is congruent with this view (reviews of self-report studies: Aldao, Nolen-Hoeksema, & Schweizer, 2010; cognitive and physiological studies: Webb, Miles, & Sheeran, 2012; electrophysiological studies: Hajcak, MacNamara, & Olvett, 2010; neuroimaging studies: Berkman & Liberman, 2009; Ochsner & Gross, 2005, 2008). In these studies a clear demonstration of this dual-process nature is also observed in the experimental manipulation in which participants are required to generate emotional responses in a relatively effortless way (e.g., viewing pictures), and most manipulations of emotion regulation have involved asking participants to deliberately instantiate effortful strategies whose aim is to modify the natural emotional responses.

ELABORATING ON THE DUAL-PROCESS ACCOUNT

While the classic dual-process account of linking emotion generation with an associative mode and emotion regulation with a reflective mode has been fruitful, in recent years it has become quite clear that emotion regulatory processes can also be initiated relatively automatically via fast, associative modes of operation (Gyurak et al., 2011; Koole, & Rothermund, 2011; Mauss et al., 2007).

As we have emphasized, our definition of what constitutes emotion regulation does not specify the nature of the underlying processes (associative or reflective). Instead, our definition holds that a process is emotion regulatory if (and only if) it is instantiated in pursuit of a goal to influence an ongoing or future emotion (Gross et al., 2011). In the following, we examine the nature of recent evidence for the existence of associative emotion regulation processes, using the aforementioned continuum of possibilities that classifies whether emotion regulation processes can be assumed to be an independent entity that is separate from emotion generation processes.

As described earlier, at one end of the continuum, there are clear signs that a stable, dominant emotion regulation goal has been activated, leading to the recruitment of regulatory processes and to the alteration of the emotion response trajectory. An example of such a case is nicely illustrated in findings by Williams, Bargh, Nocera, and Gray (2009), who have shown that unconsciously priming the goal to reappraise resulted in attenuation of experiential and physiological signatures of anxiety. Similarly influential studies on implementation intentions have shown that forming a simple if–then regulatory rule reduced behavioral and early cortical signs of fear and disgust reactions (Gallo, Keil, McCulloch, Rockstroh, & Gollwitzer, 2011) and modulated emotion generative attentional and interpretation biases of threat in socially anxious individuals (e.g., Webb, Ononaiye, Sheeran, Reidy, & Lavda, 2010). In each of these cases, it is evident from the pattern of outcomes that an associative emotion regulatory process has been engaged.

There also can be cases at the other end of the continuum, where there is no clear indication that an associative emotion regulation goal was activated or that the emotion response trajectory was altered. As stated earlier, these cases favor a parsimonious view that only includes the manifestation of emotion generative processes.

The challenge lies in the middle of the continuum, where there are clear indications that an emotion regulation goal was activated, yet we cannot detect any change in the emotion trajectory. Such situations arise in the context of studies that have manipulated goals (e.g., via unconscious priming or via the formation of implementation intentions) and observed that they were operative (e.g., via manipulation checks), yet failed to achieve a change in emotion generation processes. It is also interesting to consider cases where there is no clear sign that an emotion regulation goal was activated, yet the emotion trajectory was altered. Two such cases that fit this category are emotional conflict adaptation (e.g., Egner, Etkin, Gale, & Hirsch, 2008; Etkin, Egner, Peraza, Kandel, & Hirsch, 2006) and affect labeling (Hariri, Bookheimer, & Mazziotta, 2000; Lieberman et al., 2007; Lieberman, Hariri, Jarcho, Eisenberger, & Bookheimer, 2005); we turn now to these two cases.

Emotional conflict adaptation (e.g., Egner et al., 2008; Etkin et al., 2006) is an emotional variant of the classic Stroop task. In this task, participants are instructed to name an emotional expression (e.g., of a face displaying fear) while inhibiting the automatic reading of a superimposed emotional word (e.g., the word *sad* written on the forehead of a face displaying fear). As in the classic Stroop task, there are congruent and incongruent trial types. Importantly, the emotional conflict adaptation effect is observed when the response for an incongruent trial is faster if it is preceded by an incongruent trial than if it is preceded by a congruent trial. Related functional neuroimaging data suggest an interplay between brain regions associated with regulation (e.g., the anterior cingulate cortex and medial prefrontal cortex) and brain regions associated with emotional reactivity regions (e.g., the amygdala). The interpretation of this effect is that performing an incongruent trial activates emotional control that implicitly persists into the next trial. In this case, it is hard to determine whether a clear regulatory goal was formed (because participants try to inhibit the reading of a word), but it is clear that regulatory processes were recruited.

In a similar vein, *affect labeling* (Lieberman et al., 2005, 2007) refers to a creative task context in which the consequence of processing affective features with words recruits an emotional regulation circuitry that is different from processing affective aspects in perceptual or experiential ways. Specifically, in this task, participants are presented with a target picture (e.g., an angry face) and asked to choose either a matching word (choosing the word *angry* over the word *sad*) or a matching perceptual face (choosing an angry face over a sad face) that appear below the target face. In this context, emotional modulation is observed via the recruitment of control-related brain regions, without participants' awareness of such an effect (Lieberman, Inagaki, Tabibnia, & Crockett, 2011). Here, too, it is not clear whether an emotion regulatory goal was activated, although there are clear manifestations of emotional generation and modulation via the recruitment of regulatory brain processes.

The emerging study of associative emotion regulation has increased in volume in recent years and attracted a great deal of interest. The growing consensus is that all families of emotion regulation strategies that constitute the process model of emotion regulation (Gross, 1998a, see Figure 32.2 have associative as well as deliberate forms (for reviews, see Gross & Thompson, 2007; Mauss et al., 2007; Todd, Cunningham, Anderson, & Thompson, 2012). Nevertheless, and despite the promising potential, several definitional issues remain unclear at present. One major issue revolves around the core underlying features of the different forms of associative emotion regulation. For example, while some forms of associative regulation, such as emotional conflict adaptation and affect labeling, appear to be unconscious, studies on implementation intentions typically involve forming conscious emotion regulation if–then rules. At the same time, while implementation intentions and affect labeling require minimal cognitive effort to operate, emotional conflict adaptation engages effortful cognitive control mechanisms, and even unconscious goal pursuit appears to utilize executive control resources for its attainment (see Marien, Custers, Hassin, & Aarts, 2012).

In moving forward, the field of emotion regulation will need to find new ways to define the differences between associative and deliberate forms of emotion regulation. One important venue involves clearer empirical evaluation of the two forms of regulation. Currently, studies typically involve evaluating deliberate and associative processes using different tasks (see Hofmann et al., 2009, for a review). While informative, the use of different tasks makes it hard to separate process from measure. One promising approach that overcomes this obstacle is the quadruple-process model that provides distinct quantitative estimates of associative and deliberate processes in a single task (see Sherman et al., 2008, for a review). Insights about associative and deliberate processes in the neighboring field of self-regulation have already been utilized (e.g., Govorun & Payne, 2006; Stewart & Payne, 2008; for reviews, see Payne, 2008; Sherman et al., 2008). Therefore, their adoption in the field of emotion regulation is urgently needed.

In this chapter, we have revisited a central question in affective science that relates to whether emotion generation processes can be separated from emotion regulation processes. According to our perspective, a central consideration that justifies a separation is whether one can assume that a goal to change the emotion generation trajectory was activated. Congruent with these cases that justify a separation, conceptual models of emotion regulation have been proposed. These models have been framed in classic dual-process terms whereby emotion generation is executed via associative processes and emotion regulation via reflective processes. In this chapter, we have challenged this classic categorization by discussing the conditions that justify the existence of an additional associative emotion regulation system (in addition to the classic reflective emotion regulation system) that is separate from an associative emotion generation system.

AUTHORS' NOTE

This chapter draws upon and updates previous reviews by Gross (1998a, 2001, 2002); Gross and Thompson (2007); Gross et al. (2011a); and Sheppes and Gross (2011, 2012).

REFERENCES

Aldao, A., Nolen-Hoeksema, S., & Schweizer, S. (2010). Emotion regulation strategies across psychopathology: A meta-analytic review. *Clinical Psychology Review, 30*, 217–237.

Berkman, E., & Lieberman, M. D. (2009). Using neuroscience to broaden emotion regulation: Theoretical and methodological considerations. *Social and Personality Psychology Compass, 3*, 475–493.

Bradley, M. M., Codispoti, M., Cuthbert, B. N., & Lang, P. J. (2001). Emotion and motivation I: Defensive and appetitive reactions in picture processing. *Emotion, 1*, 276–298.

Campos, J. J., Frankel, C. B., & Camras, L. (2004). On the nature of emotion regulation. *Child Development, 75*, 377–394.

Campos, J., Walle, E., Dahl, A., & Main, A. (2011). Reconceptualizing emotion regulation. *Emotion Review, 3*(1), 26–35.

Chapman, H. A., Kim, D. A., Susskind, J. M., & Anderson, A. K. (2009). In bad taste: Evidence for the oral origins of moral disgust. *Science, 323*, 1222–1226.

Damasio, A. R. (1999). *The feeling of what happens: Body and emotion in the making of consciousness*. New York: Harcourt Brace.

Egner, T., Etkin, A., Gale, S., & Hirsch, J. (2008). Dissociable neural systems resolve conflict from emotional versus nonemotional distracters. *Cerebral Cortex, 18*, 1475–1484.

Ekman, P. (1992). Facial expressions of emotion: New findings, new questions. *Psychological Science, 3*(1), 34–38.

Etkin, A., Egner, T., Peraza, D. M., Kandel, E. R., & Hirsch, J. (2006). Resolving emotional conflict: A role for the rostral anterior cingulate cortex in modulating activity in the amygdala. *Neuron, 51*, 871–882.

Frijda, N. H. (1986). The current status of emotion theory. *Bulletin of the British Psychological Society, 39*, A75–A75.

Fujita, K., & Carnevale, J. J. (2012). Transcending temptation through abstraction: The role of construal level in self-control. *Current Directions in Psychological Science, 21*, 248–252.

Gallo, I. S., Keil, A., McCulloch, K. C., Rockstroh, B., & Gollwitzer, P. M. (2011). Strategic automation of emotion regulation. *Journal of Personality and Social Psychology, 96*, 11–31.

Govorun, O., & Payne, B. K. (2006). Ego-depletion and prejudice: Separating automatic and controlled components. *Social Cognition, 24*, 111–136.

Gross, J. J. (1998a). The emerging field of emotion regulation: An integrative review. *Review of General Psychology, 2*, 271–299.

Gross, J. J. (1998b). Antecedent and response focused emotion regulation: Divergent consequences for experience, expression and physiology. *Journal of Personality and Social Psychology, 74*, 224–237.

Gross, J. J. (2001). Emotion regulation in adulthood: Timing is everything. *Current Directions in Psychological Science, 10*, 214–219.

Gross, J. J. (2002). Emotion regulation: Affective, cognitive, and social consequences. *Psychophysiology, 39*, 281–291.

Gross, J. J., & Barrett, L. F. (2011). Emotion generation and emotion regulation: One or two depends on your point of view. *Emotion Review, 3*, 8–16.

Gross, J. J., Sheppes, G., & Urry, H. L. (2011a). Emotion generation and emotion regulation: A distinction we should make (carefully). *Cognition and Emotion, 25*, 765–781.

Gross, J. J., Sheppes, G., & Urry, H. L. (2011b). Taking one's lumps while doing the splits: A big tent perspective on emotion generation and emotion regulation. *Cognition and Emotion, 25*, 789–793.

Gross, J. J., Richards, J. M., & John, O. P. (2006). Emotion regulation in everyday life. In D. K. Snyder, J. A. Simpson, & J. N. Hughes (Eds.), *Emotion regulation in couples and families: Pathways to dysfunction and health* (pp. 12–35). Washington, DC: American Psychological Association.

Gross, J. J., & Thompson, R. A. (2007). Emotion regulation: Conceptual foundations. In J. J. Gross (Ed.), *Handbook of emotion regulation* (pp. 3–24). New York: Guilford Press.

Gyurak, A., Gross, J. J., & Etkin, A. (2011). Explicit and implicit emotion regulation: A dual process framework. *Cognition and Emotion, 25*, 400–412.

Hajcak, G., MacNamara, A., & Olvet, D. M. (2010). Event-related potentials, emotion, and emotion regulation: An integrative review.

Developmental Neuropsychology, 35, 129–155.

Hariri, A. R., Bookheimer, S. Y., & Mazziotta, J. C. (2000). Modulating emotional responses: Effects of a neocortical network on the limbic system. *NeuroReport, 11,* 43–48.

Hofmann, W., Friese, M., & Strack, F. (2009). Impulse and self-control from a dual-systems perspective. *Perspectives on Psychological Science, 4,* 162–176.

Kappas, A. (2011). Emotion is not just an alarm bell* it's the whole tootin' fire truck. *Cognition and Emotion, 25,* 785–788.

Koole, S. L. (2009). The psychology of emotion regulation: An integrative review. *Cognition and Emotion, 23,* 4–41.

Koole, S. L., & Rothermund, K. (2011). "I feel better but I don't know why": The psychology of implicit emotion regulation. *Cognition and Emotion, 25,* 389–399.

Kreibig, S. D. (2010). Autonomic nervous system activity in emotion: A review. *Biological Psychology, 84*(3), 394–421.

Levenson, R. W. (1999). The intrapersonal functions of emotion. *Cognition and Emotion, 13*(5), 481–504.

Lieberman, M. D., Eisenberger, N. I., Crockett, M. J., Tom, S. M., Pfeifer, J. H., & Way, B. M. (2007). Putting feelings into words: Affect labeling disrupts amygdala activity in response to affective stimuli. *Psychological Science, 18,* 421–428.

Lieberman, M. D., Hariri, A. R., Jarcho, J. M., Eisenberger, N. I., & Bookheimer, S. Y. (2005). An fMRI investigation of race-related amygdala activity in African-American and Caucasian-American individuals. *Nature Neuroscience, 8,* 720–722.

Lieberman, M. D., Inagaki, T. K., Tabibnia, G., & Crockett, M. J. (2011). Subjective responses to emotional stimuli during labeling, reappraisal and distraction. *Emotion, 11,* 468–480.

Macklem, G. L. (2008). *Practitioner's guide to emotion regulation in school-aged children.* New York: Springer.

Marien, H., Custers, R., Hassin, R. R., & Aarts, H. (2012). Unconscious goal activation and the hijacking of the executive function. *Journal of Personality and Social Psychology, 103,* 399–415.

Mauss, I. B., Bunge, S. A., & Gross, J. J. (2007). Automatic emotion regulation. *Social and Personality Psychology Compass, 1,* 146–167.

Mauss, I. B., Levenson, R. W., McCarter, L., Wilhelm, F. H., & Gross, J. J. (2005). The tie that binds?: Coherence among emotion experience, behavior, and physiology. *Emotion, 5,* 175–190.

Mesquita, B., & Frijda, N. H. (2011). An emotion perspective on emotion regulation. *Cognition and Emotion, 25,* 782–784.

Myrseth, K. O. R., & Fishbach, A. (2009). Self-control a function of knowing when and how to exercise restraint. *Current Directions in Psychological Science, 18,* 247–252.

Ochsner, K. N., & Gross, J. J. (2005). The cognitive control of emotion. *Trends in Cognitive Sciences, 9,* 242–249.

Ochsner, K. N., & Gross, J. J. (2008). Cognitive emotion regulation. *Current Directions in Psychological Science, 17*(2), 153–158.

Payne, B. K. (2008). What mistakes disclose: A process dissociation approach to automatic and controlled processes in social psychology. *Social and Personality Psychology Compass, 2,* 1073–1092.

Scherer, K. R., Schorr, A., & Johnstone, T. (2001). *Appraisal processes in emotion: Theory, methods, research.* New York: Oxford University Press.

Sheppes, G. (2014). Emotion regulation choice: Theory and findings. In J. J. Gross (Ed.), *Handbook of emotion regulation* (2nd ed.). New York: Guilford Press.

Sheppes, G., & Gross, J. J. (2011). Is timing everything?: Temporal considerations in emotion regulation. *Personality and Social Psychology Review, 15,* 319–331.

Sheppes, G., & Gross, J. J. (2012). Emotion regulation effectiveness: What works when. In H. A. Tennen & J. M. Suls (Eds.), *Handbook of psychology* (2nd ed., pp. 391–406). Indianapolis, IN: Wiley-Blackwell.

Sheppes, G., & Levin, Z. (2013). Emotion regulation choice: Selecting between cognitive regulation strategies to control emotion. *Frontiers in Human Neuroscience, 7,* 179.

Sheppes, G., Scheibe, S., Suri, G., & Gross, J. J. (2011). Emotion-regulation choice. *Psychological Science, 22,* 1391–1396.

Sheppes, G., Scheibe, S., Suri, G., Radu, P., Blechert, J., & Gross, J. J. (in press). Emotion regulation choice: A conceptual framework and supporting evidence. *Journal of Experimental Psychology: General.*

Sherman, J. W., Gawronski, B., Gonsalkorale, K., Hugenberg, K., Allen, T. J., & Groom,

C. J. (2008). The self-regulation of automatic associations and behavioral impulses. *Psychological Review, 115*, 314–335.

Strack, F., & Deutsch, R. (2004). Reflective and impulsive determinants of social behavior. *Personality and Social Psychology Review, 8*, 220–247.

Stewart, B. D., & Payne, B. K. (2008). Bringing automatic stereotyping under control: Implementation intentions as efficient means of thought control. *Personality and Social Psychology Bulletin*, *34*, 1332–1345.

Tamir, M. (2009). What do people want to feel and why?: Pleasure and utility in emotion regulation. *Current Directions in Psychological Science, 18*, 101–105.

Tamir, M., & Ford, B. Q. (2009). Choosing to be afraid: Preferences for fear as a function of goal pursuit. *Emotion*, *9*, 488–497.

Thompson, R. (2011). Emotion and emotion regulation: Two sides of the developing coin. *Emotion Review, 3*, 53–61.

Todd, R. M., Cunningham, W. A., Anderson, A. K., & Thompson, E. (2012). Affect-biased attention as emotion regulation. *Trends in Cognitive Sciences*, *16*, 365–372.

Webb, T. L., Miles, E., & Sheeran, P. (2012). Dealing with feeling: A meta-analysis of the effectiveness of strategies derived from the process model of emotion regulation. *Psychological Bulletin, 138*(4), 775–808.

Webb, T. L., Ononaiye, M. S. P., Sheeran, P., Reidy, J. G., & Lavda, A. (2010). Using implementation intentions to overcome the effects of social anxiety on attention and appraisals of performance. *Personality and Social Psychology Bulletin, 36*, 612–627.

Williams, L. E., Bargh, J. A., Nocera, C., & Gray, J. R. (2009). On the unconscious regulation of emotion: Nonconscious reappraisal goals modulate emotional reactivity. *Emotion, 9*, 847–854.

Wilson, T. D., & Gilbert, D. T. (2008). Explaining away: A model of affective adaptation. *Perspectives on Psychological Science, 3*, 370–386.

PART IX

CRITICISM AND ALTERNATIVES

CHAPTER 33

The Limits of Automaticity

Klaus Fiedler and Mandy Hütter

There can be no doubt that the various dual-process theories (DPTs) documented in this volume continue to have a huge impact on current research in social cognition. Dual-process ideas figure prominently in research articles, textbooks, conferences, and lecturing. Dual-process approaches solicit a huge amount of research funding, and they have been praised as major achievements in behavioral science (Evans & Frankish, 2009; Smith & DeCoster, 2000). Given the prominence and the universal claims advocated in these theories, though, it is no surprise that DPTs have been also met with criticism and skepticism. Our purpose in this chapter on limits of automaticity is to outline some of these critical arguments, with reference to both theoretical weakness and empirical counterevidence.

The chapter is organized as follows. An initial section is devoted to conceptual limits of automaticity, pointing out that the lack of a precise definition of theoretical key terms delimits and often precludes scientific progress. An empirical section then provides an overview of pertinent findings that delimit the internal and external validity of automaticity claims, with reference to the changing operational definitions of automaticity used in major research paradigms, such as evaluative conditioning, mere exposure, speeded classification tasks, semantic and evaluative priming, and behavior regulation. Research in these areas provides impressive evidence for voluntary strategic control of associative and affective processes deemed to be essentially automatic. A final section arrives at the conclusion that future progress in this prominent research area is contingent on scientists' engaging in strong inference (Platt, 1964), based on falsifiable assumptions about what outcomes DPTs exclude.

CONCEPTUAL LIMITS OF AUTOMATICITY

Precise terminology and conceptual clarity are essential preconditions of cumulative science. When different researchers and theoreticians use the same words, it is important that they refer to the same meaning. If there is no such common ground, this must be a source of permanent conflict and misunderstanding. Unfortunately, *automatic* is a prime example of a term that is used readily and abundantly, both in scientific and in ordinary language, although a commonly shared definition is lacking. Different researchers have defined *automaticity* in diverse ways, proposing different measurement procedures and experimental manipulations (see Moors & De Houwer, 2006, for a review), yet the term is presupposed to have a unitary, commonly understood meaning.

Defining Automaticity

In everyday communication, utterances such as "I turned around automatically" or "She automatically did the right thing" express how behaviors are controlled by external stimuli or that routinized behavior can be very efficient. Note that these everyday utterances hardly refer to naive theories about unconsciousness, nor do they refer to some naive distinction between (exactly) two qualitatively different processing modes or mental systems. Sticking to this ordinary language notion of automaticity, for instance, Wood and Neal (2007) interpreted habit formation as automatic in the sense that habits reflect situationally triggered action sequences that are detached from deliberate goals. Little more than the assumption of a well-learned routine is necessary to account for this modest conception of automaticity.

In contrast, Schneider and Shiffrin's (1977) definition of *automatic* versus *controlled processes* introduced strong assumptions about several correlated properties of two qualitatively distinct process types. While automatic reactions are supposed to be independent of attention and capacity, and based on parallel processing, controlled reactions rely on attention, limited capacity, and serial processing. Note that this definition includes not only falsifiable empirical assumptions about the joint appearance of capacity, attention, processing styles and related neuronal mechanisms (see Ashby, Ennis, & Spiering, 2007), but also a strong, double-barreled dichotomy. Automatic processes are not only automatic but also uncontrollable, and vice versa; controlled processes are not only controlled but also nonautomatic. The operations needed to assess or manipulate automaticity in this framework (payoffs, volition, base rates, contextual influences on strategic control) are different from the operations that distinguish overlearned habits from newly acquired, nonroutine skills (amount of learning, absence of goals).

The theoretical overload in Schneider and Shiffrin's (1977) definition was soon recognized (Ryan, 1983) or replaced by simple definitions (e.g., returning to extensive experience alone as a defining feature; Ashby et al., 2007). Nevertheless, an even more heavy-laden conception became the standard definition in social cognition. What is commonly known as the four horsemen of automaticity (Andersen, Moskowitz, Blair, & Nosek, 2007; Bargh, 1994)—independence of awareness, lack of intention, efficiency, and lack of control—renders the operational distinction of automatic versus nonautomatic processes difficult and equivocal. In addition to Schneider and Shiffrin's (1977) controllability criterion, the four horsemen include subjective and phenomenological criteria (intention, awareness), and a performance criterion (efficiency) for which hardly any absolute scale is available. Efficiency typically involves some tradeoff between speed and accuracy. It is hard to see what universal measure of efficiency can be applied to the diversity of all possible tradeoffs across all cognitive tasks.

Applying four criteria simultaneously creates a problem of overdetermination. If awareness, intention, efficiency, and control are not perfectly correlated, there will be many mixed cases that look automatic on some criteria but nonautomatic on others. The question then arises whether the four attributes should be combined conjunctively or disjunctively. Assuming the conjunctive rule that a response is only automatic if it fulfills all four criteria together, the set of automatic behaviors is very sparse, if not empty. After all, efficiency can be enhanced strategically; intention can strengthen motivation, consistency and predictability of behavior; and conscious awareness is a key to efficiency through metacognitive control. Alternatively, the disjunctive rule advocated by Bargh (1994), Moors and De Houwer (2006), or Andersen et al. (2007) renders almost every behavior automatic, though for different reasons.

Thus, depending on which and how many criteria apply jointly, phobic reactions to spiders can be classified as automatic because they are unintentional. Or they can be classified as nonautomatic because they are hardly efficient and amenable to controlled therapeutic intervention, or because awareness is essential to classical conditioning (Shanks, 2010).

Relating Automaticity to Dual-Process Theories

The equivocal status of the basic concept of automaticity is of crucial importance for any psychological conception that assumes qualitatively different processes to govern automatic and nonautomatic skills, symptoms, habits, actions, or mental procedures. This is particularly the case for DPTs, a defining feature of which is that all DPTs dichotomize the spectrum of psychic processes into exactly two basic modalities.

Notwithstanding many notable points of divergence between specific DPTs, all share the central assumption that cognition and behavior regulation involve two qualitatively different and functionally separable processing modes. DPTs state that exactly two modes or systems are required to account for psychological functioning—not three or multiple modes and, of course, not a single mode. This basic dualism is bolstered with reference to distinct anatomical brain locations or neurophysiological systems (Ashby et al., 2007), different personality types (Stanovich & West, 2002), and different implications of the two processing modes for rationality, intuition (Evans, 2010) and metacognition (Thompson, 2009).

Because most DPTs are presented in ordinary language rather than in algebraic notation or as computer algorithms (see Smith & DeCoster, 1999, for a notable exception), they often remain vague about which specific conception of automaticity they embrace and which other conceptions they refute. However, despite this noncommittal state of affairs, which is also reflected in a paucity of open debates between proponents of different DPTs, it is fair to say that virtually all DPTs refer to some notion of automaticity as a distinctive feature between the two processing modes or systems. Regardless of how the duality is conceived—as heuristic versus systematic, affective versus argumentative, impulsive versus reflective, intuitive versus deliberative, associative versus propositional, or, in neutral terms, as System 1 versus System 2—there is general agreement that the first term in each pair refers to lower levels of mental operations that are evolutionary older and less dependent on resources and higher cognitive functions than the operations covered by the second term. It is the primary, not the secondary, terms that are globally associated with automaticity or autonomy.

Given this universal status of automaticity in DPTs, the crucial question is what empirical studies on automatic behavior can contribute to scientific progress in DPTs. How can the critical discussion of conceptual limits be turned into an open discussion of empirical insights gained from automaticity research? How did proponents of DPTs, explicitly or implicitly, define and operationalize their manipulations and assessment procedures for automatic versus nonautomatic processes?

Some DPTs place an emphasis on working memory constraints (Stanovich & West, 2002; Evans, 2010; Kahneman, 2003) as a chief criterion of automaticity, assuming qualitatively different processing types, only one of which is contingent on mental resources, attention, and processing motivation. Other DPTs distinguish between associative and propositional processes (Gawronski & Bodenhausen, 2006), which are presupposed to be fundamentally different. Only associative processes are characterized by automatic affective reactions that are supposed to arise independently of the intentionally controlled assignment of truth values.

Regardless of whether DPTs allow for interactions between modes or systems (thereby sacrificing their discriminability) or whether they assume semipermeability (e.g., impulsive intrusion into reflective processes, but not vice versa), automaticity is linked to duality. "The impulsive system is conceptualized as a network in which information is processed automatically through a fast and parallel spread of activation along the associative links between contents. In contrast, processes of rule-based reasoning and of symbol manipulation are assumed to be carried out in a reflective system" (Strack, Werth, & Deutsch, 2006, p. 208). To the best of our knowledge, no DPT has explicitly refuted this automaticity link to set itself apart from rival DPTs, although some have argued for a more differentiated, disjunctive use of the automaticity concept (see Gawronski & Bodenhausen, 2007).

In their integrative review of DPTs, Sherman et al. (2008) contrast two different roles assigned to automaticity. Whereas many DPTs assume that automatic processes often intrude into and win the race with controlled processes (e.g., Schneider & Shiffrin, 1977), others advocate the reverse possibility that secondary automatic processes are only invoked when primary intentions to engage in controlled action fail (e.g., Jacoby, 1991). The quadruple-process (quad) model advocated by Sherman et al. (2008) allows for all combinations of four cognitive–process distinctions. Therefore, it dissolves the theoretical and empirical problems of dual-process models by giving up (1) the duality assumption and (2) the assumption that automaticity is confined to any subsystem or process type. Consequently, findings related to automaticity are no longer crucial; they cannot falsify the quad model.

The following synopsis of empirically obtained limits of automaticity cannot be expected to discriminate between specific DPTs. They all embrace automaticity as if it supports a seemingly natural distinction between automatic and nonautomatic processes—without, however, being explicit about what evidence might falsify this core assumption.

EMPIRICAL EVIDENCE FROM AUTOMATICITY PARADIGMS

In coping with the lack of a shared definition of automaticity, in our empirical review we take a pragmatic position and simply adopt the diverse operational definitions used in the most prominent paradigms of automaticity research. While these varying meanings of *automaticity* do not take the aforementioned problems into account, they reflect the conventional definition of the concept within the leading paradigms. We begin with the first two paradigms: evaluative conditioning and mere exposure. We then move on to speeded classifications tasks, including the implicit association test (IAT), and to priming effects as a major domain of automaticity research. We devote the final subsection to automaticity in behavior regulation. Across all paradigms, the empirical evidence converges in demonstrating much more volitional and strategic control over allegedly automatic behaviors than expected.

Evaluative Conditioning

Research on attitude formation has paid a lot of attention to evaluative conditioning (EC) and conceived of it as low-level, automatic learning of attitudes. EC is the evaluative change caused in a conditioned stimulus (CS) by pairing it with a valent, unconditioned stimulus (US). It is a paramount example of a paradigm within which evidence has been gained for all four horsemen of automaticity, resulting in evidence for both automatic and nonautomatic features.

A controversy hotly debated during the last two decades is whether evaluative conditioning necessitates contingency awareness. Early investigations that classified participants as aware versus unaware led to the conclusion that EC is independent of awareness (Baeyens, Eelen, Crombez, & Van den Bergh, 1992). Consequently, EC was conceptualized as a distinct experimental model of automatically acquired attitudes (Baeyens et al., 1992; Levey & Martin, 1975; Jones, Fazio, & Olson, 2009; Jones, Olson, & Fazio, 2010). However, as participants are typically aware of neither none nor all CS–US pairings, more recent studies employing item-based analyses concluded that EC depends on contingency awareness (Bar-Anan, De Houwer, & Nosek, 2010; Dedonder, Corneille, Yzerbyt, & Kuppens, 2010; Pleyers, Corneille, Yzerbyt, & Luminet, 2009; Stahl, Unkelbach, & Corneille, 2009), leading to the formulation of propositional accounts (De Houwer, 2007, 2009; Mitchell, De Houwer, & Lovibond, 2009; Shanks, 2010).

Subsequently, another methodological improvement introduced by Hütter, Sweldens, Stahl, Unkelbach, and Klauer (2012) demonstrated that previous studies were unfairly biased against unaware EC. They argued that participants can rely on their conditioned attitudes toward a given CS to respond correctly in memory tasks employed to measure contingency awareness. This response strategy impedes the detection of unaware EC. Based on this argument, Hütter et al. developed a process dissociation account to separate memory for pairings from conditioned attitudes without memory for the pairings to show that both aware and unaware processes are involved in EC effects. The relative proportion of these processes is moderated by the presentation schedule employed in the conditioning procedure (Sweldens, Van Osselaer, & Janiszewski, 2010). While sequential presentations of CS and US have been shown to allow for aware learning of the pairings, simultaneous presentations allow for both aware and unaware learning (Hütter & Sweldens, 2013).

The empirical evidence is mixed regarding the dependence of EC on cognitive resources, as investigated in experiments using secondary tasks to manipulate the availability of cognitive resources. The question then is whether the effect under investigation is maintained despite the reduction in accessible cognitive capacities. While the EC effect disappeared under cognitive load when using a 2-back task (Dedonder et al., 2010; Pleyers et al., 2009), the EC effect was even larger compared to the control condition when participants had to memorize an eight-digit number (Walther, 2002). Thus, the available evidence is yet not conclusive regarding the role of cognitive resources in the production of EC effects. Please also note that the numerous cognitive load tasks that exist in the literature differ in not only the demands they impose on working memory but also their potential to induce negative mood via low processing fluency (Winkielman & Cacioppo, 2001). The role of intention in EC was investigated by Corneille, Yzerbyt, Pleyers, and Mussweiler (2009). A conceptual priming task aimed at inducing a processing focus on similarities or differences. Although the processing goal moderated the EC effect, so that the EC effect was reduced in the difference condition, but not in the similarity condition, a large EC effect was still obtained in the difference condition. Thus, this initial evidence suggests that EC operates relatively independently of intentions.

The fourth horseman refers to the control exerted over the attitude acquisition. First of all, De Houwer (2006) showed that EC can be based on imagined pairings. That is, having participants merely imagine a CS paired with a positive or a negative picture can produce EC effects without ever presenting a US. These EC effects observed by De Houwer completely exclude the operation of automatic processes. In another experimental setup, Gast and De Houwer (2012) prevented the simultaneous experience of CS and US by presenting the CS covertly and revealing it only after the US was experienced. For example, the color (CS) of a sweet or bitter-tasting (US) cookie was revealed only after participants tasted the cookie. Control is also required when CS–US relations include relational qualifiers that sometimes call for a reversal of US valence. Generally, participants were able to reverse the influence of the US on the CS when they were led to believe that CS and US were enemies (as opposed to friends) or that the CS loathed (as opposed to loved) the US (Fiedler & Unkelbach, 2011; Förderer & Unkelbach, 2011; Zanon, De Houwer, & Gast, 2012).

One should be cautious not to overgeneralize these findings concerning the controllability of EC effects, because (1) so far they have been demonstrated only for designs involving stimulus–stimulus associations (Hütter & Sweldens, 2013; Sweldens et al., 2010), and (2) they presume that in conventional EC paradigms, participants make the default assumption that a positive relational qualifier links the CS to the US.

While under some conditions EC effects possess selected features of automaticity, the reviewed findings clearly show that EC can also be caused and moderated by processes that are nonautomatic in any sense of the concept. Hence, EC cannot comprise an operational definition of automaticity per se. By all standards, automaticity in terms of any one of the four horsemen is not an essential property of EC. It is rather an open empirical question for future research to specify testable conditions under which processes characterized by automatic features can or cannot contribute to EC effects (e.g., Hütter & Sweldens, 2013).

Mere Exposure

The attitudinal effects of mere exposure (Zajonc, 2001) have also been attributed to automatic mechanisms, as highlighted in Zajonc's (1980) claim that "preferences need no inferences." The mere exposure effect is the observation that neutral stimuli become more positive after repeated presentations. While theories are diverse, they share the notion of an increased familiarity due to repeated presentations. Topolinski and Strack's (2009) stimulus-specific motor simulation account is grounded in embodiment theory (e.g., Barsalou, 1999; Semin & Smith, 2008). This account assumes that motor responses associated with the presented stimulus (e.g., pronouncing a word) are triggered automatically. The mere exposure effect vanishes when the respective motor simulation is blocked by another motor task (e.g., chewing gum; Topolinski & Strack, 2010). Gillebaart, Förster, and Rotteveel (2012) assume that mere exposure increases the liking of a stimulus, if it has to be integrated into preexisting knowledge structures and if mental categories are narrow. Repeated presentations are then necessary in order to classify the stimulus. Both explanations are in line with the notion that mere exposure effects are stronger at subliminal than at supraliminal exposure durations, and in the absence of explicit recollection (Bornstein, 1989).

The mere exposure effect has frequently been linked to increases in processing fluency with repeated encounters (Bornstein & D'Agostino, 1992; Kunst-Wilson & Zajonc, 1980; Seamon, Marsh, & Brody, 1984; Zajonc, 1980). In turn, the increase in fluency is assumed to trigger positive affect automatically (Topolinski, Likowski, Weyers, & Strack, 2009). However, a meta-analysis by Bornstein (1989) revealed that too many presentations level off the mere exposure effect, which apparently led to the experience of boredom due to learning satiation (Bornstein, Kale, & Cornell, 1990). Accordingly, the mere exposure effect is contingent on an interpretation of the fluency cue as something good. However, a recent study by Briñol, Petty, and Tormala (2006) showed that the influence of fluency can be reversed by changing its interpretation. Participants were told that feelings of ease indicated many neuronal connections and high intelligence, whereas feelings of difficulty indicated few neuronal connections and low intelligence, or they were told the opposite. Similarly, the mere exposure effect can be reversed by inducing goals that are associated with growth instead of security (Gillebaart et al., 2012).

Thus, although increasing fluency and positivity is commonly attributed to an automatic exposure effect—defining automaticity as independence of cognitive inferences—its effect on liking seems to be moderated by the higher-order cognitive interpretation of the fluency cue.

Speeded Classification Tasks

Speeded classification tasks have been designed as tests of implicit attitudes that circumvent influences of voluntary control resulting from social desirability, political correctness, and self-presentation concerns that plague self-report measures. For this purpose they make use of reaction times and accuracy, comparing performance on attitude-incongruent and attitude-congruent trials. Most prominent speeded classification procedures are the emotional Stroop task (Pratto & John, 1991), the IAT (Greenwald, McGhee, & Schwartz, 1998; Greenwald, Nosek, & Banaji, 2003), the Affective Simon Task (De Houwer & Eelen, 1998), the go/no-go association task (Nosek & Banaji, 2001), and the Extrinsic Affective Simon Task (EAST; De Houwer, 2003).

The IAT is perhaps the most widely used procedure of this type. It has been proposed to "reveal attitudes and other automatic associations even for subjects who prefer not to express those attitudes" (Greenwald et al., 1998, p. 1465) and that "these automatic tendencies are closer to the 'true' attitudes than explicit self-reports" (Dasgupta, McGhee, Greenwald, & Banaji, 2000, p. 326). Indeed, IAT scores predict behavior in socially sensitive domains better than self-reported attitudes (Greenwald, Poehlman, Uhlmann, & Banaji, 2009). In general, implicit attitudes have been hypothesized to predict behavior when motivation, opportunity, or both are low (e.g., Fazio & Towles-Schwen, 1999; Strack & Deutsch, 2004), a claim that received empirical support (e.g., Friese, Hofmann, & Schmitt, 2009). However, neither an explicit psychometric model of the IAT (Blanton, Jaccard, Gonzales, & Christie, 2006) nor a testable causal model of the latency difference for compatible and incompatible trials has been specified and tested critically (Fiedler, Messner, & Bluemke, 2006). In particular, the causal origin of a significant IAT score is unclear; it may reflect a genuine attitude, extraattitudinal associative knowledge (Fazio & Olson, 2003), interindividual differences in general processing speed (Blanton et al., 2006), task-switching abilities (Mierke & Klauer, 2001), or the flexible utilization of response strategies that facilitate performance (Fiedler & Bluemke, 2005; Mitchell, 2004; Rothermund & Wentura, 2004).

The assumption that the IAT captures implicit attitudes automatically is mainly based on its reputation as an unobtrusive procedure that does not lend itself to simulation, dissimilation, and faking. In some studies, self-presentation concerns and voluntary control did not influence IAT results (Banse, Seise, & Zerbes, 2001; Egloff & Schmukle, 2002; Foroni & Mayr, 2005; Schnabel, Banse, & Asendorpf, 2006; Steffens, 2004, Study 1). Meanwhile, however, several studies have demonstrated that faking intentions and deliberate self-instructions can systematically change or even reverse IAT effects (Blair, Ma, & Lenton, 2001; Fiedler & Bluemke, 2005; Wallaert, Ward, & Mann, 2010). In a series of faking experiments by Fiedler and Bluemke (2005), German participants' ability to produce pro-German or pro-Turkish attitude scores on a German–Turk IAT was independent of strategy instructions. Regardless of whether they received an explicit strategy instruction (i.e., to slow down on compatible trials), only background information about how the IAT works, or no information whatsoever, most participants found their own strategy that enabled them to reverse their IAT scores. It is also worth noting that IAT experts were not able to discriminate between faked and nonfaked response latencies. The only precondition for successful faking was learning experience with at least one previous IAT, consistent with a strategic interpretation of IAT faking. This finding received support by Wallaert et al. (2010), who showed that after completing a practice IAT, instructions to enhance or inhibit stereotype expression on a race IAT without suggesting concrete strategies enhanced or decreased IAT effects, respectively.

A series of studies by Blair et al. (2001) demonstrates another strategy to gain control over IAT results: counterstereotypical imagery. In a gender strength IAT, imagining what a strong woman is like was sufficient to reduce the IAT effect significantly. Although one might argue that imagery itself involves potentially automatic memory functions (Bargh, 1994; Higgins, 1996), there can be no doubt that the initiation of these tools is under deliberate control.

In summary, the IAT and other speeded classification tasks are not insensitive to test knowledge and intentional control; therefore, they do not afford cogent evidence for associations supposed to be automatic in terms of independence of voluntary and strategic control. Rather, the obtained latency differences are the product of a dialectic interplay of controllable and uncontrollable processes. This notion is acknowledged in recent multinomial models of performance in speeded classification tasks (e.g., Conrey, Sherman, Gawronski, Hugenberg, & Groom, 2005; Stahl & Degner, 2007), which account for both automatic and controlled processes contributing to scores in speeded classification tasks such as the IAT or the EAST.

Priming

Priming phenomena afford another major paradigm for the study of automaticity. In semantic priming, words or pictures facilitate the responses to subsequent targets that are semantically related (e.g., *symptom–disease*), compared to unrelated pairs (*iceberg–disease*). Evaluative priming is less restrictive. To facilitate the speeded classification of the target as either positive or negative, the prime need not be closely related to the target in denotative semantic meaning. It is sufficient that the prime is of the same evaluative tone (Fazio, 2001; Hermans, Spruyt, & Eelen, 2003). Because evaluative congruence is a weaker condition than semantic relatedness, the domain of evaluative priming is broader, offering a measurement tool for attitudes, prejudice, and preferences. The rationale is simple and straightforward. If an attitude topic (brand name, food item) or social individual (defined by ethnic category, age, gender, or sexual orientation) is associated with positive or negative valence, it should be an effective prime that facilitates the classification of valence-congruent subsequent targets.

This congruity advantage in evaluative priming should be robust and automatic (Fazio, 2001). The chief criterion of automaticity here is that the measurement of attitudes must not be subject to voluntary control and strategic self-presentation. To rule out controlled responding, the stimuli are typically presented at a short presentation rate and stimulus-onset asynchrony (SOA = interval between prime onset and target onset). Traditionally, priming effects at SOA = 300 milliseconds or below were called automatic. More recently, the critical SOA has been further reduced to ensure truly unconscious priming, together with masking procedures and parafoveal presentation.

Phenomenologically, indeed, degraded primes often evade participants' awareness. Despite this phenomenological experience, however, the unconsciousness criterion of automaticity is problematic in at least two respects. First, it must be acknowledged that we are virtually never aware of the cognitive operations underlying all responses, even the clearly intentional and controlled ones. We cannot observe, introspectively, the complex parallel processes involved in perceptual constancy, memory retrieval, speech production, or moral evaluations. Only the input or results of mental processes are sometimes experienced consciously. However, second, if we do not apply the consciousness criterion to the priming process but only to the result, a critical empirical question is whether the valence of evaluative primes remains unrecognized. Research by Dijksterhuis and Aarts (2003) shows that the valence of sandwich-masked stimuli presented for 13.3 milliseconds can be guessed at a rate above chance. Similar results, with even higher accuracy rates, were found by Fiedler, Unkelbach, and Freytag (2012). Thus, there is no guarantee that even highly degraded evaluative primes remain unconscious.

With regard to lack of intention as a criterion of automaticity, a study by Teige-Mocigemba and Klauer (2008) suggests that priming effects can be controlled intentionally. Using pictures of Arabs and liked celebrities as negative and positive attitude primes presented at an SOA of 275 milliseconds, they demonstrated that both monetary payoffs (for accurate responses to incongruent pairs) and appropriate instructions (e.g., to think of positive aspects of Arabs and negative aspects of the liked celebrities) could fully eliminate priming effects.

While these faked priming effects may be due to valence shifts (e.g., positive thoughts overriding the valence of negative primes), a growing body of research on implementation intentions provides compelling evidence for voluntary control of prejudice and unwanted priming effects (Gollwitzer, Sheeran, Trötschel, & Webb, 2011). According to this theory, humans can deliberately install production rules such as "If I encounter an Arab face, I will immediately think of something positive." As soon as the condition specified in the if-phrase is met, a readily compiled action sequence will execute the goal set in the then-phrase. Ironically, although such implementation intentions constitute a volitional countermeasure to stimulus-determined priming, the execution of such a production rule was again interpreted as automatic (Bargh, Gollwitzer, Lee-Chai, Barndollar, & Trötschel, 2001).

Simply trying to suppress an upcoming reaction is certainly not a good control strategy (Wegner, 1994). Learning to control behavior—whether it is conscious or unconscious, consisting of simple reflexes or rule-based action—often involves more intelligent techniques. In systematic desensibilization, for instance, fear-incompatible approach responses are used to gain control over phobic responses. Empirical tests of automaticity should therefore focus on clever and indirect strategies and not be confined to ineffective suppression techniques.

Given this rationale, several well-known moderators of priming strength suggest themselves for controlled interventions. For example, one may reduce or eliminate priming effects by reducing cognitive load (Alexopoulos, Fiedler, & Freytag, 2012), or by attending to or overtly reacting to the prime (Fiedler, Bluemke, & Unkelbach, 2011). Another notable moderator that was shown to eliminate evaluative and semantic priming is negative mood, whereas positive mood supports priming effects (Storbeck & Clore, 2008).

Strong evidence for strategic control of allegedly automatic priming effects comes from experiments that demonstrate flexible response strategies tailored after the current stimulus series. Similar to the relatedness proportion effect in semantic priming (Neely, Keefe, & Ross, 1989), the congruity proportion effect in evaluative priming (Fiedler et al., 2011; Klauer, Rossnagel, & Musch, 1997) shows that the congruity advantage is reduced or even reversed when the list contains more incongruent than congruent prime–target pairs. Such flexible learning of an adaptive response strategy is even possible for extremely short SOAs of 0 milliseconds (Klauer et al., 1997), which are often supposed to be an exclusive domain of automaticity.

While the congruity–proportion effect testifies to strategies sensitive to the correlation between prime valence and target valence, pseudocontingency strategies are sensitive to base rates (Freytag, Bluemke, & Fiedler, 2011). When most primes are positive (negative) and most targets are also positive (negative), jointly reflecting a benevolent (malevolent) environment, a strategic response bias will support a congruity effect (i.e., fast and accurate responding on congruent trials), even though the correlation is zero. In contrast, when the more prevalent target valence is opposite to the more prevalent prime valence, then a negative pseudocontingency produces an incongruity effect in priming.

There are limits, to be sure, to all these limits of automaticity. Primes can be presented so briefly and degraded so massively, and cognitive resources can be depleted so radically that blindfolded participants can no longer exert intentional or strategic control over their performance. However, the truism that such extreme task conditions can massively reduce the efficiency and controllability holds for every performance. The crucial question from a DPT perspective, though, is whether the human mind is equipped with exactly two processing systems, only one of which shows interference under such extreme conditions.

Unlike all aforementioned priming procedures, the affect misattribution procedure (AMP; Payne, Cheng, Govorun, & Stewart, 2005) focuses on the influence of subtle valence primes (typically presented for 75 milliseconds) on evaluative responses to subsequently presented abstract symbols (e.g., Chinese pictographs). Increasing versus decreasing evaluations of the neutral symbols are considered reflections of positive versus negative attitudes toward the primed stimuli, respectively. The AMP has been praised for many advantages, including large effect sizes, high reliability, ease of use, and resistance to correction attempts. AMP effects were unaffected by volitional attempts to conceal one's true attitude (Payne et al., 2005), consistent with the principle that merely suppressive or compulsive control attempts are inefficient. This evidence testifies to the AMP as an automatic procedure, according to the unobtrusiveness and uncontrollability criteria.

Drawing on the criteria of presentation speed and independence of mental resources, Deutsch, Kordts-Freudinger, Gawronski, and Strack (2009) recently found that in the absence of a distracter task, the AMP was sensitive to prime negation. When a 200-millisecond positive prime (friend) was negated syntactically (no friend), a reversed AMP effect was evident in more negative, rather than in more positive evaluations. Only under cognitive load was the AMP as unaffected by negation priming as a latency-based measure of evaluative priming. In a previous article by Deutsch, Gawronski, and Strack (2006), insensitivity to negation had been introduced as a crucial check on automaticity in the context of the impulsive–reflective DPT.

So what does this AMP evidence reveal about automaticity, and what is the latter construct worth if different criteria lead to opposite conclusions? Are AMP effects automatic because they resist intentional correction attempts, or does the influence of higher syntactic processing indicate that they are not automatic? In any case, references to automaticity must not be circular, or output-bound; that is, one cannot classify the AMP as automatic whenever negation is ignored but as nonautomatic whenever negation moderates the priming effect.

No particular task setting per se, such as prime negation, affords a process-pure measure of automaticity, or of only one system in DPTs. Closer inspection of the empirical basis of the role assigned to prime negation reveals that Deutsch et al. (2006) had used valenced words as primes or as targets that were either negated or not. Over several trial blocks, responses to all stimuli became substantially faster, and the latency difference between negated (slower) and unqualified (faster) words remained roughly constant across blocks. Rather than inferring from the regularly decreasing parallel slopes that all performance was far from being automatized at the beginning, the authors inferred from the parallel slope that only the syntactic negation operation was not amenable to automaticity. We reckon that no single experimental task provides unambiguous evidence for only one processing mode.

Adaptive Regulation and Automatic Reactions to the Environment

Remarkably little priming research is directly concerned with the basic premise that priming must serve an adaptive function that enables organisms to predict and prepare for environmental stimuli, threats, and affordances. This basic adaptive notion is, however, central to the research program on goal priming and action priming (Aarts, Custers, & Marien, 2008; Bargh, Chen, & Burrows, 1996). According to this neobehaviorist idea, environmental stimuli automatically determine diverse behaviors such as aggression, phobic responses, cooperation, independence, trust, and even intellectual performance (Dijksterhuis & van Knippenberg, 1998; Todorov & Bargh, 2002; Schul, Mayo, & Burnstein, 2008; Vohs, Mead, & Goode, 2006).

For instance, money primes have been shown to trigger independence, reducing the help one offers to others and requests for oneself (Vohs et al., 2006). Dijksterhuis et al. (1998) demonstrated improved intellectual performance of participants exposed to the prime word *professor,* or enhanced self-ratings of attractiveness in women exposed to a *model* prime. These demonstrations are fundamentally different from semantic or evaluative priming with only two response options (e.g., positive vs. negative). Action priming instead entails the strong assumption that environmental primes alone determine seemingly spontaneous actions chosen from an unrestricted repertoire. As expressed by Dijksterhuis, Bargh, and Miedema (2000), "People and mackerels are similar in the sense that there is a direct and express connection between our perception and our behavior" (p. 37). Like instincts in animals, these direct pathways can apparently serve important adaptive functions, preparing the organism for fast, efficient, and ecologically prudent behavior, without taxing attention and resources.

However, first of all, note that still another meaning of automaticity has been introduced silently: *Automatic* now means stimulus-determined. Individuals are automatically supposed to follow directions given by the environment, calling the notion of free will and self-determined behavior into question. The term *automatic* no longer refers to a short SOA, to lack of awareness, or to an unobtrusive relation between stimulus and behavior. For action priming to explain expressway connections from perception to real behaviors, it has to allow for a wide range of SOAs. Unobtrusiveness is hardly possible when weapons or other aggression cues solicit aggressive reactions in ambiguous situations. Intellectual performance is hardly experienced as unintentional, or detached from intentional goal settings.

Note also how reflex-like and preprogrammed the prime–action cycle really is. Opposite to the action consequences of the *professor* and *model* primes used by Dijksterhuis and van Knippenberg (1998), an *Albert Einstein* prime reduced intellectual performance, and *Claudia Schiffer* led to decreased self-ratings of attractiveness. Epistemic constraints (e.g., the higher inclusiveness of *professor* than *Einstein*) moderated the outcome. In the same article as the expressway metaphor, Dijksterhuis et al. (2000) also hypothesized that "any shift in attention toward one's current functioning has the ability to override automatic behavior" (p. 37). Apparently, "automatic" behaviors shared by humans and mackerels can be easily overridden by metacognitive shifts of attention.

A recently published defense by Bargh (2012) in response to an empirical critique by Doyen, Klein, Pichon, and Cleeremans (2012) also raises the impression of action priming as a rather labile phenomenon. Doyen and colleagues had failed to replicate the seminal findings by Bargh et al. (1996) that priming the concept "older adult" decreases participants' walking speed. In his response, Bargh (2012) drew heavily on a number of very subtle side conditions that must be met to solicit the original effect, which apparently is contingent on various subtle, extra conditions that are not "automatically" fulfilled.

A growing body of evidence on flexible behavior regulation highlights the possibility to gain internal control over seemingly autonomous reactions. When coping with unpleasant affective states, people succeed in emotion regulation (Gross, 2008; Koole, 2010). When recognizing upcoming primes, flexible correction processes can undo or even reverse the normal priming effect (Bless & Schwarz, 2010). By reacting actively to a prime, people can functionally separate the prime from the target, as if they were pressing a reset button that deletes all priming influences (Fiedler et al., 2011; Martin, 1986).

From an adaptive behavior perspective, the possibility to regulate and undo priming effects is of obvious significance. Getting rid of old and obsolete priming effects can be as important for adaptive responding as high sensitivity to new signals and priming effects. Memory decay alone is hardly sufficient to terminate all previous stimuli in a sequential priming experiment with hundreds of trials. If there were no active inhibition, organisms would be overwhelmed in a sea of environmental or proprioceptive primes.

The necessity to consider both the facilitative and inhibitory component in the priming process is vividly apparent from the phenomenon of negative priming (Tipper, 1985). When two words or figures appear together in different colors and the task is to attend to and respond to the green rather than the red one, selective attention produces not only facilitation of the task-relevant (green) stimuli but also inhibition of the task-irrelevant (red) stimuli. Consequently, when the inhibited red stimuli are later presented in green, the response latency will be slower. In several studies, active inhibition was accompanied by devaluation of non-attended-to stimuli (e.g., Raymond, Fenske, & Tavassoli, 2003). Actively excluding a stimulus from one's focus of attention may not only counteract typical priming effects but also reverse a common mere exposure effect (i.e., less positive evaluation after non-attended-to exposure).

Like flexible strategy changes induced by the list context, selective attention induced by deliberate instructions can strongly moderate allegedly automatic stimulus influences. From an adaptive behavior standpoint, indeed, such flexibility or malleability is not surprising. Why should inflexibly determined, fast execution of stimulus–response sequences benefit organisms whose adaptive success depends on the ability to change their strategy in changing environments? Why should determinism in general constitute an adaptive advantage? Even though organisms certainly profit from a rich repertoire of well-exercised defaults and routine behaviors, an adaptive organism must also have learned to regulate the execution of these routines and to prevent them from becoming perfectly automatic.

CONCLUSIONS

Our concern in this chapter has been the conceptual and empirical limits of automaticity. At the conceptual level, we have criticized use of the term *automatic* in ever-changing ways, and the way that the various defining features (routinization, efficiency, unintentionality, lack of control, lack of awareness, resource independence, subliminality, stimulus control), and combinations thereof (conjunctive, disjunctive, selective) call for heterogeneous measures and manipulations of automaticity. It is therefore impossible to determine automaticity as a unique theoretical construct.

Given this lack of a solid conceptual ground, the pertinent empirical evidence is necessarily equivocal, missing the ultimate scientific goal of what Platt (1964) called "strong inference," which means devising and testing falsifiable hypotheses. In spite of a good deal of disconfirming evidence showing that many allegedly automatic behaviors are not independent of intention, voluntary control, and consciousness, and are hardly efficient, researchers continue to call them "automatic" just because some of the criteria may apply some of the time. With reference to Platt's (1964, p. 350) Popperian claim that "science advances only by disproofs," it is extremely important that DPTs explicitly specify precise conditions that could exclude or falsify a non-empty notion of automaticity.

Dealing with the fuzziness of the automaticity concept, we have taken a pragmatic stance in reviewing empirical evidence, adopting whatever operational meaning of automaticity is used in leading paradigms: evaluative conditioning, mere exposure, speeded classification tasks, priming, and behavior regulation. Across all paradigms, the evidence reveals distinct limits of all kinds of automaticity:

1. Rather than being independent of attention and cognitive resources, many so-called "automatic" behaviors depend on or are influenced by participants' cooperation and volitional goal settings and their meta-cognitive correction processes.
2. Awareness may strongly moderate effects of mere exposure, evaluative conditioning, speeded classifications, priming, and behavior regulation effects that are supposed to be automatic.
3. What are commonly considered automatic results of purely associative, reflexive, nondeliberative processes turn out to be amenable to flexible response strategies tailored to the task at hand.
4. Finally, the dependence on optimal stimuli, task parameters, and procedural details is often so strong that supposedly automatic phenomena turn out to be labile and hard to replicate.

To be sure, there are also limits to the limits of automaticity. Stimuli can be presented so briefly, in such a degraded and seriously masked format, and involve such abundant parallel processing that no faking, deliberate processing, or conscious experience is possible. However, granting that many behaviors break down under such extreme conditions, the crucial question from a DPT perspective is whether such extreme treatments interfere with only one processing mode (i.e., the one called *nonautomatic*) but leave the other processing mode (called *automatic*) fully intact. Speaking of strong inference, it would be interesting to see whether proponents of DPTs admit that their theories failed if priming, evaluative conditioning, and speeded-classification performance can be shown to depend on attention and working memory resources.

We believe that in this situation—facing the limits of *automaticity* and the weakness of crucial evidence—it is only appropriate to use the term cautiously and modestly. Given its place in ordinary language, we do not want to ban it from scientific communication. However, researchers should make it crystal clear whether they are using their own concept of automaticity or they mean it to be a technical term, and they should refrain from too strong assumptions about unique properties of a reference class called *automatic behavior*. One example of a realistic position can be found in Ashby et al. (2007): "We use the terms automaticity and expertise interchangeably. In both cases, we simply mean a state that is acquired following extensive experience with a particular task" (p. 632). Such a modest definition may turn out to be sufficient to explain speed and accuracy on implicit categorization tasks, as well as the corresponding evidence from neuroscience. There is no need, and hardly any empirical justification, to link automaticity to the introspective and ill-defined criterion of conscious awareness, to efficiency as a hardly quantifiable yardstick, or to only one of two processing modes or systems that confound several correlated criteria (cf. Keren & Schul, 2009).

Despite all these reservations, though, future researchers should continue to investigate the fascinating phenomena that have been attached the label *automatic*, along with their enormous theoretical and practical implications. Realizing the limits and the nonviability of too strong a notion of automaticity should not reduce this fascination but rather should facilitate progress and strong inference (Platt, 1964) in a virulent area of behavioral science.

ACKNOWLEDGMENTS

The research underlying this chapter was supported by a Koselleck grant awarded by the Deutsche Forschungsgemeinschaft to Klaus Fiedler. Helpful and constructive comments on a draft of this chapter by Herbert Bless, Steven Sweldens, and Olivier Corneille are gratefully acknowledged.

REFERENCES

Aarts, H., Custers, R., & Marien, H. (2008). Preparing and motivating behavior outside of awareness. *Science*, *319*, 1639.

Alexopoulos. T., Fiedler, K., & Freytag, P. (2012). The impact of open and closed mindsets on evaluative priming. *Cognition and Emotion*, *26*(6), 978–994.

Andersen, S. M., Moskowitz, G. B., Blair, I. V., & Nosek, B. A. (2007). Automatic thought. In A. W. Kruglanski & E. Higgins (Eds.), *Social psychology: Handbook of basic principles*

(2nd ed., pp. 138–175). New York: Guilford Press.

Ashby, F., Ennis, J. M., & Spiering, B. J. (2007). A neurobiological theory of automaticity in perceptual categorization. *Psychological Review, 114*, 632–656.

Baeyens, F., Eelen, P., Crombez, G., Van den Bergh, O. (1992). Human evaluative conditioning: Acquisition trials, presentation schedule, evaluative style and contingency awareness. *Behaviour Research and Therapy, 30*, 133–142.

Banse, R., Seise, J., & Zerbes, N. (2001). Implicit attitudes toward homosexuality: Reliability, validity, and controllability of the IAT. *Zeitschrift für Experimentelle Psychologie, 48*, 145–160.

Bar-Anan, Y., De Houwer, J., & Nosek, B. A. (2010). Evaluative conditioning and conscious knowledge of contingencies: A correlational investigation with large samples. *Quarterly Journal of Experimental Psychology, 63*, 2313–2335.

Bargh, J. A. (1994). The four horsemen of automaticity: Awareness, intention, efficiency, and control in social cognition. In R. S. Wyer, Jr. & T. K. Srull (Eds.), *Handbook of social cognition: Vol. 2. Applications* (2nd ed., pp. 1–40). Hillsdale, NJ: Erlbaum.

Bargh, J. A. (2012). Nothing in their heads. *Psychology Today*. Retrieved April 17, 2012, from *www.psychologytoday.com/blog/the-natural-unconscious/201203/nothing-in-their-heads*.

Bargh, J. A., Chen, M., & Burrows, L. (1996). Automaticity of social behavior: Direct effects of trait construct and stereotype activation on action. *Journal of Personality and Social Psychology, 71*, 230–244.

Bargh, J. A., Gollwitzer, P. M., Lee-Chai, A., Barndollar, K., & Trötschel, R. (2001). The automated will: Nonconscious activation and pursuit of behavioral goals. *Journal of Personality and Social Psychology, 81*, 1014–1027.

Barsalou, L. W. (1999). Perceptual symbol systems. *Behavioral and Brain Sciences, 22*, 577–609.

Blair, I. V., Ma, J. E., & Lenton, A. P. (2001). Imagining stereotypes away: The moderation of implicit stereotypes through mental imagery. *Journal of Personality and Social Psychology, 81*, 828–841.

Blanton, H., Jaccard, J., Gonzales, P., & Christie, C. (2006). Decoding the Implicit Association Test: Implications for criterion prediction. *Journal of Experimental Social Psychology, 42*, 192–212.

Bless, H., & Schwarz, N. (2010). Mental construal and the emergence of assimilation and contrast effects: The inclusion/exclusion model. *Advances in Experimental Social Psychology, 42*, 319–374.

Bornstein, R. F. (1989) Exposure and affect: Overview and meta-analysis of research, 1968–1987. *Psychological Bulletin, 106*, 265–289.

Bornstein, R. F., & D'Agostino, P. R. (1992). Stimulus recognition and the mere exposure effect. *Journal of Personality and Social Psychology, 63*, 545–552.

Bornstein, R. F., Kale, A. R., & Cornell, K. R. (1990). Boredom as a limiting condition on the mere exposure effect. *Journal of Personality and Social Psychology, 58*, 791–800.

Briñol, P., Petty, R. E., & Tormala, Z. L. (2006). The malleable meaning of subjective ease. *Psychological Science, 17*, 200–206.

Conrey, F. R., Sherman, J. W., Gawronski, B., Hugenberg, K., & Groom, C. (2005). Separating multiple processes in implicit social cognition: The Quad model of implicit task performance. *Journal of Personality and Social Psychology, 89*, 469–487.

Corneille, O., Yzerbyt, V., Pleyers, G., & Mussweiler, T. (2009). Beyond awareness and resources: Evaluative conditioning may be sensitive to processing goals. *Journal of Experimental Social Psychology, 45*, 279–282.

Dasgupta, N., McGhee, D. E., Greenwald, A. G., & Banaji, M. R. (2000). Automatic preference for White Americans: Eliminating the familiarity explanation. *Journal of Experimental Social Psychology, 36*, 316–328.

De Houwer, J. (2003). The Extrinsic Affective Simon Task. *Experimental Psychology, 50*, 77–85.

De Houwer, J. (2006). Using the Implicit Association Test does not rule out an impact of conscious propositional knowledge on evaluative conditioning. *Learning and Motivation, 37*, 176–187.

De Houwer, J. (2007). A conceptual and theoretical analysis of evaluative conditioning. *Spanish Journal of Psychology, 10*, 230–241.

De Houwer, J. (2009). The propositional approach to associative learning as an alternative for association formation models. *Learning and Behavior, 37*, 1–20.

De Houwer, J., & Eelen, P. (1998). An affective

variant of the Simon paradigm. *Cognition and Emotion, 12,* 45–61.

Dedonder, J., Corneille, O., Yzerbyt, V., & Kuppens, T. (2010). Evaluative conditioning of high-novelty stimuli does not seem to be based on an automatic form of associative learning. *Journal of Experimental Social Psychology, 45,* 279–282.

Deutsch, R., Gawronski, B., & Strack, F. (2006). At the boundaries of automaticity: Negation as reflective operation. *Journal of Personality and Social Psychology, 91,* 385–405.

Deutsch, R., Kordts-Freudinger, R., Gawronski, B., & Strack, F. (2009). Fast and fragile: A new look at the automaticity of negation processing. *Experimental Psychology, 56,* 434–446.

Dijksterhuis, A., & Aarts, H. (2003). On wildebeests and humans: The preferential detection of negative stimuli. *Psychological Science, 14,* 14–18.

Dijksterhuis, A., Bargh, J. A., & Miedema, J. (2000). Of men and mackerels: Attention, subjective experience, and automatic social behavior. In H. Bless, J. P. Forgas, H. Bless, & J. P. Forgas (Eds.), *The message within: The role of subjective experience in social cognition and behavior* (pp. 37–51). New York: Psychology Press.

Dijksterhuis, A., & van Knippenberg, A. (1998). The relation between perception and behavior, or how to win a game of Trivial Pursuit. *Journal of Personality and Social Psychology, 74,* 865–877.

Dijksterhuis, A., Spears, R., Postmes, T., Stapel, D. A., Koomen, W., van Knippenberg, A., et al. (1998). Seeing one thing and doing another: Contrast effects in automatic behavior. *Journal of Personality and Social Psychology, 75,* 862–871.

Doyen, S., Klein, O., Pichon, C., Cleeremans, A. (2012). Subliminal behavioral priming: It is all in the brain, but whose brain? *PLoS ONE, 7,* e29081.

Egloff, B., & Schmukle, S. C. (2002). Predictive validity of an Implicit Association Test for assessing anxiety. *Journal of Personality and Social Psychology, 83,* 1441–1455.

Evans, J. St. B. T. (2010). Intuition and reasoning: A dual-process perspective. *Psychological Inquiry, 21,* 313–326.

Evans, J. St. B. T., & Frankish, K. (2009). *In two minds: Dual processes and beyond.* New York: Oxford University Press.

Fazio, R. H. (2001). On the automatic activation of associated evaluations: An overview. *Cognition and Emotion, 15,* 115–141.

Fazio, R. H., & Olson, M. A. (2003). Implicit measures in social cognition research: Their meaning and use. *Annual Review of Psychology, 54,* 297–327.

Fazio, R. H., & Towles-Schwen, T. (1999). The MODE model of attitude-behavior processes. In S. Chaiken & Y. Trope (Eds.), *Dual process theories in social psychology* (pp. 97–116). New York: Guilford Press.

Fiedler, K., & Bluemke, M. (2005). Faking the IAT: Aided and unaided response control on the Implicit Association Test. *Basic and Applied Social Psychology, 27,* 307–316.

Fiedler, K., Bluemke, M., & Unkelbach, C. (2011). On the adaptive flexibility of evaluative priming. *Memory and Cognition, 39,* 557–572.

Fiedler, K., Messner, C., & Bluemke, M. (2006). Unresolved problems with the "I," the "A" and the "T": Logical and psychometric critique of the Implicit Association Test (IAT). *European Review of Social Psychology, 17,* 74–147.

Fiedler, K., & Unkelbach, C. (2011). Evaluative conditioning depends on higher-order encoding processes. *Cognition and Emotion, 25,* 639–656.

Fiedler, K., Unkelbach, C., & Freytag, P. (2012). *Reactions to primes: Implications for evaluative priming processes.* Unpublished manuscript, University of Heidelberg, Heidelberg, Germany.

Förderer, S., & Unkelbach, C. (2011). Hating the cute kitten or loving the aggressive pit-bull: EC effects depend on CS–US relations. *Cognition and Emotion, 26,* 534–540.

Foroni, F., & Mayr, U. (2005). The power of a story: New, automatic associations from a single reading of a short scenario. *Psychonomic Bulletin and Review, 12,* 139–144.

Freytag, P., Bluemke, M., & Fiedler, K. (2011). An adaptive-learning approach to affect regulation: Strategic influences on evaluative priming. *Cognition and Emotion, 25,* 426–439.

Friese, M., Hofmann, W., & Schmitt, M. (2009). When and why do implicit measures predict behavior?: Empirical evidence for the moderating role of opportunity, motivation, and process reliance. *European Review of Social Psychology, 19,* 285–338.

Gast, A., & De Houwer, J. (2012). Evaluative conditioning without directly experienced pairings of the conditioned and unconditioned stimuli. *Quarterly Journal of Experimental Psychology, 65*(9), 1657–1674.

Gawronski, B., & Bodenhausen, G. V. (2006). Associative and propositional processes in evaluation: An integrative review of implicit and explicit attitude change. *Psychological Bulletin, 132*, 692–731.

Gillebaart, M., Förster, J., & Rotteveel, M. (2012). Mere exposure revisited: The influence of growth versus security cues on evaluations of novel and familiar stimuli. *Journal of Experimental Psychology: General, 141*(4), 699–714.

Gollwitzer, P. M., Sheeran, P., Trötschel, R., & Webb, T. L. (2011). Self-regulation of priming effects on behavior. *Psychological Science, 22*, 901–907.

Greenwald, A. G., McGhee, D. E., & Schwartz, J. L. K. (1998). Measuring individual differences in implicit cognition: The Implicit Association Test. *Journal of Personality and Social Psychology, 74,* 1464–1480.

Greenwald, A. G., Nosek, B. A., & Banaji, M. R. (2003). Understanding and using the Implicit Association Test: I. An improved scoring algorithm. *Journal of Personality and Social Psychology, 85*, 197–216.

Greenwald, A. G., Poehlman, T. A., Uhlmann, E., & Banaji, M. R. (2009). Understanding and using the Implicit Association Test: III. Meta-analysis of predictive validity. *Journal of Personality and Social Psychology, 97*, 17–41.

Gross, J. J. (2008). Emotion and emotion regulation: Personality processes and individual differences. In O. P. John, R. W. Robins, & L. A. Pervin (Eds.), *Handbook of personality: Theory and research* (3rd ed., pp. 701–724). New York: Guilford Press.

Hermans, D., Spruyt, A., & Eelen, P. (2003). Automatic affective priming of recently acquired stimulus valence: Priming at SOA 300 but not at SOA 1000. *Cognition and Emotion, 17*, 83–99.

Higgins, E. T. (1996). Knowledge activation: Accessibility, applicability, and salience. In E. T. Higgins & A. W. Kruglanski (Eds.), *Social psychology: Handbook of basic principles* (pp. 133–168). New York: Guilford Press.

Hütter, M., & Sweldens, S. (2013). Implicit misattribution of evaluative responses: Contingency-unaware evaluative conditioning requires simultaneous stimulus presentations. *Journal of Experimental Psychology: General, 142*(3), 638–643.

Hütter, M., Sweldens, S., Stahl, C., Unkelbach, C., & Klauer, K. C. (2012). Dissociating contingency awareness and conditioned attitudes: Evidence of contingency-unaware evaluative conditioning. *Journal of Experimental Psychology: General, 141*, 539–557.

Jacoby, L. L. (1991). A process dissociation framework: Separating automatic from intentional uses of memory. *Journal of Memory and Language, 30*, 513–541.

Jones, C. R., Fazio, R. H., & Olson, M. A. (2009). Implicit misattribution as a mechanism underlying evaluative conditioning. *Journal of Personality and Social Psychology, 96*, 933–948.

Jones, C. R., Olson, M. A., & Fazio, R. H. (2010). Evaluative conditioning: The "How" question. In M. P. Zanna & J. M. Olson (Eds.), *Advances in experimental social psychology* (Vol. 43, pp. 205–255). San Diego: Academic Press.

Kahneman, D. (2003). A perspective on judgement and choice: Mapping bounded rationality. *American Psychologist, 58*, 697–720.

Keren, G., & Schul, Y. (2009). Two is not always better than one: A critical evaluation of two-system theories. *Perspectives on Psychological Science, 4*, 533–550.

Klauer, K. C., Rossnagel, C., & Musch, J. (1997). List-context effects in evaluative priming. *Journal of Experimental Psychology: Learning, Memory, and Cognition, 23*, 246–255.

Koole, S. L. (2010). The psychology of emotion regulation: An integrative review. In J. De Houwer & D. Hermans (Eds.), *Cognition and emotion: Reviews of current research and theories* (pp. 128–167). New York: Psychology Press.

Kunst-Wilson, W. R., & Zajonc, R. B. (1980). Affective discrimination of stimuli that cannot be recognized. *Science, 207*, 557–558.

Levey, A. B., & Martin, I. (1975). Classical conditioning of human "evaluation" responses. *Behaviour Research and Therapy, 13*, 221–226.

Martin, L. L. (1986). Set/reset: The use and disuse of concepts in impression formation. *Journal of Personality and Social Psychology, 51*, 493–504.

Mierke, J., & Klauer, K. C. (2001). Implicit association measurement with the IAT: Evidence for effects of executive control processes. *Zeitschrift für Experimentelle Psychologie, 48*, 107–122.

Mitchell, C. J. (2004). Mere acceptance produces apparent attitude in the Implicit Association Test (IAT). *Journal of Experimental Social Psychology, 40*, 366–373.

Mitchell, C. J., De Houwer, J., & Lovibond, P. F. (2009). The propositional nature of human associative learning. *Behavioral and Brain Sciences, 32*, 183–198.

Moors, A., & De Houwer, J. (2006). Automaticity: A conceptual and theoretical analysis. *Psychological Bulletin, 132*, 297–326.

Neely, J. H., Keefe, D. E., & Ross, K. L. (1989). Semantic priming in the lexical decision task: Roles of prospective prime-generated expectancies and retrospective semantic matching. *Journal of Experimental Psychology: Learning, Memory, and Cognition, 15*, 1003–1019.

Nosek, B. A., & Banaji, M. R. (2001). The go/no-go association task. *Social Cognition, 19*, 625–666.

Payne, B., Cheng, C., Govorun, O., & Stewart, B. D. (2005). An inkblot for attitudes: Affect misattribution as implicit measurement. *Journal of Personality and Social Psychology, 89*, 277–293.

Platt, J. R. (1964). Strong inference. *Science, 146*, 347–353.

Pleyers, G., Corneille, O., Yzerbyt, V., & Luminet, O. (2009). Evaluative conditioning may incur attentional costs. *Journal of Experimental Psychology: Animal Behavior Processes, 35*, 279–285.

Pratto, F., & John, O. P. (1991). Automatic vigilance: The attention-grabbing power of negative social information. *Journal of Personality and Social Psychology, 61*, 380–391.

Raymond, J. E., Fenske, M. J., & Tavassoli, N. T. (2003). Selective attention determines emotional responses to novel visual stimuli. *Psychological Science, 14*, 537–542.

Rothermund, K., & Wentura, D. (2004). Underlying processes in the Implicit Association Test: Dissociating salience from associations. *Journal of Experimental Psychology: General, 133*, 139–165.

Ryan, C. (1983). Reassessing the automaticity–control distinction: Item recognition as a paradigm case. *Psychological Review, 90*, 171–178.

Schnabel, K., Banse, R., & Asendorpf, J. B. (2006). Employing automatic approach and avoidance tendencies for the assessment of implicit personality self-concept: The Implicit Association Procedure (IAP). *Experimental Psychology, 53*, 69–76.

Schneider, W., & Shiffrin, R. M. (1977). Controlled and automatic human information processing: II. Perceptual learning, automatic attending, and a general theory. *Psychological Review, 84*, 127–190.

Schul, Y., Mayo, R., & Burnstein, E. (2008). The value of distrust. *Journal of Experimental Social Psychology, 44*, 1293–1302.

Seamon, J. G., Marsh, R. L., & Brody, N. (1984). Critical importance of exposure duration for affective discrimination of stimuli that cannot be recognized. *Journal of Experimental Psychology: Learning, Memory, and Cognition, 10*, 465–469.

Semin, G. R., & Smith, E. R. (2008). Introducing embodied grounding. In G. R. Semin & E. R. Smith (Eds.), *Embodied grounding: Social, cognitive, affective, and neuroscientific approaches* (pp. 1–8). New York: Cambridge University Press.

Shanks, D. R. (2010). Learning: From association to cognition. *Annual Review of Psychology, 61*, 273–301.

Sherman, J. W., Gawronski, B., Gonsalkorale, K., Hugenberg, K., Allen, T. J., & Groom, C. J. (2008). The self-regulation of automatic associations and behavioral impulses. *Psychological Review, 115*, 314–335.

Smith, E. R., & DeCoster, J. (1999). Associative and rule-based processing: A connectionist interpretation of dual-process models. In S. Chaiken & Y. Trope (Eds.), *Dual-process theories in social psychology* (pp. 323–336). New York: Guilford Press.

Smith, E. R., & DeCoster, J. (2000). Dual-process models in social and cognitive psychology: Conceptual integration and links to underlying memory systems. *Personality and Social Psychology Review, 4*, 108–131.

Stahl, C., & Degner, J. (2007). Assessing automatic activation of valence: A multinomial model of EAST performance. *Experimental Psychology, 54*, 99–112.

Stahl, C., Unkelbach, C., & Corneille, O. (2009). On the respective contributions of awareness of US valence and US identity in valence acquisition through evaluative conditioning. *Journal of Personality and Social Psychology, 97*, 404–420.

Stanovich, K. E., & West, R. F. (2002). Individual differences in reasoning: Implications for the rationality debate? In T. Gilovich, D. Griffin, & D. Kahneman (Eds.), *Heuristics and biases: The psychology of intuitive judgment* (pp. 421–440). New York: Cambridge University Press.

Steffens, M. C. (2004). Is the Implicit Association Test immune to faking? *Experimental Psychology, 51,* 165–179.

Storbeck, J., & Clore, G. L. (2008). The affective regulation of cognitive priming. *Emotion, 8,* 208–215.

Strack, F., & Deutsch, R. (2004). Reflective and impulsive determinants of social behavior. *Personality and Social Psychology Review, 8,* 220–247.

Strack, F., Werth, L., & Deutsch, R. (2006). Reflective and impulsive determinants of consumer behavior. *Journal of Consumer Psychology, 16,* 205–216.

Sweldens, S., van Osselaer, S. M. J., & Janiszewski, C. (2010). Evaluative conditioning procedures and the resilience of conditioned brand attitudes. *Journal of Consumer Research, 37,* 473–489.

Teige-Mocigemba, S., & Klauer, K. (2008). "Automatic" evaluation?: Strategic effects on affective priming. *Journal of Experimental Social Psychology, 44,* 1414–1417.

Thompson, V. A. (2009). Dual-process theories: A metacognitive perspective. In J. T. Evans & K. Frankish (Eds.), *In two minds: Dual processes and beyond* (pp. 171–195). New York: Oxford University Press.

Tipper, S. P. (1985). The negative priming effect: Inhibitory priming by ignored objects. *Quarterly Journal of Experimental Psychology: Human Experimental Psychology, 37A,* 571–590.

Todorov, A., & Bargh, J. A. (2002). Automatic sources of aggression. *Aggression and Violent Behavior, 7,* 53–68.

Topolinski, S., Likowski, K. U., Weyers, P., & Strack, F. (2009). The face of fluency: Semantic coherence automatically elicits a specific pattern of facial muscle reactions. *Cognition and Emotion, 23,* 260–271.

Topolinski, S., & Strack, F. (2009). The architecture of intuition: Fluency and affect determine intuitive judgments of semantic and visual coherence, and of grammaticality in artificial grammar learning. *Journal of Experimental Psychology: General, 138,* 39–63.

Topolinski, S., & Strack, F. (2010). False fame prevented: Avoiding fluency effects without judgmental correction. *Journal of Personality and Social Psychology, 98,* 721–733.

Vohs, K. D., Mead, N. L., & Goode, M. R. (2006). The psychological consequences of money. *Science, 314,* 1154–1156.

Wallaert, M., Ward, A., & Mann, T. (2010). Explicit control of implicit responses: Simple directives can alter IAT performance. *Social Psychology, 41,* 152–157.

Walther, E. (2002). Guilty by mere association: Evaluative conditioning and the spreading attitude effect. *Journal of Personality and Social Psychology, 82,* 919–934.

Wegner, D. M. (1994). Ironic processes of mental control. *Psychological Review, 101,* 34–52.

Winkielman, P., & Cacioppo, J. T. (2001). Mind at ease puts a smile on the face: Psychophysiological evidence that processing facilitation increases positive affect. *Journal of Personality and Social Psychology, 81,* 989–1000.

Wood, W., & Neal, D. T. (2007). A new look at habits and the habit–goal interface. *Psychological Review, 114,* 843–863.

Zajonc, R. B. (1980). Feeling and thinking: Preferences need no inferences. *American Psychologist, 35,* 151–175.

Zajonc, R. B. (2001). Mere exposure: A gateway to the subliminal. *Current Directions in Psychological Science, 10,* 224–228.

Zanon, R., De Houwer, J., & Gast, A. (2012). Context effects in evaluative conditioning of implicit evaluations. *Learning and Motivation, 43,* 155–165.

CHAPTER 34

The Unimodel Unfolding

Arie W. Kruglanski, Kristen M. Klein, Antonio Pierro,
and Lucia Mannetti

THE MAGICAL NUMBER TWO

Dichotomies and dualisms carry an uncanny epistemic appeal. They simplify experience and offer guidance for one's actions. They manage a "confusing buzz" of stimuli that clamor for attention and distill reassuring order out of chaos. Distinctions between good and evil, heaven and hell, right and wrong, life and death, body and soul, and God and Satan lend meaning and direction to our lives and delineate our fundamental choices.

The intuitive appeal of dichotomies has not been lost on psychological theorists. Early on William James (1890) in his classic *Principles of Psychology* posited two distinct types of thought. The first was portrayed as associative or empirical and was assumed to be governed by the principles of contiguity and conditioning. The second, assumed to apply to higher mental processes, was labeled as "true reasoning" and depicted as the drawing of novel inferences from the information given. But not until a century later did dualistic theorizing come to its own as the dominant conceptual paradigm in cognitive and social cognitive psychology. At that time, Kelley (1971) distinguished between attributions arrived at through the application of causal schemas, and ones based on a laborious analysis of variance (ANOVA)-like process (Kelley, 1967); Tversky and Kahneman (1974; Kahneman & Tversky, 1973) drew the distinction between *heuristic* and *extensional* reasoning; Anderson (1976) identified two types of long-term memory: *implicit* or *procedural* and *explicit* or *declarative* (the latter cascading into a further dichotomy between *semantic* and *episodic* memory); Petty and Cacioppo (1986) outlined a two-route model of persuasion that sets apart *central* and *peripheral* persuasion processes; and Chaiken, Liberman, and Eagly (1989) proposed a dualistic model of attitude change resting on the distinction between *heuristic* and *systematic* information processing. Other dualistic models proliferated. Many were featured in a sourcebook on dual-process models, edited by Chaiken and Trope (1999). That volume contained 31 chapters, most of which featured their own versions of cognitive dualism, with each identifying a distinct dichotomous way of reasoning and judging.

Popularity is no vice, and just because the dual-mode paradigm has been accepted widely by social and cognitive researchers does not render it necessarily wrong. Indeed, its popularity likely stems from its heuristic value and generative potential, which have led to important insights and testable ideas about the limitations, strengths, and very nature of human information-processing mechanisms. However, the popularity of the dual-mode paradigm does not make it necessarily right either. As with any conceptual paradigm, its validity is to be decided on basis of its critical examination in light of available evidence and its comparison with alternative theories and models. In the last 15 years, several critiques of and alternatives to dual-mode frameworks have appeared in print (among others, Conrey, Sherman, Gawronski, Hugenberg, & Groom, 2005; Gigerenzer & Regier, 1996; Keren & Schul, 2009; Kruglanski & Thompson, 1999; Kruglanski & Gigerenzer, 2011; Kruglanski et al., 2012; Osman, 2004). Cumulatively, they suggest that, its contributions notwithstanding, the cognitive duality paradigm is not as coherent and compelling as its pervasive popularity might suggest.

In this chapter, we come neither "to bury the dual-process models nor to praise them." Indeed, we eschew (for the most part) yet another critical evaluation of dualistic frameworks. Instead, we focus on a general alternative to these formulations, known as the *unimodel*. The unimodel offers a single-mode theory of human judgment. Its message is that all instances of judgment are mediated by the same underlying process, whose parameters may assume different values.

Over the years, the unimodel has evolved in various ways. It has gone through several phases, each with a different conceptual focus and a somewhat different set of concerns. The *first* phase of the unimodel centered exclusively on *persuasion*. The *second* phase expanded the unimodel to additional dual-process models, concerned with *causal attribution*, *impression formation*, and *judgment under uncertainty*. The *third* phase extended the unimodel to "intuitive," "associative," and "implicit" judgments that, according to some *dual-systems* models, are driven by a qualitatively different process than "deliberative," "rule-following" and "explicit" judgments. Finally, the *fourth* phase translated some of the unimodel's major insights into a theory of *cognitive energetics* that highlights the role of motivational and cognitive resources in human judgment. Our purpose here is to portray the unimodel's evolution through its various phases.

PHASE 1: THE UNIMODEL ASCENDING

Persuasion by a Single Route

From the early 1980s onward, the field of persuasion and attitude change has been virtually dominated by two dual-process models: Petty and Cacioppo's (1986) elaboration likelihood model (ELM) and Chaiken et al.'s (1989) heuristic systematic model (HSM). The ELM suggested that persuasion is carried out via two alternative routes: the central route and the peripheral route. Extensive elaboration of the message information was labeled as persuasion via the *central route*, whereas reliance on message-unrelated cues (e.g., expertise or attractiveness of the communicator) was referred to as persuasion via the *peripheral route*.

The HSM similarly distinguished between two distinct ways of processing persuasively relevant information, this time referred to as *systematic* and *heuristic*. Systematic processing was defined as "comprehensive, analytic orientation in which perceivers access all informational input for its relevance and importance to the judgment task, and integrate all useful information in forming their judgments" (Chaiken et al., 1989, p. 212). Heuristic processing, in contrast, was depicted as reliance on general informational "rules of thumb," schemas, and cognitive heuristics in reaching one's judgments and decisions.

The ELM and the HSM made significant contributions to understanding persuasion and generated a considerable body of research findings on attitude change. But in 1999, Kruglanski and Thompson published a target article in *Psychological Inquiry*, in which they reinterpreted these findings in terms of a "unimodel," a theoretical framework that dispensed with the qualitative dichotomy of process assumed by the ELM and HSM formulations. The unimodel's basic argument was simple. It stated that the crucial distinction between *peripheral* or *heuristic* cues on one hand and *message arguments* on the other pertained to informational *contents* relevant to a conclusion rather than to a principled difference in the persuasion process as such.

Cues and message arguments both are *evidence* for a given conclusion. Both function similarly in instantiating the antecedent condition of a preexisting "if *x*, then *y*" rule to which the individual subscribed, hence functioning as a minor premise in a syllogism whose major premise was *that rule*. Thus, a *singular*, syllogistic process was assumed to govern the path from cues or arguments and a conclusion, warranting the "unimodel" label.

For instance, a voter might subscribe to the rule "If a political candidate was a successful governor of a state, then he or she would be a successful U.S. President as well" (major premise) and proceed to note that "Mitt Romney was a successful governor of Massachusetts" (minor premise) and conclude that "Romney would be a successful President." Alternatively, a voter might subscribe to the rule "If Chris Christie endorses a presidential candidate, then he or she would make a successful President" (major premise), and note that "Chris Christie endorsed Mitt Romney" (minor premise), so "Romney would make a successful President." Note that the former example can be considered as issue-relevant, or part of a "message," and hence to represent *central or systematic* processing. In contrast, the latter example is irrelevant to the issue and based on the presumed authority of the endorsing source, hence representing peripheral or heuristic processing. Yet both reasoning instances follow the same syllogistic structure contrary to the notion of a qualitative difference separating *central or systematic* from *peripheral or heuristic* types of processing.

The structure of the major premise implies a *quantitative* continuum reflecting degrees of *evidential relevance*. Specifically, information *x* is considered highly relevant to conclusion *y* if the individual has high confidence (subjective probability) that *y* will follow if *x* occurs, and less relevant if the individual's confidence in that relation is lower. So, for example, one may have a high confidence in the premise linking a successful governorship to a successful presidency, and lower confidence in the premise linking Christie's endorsement to a successful presidency. This would render a successful governorship to be more relevant evidence for a successful presidency than Christie's endorsement. Note, however, that the present notion of relevance is subjective and in the eye of the beholder. Whereas for a given individual, *x* may be more relevant to *y* than *z*, for a different person their relative relevance may be reversed. Thus, it is not universally the case that "heuristic" premises (e.g., concerning a given communicator's expertise) are less relevant evidence for some conclusions than "issue-related" premises. This would all depend on the conditional (if–then) beliefs of different individuals, and would be specific to a given heuristic rule and a given message argument.

So What?

Assuming that reliance on heuristics (or peripheral cues) and on arguments about the issue itself (the so-called "message arguments") are mediated by syllogistic reasoning as proposed, one could still pose the inveterately skeptical "So *what*?" question concerning its implications, if any, for the intriguing phenomena uncovered by ELM and the HSM research. Such a major phenomenon is the differential use of heuristic or peripheral cues versus issue-relevant arguments under different conditions of cognitive resources and motivational magnitude. Specifically, it was found in numerous experiments that reliance on heuristic and peripheral cues is particularly likely under conditions of low capacity and low motivational involvement on the part of the judging individual. In contrast, use of issue-relevant (message) arguments is particularly likely under conditions of high capacity and motivational involvement. These findings were generally considered as evidence that reliance on cues/heuristics versus issue-relevant arguments is mediated by two qualitatively different processes. How can the unimodel differentially explain such evidence?

The answer lies in three additional parameters that determine what information is relied upon as evidence for judgments: (1) the magnitude of the individual's motivational investment in the judgmental topic; (2) the mental resources available at a given moment; and (3) the difficulty of the cognitive task confronting the individual, which involves the gleaning of relevant information (minor premise of the syllogism) from the general stimulus array available to the person, retrieving the inference rule (major premise) that the information would fit, and so forth. It turns out that these parameters were typically confounded in much dual-process research.

Specifically, in most dual-process persuasion studies, information concerning the peripheral (heuristic) cues was presented to research participants briefly and early on in the informational sequence; this made them rather easy to process. In contrast, the issue-related message–argument information was presented in a lengthy format and late in the sequence, which could have made it much more difficult to process. Kruglanski and Thompson (1999) hypothesized, therefore, that the reason issue-related information had an impact under ample motivation and resources, whereas the peripheral/heuristic information had an impact under limited motivation and resources, was that the former was more difficult in most studies, hence more resource demanding, whereas the latter was much easier, hence relatively undemanding.

This hypothesis was supported by several studies that uncoupled informational contents from ease of processing and showed that irrespective of whether the information is issue-related, when presented in an easy-to-process format it tends to be relied upon in the absence of high motivational involvement in the topic or ample resources, and when it is presented in a difficult-to-process format it is relied upon in the presence of high motivational involvement and ample resources (Erb, Pierro, Mannetti, Spiegel, & Kruglanski, 2007; Kruglanski, Pierro, & Sheveland, 2011; Pierro, Mannetti, Kruglanski, & Sleeth-Keppler, 2004; Pierro, Mannetti, Kruglanski, Klein, & Orehek, 2012).[1]

PHASE 2: THE UNIMODEL EXPANDING

The ELM and HSM were arguably the first harbingers of the dual-mode wave to inundate the shores of social cognition. Further dualistic models were being put forth in a quick succession, in domains of attribution, impression formation, and judgment under uncertainty, among others. The next phase of the unimodel program, therefore, comprised an analysis of those formulations and a consideration of their evidential base in light of our own assumptions and postulates (for discussions, see Erb et al., 2003; Kruglanski et al., 2003).

This analysis suggested that, across judgmental domains, people use information of varying contents as evidence, in accordance with the same general inference mechanism (based on syllogistic reasoning from evidence to conclusions). Research on dual-process, -system, or -mode models that found differences in conditions under which given contents are utilized typically has confounded informational contents with other parameters such as ease of information processing, informational accessibility, and so forth. Once researchers control for these confounds, the evidence is consistent across contents that attests to the uniformity of process whereby judgments are rendered. We present here two illustrative examples of the unimodel's research on this point, in the areas of attribution and base rate neglect.

Dispositional Attributions

A major question posed by attribution researchers concerns conditions in which a behavior emitted by an actor is causally ascribed to the situational context rather than the actor's disposition.In this vein, Trope (1986) proposed an elegant two-phase attributional model in which each phase is governed by a different process. The first phase, *identification* of the enacted behavior, was assumed to be automatic, hence independent of individuals' cognitive resources. The second phase, assumed to be controlled and resource dependent, causally attributed the behavior to the appropriate causal entity (i.e., the person or the situation).

In the present context, the question is whether Trope's intriguing formulation needs to be viewed as a *dual-process* model whereby the process that mediates *action identification* qualitatively differs from that which mediates *causal attribution*. In an initial set of studies, interpreted as supportive of process duality, Trope and Alfieri (1997) found that the phase of behavior identification was independent of cognitive load, whereas that of dispositional attribution was undermined by load. These investigators also found that *invalidating* the contextual information did not manage to eliminate its effect on the behavioral identification, whereas it did eliminate it on dispositional attributions. Do these findings establish a *qualitative* duality of the identification and attribution processes? Not necessarily, because there exists a plausible *quantitative* reinterpretation of these data, specifically, that for some reason the behavior identification task in Trope and Alfieri's studies was less demanding than the dispositional attribution task; hence, it was less sensitive to load and perhaps it was carried out more automatically and unconsciously, and therefore was less impacted by subsequent invalidating information.

Consistent with the latter possibility, Trope and Gaunt (2000) discovered that when demands associated with the dispositional attribution task were lowered (e.g., by increasing the salience of the information given), the dispositional attributions phase was no longer affected by load. Furthermore, Chun, Spiegel, and Kruglanski (2002) found that when the behavior identification task was made more difficult (e.g., by decreasing the salience of the information given) it, too, was undermined by load. Moreover, under those conditions, invalidating the information on which the behavioral identifications were based, managed to undo those identifications.

These findings are consistent with the notion that when a judgmental task (e.g., of "behavior identification" or of "dispositional attribution") is sufficiently demanding, its adequate performance requires cognitive resources and can be undermined by load. Furthermore, addressing such a task can be a conscious, deliberative process registered in awareness. Consequently, invalidating the informational input into this process is likely to be taken into account, resulting in appropriate adjustments to the judgments rendered. When the task is substantially less demanding, however, it requires correspondingly less resources, possibly to the point of immunity from interference by (some degrees of) load. Furthermore, under such conditions the process may occur so quickly and subconsciously that its details are not fully encoded. Hence, invalidating the informational input into this process may not occasion corrective adjustments to the pertinent judgments.

Base Rate Neglect

Confounding of informational contents with processing ease may have played a role in demonstrating conditions under which a cognitive heuristic may be preferred over an "extensional" analysis of available information (e.g., Kahneman, 2003; Sloman, 1996). In what follows, we address such confounding in research juxtaposing the use of the *representativeness heuristic* with an "extensional" use of *base rate* information.

In the original demonstrations of base rate neglect (Kahneman & Tversky, 1973) the base rate information was typically presented briefly, via a single sentence, and up front. By contrast, the individuating ("representativeness") information was presented subsequently via a relatively lengthy vignette. If one assumes that participants in such studies had sufficient motivation and cognitive capacity to wade through the entire informational package with which they were presented, then they might have managed to process fully the later, lengthier, and hence more demanding vignette information, and consequently to have given it considerable weight in the ultimate judgment. This is analogous to the finding in persuasion studies that the lengthier, later appearing, message argument information but not the brief, up front appearing, "cue" information typically had impact under ample processing resources. If the aforementioned holds true, we should be able to "move" base rate neglect around by reversing the relative length and ordinal position of the base rate and the individuating ("representativeness") information. A series of studies by Chun and Kruglanski (2006) attempted just that.

In one condition of their first study, the typical lawyer–engineer paradigm (Kahneman & Tversky, 1973) was replicated via presentation of brief and up front base rate information, followed by lengthier individuating information. In another condition, these relations were reversed by presenting brief individuating information first, followed by lengthier and more complex base rate information (in which the overall base rate of lawyers and engineers was decomposed into base rates of the various subcategories of lawyers and engineers). As predicted, the former condition replicated the typical finding of base rate neglect, whereas the latter condition evinced considerable base rate utilization.

Several additional studies of this genre manipulating type of information, cognitive load, and so forth (for details, see Chun & Kruglanski, 2006) supported the notion that base rates and category information are but alternative contents of evidence for likelihood judgments, plugged into inference rules of the same "if–then" format. Of particular interest, it appears that the prior differences found in their relative use or neglect of base rate information do not reflect qualitative distinction in their manner of processing but instead could arise due to differences in their relative ease of processing in certain circumstances and participants' corresponding degree of processing motivation or cognitive resources.[2] As with the unimodel research on attributions, then, work on base rate neglect demonstrated the importance of quantitative differences along key parameters rather than qualitative differences in informational types, in the judgment process.

PHASE 3: THE UNIMODEL EXTENDING

Rules or Associations?

Not all dual-process models were tied to *informational contents.* Some revolved on the distinction between two fundamental mechanisms of judgment, namely, *rules* and *associations* (e.g., Sloman, 1996; Strack & Deutsch, 2004). Rules were typically assumed to be "rational," "conscious," "explicit," and therefore distinct from associative judgments, portrayed as "intuitive," "implicit," or "automatic." In two recent articles (Kruglanski, Pierro, Mannetti, Erb, & Chun, 2007; Kruglanski & Gigerenzer, 2011) we examined the distinction between rules and associations[3] and found it wanting.

Consider classical conditioning, a paradigmatic example of associative learning. Researchers in this domain have generally agreed that conditioning is a matter of *rule learning* (Holyoak, Koh, & Nisbett, 1989). According to their view, an animal, rather than responding mechanistically to contiguous pairings of stimuli over repeated occasions (representing the "associative" account) is attempting to learn *environmental contingencies* in which the occurrence of one event (e.g., shock) is conditional on the occurrence of another (e.g., noise).

The notion that even the basic, unconsciously made, perceptual judgments are rule-based receives support from research in psychophysics (Pizlo, 2001). Similar views have been articulated by Rock (1983), who discussed perceptual phenomena as inferences from premises (p. 3). A recent *Annual Review of Psychology* issue "treats object perception as a visual *inference* problem" (Kersten, Mammassian, & Yuille, 2004, p. 272, emphasis added) and proposes that "the visual system resolves ambiguity through built in knowledge of how retinal images are formed and uses this knowledge to automatically and unconsciously *infer* the properties of objects" (p. 273, emphasis added).

Kruglanski et al. (2007) further analyzed mechanisms such as *pattern recognition*, or *attribute matching*, occasionally juxtaposed to rules, and showed that these, too, represent rule following. For instance, *pattern recognition* is often said to depend on constraint satisfaction, a relative fit between (1) external input stimuli, and (2) a preexisting structure of associations in memory. The activation of a concept is said to occur whenever such fit obtains. Although the language here may differ from the syllogistic terminology of if–then rules, the substance is remarkably similar. The "pre-existing structure of associations in memory" represents a compound *X* that *if* affirmed in a given instance by the "external input stimuli" indicates concept *Y*, that is, a given inference or conclusion. For instance, a conjunctive presence of "elegant attire," "interest in politics," and "high degree of articulateness" may be assumed to indicate a "lawyer" to an individual holding the appropriate if–then rule. If a newly encountered individual presented this particular "association" of characteristics, this could be regarded as an "external input stimulus" that fits the antecedent term of the rule, warranting the "lawyer" inference.

Heuristics Are Rules

These notions were further developed by Kruglanski and Gigerenzer (2011) into a unified theory of judgment. This theory integrates the unimodel with Gigerenzer's work on cognitive heuristics; it proposes that judgments referred to as *intuitive*, comprising the mainstay of System 1 processing (Kahneman, 2003, 2011) and those called *deliberative*, essential to System 2 processing, are based on common principles. On the surface, intuitive and deliberative judgments could not seem more different. The former come to mind quickly and effortlessly; they pop out, as if from nowhere, unaccompanied by a conscious awareness of their origins or of the manner of their formation. The latter seem just the opposite: They arise from a lengthy and painstaking thought process that is transparent and accessible to awareness. Yet these superficial differences conceal profound similarities.

Specifically, Kruglanski and Gigerenzer's (2011) unified theory of judgment asserts the following:

1. Judgments called "intuitive" and "deliberative" are both based on rules.[4] Moreover, intuitive and deliberative judgments need not be based on different rules: The very same rules can underlie both.

2. Whereas some inference rules that humans use (e.g., in the realm of perception) may have been acquired in the course of evolution and are universal across our species, other rules may have been acquired in the course of learning, socialization, and acculturation in specific social circumstances, and a given time and place.

3. There exists a rule selection problem for both intuitive and deliberative judgments. The task itself and individual memory constrain the set of applicable rules, whereas individual processing potential and (perceived) ecological rationality of the rule, given the task, guide the final selection from that set.

4. .When two or more rules have nearly equal ecological rationality, rule conflict may ensue. In such a case, proper application of a given rule may suffer interference from other competing rules.

5. Rules are based on core cognitive capacities, such as recognition memory. Individual differences in these capacities, trait or state, influence the speed and the accuracy with which a rule is executed. There is no general relation between the type or content of a rule and its difficulty of application. Rules typically characterized as intuitive (e.g., heuristics based on learned stereotypes) may be easy or difficult to apply, depending on their degree of routinization and their momentary accessibility; so may rules considered deliberative (e.g., rules of logic or mathematics).

6. There is a reciprocal relation between individuals' processing potential (related to their motivation and cognitive capacity) and their use of difficult to implement rules: The greater such difficulty, the more processing potential is needed for application. Consequently, when processing potential is limited, only easy-to-apply rules will mediate judgments. In contrast, when processing potential is high, both easy and difficult rules will be considered and selected in accordance with their (perceived) ecological rationality.

7. The accuracy of both deliberate and intuitive judgments depends on the ecological rationality of the rule for a given class of problems, that is, the extent to which a rule works in a given context. More complex rules are not necessarily more accurate than simpler ones, nor are statistical rules necessarily more accurate than heuristic rules. A rule would not be adopted unless it was "proven" as (subjectively) valid in a given ecology. But a once "proven" rule may not remain so forever. The ecology might change and a rule supported in a given context might not "work" anymore (i.e., fail to receive support) once the context has changed.

A Note on Automaticity

The unimodel views *automaticity* as a continuum (of the extent of routinization) rather than as a dichotomy (of automatic vs. control processes). Furthermore, within the unimodel, automaticity is closely tied to the parameter of task demand: The more automatized the inference, the stronger the connection between *x* and *y* in the inferential rule, and the easier and hence less resource demanding the inference. That is why highly automatized processes are less likely to be affected by reduction in cognitive resources (e.g., their depletion by prior fatiguing experiences or by concomitant cognitive load), whereas less automatic inferences may require cognitive resources and hence be disrupted by their depletion. Although to date the unimodel has not explicitly outlined the conditions under which various "qualities" of automatic processing (e.g., efficiency, control, awareness, intentionality; Bargh, 1994) should manifest, considering the role of these features in the unimodel's analysis could prove a fruitful new research direction.

THE UNIMODEL AND EVIDENCE FOR DUAL-SYSTEMS APPROACHES

Space constraints do not permit a detailed consideration of evidence for the unimodel's postulates (for summaries of such evidence, see Erb et al., 2003; Kruglanski et al., 2007). Yet insofar as the theory of Kruglanski and Gigerenzer (2011) was offered as an alternative to the dual-systems formulations, it is important to show how it is able to account for the varied empirical base adduced in their support. By and large, the evidence to date suggests that judgments are mediated by inference rules that can be consciously or unconsciously applied, that can be easier or more difficult to process, and that (therefore) may require lesser or greater amounts of effort and resources on the part of judging individuals. The evidence to date is also consistent with the notion that associations constitute "if *x*, then *y*" premises,[5] that is *rules*, and that pattern matching and similarity judgments are also rule based. Consider the following:

Criterion S

In a well-known article, Sloman (1996) drew a qualitative distinction between *associative* and *rule-following* judgmental processes, and elaborated a case for this dichotomy. Yet his criteria for processing duality seem readily explicable in terms of the unimodel. As Sloman admits, rapidity, lack of awareness, or automaticity more generally may reflect degrees of routinization (hence, processing difficulty) rather than a qualitative duality. And the "Criterion S" on which he settles, of incompatible, strongly held beliefs is highly compatible, in fact, with the unimodel notion whereby different rules (major premises) applied to the same evidence (minor premises) may clash and yield completely different conclusions. Take Sloman's example, the statement that a "whale is a mammal" (see discussion on p. 11 of Sloman, 1996). Whales are commonly perceived to resemble fish more than typical mammals, such as a cow or a horse. Thus, a knower may need to deal in this case with two contradictory beliefs, one derived from the whale's outward similarity to fish and the other from the "academic" knowledge that classifies whales as mammals. But from the unimodel's perspective, all we have here are two distinct *rules* yielding opposite conclusions. One rule is based on similarity, or the "representativeness" heuristic (and heuristics, after all, constitute rules by definition), for example, "If *x* looks like a fish, swims like a fish, and lives like a fish, *x is* a fish." The other rule may be based on other criteria for classification in the mammal category, for example, "breastfeeding of offspring" or, indeed, the source *heuristic* "If a biology text claims *x* (e.g., that whales are mammals) then *x* is the case."

The "Default Interventionist" Perspective

Evans (2008, 2010) advocated a dualistic "default interventionist" approach, according to which some response would occur as a *default,* representing "Type 1" processing. This response could be then overridden by further information processing and elaboration, assumed to constitute "Type 2" processing. A big question, however, is what constitutes that "default response" anyway? Research on knowledge activation (see Higgins, 1996) shows that it is the response that was made momentarily accessible to the individual via recent priming, or was chronically accessible by virtue of having been practiced and routinized to automaticity.

But the idea that a given rule comes early to mind hardly means that it is processed differently. After all, something has to come to mind first, and it is typically the accessible, highly routinized idea; this initial thought can then be overridden if the individual possessed sufficient cognitive resources and/or the motivation to keep on looking and invoking different schemas and inference rules. This is precisely what the *unimodel* suggests, namely, looking for the best, most appropriate inference given one's available resources.

Belief Bias and Four-Card Selection

Consider now, the empirical evidence that Evans (2008, 2010) cites in support of his dual-process framework. First, consider the finding that the *belief bias* (Evans, Barston, & Pollard, 1983), or the tendency for judgments to support *prior beliefs* and discard inconsistent novel information, is strengthened under time pressure (Evans & Curtis-Holmes, 2005) or cognitive load (De Neys, 2006). This finding is readily explicable via an account whereby the first rule that comes to mind (often an accessible prior belief) is relied on in the absence of the motivation and/or resources to engage in further rule search.

Similarly, performance on the Wason's (1966) four-card selection task, a rather *difficult*, activity that operates on abstract inferential rules, is typically poor (except for rare participants with exceptional cognitive abilities; Stanovich & West, 1998). Such performance deficits have been interpreted as reflecting dual processes resulting in erroneous versus correct responses. However, when researchers make it *easier* for participants to use the inferential rules necessary for success on the task (e.g., by making the premise more ecologically relevant or familiar; Griggs & Cox, 1982), the success rate is considerably improved. Thus, as Kruglanski and Gigerenzer (2011) theorized, any rule can be rendered easier (or more difficult) to process, and what determines its use is not the operation of one system or another but rather the amount of available resources (motivational and cognitive) that allow people to keep searching for the best inferential rule under the circumstances.

Processing Negations

Strack and Deutsch (2004) suggested that the processing of negations differs qualitatively from the processing of affirmations. Specifically, whereas *affirmations* were assumed to be amenable to processing both in the controlled, deliberative (or what Strack and Deutsch called the "reflective" system), and in the intuitive, associative (or in Strack and Deutsch's terms the "impulsive" system), *negations* were assumed to be capable of being processed only in the controlled system, not in the automatic system.

Early research on this issue appeared to confirm the foregoing distinction in suggesting that the processing of verbal negations requires cognitive control and may produce slow or erroneous responses (e.g., Deutsch, Gawronski, & Strack, 2006; Gawronski, Deutsch, Mbirkou, Selbt, & Strack, 2008). These findings were considered as evidence for a qualitative distinction between the "reflective" and the "impulsive" systems. Yet more recent studies by Deutsch, Kordts-Freudinger, Gawronski, and Strack (2009) show that, contrary to the prior view, negations may be processed unintentionally and very quickly, but they do depend, nonetheless, on working memory resources. Consequently, Deutsch et al. refer to negation processing as "fast and fragile" and propose that it is "best characterized as a semiautomatic" (p. 445).

It is quite possible that, all else being equal, negations are inherently more difficult to process than affirmations; hence, they require more resources. But this does not constitute compelling evidence for qualitatively distinct judgmental processes. Some informational stimuli (e.g., those containing a negation, or compound vs. unitary stimuli) may be more difficult to process than others, and need therefore to be processed only under sufficient resources (Kruglanski & Thompson, 1999). Yet the extraction of judgmental conclusions from such stimuli may still proceed in a syllogistic manner (e.g., in accordance with a premise such as "*If* x is not friendly, *then* x is unfriendly").

Moreover, work by Deutsch et al. (2006) suggests that efficient negation processing may occur when the negation has been practiced extensively, such as in the expression *no problem* (Deutsch et al., 2006), or when the negated term implies a clear opposite such as *not rich* (i.e., poor) or *not active* (i.e., inactive) (Hasson, Simmons, & Todorov, 2005). This suggests that, as with other inference rules, the applications of negation-based rules (e.g., if *not rich,* then *poor*) can be routinized or "automatized" with repeated applications, rendering them less resource-dependent.

PHASE 4: THE UNIMODEL TRANSCENDING

Leaving Controversy Behind

It is, perhaps, time to step back from fiery debates and explore in depth unimodel's unique perspective on the process of human judgment. A recent article (Kruglanski et al., 2012) represents a step in that direction. It features a novel integrative theory, cognitive energetics theory (CET), that grows out of the unimodel and highlights the energetic aspects of motivated cognition.

The CET

As our earlier review has shown, an important emphasis of the unimodel has been the role in the judgmental process of *energy* and *effort* invested in the elaboration of information. These have been deemed crucial in determining the use of some information in some circumstances and other information in other circumstances (e.g., see Kruglanski & Thompson, 1999; Chun & Kruglanski, 2006; Chun, Spiegel, & Kruglanski, 2002).

The CET formalized these considerations by positing the action of a *force field* on a judging individual at a given moment in time. In this formulation, the *potential* driving force represents the maximal amount of energy the individual is *prepared* to invest in a cognitive goal pursuit. Its overall magnitude is assumed to be multiplicatively determined by magnitudes of its two constitutive elements: *goal importance* and the available *pool of mental resources*. The *effective* driving force represents the *actual* amount of energy the individual invests in the cognitive activity. The *restraining force* represents resistance to a given pursuit; such resistance arises cumulatively from task demands, the pull of competing goals, and one's inclination toward resource conservation (or cognitive "miserliness"). The CET assumes that elements of the driving force (goal importance and amount of resources) combine *multiplicatively* to determine overall force magnitude. Thus, increasing or decreasing by a given amount one of the elements (say, goal importance) has the same effect on magnitude of the potential driving force as decreasing or increasing by the same amount the extent of its counterpart (say, available resources).

Elements of the restraining force (task demands, competing goals, and resource conservation) are assumed to combine *additively*. They, too, are functionally interchangeable: Increasing or decreasing the magnitudes of each is tantamount, as far as the overall restraint magnitude is concerned, to proportionately increasing or decreasing the magnitude(s) of the remaining elements.

The CET maintains that elements of the *effective driving* force and those of the *restraining* force are *compensatory*: Specifically, to keep the activity going, increase in the magnitude of a restraining element, say task demands, must be offset by an equivalent increase in driving element(s), that is, goal importance or resource availability. The larger the magnitude of one's potential driving force, the broader the *range* of restraining forces that could be overcome. As an important implication, given a high potential driving force, one could choose highly demanding tasks as means of goal attainment; these could not be implemented if one's potential driving force was low. Because some demanding (vs. less demanding) tasks might seem to be more effective means to goal attainment, CET implies that individuals' have a greater tendency to elect low-demand informational means to their cognitive goals when their potential driving force is low, and to elect means seen to be highly effective (even if demanding) when their potential driving force is high.A choice of tasks according to their level of demand represents an adjustment of one's restraining force to affordances of one's driving force, but opposite dynamic may be at play as well: One typically adjusts one's actual energy expenditures, that is, one's effective driving force, to the restraining force at hand. For instance, more of one's energy supply is typically invested if the (chosen or assigned) task is more demanding. These various implications have received considerable support from a wide variety of research findings in social cognition and self-regulation. In what follows we summarize them briefly (for a full discussion, see Kruglanski et al., 2012).

Interchangeability of Elements within the Driving Force

Evidence that goal *importance* and *resource pool* contribute similarly to driving force magnitude and in this sense are interchangeable comes from the work of Muraven and Slessareva (2003), who showed that the performance decrement of initially depleted individuals is eliminated when they are led to believe that their success is of high importance. DeWall, Baumeister, Schurtz, and Gailliot (2010) similarly showed that depletion effects can be erased when goal importance is heightened.

Interchangeability of Elements within the Restraining Force

The CET affirms a functional interchangeability between elements of the restraining force. For instance, we predict a positive, compensatory relation between the tendency to conserve one's mental resources and choice of relatively undemanding means to one's cognitive ends. Accordingly, in the realm of persuasion, it was found that the lower individuals' need for cognition (i.e., the higher their reluctance to expend cognitive resources), the stronger their tendency to base their attitudes on easy-to-process "peripheral" or "heuristic" cues, and the weaker their tendency to base them on the more laborious processing of message arguments (Cacioppo, Petty, & Morris, 1983). Moreover, individuals with a low need for cognition have been found to succumb to various cognitive biases resulting from employment of "ready-made" inferential shortcuts afforded by heuristic cues (Dudley & Harris, 2003).

Proportionality of Effort Investment

The CET suggests that individuals' investment of mental resources in an activity is proportionate to the estimated amount of resources it requires. Extensive evidence for this proposition has been furnished by the pioneering work of Brehm and his colleagues (e.g., Brehm & Self, 1989; Wright, 2008). In this work, which suggests that the amount of effort invested in a cognitive activity is proportionate to relevant task demands, effort was assessed via a wide range of physiological indices (e.g., systolic blood pressure [SBP], pupil size, or blood glucose).

Adjusting Restraint Level to Energetic Potential

Research reviewed earlier suggests that magnitude of the driving force determines the level of the restraining force individuals choose to confront. This is reflected in individuals' differential reliance on easy- versus difficult-to-process information (of varied contents) when their motivation (i.e., goal importance) is high and/or their cognitive resources are ample versus limited (for reviews see, e.g., Kruglanski et al., 2007; Kruglanski & Gigerenzer, 2011). These findings attest that the magnitude of one's potential driving force limits the restraint level with which one feels comfortable, and additionally that the two elements of the potential driving force (i.e., goal importance, and resource pool) are interchangeable. The findings of Pierro et al. (2004) show, additionally, that given sufficient resources, individuals choose the most relevant evidence (i.e., the most effective cognitive means) for a given judgment irrespective of whether such information is easy or difficult to process.

Magnitude of the Driving Force and Goal Attainment

Because some effective means to requisite judgments may require considerable cognitive resources, the likelihood of attaining one's cognitive objectives may vary positively with magnitude of one's potential driving force. For instance, replenishment of depleted resources (i.e., expanding the resource pool component of one's driving force) has been shown to result in performance improvements (Martin & Benton, 1999). In parallel, studies have revealed that a depletion of resources results in impaired cognitive performance on tasks of logic and reasoning, cognitive extrapolation, and reading comprehension (e.g., Vohs et al., 2008).

Overcoming "Reality Constraints"

Research on motivated biases (e.g., Kunda, 1990; Kunda & Sinclair, 1999; Dunning, 1999) reveals that they are more likely where the cognitive stimulus is ambiguous, hence more "elastic" or malleable. Accordingly, Kunda (1990) proposed that motivational biases are limited by "reality constraints" and will fail to occur if the stimulus information is clear and unambiguous. Rather than regarding "reality constraints" in absolute terms, however, the CET represents them as high, though not insurmountable, *demands* of the cognitive task of forming a motivationally desirable conclusion. In other words, "reality constraints" represent a *restraining force* that needs to be overcome if the desirable conclusion is to be reached. Increasing the magnitude of the driving force by augmenting the importance and/or salience of the biasing goal, or augmenting individuals' pool of available resources, should increase the likelihood of overcoming the "reality constraints" and reaching motivationally biased conclusions. Several recent studies have investigated these possibilities.

In one experiment (see Bélanger, Orehek, Chen, & Kruglanski, 2011) participants were deciding which of two brands of tea was tastier. One tea was labeled "everyday smooth tea"; the other, carrying the implication of healthfulness, was labeled a "nutrition essential tea." In one experimental condition, the two teas were essentially identical in taste. This made for a highly ambiguous informational stimulus that readily lent itself to a motivational distortion, representing a case of low "reality constraints" (Kunda, 1990). In another condition, the "nutrition essential tea" was substantially diluted (20% water was added) making it appreciably less tasty than the undiluted "everyday smooth tea." This manipulation rendered the informational stimulus relatively unambiguous, defining high "reality constraints" and making it difficult to bias one's tastiness judgments in favor of the "nutrition essential tea" should one so desire.

Crosscutting the stimulus ambiguity manipulation, we implemented a goal activation manipulation in which half the participants were primed with a *health goal* (via a scrambled sentence technique), and the other half, those in the *neutral prime* condition, were not. In the neutral goal condition, the "nutrition essential tea" was chosen to a significantly lesser degree in the unambiguous (vs. ambiguous) stimulus condition (where it was selected, appropriately, about 50% of the time); this attests to the efficacy of our manipulation and the operation of appreciable "reality constraints." Of greater interest, where the health goal was primed, the "nutrition essential tea" was chosen preponderantly not only in the ambiguous, low-reality constraint condition, but also in the unambiguous, high-reality constraint condition. This suggests that when goal importance is sufficiently high (namely, the goal of viewing the healthful tea as tastier, hence more likely to be selected for use), reality constraints can be overcome and the biasing goal may be achieved. Additional studies in the Bélanger et al. (2011) research replicated these results with other biasing motivations and alternative contents of judgment. They also attested that when the "reality constraints" are relatively strong, availability of cognitive resources (augmenting the driving force in favor of a desired judgment) appropriately increases the likelihood of the motivated bias.

CONCLUSION

The research program within the unimodel framework has come a long way from its narrow beginnings as a single-route theory of persuasion to the overarching CET framework whose scope covers motivated thought in all of its domains. Because its different incarnations focused on different aspects of cognitive activity, it may be well to restate here the unimodel's core assumptions. First, it portrays human judgments, the fruits of human thought, as fundamentally *evidence-based*. Humans may vehemently disagree in their conclusions, they may have opposing "intuitions" about a multitude of issues, yet all such discrepant judgments are subjectively warranted rather than arbitrary, and are reasonably derived from rules to which people subscribe.

Second, variables that affect our thought processes represent *continuous* "shades of gray" rather than *dichotomous* types in "black and white." Our subscription to various inference rules is a matter of degree; so is the magnitude of our processing motivation, the cognitive resources at our disposal, our readiness to engage in deep-cutting thought, or the demandingness of cognitive tasks we confront. Third, the way we think crucially depends on our reservoirs of energy and felt vitality, and this may vary widely depending on time of day, nutrition, age, or state of health. Yet even when down on our resources, we might be able to rise to the occasion and mobilize the requisite mental effort where it critically matters.This is where the cognitive task at hand is felt to serve a supremely important purpose of some kind. These core properties of the unimodel are assumed to apply to all instances of judgment, however different they appear on the surface.

Because thinking, judging, and decision making are centrally implicated in all realms of human behavior, their depiction within a unitary framework may offer useful insights into a broad range of issues that matter to society, including health-related attitudes and behavior, culture and thought, conflict and political ideology, or the effects of aging on judgment and decision making. From this perspective, research in the unimodel paradigm may have a promising future and afford exciting further discoveries in days ahead.

NOTES

1. The debate between proponents of the unimodel and the dual-mode theorists of persuasion entered into numerous further issues too numerous and detailed to cover here. The interested reader is referred to two issues of *Psychological Inquiry* devoted to these topics, including the target articles, commentaries, and rebuttals (Kruglanski & Thompson, 1999; Kruglanski et al., 2006).
2. We note here that other research on the role of subjective relevance in base rate neglect (e.g., Bar-Hillel, 1980, 1990) is actually consistent with the unimodel. It simply suggests that the base rate likelihood rule is not equally available or accessible to all persons (i.e., that base rates are not perceived as equally subjectively relevant to likelihood judgments for all persons), and that some persons or most persons in some situations are therefore more likely to neglect the base rates as a source of information about likelihood than other persons in other situations (see Kruglanski et al., 2006).
3. Some commentators (Strack, personal communication, March 12, 2012) have suggested that whereas rules are unidirectional, running from the antecedent to the consequent, associations are bidirectional—hence, the qualitative difference between them. But bidirectionality hardly vitiates the rule-like property of associations. In fact, in logic, bidirectionality is referred to as *bi-implication* (or logical equivalence), suggesting simply that the rule-like "if–then" structure of a simple implication is doubled up in reverse.
4. Our suggestion that judgments are rule based is not unique. Other authors across diverse domains of psychology and cognitive science have been making similar proposals (for a review, see, e.g., Hahn & Chater, 1998). Rule following has been assumed to play a key rold in linguistic behavior (e.g., Chomsky, 1986) and animal learning, as noted earlier (e.g., Holyoak et al., 1989).
5. Some associations may constitute bidirectional premises of the "If *x*, then *y*" and"If *y*, then *x*" variety.

REFERENCES

Anderson, J. R. (1976). *Language, memory, and thought.* Hillsdale, NJ: Erlbaum.

Bargh, J. A. (1994). The four horsemen of automaticity: Awareness, efficiency, intention, and control in social cognition. In R. S. Wyer, Jr., & T. K. Srull (Eds.), *Handbook of social cognition* (2nd ed., pp. 1–40). Hillsdale, NJ: Erlbaum.

Bar-Hillel, M. (1980). The base-rate fallacy in probability judgments. *Acta Psychologica, 44,* 211–233.

Bar-Hillel, M. (1990). Back to base rates. In R. M. Hogarth (Ed.), *Insights in decision making: A tribute to Hillel J. Einhorn* (pp. 200–216). Chicago: University of Chicago Press.

Bélanger, J. J., Orehek, E., Chen, X., & Kruglanski, A. W. (2011). *Bending "reality" to desire: The role of biasing difficulty and cognitive resources.* Unpublished manuscript, Department of Psychology, University of Maryland, College Park.

Brehm, J. W., & Self, E. (1989). The intensity of motivation. *Annual Review of Psychology, 40,* 109–131.

Cacioppo, J. T., Petty, R. E., & Morris, K. J. (1983). Effects of need for cognition and message evaluation, recall, and persuasion. *Journal of Personality and Social Psychology, 45*(4), 805–818.

Chaiken, S., Liberman, A., & Eagly, A. H. (1989). Heuristic and systematic information processing within and beyond the persuasion context. In J. S. Uleman & J. A. Bargh (Eds.), *Unintended thought* (pp. 212–252). New York: Guilford Press.

Chaiken, S., & Trope, Y. (1999). *Dual-process theories in social psychology*. New York: Guilford Press.

Chomsky, N. (1986). *Knowledge of language: Its nature, origin, and use*. Westport, CT: Praeger.

Chun, W. Y., & Kruglanski, A. W. (2006). The role of task demands and processing resources in the use of base-rate and individuating information. *Journal of Personality and Social Psychology, 91*(2), 205–217.

Chun, W. Y., Spiegel, S., & Kruglanski, A. W. (2002). Assimilative behavior identification can also be resource dependent: The unimodel perspective on personal-attribution phases. *Journal of Personality and Social Psychology, 83*(3), 542–555.

Conrey, F. R., Sherman, J. W., Gawronski, B., Hugenberg, K., & Groom, C. (2005). Separating multiple processes in implicit social cognition: The quad model of implicit task performance. *Journal of Personality and Social Psychology, 89*(4), 469–487.

De Neys, W. (2006). Dual processing in reasoning: Two systems but one reasoner. *Psychological Science, 17*(5), 428–433.

Deutsch, R., Gawronski, B., & Strack, F. (2006). At the boundaries of automaticity: Negation as reflective operation. *Journal of Personality and Social Psychology, 91*(3), 385–405.

Deutsch, R., Kordts-Freudinger, R., Gawronski, B., & Strack, F. (2009). Fast and fragile: A new look at the automaticity of negation processing. *Experimental Psychology, 56*(6), 434–446.

DeWall, C. N., Baumeister, R. F., Schurtz, D. R., & Gailliot, M. T. (2010). Acting on limited resources: Self-regulatory depletion and personality. In R. Hoyle (Ed.), *Handbook of personality and self-regulation* (pp. 243–262). Oxford, UK: Wiley-Blackwell.

Dudley, M. G., & Harris, M. J. (2003). To think or not to think: The moderating role of need for cognition in expectancy-consistent impression formation. *Personality and Individual Differences, 35*(7), 1657–1667.

Dunning, D. (1999). A new look: Motivated social cognition and the schematic representation of social concepts. *Psychological Inquiry, 10*(1), 1–11.

Erb, H. P., Kruglanski, A. W., Chun, Y. W., Pierro, A., Mannetti, L., & Spiegel, S. (2003). Searching for commonalities in human judgment: The parametric unimodel and its dual-model alternatives. *European Review of Social Psychology, 14*, 1–48.

Erb, H. P., Pierro, A., Mannetti, L., Spiegel, S., & Kruglanski, A. W. (2007). Biased processing of persuasive information: On the functional equivalence of cues and message arguments. *European Journal of Social Psychology, 37*(5), 1057–1075.

Evans, J. St. B. T. (2008). Dual-processing accounts of reasoning, judgment, and social cognition. *Annual Review of Psychology, 59*, 255–278.

Evans, J. St. B. T. (2010). Intuition and reasoning: A dual-process perspective. *Psychological Inquiry, 21*(4), 313–326.

Evans, J. St. B. T., Barston, J. L., & Pollard, P. (1983). On the conflict between logic and belief in syllogistic reasoning. *Memory and Cognition, 11*(3), 295–306.

Evans, J. St. B. T., & Curtis-Holmes, J. (2005). Rapid responding increases belief bias: Evidence for the dual-process theory of reasoning. *Thinking and Reasoning, 11*(4), 382–389.

Gawronski, B., Deutsch, R., Mbirkou, S., Selbt, B., & Strack, F. (2008). When "just say no" is not enough: Affirmation versus negation training and the reduction of automatic stereotype activation. *Journal of Experimental Social Psychology, 44*(2), 370–377.

Gigerenzer, G., & Regier, T. (1996). How do we tell an association from a rule?: Comment on Sloman (1996). *Psychological Bulletin, 119*(1), 23–26.

Griggs, R. A., & Cox, J. R. (1982). The elusive thematic-materials effect in Wason's selection task. *British Journal of Psychology, 73*(3), 407–420.

Hahn, U., & Chater, N. (1998). Similarity and rules: Distinct? Exhaustive? Empirically distinguishable? *Cognition, 65*(2–3), 197–230.

Hasson, U., Simmons, J. P., & Todorov, A. (2005). Believe it or not: On the possibility of suspending belief. *Psychological Science, 16*(7), 566–571.

Higgins, E. T. (1996). Knowledge activation: Accessibility, applicability and salience. In E. T. Higgins & A. W. Kruglanski (Eds.), *Social psychology: A handbook of basic processes* (pp. 133–168). New York: Guilford Press.

Holyoak, K. J., Koh, K., & Nisbett, R. E. (1989). A theory of conditioning: Inductive learning within rule-based default hierarchies. *Psychological Review, 96*(2), 315–340.

James, W. (1890). *The principles of psychology.* New York: Holt.

Kahneman, D. (2003). A perspective on judgment and choice: Mapping bounded rationality. *American Psychologist, 58*(9), 697–720.

Kahneman, D. (2011). *Thinking, fast and slow.* New York: Farrar, Straus & Giroux.

Kahneman, D., & Tversky, A. (1973). On the psychology of prediction. *Psychological Review, 80*(4), 237–251.

Kelley, H. H. (1967). Attribution theory in social psychology. In D. Levine (Ed.), *Nebraska Symposium on Motivation* (Vol. 15, pp. 192–238). Lincoln: University of Nebraska Press.

Kelley, H. H. (1971). *Attribution in social interaction.* New York: General Learning Press.

Keren, G., & Schul, Y. (2009). Two is not always better than one: A critical evaluation of two-system theories. *Perspectives on Psychological Science, 4*(6), 533–550.

Kersten, D., Mammassian, P., & Yuille, A. (2004). Object perception as Bayesian inference. *Annual Review of Psychology, 55,* 271–304.

Kruglanski, A. W., Bélanger, J. J., Chen, X., Kopetz, C., Pierro, A., & Mannetti, L. (2012). The energetic of motivated cognition: A force field analysis. *Psychological Review, 119*(1), 1–20.

Kruglanski, A. W., Chun, W. Y., Erb, H. P., Pierro, A., Mannetti, L., & Spiegel, S. (2003) A parametric unimodel of human judgment: Integrating dual-process frameworks in social cognition from a single-mode perspective. In J. P. Forgas, K. D. Williams, & W. von Hippel (Eds.), *Social judgments: Implicit and explicit processes* (pp. 137–161). New York: Cambridge University Press.

Kruglanski, A. W., Dechesne, M., Erb, H. P., Pierro, A., Mannetti, L., & Chun, W. Y. (2006). Modes, systems and the sirens of specificity: The issues in gist. *Psychological Inquiry* (Authors' Response to Commentaries), *17*(3), 256–264.

Kruglanski, A. W., & Gigerenzer, G. (2011). Intuitive and deliberate judgments are based on common principles. *Psychological Review, 118*(1), 97–109.

Kruglanski, A. W., Pierro, A., Mannetti, L., Erb, H.-P., & Chun, W. Y. (2007). On the parameters of human judgment. In M. P. Zanna (Ed.), *Advances in experimental social psychology* (Vol. 39, pp. 255–303). New York: Academic Press.

Kruglanski, A. W., Pierro, A., & Sheveland, A. (2011). How many roads lead to Rome?: Equifinality set-size and commitment to goals and means. *European Journal of Social Psychology, 41*(3), 344–352.

Kruglanski, A. W., & Thompson, E. P. (1999). Persuasion by a single route: A view from the unimodel. *Psychological Inquiry, 10*(2), 83–109.

Kunda, Z. (1990). The case for motivated reasoning. *Psychology Bulletin, 108*(3), 480–498.

Kunda, Z., & Sinclair, L. (1999). Motivated reasoning with stereotypes: Activation, application, and inhibition. *Psychological Inquiry, 10*(1), 12–22.

Martin, P. Y., & Benton, D. (1999). The influence of a glucose drink on a demanding working memory task. *Physiology and Behaviour, 67*(1), 69–74.

Muraven, M., & Slessareva, E. (2003). Mechanism of self-control failure: Motivation and limited resources. *Personality and Social Psychology Bulletin, 29*(7), 894–906.

Osman, M. (2004). An evaluation of dual-process theories of reasoning. *Psychonomic Bulletin and Review, 11*(6), 988–1010.

Petty, R. E., & Cacioppo, J. T. (1986). The elaboration likelihood model of persuasion. In L. Berkowitz (Ed.), *Advances in experimental social psychology* (Vol. 19, pp. 123–205). New York: Academic Press.

Pierro, A., Mannetti, L., Kruglanski, A. W., Klein, K., & Orehek, E. (2012). Persistence of attitude change and attitude–behavior correspondence based on extensive processing of source information. *European Journal of Social Psychology, 42*(1), 103–111.

Pierro, A., Mannetti, L., Kruglanski, A. W., & Sleeth-Keppler, D. (2004). Relevance override: On the reduced impact of "cues" under high motivation conditions of persuasion studies. *Journal of Personality and Social Psychology, 86*(2), 251–264.

Pizlo, Z. (2001). Perception viewed as an inverse problem. *Vision Research, 41*(24), 3145–3161.

Rock, I. (1983). *The logic of perception.* Cambridge, MA: MIT Press.

Sloman, S. A. (1996). The empirical case for two systems of reasoning. *Psychological Bulletin, 119*(1), 3–22.

Stanovich, K. E., & West, R. F. (1998). Cognitive ability and variation in selection task performance. *Thinking and Reasoning*, *4*(3), 193–230.

Strack, F., & Deutsch, R. (2004). Reflective and impulsive determinants of social behavior. *Personality and Social Psychology Review*, *8*(3), 220–247.

Trope, Y. (1986). Self-assessment and self-enhancement in achievement motivation. In R. M. Sorrentino & E. T. Higgins (Eds.), *Handbook of motivation and cognition: Foundations of social behavior* (Vol. 1, pp. 350–378). New York: Guilford Press.

Trope, Y., & Alfieri, T. (1997). Effortfulness and flexibility of dispositional judgment processes. *Journal of Personality and Social Psychology*, *73*(4), 662–674.

Trope, Y., & Gaunt, R. (2000). Processing alternative explanations of behavior: Correction of integration? *Journal of Personality and Social Psychology*, *79*(3), 344–354.

Tversky, A., & Kahneman, D. (1974). Judgment under uncertainty: Heuristics and biases. *Science, 185*(4157), 1124–1131.

Vohs, K. D., Baumeister, R. F., Schmeichel, B. J., Twenge, J. M., Nelson, N. M., & Tice, D. M. (2008). Making choices impairs subsequent self-control: A limited-resource account of decision making, self-regulation, and active initiative. *Journal of Personality and Social Psychology, 94*(5), 883–898.

Wason, P. C. (1966). Reasoning. In B. M. Foss (Ed.), *New horizons in psychology* (pp. 113–135). Harmondsworth, UK: Penguin.

Wright, R. A. (2008). Refining the prediction of effort: Brehm's distinction between potential motivation and motivation intensity. *Social and Personality Psychology Compass*, *2*(2), 682–701.

CHAPTER 35

Why a Propositional Single-Process Model of Associative Learning Deserves to Be Defended

Jan De Houwer

During the past 40 years or so, research on associative learning has been dominated by cognitive association formation theories. These models postulate that the effect of relations between events in the world on behavior is mediated by the formation of associations between the mental representations of those events (for reviews, see Bouton, 2007; Pearce & Bouton, 2001). Recently, however, it has been proposed that associative learning might be mediated by the formation and truth evaluation of propositions about relations in the world (e.g., De Houwer, 2009; Mitchell, De Houwer, & Lovibond, 2009a; Waldmann, 2000). Although most learning researchers now accept that associative learning can reflect the operation of propositional processes (e.g., Shanks, 2007; Mitchell, De Houwer, & Lovibond, 2009b), many believe that at least some instances of associative learning are mediated by the formation of associations (e.g., McLaren, Green, & Mackintosh, 1994; Sternberg & McClelland, 2012). As such, most learning researches endorse a dual-process model of associative learning (see Mitchell et al., 2009b, p. 230).

In this chapter, I argue that there is merit in defending the position that all instances of associative learning are due to the formation and truth evaluation of propositions about relations in the environment. I first provide a functional definition of *associative learning* that is neutral with regard to the mediating processes, allowing for both associative and propositional accounts of associative learning. After explaining the core assumptions of these accounts, I consider and dismiss several arguments for postulating the existence of an association formation mechanism in addition to a propositional learning mechanism. I then offer several reasons why it is actually better to avoid a dual-process account of associative learning. Finally, I discuss what the debate on the mechanisms of associative learning teaches us about the merits of dual-process models in general.

WHAT IS ASSOCIATIVE LEARNING?

I define *associative learning* as an effect, that is, as the impact of relations between events in the environment on behavior (De Houwer, 2007; De Houwer, Barnes-Holmes, & Moors, 2013). Whereas some relations involve two stimuli (e.g., a bell and food), others involve a stimulus and a behavior (e.g., pressing a lever and food). Labeling a change in behavior as an instance of associative learning therefore implies a hypothesis about the environmental causes of the behavior. In other words, the learned behavior is considered to be an effect of a particular relation in the environment. Importantly, this functional definition of learning does not contain any assumptions about the mental mechanisms by which the relation in the environment causes the change in behavior. Hence, associative learning is an effect that could in principle be due to different types of mental processes. Distinguishing between associative learning as an effect on the one hand, and as a mental mechanism on the other not only maximizes theoretical freedom but also allows one to verify the presence of associative learning without having to verify the presence of a particular mental mechanism (De Houwer, 2007, 2011). To determine whether associative learning has taken place, it suffices to test whether an observed change in behavior is caused by a particular relation in the environment. In laboratory settings, this can be achieved by manipulating the presence of the relation while controlling for other environmental differences. If the manipulation affects the target behavior, one can infer that the behavior was caused by the relation, and in that way conclude that associative learning has taken place.

MODELS OF ASSOCIATIVE LEARNING

Association Formation Models

All cognitive association formation models postulate that, under certain conditions, relations in the world result in the formation and adaptation of associations in memory that in turn influence behavior under certain conditions. Association formation models differ with regard to their assumptions about the conditions under which associations are formed and adjusted, the nature of the representations that are linked via associations (e.g., stimulus or response representations), and the conditions under which associations in memory influence behavior (for reviews, see Bouton, 2007; Pearce & Bouton, 2001).

Although association formation and the impact of associations on behavior are assumed to occur only under certain conditions (e.g., when the presence of stimuli is unexpected; e.g., Rescorla & Wagner, 1972), these mechanisms are often conceived of as being relatively automatic and stimulus-driven (see Mitchell et al., 2009b, p. 231, for a discussion). For instance, it is often assumed that association formation is automatic, in that it can occur even when participants are unaware of the relations in the world that drive the formation of those associations, or when they have the goal to prevent the formation of associations. Moreover, association formation is stimulus-driven, in that it is determined by objective events as they occur in environment. Most models do assign an active role to the organism, but this active role is explained also in terms of objective events that the organism recently experienced. For instance, several models postulate that the effect of a single pairing of two stimuli on the strength of the association between the representations of those stimuli depends on the extent to which the organism pays attention to the stimuli. However, attention is assumed to be a function of the way in which stimuli have co-occurred in the past (e.g., Mackintosh, 1975; Pearce & Hall, 1980; Rescorla & Wagner, 1972). In summary, although there are important differences between association formation models, it is safe to say that these models tend to view learning as fairly automatic and stimulus-driven.

Propositional Models

Propositional models of associative learning postulate that the impact of relations in the environment on behavior is mediated by the formation and truth evaluation of propositions about those relations. A *proposition* is a belief about a state of affairs in the world. Hence, a proposition about a relation between events in the world is a belief about the relation between those events. As such, propositions have an objective *truth value;* that is, they can correspond in different degrees to the actual state of the environment. Associations between mental representations, on the other hand, do not imply a claim about events in the world and therefore do not have truth value (also see Moors, Chapter 2, this volume).

A second difference between propositions and associations is that only propositions can contain information about the type of relation between events (see Lagnado, Waldmann, Hagmayer, & Sloman, 2007, for an excellent discussion of this issue). Events in the world can be related in many different ways. For instance, a substance in the blood of a patient can be either a cause or an effect of a disease. Knowing the type of relation between events is vital for our understanding and control of the world. For instance, knowing whether a substance in the blood is a cause or effect of a disease determines how useful it is to try to remove the substance from the blood of the patient (Lagnado et al., 2007). This crucial information can be contained within propositions (e.g., "The substance causes the disease") but not associations. The fact that propositions have a truth value and specify the way in which events are related, opens the possibility to generate and truth evaluate novel propositions based on existing propositions, that is, to make inferences.

Current propositional models incorporate the assumption that the formation and truth evaluation of propositions is a nonautomatic process (De Houwer, 2009; Mitchell et al., 2009a). It is thought to involve active problem solving that organisms undertake in order to discover the structure of the world in which they live. Like problem solving, learning can make use of all the mental capacities that organisms have at their disposal. Given that problem solving is typically an intentional, time-consuming, and effortful process, one can envisage that associative learning is facilitated when organisms have the goal, the time, and the resources to engage in the formation and truth evaluation of propositions about relations in the world. However, just as problem solving can become more automatic in certain situations as a result of practice, associative learning might also be unintentional, fast, and efficient in certain situations. Nevertheless, current propositional models postulate that associative learning always depends on awareness. More specifically, it is assumed that a relation in the world can influence behavior only after a proposition about that relation has been consciously entertained as being true. Although this assumption is not a logical implication of the idea that associative learning is mediated by the formation of propositions, it does seem reasonable to assume that a belief about the world can only be considered to be a belief once it has been entertained consciously. The processes by which the proposition arises into consciousness, or the processes by which it is evaluated as true, might well be unconscious, but the proposition itself at some point in time needs to be entertained consciously. The emphasis on consciousness also strengthens the constructive nature of propositional models, that is, their emphasis on the active role of the organism. According to these models, (learned) behavior is determined not by the objective (co-)occurrence of events but by whether and how the (co-)occurrences are constructed and interpreted by the organism. Whereas it is generally accepted that perception and memory involve constructive processes (Bruner, 1992), propositional models emphasize the idea that associative learning is also based on constructive processes. A contingency between events in the world is psychologically inert until the contingency is consciously appraised as some type of relation between the events (see Hayes, Barnes-Holmes, & Roche, 2001, for related ideas).

DO WE NEED A SECOND MECHANISM FOR ASSOCIATIVE LEARNING?

Although propositional models have not (yet) been formalized, they are able to explain a wide range of empirical findings and have generated many new predictions that have been verified empirically (for reviews, see De Houwer, 2009; Mitchell et al., 2009a, 2009b). As a result, most learning researchers now accept the idea that at least some instances of associative learning are mediated by propositional processes (e.g., Mitchell et al., 2009b, p. 230; Shanks, 2007, p. 297). However, very few researchers seem to believe that associative learning always involves the formation and truth evaluation of propositions (see Mitchell et al., 2009b). In this section, I discuss three types of associative learning that are alleged to fall outside the scope of propositional models: automatic associative learning, irrational associative learning, and associative learning in (certain) nonhuman organisms. Before I evaluate these proposals, I would like to point out that their validity does not necessarily inform us about the validity of association formation models. Associative learning effects that cannot be explained by propositional models are not necessarily due to association formation processes. The only conclusion would be that a second, nonpropositional process needs to be assumed in order to provide a full account of associative learning. In principle, this can be a mechanism other than the formation of associations (see Jamieson, Crump, & Hannah, 2012, for an example).

Association Formation Mechanisms Are Needed to Explain Automatic Associative Learning Effects

Automaticity is an umbrella term that refers to the conditions under which an effect or process can occur (De Houwer & Moors, 2012; Moors & De Houwer, 2006a). For instance, associative learning can be described as automatic if it occurs independently of certain goals of the organism that learns, even when the organism is not aware of what is learned or that learning takes place, even when the organism is engaged in other tasks or has little time. It is reasonable to assume that associative learning can have features of automaticity. For instance, a light that is paired with a painful electric shock is likely to evoke an involuntary galvanic skin conductance response that, by definition, is hard to control consciously.

Some have argued that automatic instances of associative learning cannot be due to propositional processes, simply because these processes are assumed to operate in a nonautomatic manner. There are two reasons why this argument is incorrect. First, behavior is always the product of multiple underlying processes. Associative learning, for instance, requires not only the formation of representations but also processes by which these representations influence behavior. Although propositional models do specify that the formation of propositions has certain features of nonautomaticity, they do not stipulate that the impact of propositions on behavior is nonautomatic. In fact, there are good reasons to assume that propositional knowledge can have uncontrolled effects on behavior. Imagine, for instance, that someone tells you that a tiger is lurking behind your back. If you evaluate this proposition as being true, you are bound to experience all kinds of uncontrolled changes in behavior (e.g., increased heart rate, sweating). Likewise, entertaining the belief that a light will be followed by an electric shock is likely to cause uncontrolled changes in behavior. In fact, providing verbal instructions about the relation between a light and an electric shock has been shown to produce conditioned galvanic skin responses even when light and shock never co-occurred (Cook & Harris, 1937). The effects of consciously entertained propositions on behavior can be automatic also in the sense of being fast and efficient. Hence, contrary to what is sometimes assumed, learning effects that arise in speeded response tasks (e.g., priming tasks) or tasks in which responding occurs under considerable mental load (e.g., when engaging in difficult secondary task) could also be due to propositional processes (for evidence supporting this argument, see De Houwer & Vandorpe, 2010; Peters & Gawronski, 2011).

Also propositions that are no longer consciously entertained might influence behavior in an automatic manner. Once a proposition has been formed, it can be stored in memory. Memory research has shown that information can be retrieved from memory automatically, that is, without intention or consciousness (e.g., Richardson-Klavehn, Lee, Joubran, & Bjork, 1994). Hence, a proposition about the relation between events in the world (e.g., that a light is followed by an electric shock) could be retrieved from memory automatically and in that way influence behavior in a fast, efficient, and uncontrolled manner (see Moors, Chapter 2, this volume, for an insightful discussion about the conceptual implications of this assumption). An automatically activated proposition might influence behavior even when the proposition can no longer be consciously recalled or when a conflicting proposition is consciously entertained (e.g., that the light will no longer be followed by an electric shock). Hence, propositional models are compatible with instances of associative learning that seem to go beyond or even to contradict currently held beliefs. Note, however, that these models are currently silent about when automatically retrieved propositions can overrule currently held beliefs. Without specific assumptions about this issue, propositional models can become impossible to falsify.

There is also a second reason why the existence of automatic associative learning effects does not invalidate propositional models: Very few, if any, processes are fully automatic. It is now generally accepted that different features of (non)automaticity do not always co-occur (Bargh, 1992; Moors & De Houwer, 2006a). Instead, all processes are likely to possess features of both automaticity and nonautomaticity. Propositional models emphasize the fact that a relation between events in the world can have an impact on behavior only after a proposition about those events has been entertained consciously, but it is less clear whether the formation of propositions also requires other features of automaticity. Just as problems can sometimes be solved in a nonintentional, efficient, and fast manner, propositions about relations in the world sometimes appear to pop up very quickly and without much effort in our conscious minds when we do not have the intention to detect a relation. Although, in most cases, the formation of propositions, just like problem solving, is hampered by the absence of motivation, time, and mental resources, it seems reasonable to assume that propositions can sometimes be formed in an unintentional, fast, and efficient manner. Hence, evidence for unintentional, fast, or efficient associative learning effects does not necessarily contradict propositional models.

Because proponents of propositional models emphasize the assumption that the formation of propositions requires consciousness, much of the debate about the validity of propositional models has focused on whether there are instances of unconscious associative learning. Although there have been repeated reports of the impact of relations between events on behavior in the absence of awareness of these relations, many of these reports have been criticized because (1) the reported effects cannot be replicated, (2) the observed changes in behavior were not instances of associative learning (i.e., were not due to relations between events), or (3) consciousness of the relations was not assessed properly (for reviews, see Lovibond & Shanks, 2002; Mitchell et al., 2009a, 2009b). It is beyond the scope of this chapter to revisit this debate in detail. However, it might be possible to draw two conclusions on the basis of the existing literature. First, it is striking that there is so little undisputed evidence for unconscious learning in the literature. In contrast, there is clear evidence that awareness of relations does strengthen learning (e.g., Dawson & Biferno, 1973; Hoffmann & Sebald, 2004; Hofmann, De Houwer, Perugini, Baeyens, & Crombez, 2010). This suggests that if a nonpropositional learning mechanism does underlie associative learning, it does so only under very limited conditions. Second, there are some striking demonstrations of unconscious learning that do appear to challenge propositional models (see Custers & Aarts, 2011, for recent intriguing findings). If it can be verified that these demonstrations involve genuine instances of unconscious associative learning, there are only two ways that propositional models can deal with this challenge: (1) Concede that a second nonpropositional mechanism produces certain instances of associative learning or (2) drop the assumption that propositions must be entertained consciously before they can influence behavior. Although the latter option would require a post hoc assumption and further reduce the falsifiability of propositional models, it could lead to interesting new predictions. For instance, if unconscious propositions mediate unconscious associative learning, then even unconscious associative learning effects might depend on the way in which events are related (e.g., *A* causes *B*, or *A* is an effect of *B*). To the best of my knowledge, this hypothesis has not yet been considered in the literature. Finally, I would like to point out that the current emphasis of propositional models on consciousness relates only to the formation of propositions. Once a proposition has been stored in memory, it can be retrieved from memory and influence behavior even if the organism is not aware of the proposition itself, the origins of the proposition, or the impact of the proposition on behavior (also see Gast, De Houwer, & De Schryver, 2012; Gawronski & Walther, 2012).

Association Formation Mechanisms Are Needed to Explain Irrational Associative Learning Effects

It has been proposed that associative learning effects can be irrational in at least one of two ways: (1) The changes in behavior are not in line with the actual relations in the world, or (2) the changes in behavior are not in line with the conscious propositions that people report. Several distinguished researchers have documented such irrational associative learning effects and argue that they invalidate a propositional account of associative learning (e.g., Karazinov & Boakes, 2007; Sternberg & McClelland, 2012; see Mitchell et al., 2009a, pp. 192–193, for a discussion). It is, however, difficult to see why so-called "irrational" learning effects would pose a serious problem for propositional models. One might perhaps argue that propositional models are "rational" in that the formation and transformation of propositions is probably involved in rational thinking and behavior. However, this does not imply that the propositional processes themselves or their effects are always rational.

First, people can make errors in forming propositions about the world. Making errors in their propositions about relations in the world (e.g., they see relations where there are none) would produce irrational associative learning effects. Second, as I pointed out in the previous section, propositional processes can result in automatic associative learning effects. Some of these effects can be described as being irrational, for instance, when the change in behavior cannot be controlled, or when automatic retrieval of old propositions from memory leads to effects that run counter to currently held propositions. Third, retrieval of propositions from memory might be incomplete. For instance, after forming and memorizing the proposition "*A* is opposite to *B*," subsequent presentations of *A* might result in the recollection that *A* is somehow related to *B*, without retrieving the information that *A* is the opposite of *B*. Such partial retrieval of propositions is functionally very similar to the operation of associations in memory and therefore allows propositional models to mimic the operation of association formation models, including irrational learning effects.

A propositional single-process model of associative learning is also compatible with the existence of dissociations between different effects of a single relation in the world. For instance, Sternberg and McClelland (2012) recently showed that information about the nature of relations between events (i.e., whether some stimuli are causes of other stimuli) influences learning as indexed by predictions about the presence of a stimulus, but not learning as indexed by the speed of responding to the presence of a stimulus. Such dissociations are often interpreted as strong evidence for the operation of multiple learning mechanisms. Assuming that there is only one rational way in which a particular relation in the world influences behavior, dissociations can also be seen as evidence for irrational learning. However, dissociations might result also from the operation of a single propositional learning mechanism. For instance, they might arise because different types of behavior depend on different propositions about the same relation (e.g., see De Houwer, 2009, pp. 6–7). It is also possible that some types of behavior (e.g., fast responses in a reaction time task) are more likely to be influenced by the partial retrieval of propositions from memory than other types of behavior (e.g., predictions that are made without time pressure).

Although irrational learning effects, by definition, are not incompatible with propositional learning models, it is true that these models need auxiliary post hoc assumptions in order to explain them (see Mitchell et al., 2009a, pp. 192–193, for examples). Adding post hoc assumptions to a model is often regarded as undesirable. However, extending models with post hoc assumptions is scientifically valuable if it generates new predictions that can be verified or disconfirmed in subsequent studies. Therefore, if proponents of propositional models want to maintain that irrational learning effects do not challenge their models, then they must specify the auxiliary assumptions that need to be made and test new predictions that can be derived from these adapted models. If new predictions cannot be derived or verified, one should concede that the observed learning effect is beyond the scope of propositional models and therefore accept that a second, nonpropositional learning mechanism drives associative learning.

Association Formation Mechanisms Are Needed to Explain Associative Learning Effects in Nonhuman Animals

Propositional models focus on the role of complex cognitive processes in associative learning. Assuming that (some of) these cognitive processes are uniquely human, one has to conclude that propositional models cannot account for associative learning as it is observed in nonhuman animals. One should, however, not underestimate the cognitive capabilities of certain nonhuman animals. There are good reasons to believe that many species of nonhuman animals do form propositions about relations in the world using complex cognitive processes akin to those used during problem solving. More and more empirical studies reveal that nonhuman animals possess a wide range of complex cognitive capabilities, including reasoning and problem solving (e.g., Clayton & Dickinson, 1998; Wass et al., 2012). Some studies strongly suggest that they use these capacities when learning about relations between events in the world (e.g., Beckers, Miller, De Houwer, & Urushihara, 2006; Blaisdell, Sawa, Leising, & Waldmann, 2006). It does indeed make sense to assume that cognitive capabilities developed gradually throughout the evolution of animal life rather than rise out of thin air with the dawn of humankind. Moreover, differences that are observed between associative learning in human and in nonhuman animals may be related to quantitative differences (e.g., in working memory capacity) rather than to qualitative differences in the nature of the representations and processes involved.

One could argue that the formation and truth evaluation of propositions does depend on one cognitive capacity that is uniquely human: the use of language. This assumption can, however, be contested. Propositions are in essence beliefs about the state of the world. Such beliefs might well be nonverbal and could involve embodied, grounded representations (Barsalou, 2008). In fact, tool use such as seen in many nonhuman species seems to require propositional beliefs, that is, beliefs about how events in the world are related.

Even if one were to concede that some nonhuman animals are capable of associative learning by forming and testing propositions about relations in the world, it still seems highly unlikely that all animals possess such capabilities. Nevertheless, very simple organisms, such as honeybees and snails, also show associative learning effects that are functionally quite similar to learning that is observed in more complex organisms, such as humans (e.g., Deisig, Sandoz, Giurfa, & Lachnit, 2007). It is highly improbable that learning in these simple organisms is based on the formation and testing of propositions, which leads to the conclusion that these organisms rely on a nonpropositional learning mechanism. This does not mean, however, that one should accept the existence of a nonpropositional learning mechanism in humans.

First, even if association formation as a mental mechanism had evolved first during the evolution of life on our planet, it is not necessarily the case that this mechanism would have remained active when a second, propositional mechanism came into being. Instead, the association formation mechanism might have been transformed into a propositional mechanism rather than that a propositional mechanism was suddenly added to the association formation mechanism (Mitchell et al., 2009b).

Second, learning in very simple organisms probably tells us little about how mental processes mediate learning in humans. Whereas the formation of both propositions and associations belongs to the nonphysical realm of mental representations and information processing (Gardner, 1987), learning that occurs in simple organisms or man-made cell assemblies is most likely not mediated by mental processes. It could be argued that learning in simple organisms and cell assemblies tells us something about how neural links are formed in the human brain. However, this does not mean that it also informs us about the mental processes that mediate learning in humans. To understand this point, it is important to realize that there is a many-to-many relation between the physical neural level and the nonphysical mental level of scientific inquiry. That is, one physical (neural) system can in principle implement many nonphysical mental processes, whereas one nonphysical mental process can in principle be implemented in many physical (neural) systems (Gardner, 1987). Although knowledge about the neural level certainly constrains theories at the mental level, one cannot simply confound the two levels of inquiry.

Third, Mitchell et al. (2009b) pointed out that there is little to be gained by having a second, association-based learning mechanism. One might argue that the principle of spreading of activation that is incorporated into association formation models is highly adaptive, because it allows for quick responses to stimuli in the environment via the process of spreading of activation through associations once they have been formed. The formation of propositions, on the other hand, is assumed to be a slow and effortful mechanism. However, this argument is flawed, because it compares properties of the *activation* of associations with properties of the *formation* of propositions. It is indeed true that the formation of propositions is typically a slow and effortful process. But the formation of associations is typically assumed to also require many pairings of events before activation can spread automatically between the representations of those events (e.g., Fazio, Sanbonmatsu, Powell, & Kardes, 1986). If anything, the formation of propositions is more flexible and fast, because it can be based on all the knowledge and cognitive capacities of an organism. Therefore, even a single experience may be enough to form a proposition about relations between events. In fact, the organism might discover relations purely on the basis of inferences, even before experiencing the relevant events. From this perspective, learning via the formation of propositions has huge evolutionary benefits. Moreover, once a proposition has been formed and stored in memory, it can be retrieved from memory very quickly, therefore allowing fast and efficient responses to objects in the environment. In summary, there are few, if any, compelling evolutionary reasons for accepting the existence of a nonpropositional learning mechanism in humans.

ARGUMENTS FOR RESISTING DUAL-PROCESS MODELS OF ASSOCIATIVE LEARNING

Until now, I have argued that there is little to be gained by postulating the existence of a nonpropositional learning mechanism in addition to the existence of a propositional learning mechanism. Now I point out that there are also costs attached to proposing a dual-process account of associative learning.

First, dual-process models tend to be less parsimonious than single-process models. Although parsimony is perhaps not the primary criterion on which to evaluate mental process theories, the most parsimonious model should be preferred until it is absolutely clear that it has less heuristic and predictive value than more complex models. This provides a first justification to defend the idea that all associative learning is mediated by propositional processes. One should note, however, that single-process models might become less parsimonious than dual-process models if the former need to be supplemented with more auxiliary assumptions in order to account for the properties of the to-be-explained effects.

Second, dual-process theories tend to be more difficult to falsify than single-process theories. As a class, both propositional and association formation models of associative learning are already virtually impossible to falsify. Whereas propositional models are not yet formalized and are therefore to a large extent unconstrained in their predictions, association formation models can vary on such wide range of parameters that they can be made to predict almost any pattern of results (e.g., De Houwer, 2009; Miller & Escobar, 2001). When these levels of freedom are combined in a dual-process model that allows for the operation of both classes of mechanisms, there is even less hope of ever falsifying such a model. Without further constraints, it would often be difficult to derive a single, clear prediction about learning in a particular situation. Because of this loss in falsifiability and predictive value, there is little scientific merit in simply claiming that associative learning can be due to both propositional and association formation processes.

Dual-process models can contribute to our understanding of associative learning only if they specify (1) the nature of the association formation mechanism, (2) the nature of the propositional mechanism, (3) the conditions under which each process operates, and (4) the ways in which both mechanisms interact. With regard to (1), researchers have to decide which kind of association formation mechanism they actually want to include in their dual-process model. Whereas some seem to favor a very simple mechanism that forms stimulus–response associations in a highly automatic, almost unconditional manner, others favor a complex mechanism that forms stimulus–stimulus associations in a complex, somewhat nonautomatic manner (see Mitchell et al., 2009b, p. 237). Accepting more than one association formation mechanism is possible but further decreases parsimony and requires additional assumptions about how each association formation mechanism interacts with the other association formation mechanism(s) and with the propositional mechanism. Specifying these interactions implies assumptions about not only when which mechanism controls behavior but also how the operation of one mechanism influences the operation of the other mechanism(s). Although it might be feasible to construct dual-process models that possess this level of detail (see Gawronski & Bodenhausen, 2011, for an example), until now most researchers who argued in favor of dual-process models of associative learning have remained silent about these essential assumptions (Mitchell et al., 2009a, 2009b). Until dual-process models are proposed that provide a full-fledged alternative for a propositional single-process model of associative learning, it remains sensible to adhere to the latter type of model.

LESSONS FOR DUAL-PROCESS MODELS IN GENERAL

As is evidenced by the mere existence of this book, a call for dual- or multiple-process models has been launched in many areas of psychological inquiry. In this section, I have discussed how the debate between proponents of propositional and dual-process models of associative learning might be relevant for the debate between single- and dual-process models in general. In my opinion, the arguments for upholding a propositional single model of associative learning reveal some reasons for why single models in general should not be dismissed too easily.

First, any mental process theory of behavior needs to specify not only the nature of the representations that mediate the impact of the environment on behavior but also the processes by which those representations are formed or activated, and the processes by which they influence behavior. When researchers focus on one step in the chain of mental processes that mediate behavior, they might be inclined to explain all the complexity of behavior at that step in the chain of mental events. For instance, in order to explain both automatic and nonautomatic instances of associative learning, one might postulate both an automatic (associative) and a nonautomatic (propositional) mechanism for forming representations. However, the existence of both automatic and nonautomatic associative learning effects could result from the operation of one (nonautomatic propositional) mechanism for forming representations if those representations can influence behavior in different (automatic and nonautomatic) ways. More generally, before doubling the number of processes that perform a single mental function (e.g., the formation of representations) or before doubling the number of representations, one should consider whether similar explanatory power can be achieved by mental processes that perform another mental function (e.g., the retrieval of information) within the chain of processes that is assumed to determine behavior. Note that from this perspective, the expressions *single-process model* and *dual-process model* are misleading, because there cannot be any behavior that depends on just one or two processes. Instead, these expressions make sense only when applied to one step in a chain of multiple processes that mediate the impact of environment on behavior.

Second, the proposal of dual-process theories is often motivated by the observation of instances of behavior that seem to fall beyond the scope of existing single-process models. This typically leads to the proposal of a criterion for differentiating the behaviors that can and cannot be accounted for on the basis of a single process. In learning research, for instance, we have seen that instances of associative learning were dichotomized in terms of automaticity, rationality, or the type of organism that is involved. The merit of this approach, however, depends on the extent to which (1) the criterion can be actually used to differentiate between the two types of behavior and (2) the two types of behavior actually overlap with the two types of processes in the dual-process account. With regard to the first point, few criteria for distinguishing between types of behavior are unambiguous (also see Moors, Chapter 2, this volume). Most importantly, the automaticity criterion that is often central in dual-process accounts does not allow one to dichotomize behavioral effects. As I noted earlier, all effects probably have features of both automaticity and nonautomaticity (Bargh, 1992; Moors & De Houwer, 2006a). Moreover, several automaticity features are continuous and therefore do not allow for a straightforward dichotomization. Likewise, the distinction between rational and irrational behavior or complex and simple organisms is not always easy to make. With regard to the second point, it is unlikely that any behavioral dichotomy (if one can be found) overlaps perfectly with a dichotomy between two types of processes (e.g., Keren & Schul, 2009; Moors & De Houwer, 2006b). All behavioral effects are determined by multiple processes. Hence, the features of behavior (e.g., whether learned behavior is irrational) are unlikely to provide a perfect index of whether a particular process determined that behavior (e.g., the formation of associations; De Houwer, 2011).

Third, competing single- and dual-process models should be formulated and compared at the same level of explanation. Deviations from this principle could bias the scientific debate. For instance, evidence for learning in organisms that are unlikely to possess mental capacities (e.g., worms or man-made cell assemblies) or evidence for plasticity in the physical brain (i.e., dendrites that form between neurons) is often seen as providing unique support for association formation models. This point of view is incorrect, because neural and mental processes are not related in a one-to-one manner. Although information about neural processes and structures does constrain mental process theories, one should avoid a conflation of the two levels of analysis (Poldrack, 2006).

Finally, the scientific merit of dual-process models depends on the extent to which they incorporate specific assumptions about the nature of the two types of processes and the way in which they interact. Although a model with two processes can probably explain more effects than a model with just one of those processes, this potential benefit in heuristic value can be offset by a decrease in parsimony, falsifiability, and predictive validity. Dual-process models therefore have merit only if the nature of the processes and their interactions are specified in sufficient detail.

CONCLUSION

Although it is now generally accepted that associative learning can be due to propositional processes, many researchers still believe that at least some instances of associative learning are due to the formation of associations. The idea that all associative learning is propositionally mediated should, however, not be dismissed too easily. I have argued that many of the arguments against a propositional single-process model are misguided. Moreover, there are also downsides to accepting a dual-process account of associative learning. In addition to evaluating the merits of a propositional single-process model of associative learning, I hope to have revealed the implications of this particular debate for the more general debate on the usefulness of dual-process models in general.

ACKNOWLEDGMENTS

The preparation of this chapter was made possible by Grant Nos. BOF/GOA2006/001 and BOF09/01M00209 of Ghent University to Jan De Houwer. Thanks to Agnes Moors for her comments on an earlier version of this chapter.

REFERENCES

Bargh, J. A. (1992). The ecology of automaticity. Toward establishing the conditions needed to produce automatic processing effects. *American Journal of Psychology, 105*, 181–199.

Barsalou, L. W. (2008). Grounded cognition. *Annual Review of Psychology, 59*, 617–645.

Beckers, T., Miller, R. R., De Houwer, J., & Urushihara, K. (2006). Reasoning rats: Forward blocking in Pavlovian animal conditioning is sensitive to constraints of causal inference. *Journal of Experimental Psychology: General, 135*, 92–102.

Blaisdell, A., Sawa, K., Leising, K. J., & Waldmann, M. R. (2006). Causal reasoning in rats. *Science, 311*, 1020–1022.

Bouton, M. E. (2007). *Learning and behavior.* Sunderland, MA: Sinauer.

Bruner, J. S. (1992). Another look at New Look I. *American Psychologist, 47*, 780–783.

Clayton, N. S., & Dickinson, A. (1998). Episodic-like memory during cache recovery by scrub jays. *Nature, 395*, 272–274.

Cook, S. W., & Harris, R. E. (1937). The verbal conditioning of the galvanic skin reflex. *Journal of Experimental Psychology, 21*, 202–210.

Custers, R., & Aarts, H. (2011). Learning of predictive relations between events depends on attention, not on awareness. *Consciousness and Cognition, 20*, 368–378.

Dawson, M. E., & Biferno, M. A. (1973). Concurrent measurement of awareness and electrodermal classical conditioning. *Journal of Experimental Psychology, 101*, 55–62.

De Houwer, J. (2007). A conceptual and theoretical analysis of evaluative conditioning. *Spanish Journal of Psychology, 10*, 230–241.

De Houwer, J. (2009). The propositional approach to associative learning as an alternative for association formation models. *Learning and Behavior, 37*, 1–20.

De Houwer, J. (2011). Why the cognitive approach in psychology would profit from a functional approach and vice versa. *Perspectives on Psychological Science, 6*, 202–209.

De Houwer, J., Barnes-Holmes, D., & Moors, A. (2013). What is learning?: On the nature and merits of a functional definition of learning. *Psychonomic Bulletin and Review, 20*(4), 631–642.

De Houwer, J., & Moors, A. (2012). How to define and examine implicit processes? In R. Proctor & J. Capaldi (Eds.), *Psychology of science: Implicit and explicit processes* (pp. 183–198). New York: Oxford University Press.

De Houwer, J., & Vandorpe, S. (2010). Using the Implicit Association Test as a measure of causal learning does not eliminate effects of rule learning. *Experimental Psychology, 57*, 61–67.

Deisig, N., Sandoz, J.-C., Giurfa, M., & Lachnit, H. (2007). The trial spacing effect in olfactory patterning discriminations in honeybees. *Behavioural Brain Research, 176*, 314–322.

Fazio, R. H., Sanbonmatsu, D. M., Powell, M. C., & Kardes, F. R. (1986). On the automatic activation of attitudes. *Journal of Personality and Social Psychology, 50*, 229–238.

Gardner, H. (1987). *The mind's new science: A history of the cognitive revolution.* New York: Basic Books.

Gast, A., De Houwer, J., & De Schryver, M. (2012). Evaluative conditioning can be modulated by memory of the CS–US pairings at the time of testing. *Learning and Motivation, 43*, 116–126.

Gawronski, B., & Bodenhausen, G. V. (2011). The associative–propositional evaluation model: Theory, evidence, and open questions. *Advances in Experimental Social Psychology, 44*, 59–127.

Gawronski, B., & Walther, E. (2012). What do memory data tell us about the role of contingency awareness in evaluative conditioning? *Journal of Experimental Social Psychology, 48*, 617–623.

Hayes, S. C., Barnes-Holmes, D., & Roche, B. (Eds.). (2001). *Relational frame theory: A post-Skinnerian account of human language and cognition.* New York: Plenum.

Hoffmann, J., & Sebald, A. (2005). When obvious covariations are not even learned implicitly. *European Journal of Cognitive Psychology, 17*, 449–480.

Hofmann, W., De Houwer, J., Perugini, M., Baeyens, F., & Crombez, G. (2010). Evaluative conditioning in humans: A meta-analysis. *Psychological Bulletin, 136*, 390–421.

Jamieson, R. K., Crump, M. J. C., & Hannah, S. D. (2012). An instance theory of associative learning. *Learning and Behavior, 40*, 61–82.

Karazinov, D. M., & Boakes, R. A. (2007). Second order conditioning in human predictive judgments when there is little time to think. *Quarterly Journal of Experimental Psychology, 60*, 448–460.

Keren, G. B., & Schul, Y. (2009). Two is not always better than one: A critical evaluation of two-systems theories. *Perspectives on Psychological Sciences, 4*, 533–550.

Lagnado, D. A., Waldmann, M. R., Hagmayer, Y., & Sloman, S. A. (2007). Beyond covariation: Cues to causal structure. In A. Gopnik & L. Schulz (Eds.), *Causal learning: Psychology, philosophy, and computation* (pp. 154–172). Oxford, UK: Oxford University Press.

Lovibond, P. F., & Shanks, D. R. (2002). The role of awareness in Pavlovian conditioning: Empirical evidence and theoretical implications. *Journal of Experimental Psychology: Animal Behavior Processes, 28*, 3–26.

Mackintosh, N. (1975). A theory of attention: Variations in the associability of stimuli with reinforcement. *Psychological Review, 82*, 276–298.

McLaren, I. P. L., Green, R. E. A., & Mackintosh, N. J. (1994). Animal learning and the implicit/explicit distinction. In N. C. Ellis (Ed.), *Implicit and explicit learning of languages* (pp. 313–332). New York: Academic Press.

Miller, R. R., & Escobar, M. (2001). Contrasting acquisition-focused and performance-focused models of acquired behavior. *Current Directions in Psychological Science, 10*, 141–145.

Mitchell, C. J., De Houwer, J., & Lovibond, P. F. (2009a). The propositional nature of human associative learning. *Behavioral and Brain Sciences, 32*, 183–198.

Mitchell, C. J., De Houwer, J., & Lovibond, P. F. (2009b). Link-based learning theory creates more problems than it solves. *Behavioral and Brain Sciences, 32*, 230–246.

Moors, A., & De Houwer, J. (2006a). Automaticity: A conceptual and theoretical analysis. *Psychological Bulletin, 132*, 297–326.

Moors, A., & De Houwer, J. (2006b). Problems with dividing the realm of cognitive processes. *Psychological Inquiry, 17*, 199–204.

Pearce, J. M., & Bouton, M. E. (2001). Theories of associative learning in animals. *Annual Review of Psychology, 52*, 111–139.

Pearce, J. M., & Hall, G. (1980). A model for Pavlovian learning: Variations in the effectiveness of conditioned but not of unconditioned stimuli. *Psychological Review, 87*, 532–552.

Peters, K. R., & Gawronski, B. (2011). Are we puppets on a string?: Comparing the impact of contingency and validity on implicit and explicit evaluations. *Personality and Social Psychology Bulletin, 37*, 557–569.

Poldrack, R. A. (2006). Can cognitive processes be inferred from neuroimaging data? *Trends in Cognitive Sciences, 10*, 59–63.

Rescorla, R. A., & Wagner, A. R. (1972). A theory of Pavlovian conditioning: Variations in the effectiveness of reinforcement and nonreinforcement. In A. H. Black & W. F. Prokasy (Eds.), *Classical conditioning II: Current research and theory* (pp. 64–99). New York: Appleton.

Richardson-Klavehn, A., Lee, M. G., Joubran, R., & Bjork, R. A. (1994). Intention and awareness in perceptual identification priming. *Memory and Cognition, 22*, 293–312.

Shanks, D. R. (2007). Associationism and cognition: Human contingency learning at 25. *Quarterly Journal of Experimental Psychology, 60*, 291–309.

Sternberg, D. A., & McClelland, J. L. (2012). Two mechanisms of human contingency learning. *Psychological Science, 23*, 59–68.

Waldmann, M. R. (2000). Competition among causes but not effects in predictive and diagnostic learning. *Journal of Experimental Psychology: Learning, Memory, and Cognition, 26*, 53–76.

Wass, C., Denman-Brice, A., Rios, C., Light, K. R., Kolata, S., Smith, A. M., et al. (2012). Covariation of learning and "reasoning" abilities in mice: Evolutionary conservation of the operations of intelligence. *Journal of Experimental Psychology: Animal Behavior Processes, 38*(2), 109–124.

CHAPTER 36

How Many Processes Does It Take to Ground a Concept?

Gün R. Semin, Margarida V. Garrido, and Ana Rita Farias

The idea that true knowledge is disembodied or "amodal" can be traced back to the origins of Western thought. For instance, Plato argues in *Phaedo* that true knowledge is attained by freeing one's self from the body, the source of passions and appetites, and therefore an obstacle to the acquisition of truth. An analogous focus on the disembodied nature of knowledge is the hallmark of the cognitive sciences in the second half of the 20th century. This period marks the resurgence of investigations of the mind, driven by the disembodied computer metaphor across the cognitive sciences. The drawbacks of disregarding the constraints imposed by the body on knowledge became increasingly apparent toward the last decade of the 20th century (e.g., Harnad, 1990) with the emergence of the situated cognition "movement"' with precursors such as Vygotsky, Bartlett, and Dewey, who also emphasized the significance of the contexts in which cognitive activity takes place (for overviews, cf. Semin, Garrido, & Palma, 2012, 2013; Semin & Smith, 2013).

Harnad (1990) eloquently illustrated the fundamental problem with amodal representational systems using Searle's (1980) Chinese room argument. It is impossible to ground the meaning of words by defining them with other words, as is illustrated when you try to learn a language you do not know, armed only with a dictionary. Assume that you are confronted with a Chinese symbol and want to understand what it means. You look up the symbol and find other symbols. You look up these symbols and find yet another array of symbols, and so on. There is no way you are going to learn Chinese this way. The only way you can start learning the meaning of the symbol is by grounding it with something else other than symbols.

Embodied cognition is regarded as a solution for Harnad's problem, highlighting the importance of action for cognition and the role played by bodily states in grounding concepts. The significance of sensorimotor grounding was taken seriously for some time in philosophy and linguistics but only gained importance in cognitive psychology after a set of influential psychological articles appeared in the late 1990s (Barsalou, 1999a; Glenberg, 1997; Pulvermüller, 1999; Zwaan & Radvansky, 1998). Since then, the idea of cognitive processes being grounded in the same systems employed by perception and action has become a burgeoning field of theorizing, debate, and considerable empirical research that has given rise to a new set of assumptions about how psychological processes are represented. As Barsalou (2008) states: "Grounded cognition reflects the assumption that cognition is typically grounded in multiple ways, including simulations, situated action, and, on occasion, bodily states" (p. 619). Not surprisingly, embodied cognition comes in diverse guises. Some focus on the body and its dynamic architecture, and how it shapes cognition (e.g., Lakoff & Johnson 1980; Tversky, Morrison, Franklin, & Bryant, 1999). Others emphasize simulation, namely, the reactivation of perceptual, motor, and introspective states obtained when experiencing the world (e.g., Barsalou, 1999a; Decety & Grèzes, 2006; Goldman, 2006). Still other versions of embodied cognition regard situated action and the processes involved in the action and perception link as grounding cognition (e.g., Glenberg, 1997). In this view, cognition is for the adaptive regulation of action, and that mental representations are action-oriented (e.g., Smith & Semin, 2004). Today, embodied cognition constitutes an increasingly fertile field, with a rich range of theories across a variety of disciplinary perspectives in cognitive sciences spanning artificial intelligence, robotics, psychology, cognitive neuroscience, philosophy, linguistics, and cognitive anthropology. The wealth of nonintersecting interests in embodied cognition has inevitably paved multiple roads toward the possible resolution of the symbol-grounding problem and have achieved increased acceptance throughout the cognitive sciences.

The common denominator to these approaches is that thinking is not driven by symbols but rather by multimodal images that activate the sensorimotor system. For instance, thinking about a "Granny Smith" is assumed to activate the multimodal neural patterns shaped in earlier experiences with "Granny Smiths," namely, motor, gustatory, tactile, olfactory, visual, and auditory systems all at the same time, and to different degrees. Thus, thinking about an apple activates the perceptual coding of its color, its inviting smell, the crunch of the bite, the juicy taste, and so on.

Within this broader perspective, this chapter has a very specific purview and attempts to answer a set of related questions: How are concepts grounded? The issue that arises in answering this question is whether one can assume that the very same processes involved in grounding concepts that are concrete, such as apple, dog, or chair, are also involved in grounding abstract concepts, which we cannot touch, see, or smell, such as democracy, truth, or time. Obviously, we do not have direct sensorimotor experiences with abstract concepts. Can sensorimotor simulations nevertheless represent such concepts? Or are there two or more processes that are coactivated to varying degrees in the grounding of concepts, depending on the nature of the concept? Are some concepts grounded modally (e.g., concrete terms) and others representationally (e.g., abstract terms)? The research to date does not furnish a unified theoretical perspective on how the processes involved in grounding concrete and abstract concepts are possibly integrated. As will be evident from the following review of this area, it can be argued that semantic processes largely drive abstract concepts, whereas perceptual processes drive concrete concepts. This invites the possible argument that there are two processes driving the grounding of concepts.

A substantial amount of the empirical work on how concepts are grounded has been done with concrete concepts. This research has furnished evidence for the idea that the processing mechanisms involved are shared with those involved in perception and action. In the next section we review this research reported predominantly in cognitive psychology (e.g., Borghi, 2005; Borghi, Glenberg, & Kaschak, 2004; Glenberg & Kaschak, 2002, Kaschak & Glenberg, 2004; Stanfield & Zwaan, 2001) and neuropsychology (e.g., Hauk, Johnsrude, & Pulvermüller, 2004), along with the accompanying theories. We also report the critiques marshaled against this research, from both a neuropsychological perspective (e.g., Mahon & Caramazza, 2008) and a computational linguistics perspective (e.g., Burgess & Lund, 2000; Louwerse & Jeuniaux, 2008).

The second section examines the research on abstract concepts (e.g., morality, affect, valence, power). Those attempting to understand how these concepts are grounded have examined whether the embodied, sensorimotor domains that we use to *describe* them are responsible for how they are structured. In other words, this research has examined the metaphors that are available in language with a view toward understanding whether these constitute manifestations of "mappings of mind to body through which we grasp the world" (Crawford, 2009, p. 129). There is an increasing body of research, in line with conceptual metaphor theory (Lakoff & Johnson, 1980, 1999), showing that the characteristic associations between concrete domains (e.g., space) and abstract concepts shape performance on a number of cognitive tasks, such as reaction times (e.g., Meier & Robinson, 2004), attentional processes (e.g., Meier & Robinson, 2006), and memory (e.g., Crawford, Margolies, Drake, & Murphy, 2006; Palma, Garrido, & Semin, 2011). In the third section, we present a possible resolution for the apparent tension between concrete and abstract concepts.

GROUNDING CONCEPTS

Grounding cognition has inspired innovative research largely because the idea of an embodied component to concepts has opened a hitherto unexplored perspective on human functioning that has yielded a very fruitful harvest. Notably, the explosive growth of grounded cognition has taken place across different disciplinary perspectives ranging from cognitive psychology to social psychology, and from computational linguistics to neuropsychology and neurophysiology. The theories guiding this research are connected with each other by family resemblance rather than any systematically shared conceptual premises. It can be argued that the field consists of an abundance of demonstration experiments and a paucity of well-developed integrative theories. Different theorists anchor even the term *embodiment* differently. Just to illustrate, it can refer to bodily constraints, situational constraints, and a generic perceptual dimension, among other meanings.

Notably, one of the challenges that diverse embodied theories have faced is whether the same systems (e.g., action or perception systems) and processes (e.g., simulation) ground abstract and concrete concepts. Some view both abstract and concrete concepts as grounded in perception–action systems; other accounts suggest that abstract concepts are represented by means of metaphoric mappings, or by activating simulations of situations, and introspection, and so on. In the following, we review the diverse theories and research surrounding the grounding of concrete concepts first and abstract concepts next.

GROUNDING CONCRETE CONCEPTS

In the following we proceed by representing the different conceptual approaches that have been primarily tested in domains entailing concrete objects, or events.

The Perceptual Simulation Hypothesis

A prominent account of grounded cognition is Barsalou's (1999a) approach, perceptual symbol systems, which emphasizes the role of simulation in cognition, a process that can also be found in other conceptualizations of cognition (e.g., Decety & Grèzes, 2006; Goldman, 2006). Accordingly, during the process of experiencing an object or an event, the brain captures this event in multimodal states that are then stored in memory. Thus, experiencing an apple engages visual (e.g., color and shape), tactical (e.g., the rounded and hard feel), auditory (e.g., the sound of the crunch when we bite into it), olfactory (e.g., the particular smell), and gustatory (e.g., the taste) modalities. This multimodal representation is integrated and captured in the brain and stored. At any later point in time, when we need to represent an apple, we reenact these introspective multimodal states. In other words, we simulate the multimodal representation we acquired in our experience of that object or event. Neurally, the simulation model adopts Damasio's (1989) idea of convergence zone architecture, or probably, more appropriately, its recent formulation (Damasio, 2010) of convergence–divergence zones that consist of neuron ensembles within which many feedforward–feedback loops make contact. These zones are assumed to re-create separate sets of neural activity that were once approximately simultaneous during perception.

The assumption is that these sensorimotor systems are actively engaged in offline cognitive processes that involve, for instance, *language comprehension*, or *categorization*, as well as *retrieval* processes. Feature verification tasks play a prominent part in behavioral demonstrations of these processes.

One argument derived from the simulation assumption is that concepts retain multimodal perceptual features of objects. Consequently, conceptual processing involves the activation of modality-specific sensory brain areas (cf. Martin, 2007). To continue with the apple example: Verifying that a Granny Smith is green should activate the visual area; verifying its slightly sour, juicy taste should activate the gustatory area, and so on (cf. Goldberg, Perfetti, & Schneider, 2006; Kan, Barsalou, Solomon, Minor, & Thompson-Schill, 2003).

The reasoning behind the activation of different sensory brain areas has an interesting implication that has been exploited in the investigation of the costs incurred while switching from one modality to another during a property verification task. Thus, verifying a property in a modality (e.g., auditory: blender–loud) after having verified a property in a different modality (e.g., gustatory: cranberry–tart) should be slower than if it has been preceded by verifying a property in the same modality (e.g., leaves–rustling) (see Pecher, Zeelenberg, & Barsalou, 2003). Thus, a number of subsequent studies (cf. Van Dantzig, Pecher, Zeelenberg, & Barsalou, 2008; Marques, 2006; Vermeulen, Niedenthal, & Luminet, 2007) that have investigated switching costs in property verification tasks have been regarded as providing support for the argument that perceptual simulation underlies conceptual processing. More recently, Collins, Pecher, Zeelenberg, and Coulson (2011) furnished support for the claim that brain systems for perception and action subserve the representation of concepts in a modality switch study with event-related potentials (ERPs). They report that modality switching for visual property verifications is associated with increased N400 amplitude. Furthermore, their findings suggest that perceptual systems impact the decision-making stage in the verification of auditory properties, and the semantic stage in the verification of visual properties.

Simulations involve representations that engage processing in sensorimotor systems. If this is the case, then perceptual processes should interact with representational processes. Stanfield and Zwaan (2001) gave participants a task in which they had to judge whether the picture that they saw contained an object mentioned in a sentence preceding the picture. If the visual features (picture) overlap with those induced in the mental representation, then there should be a speedup in the verification process. The sentences implied the horizontal (John put the pencil in *the drawer*) or vertical (John put the pencil *in the cup*) orientation of an object. A picture with the object followed the sentence and was depicted in either the implied orientation or not. Participants were faster and more accurate in the congruent cases than in the incongruent ones. These findings have been replicated under a variety of different conditions (Connell, 2007; Pecher, Van Dantzig, Zwaan, & Zeelenberg, 2009; Van Dantzig et al., 2008; Zwaan, Stanfield, & Yaxley, 2002) showing the generality of the systematic interaction between perceptual and representational processes.

Other studies have explored the effects of visual perspective (Borghi et al., 2004; Solomon & Barsalou, 2004; Wu & Barsalou, 2009) upon property verification. For instance, Borghi et al., (2004) experimentally induced the inside or outside perspective of a car and showed a speedup in the verification of perspective-congruent properties. Thus, participants were faster in verifying "steering wheel" or "horn" as properties of the car if they had an inside perspective (driving the car) rather than an outside perspective (washing the car). The results are regarded as supportive of the simulated perspective used during a property verification task.

Grounding Concepts via Action

A distinctive idea about how concepts are grounded rests on the argument that cognition evolved for the control of adaptive action, not for its own sake (cf. Smith & Semin, 2004; Semin & Smith, 2013) an insight that dates back to William James (1890/1950). It is with this argument that Glenberg (1997) proposes meaning to be grounded by the set of actions that can be undertaken in a situation (e.g., Glenberg, 2008). One line of research to which this framework has led is whether the comprehension of an action depicted in a sentence is facilitated when an action that the participant performs is compatible. This so-called *action compatibility effect* (ACE) involves participants judging the sensibility of sentences, such as "You gave Andy the pizza" or "Andy gave you the pizza," by moving the hand from a start button to a "yes" button (Glenberg & Kaschak, 2002). The position of the "yes" button was counterbalanced so that a response could be performed by a movement either toward the or away from the body. As the ACE would have predicted, movements consistent with the action implied in the sentence were faster than movements that were incongruent. More recently, Glenberg et al. (2008) performed two experiments with comparable sentences, this time, however, with concrete (e.g., "You give Marco the papers") or abstract sentences (e.g., "Anna delegates the responsibilities to you"). The same ACE pattern emerged. Movements congruent with the action implied with the sentence were faster than incongruent ones for both concrete and abstract sentences. The second study used a single-pulse transcranial magnetic stimulation with the same sentences and indicated that modulation of activity in the hand muscles is greater when reading sentences describing transfer (abstract and concrete) relative to sentences that do not describe transfer. These results are seen as providing neurophysiological evidence for modulation of motor system activity during the comprehension of both concrete and abstract language. These results and comparable ones from other studies (e.g., Bub & Masson, 2010; Girardi, Lindemann, & Bekkering, 2010; Klatzky, Pellegrino, McCloskey, & Doherty, 1989; Masson, Bub, & Warren, 2008; Pezzulo, Barca, Bocconi, & Borghi, 2010; Taylor & Zwann, 2008; Zwaan & Taylor, 2006) are taken to indicate that sentences entailing action call on the same neural states involved in the actual movement.

Neuroscientific Grounding

A large number of studies has examined the interface between brain processes and language. However, a particular functional magnetic resonance imagery (fMRI) study by Hauk et al. (2004) was pivotal in opening up our understanding of how concrete concepts are neurally represented. They used event-related fMRI to record brain activity while people were passively reading a number of action verbs (e.g., *lick, pick,* or *kick*). They discovered that areas along the motor strip that were either directly adjacent to or that overlapped with areas activated by the actual movement of the tongue, fingers, or feet were activated during this passive reading task. Following up on these is an fMRI study by Tettamanti, Buccino, Saccuman, Gallese, Danna, et al. (2005), who showed that listening to sentences describing actions (e.g., "I eat an apple," "I grasp the knife," "I kick the ball") performed with different body parts (mouth, hand, or leg, respectively) induces the activation of a left frontal–parietotemporal circuit with somatotopic organization in the premotor cortex. Buccino et al. (2005) reported related findings for whole sentences. That is, when people listened to sentences describing leg (or arm) movements while transcranial magnetic stimulation (TMS) was applied to leg (or arm) motor centers, there was differential modulation of electrical activity recorded in the legs (or arms). These studies, along with other evidence (e.g., Aziz-Zadeh, Wilson, Rizzolatti, & Iacoboni, 2006), indicate that the meaning of action concepts is reflected in the somatotopic activation of motor circuits.

The problematic issue surrounding these studies arises from the poor temporal resolution of fMRI studies, leaving considerable room for different processes to take place between stimulus presentation and image recording, thus opening the studies to criticism suggesting that the evidence may not be as conclusive as desired (e.g., Mahon & Caramazza, 2008; see the next section for details). It is possible that amodal representations are formed first, which then lead to the type of neural activation noted in these studies. The complementary evidence comes from studies relying on techniques with high temporal resolution. For instance, Hauk, Shtyrov, and Pulvermüller (2006) revealed that motor areas are involved early on for the recognition and processing of action related words. Other studies by Pulvermüller and colleagues (Hauk & Pulvermüller, 2004; Pulvermüller, Härle, & Hummel, 2000) using ERP during silent reading of face-, hand-, and leg-related words showed category-specific activations at 200 milliseconds after words onset. These findings indicate the existence of shared neural substrates for action and language, and that the activation of action-related neural networks is very rapid (see also Pulvermüller, Shtyrov, & Ilmoniemi, 2005; Shtyrov, Hauk, & Pulvermüller, 2004).

Concluding Notes to Concrete Concepts and the Evidence

The "embodied" account of how concrete concepts are grounded relies on the argument that the sensorimotor systems that form them are integral components to concepts. This integral component remains the common denominator in the diverse, overlapping research traditions while the nature of how the sensorimotor system is integrated reveals subtle variations between the different approaches we have noted, namely, simulations, actions and interactions, and neural structures that are shared with perception and action, and so on. Obviously, these approaches are not without their critics. We briefly note these criticisms and some concerns that have been raised before we turn to the second major section on this contribution, namely, the research that addresses how abstract concepts are grounded.

Problems

The different approaches taken to elucidate how concepts are grounded vary with respect to their reliance on the role of sensorimotor processes. As Wilson (2002) noted, the different theories in this domain can be placed on a continuum from purely embodied accounts of cognition to purely disembodied accounts. The former argue that cognition is completely grounded in the sensorimotor system. The claim advanced for the latter position is that cognition is completely symbolic and amodal. And, of course, there are theories that occupy the middle range on this continuum.

An example of the former are theories arguing that sensorimotor processes ground all concepts and cognition, as for instance: "Perceptual symbol systems can implement all of the critical cognitive functions that amodal symbol systems have implemented traditionally. If so, then why did evolution add a redundant layer of amodal symbols?" (Barsalou, 1999b, pp. 75–76). The opposite view is the traditional representational perspective against which the "embodiment" movement grew. In this perspective, concepts and cognitive processes are based on amodal symbols that are transduced from perceptual states. This amodal symbolic system is akin to language (e.g., Dennett, 1969; Fodor, 1975).

In assessing the import of the substantial research that has emerged, a number of critical issues have been identified by philosophers (e.g., Dove, 2009, 2011; Machery, 2007, 2010) and some neuroscientists (e.g., Mahon & Caramazza, 2008), along with proposed solutions that occupy the middle range on the continuum from purely "embodied" to purely "amodal and representational." The debate taking place in the middle ground is chiefly about the degree to which cognition is amodal and the degree to which it is modal. This is related to the so-called "scope" problem noted by Machery (2007), according to whom the critical question should not revolve around whether concepts are modal or amodal, but rather: "To what extent do we use reenacted perceptual representations in cognition and to what extent do we use amodal representations?" (p. 42). Machery refers to this as the "scope" issue, and it is based in part on the argument that the embodiment findings cannot be generalized readily. On this issue, different proponents take different positions. Dove (2011), for instance, suggests that symbolic processing complements sensorimotor processing:

> My proposal is that the human conceptual system is characterized by a representational division of labor in which modal and amodal representations handle different aspects of our concepts. Although many of our concepts may be grounded in perception, the existence of amodal codes provides a partial explanation of how we are able to acquire semantic content that goes beyond perceptual experience. This capacity to go beyond experience may reflect a fundamental design feature of human minds. (Dove, 2009, p. 413)

A different perspective is advanced by Mahon and Caramazza (2008), who question the conclusiveness of neurophysiological studies. For instance, they argue that the demonstration of a 200-millisecond interval between reading an action word and the activation of the motor system (e.g., Boulenger et al., 2006; Hauk & Pulvermüller, 2004; Pulvermüller et al., 2000) as an unequivocal indication that amodal processes are not involved is, at best, questionable. The 200-millisecond interval leaves the operation of different cognitive processes open, and Mahon and Caramazza (2008) argue that "it would have to be known that the activation of the motor system was not mediated by the retrieval of 'abstract' conceptual content. Of course, this is precisely the 'unknown' that is at issue" (p. 61). The alternative model they advance, namely, the grounding by interaction framework, posits that concepts partially consist of amodal symbols and partially of sensorimotor information. In this view, the core of a concept is amodal or symbolic and sensorimotor information is an embellishment that "colors conceptual processing, enriches it, and provides it with a relational context" (p. 168).

Barsalou, Santos, Simmons, and Wilson (2008; see also Simmons, Hamann, Harenski, Hu, & Barsalou, 2008; Solomon & Barsalou, 2004) advance a similar modal theory: language and situated simulation (LASS) theory. This theory's take is that concepts are represented in terms of both linguistic representations and sensorimotor simulations. Their joint operation contributes to the representation of concepts, with the former, linguistic system, assumed to induce superficial processing, and the latter, deeper conceptual processing via the simulation system.

It is the representation of abstract concepts such as truth, democracy, and morality that arguably present interesting challenges to embodied approaches. We now turn to abstract concepts and their grounding.

GROUNDING ABSTRACT CONCEPTS

Abstract concepts pose a major hurdle for simulation or action theories, or neuropsychological ones. These accounts of how concepts are grounded rely on some form of stored perceptual state as argued by, for instance, perceptual symbol systems, according to which human conceptual knowledge is built from stored perceptual states (Barsalou, 1999a). However, abstract concepts do not have a shared appearance like concrete concepts ("apples" do but "law" does not). Andy Clark (1999) drew attention to the difficulty of accounting for the complexity of, for example, moral and abstract reasoning by means of sensorimotor simulation: "It does seem that the more decoupled and abstract the target contents become, either the less applicable the sensory–motor simulation strategy is, or the less clearly it can then be differentiated from the more traditional approaches it seeks to displace" (p. 348). So, we are left with the puzzle of how we represent and reason about abstract domains, such as love, justice, time, morality. Yet precisely these domains are the hallmark of what it means to be human.

A general strategy for grounding abstract concepts was advanced in cognitive linguistics, which arose in reaction to the amodal linguistic theories (e.g., theories of syntax; Chomsky 1957). Prominent among these is Lakoff and Johnson's (1980, 1999) proposal that abstract concepts are grounded metaphorically in embodied and situated knowledge (also see Gibbs, 1994). In the following, we review the work that has been inspired by *conceptual metaphor theory* (CMT, Lakoff & Johnson, 1980, 1999). In the concluding portion of this section we draw attention to a number of problematic issues with this perspective (e.g., Murphy, 1997).

Conceptual Metaphor Theory

Metaphors facilitate our understanding of concepts that we cannot touch, smell, or see by associating them with concepts based on primary sensorimotor experiences, such as space, gravity, and so forth (e.g., Lakoff & Johnson, 1980). Metaphors, in this view, constitute mental associations between basic *source concepts* derived from interactions with the physical and social world and *target concepts* that represent abstract referents. Abstract domains are thus understood through analogical extensions from more experience-based domains. For instance, the abstract concept of *argument* is linked to *war* (Lakoff & Johnson, 1980), as can be seen in the metaphors we use:

> He attacked every weak point in my argument.
>
> His criticisms were right on target.
>
> If you use this strategy, he'll wipe you out.

Notably, more than one concrete domain can be used to define an abstract concept—for example, *life is a journey* but also *life is a gambling game*, and so forth. Although a chief function of metaphors is to facilitate understanding and reasoning with abstract concepts, they also structure a domain. For instance, space acts as a source domain to conceptualize the abstract domain of time. As a result, by means of a metaphor, time becomes not only spatially ordered but it also acquires other features of space, namely, stability and measurability. CMT has led to a wealth of demonstration experiments in cognitive psychology, as well as social psychology (see Landau, Meier, & Keefer, 2010, for a review). We next provide an overview of the research inspired by CMT.

Affect, Spatial Position, and Motor Actions

Empirical evidence investigating the relation between affect and verticality (cf. Crawford, 2009) supports the argument that metaphors referring to the vertical spatial orientation such as "I'm feeling up" or "I'm feeling down" structure the way people think and represent affect-related concepts. For example, Meier and Robinson (2004) have shown (Experiment 1) that positive words (e.g., *ethical, friendly*) were classified more rapidly as positive when they were presented on the upper half rather than the lower half of a monitor, while the opposite was true for negative words. However, the activation of spatial areas (Experiment 3) does not prime evaluations (e.g., "up" does not activate "good"), suggesting the asymmetrical nature of this relationship.

This idea of grounding affect in vertical space was subsequently extended to spatial memory. For instance, Crawford et al. (2006), observed that the association between valence and verticality influences memory for the locations of emotionally evocative stimuli. By presenting positive and negative images in various locations, the authors observed that memories of location were influenced by stimulus valence. Positive items were biased upward relative to negative items. In a third experiment, yearbook photos were paired with positive or negative behavioral descriptions, and participants were asked to rate how they felt about the person they had just seen and to move the picture back to its remembered location. On average, pictures that were rated as more positive were shifted upward, and pictures that were rated as more negative were shifted downward.

Casasanto and Dijkstra (2010) reported two experiments demonstrating bidirectional influences between motor actions and the retrieval of autobiographical memories with emotional content. In the first experiment, participants were asked to retell either positively or negatively valenced memories while moving marbles either upward or downward. Results indicate that they retrieved memories faster and moved marbles at a higher rate when the direction of movement was congruent with the valence of the memory (i.e., upward for positive memories, downward for negative memories). In a second experiment, the authors also demonstrated that the repetitive motor actions also partly determined the emotional content of the retrieved memories. After being provided with neutral-valence prompts (e.g., "Tell me about an event that happened yesterday"), participants retrieved more positive memories when instructed to move marbles upward, and more negative memories when instructed to move them downward.

In two experiments, Palma, Garrido, and Semin (2011) further documented the role of spatial position and valence in the processes involved in person memory. They examined the general hypothesis that a vertical spatial dimension anchors memory for affectively charged social information about persons. The obtained results indicated that participants' recall of positive and negative target person's behaviors is enhanced when they are presented in or moved to compatible vertical spatial locations (up and down, respectively). Similar lines of research have explored the link between affect and other concrete domains, such as size and brightness. As the results of Meier, Robinson, and Caven (2008) indicate, participants were faster and more accurate in evaluating positive words presented in a large font than in a small font, whereas the reverse pattern was true for negative words. The metaphorical use of *bright* (e.g., "bright ideas") or *dark* ("dark days") to refer to positive or negative aspects, finds support in the observation that participants' responses were facilitated when the word meaning (e.g., *gentle*) and the font color (white) were congruent with the metaphor (Meier, Robinson, & Clore, 2004). Related research further supports this metaphor by indicating that squares are seen as lighter after the evaluation of positive rather than negative words (Meier, Robinson, Crawford, & Ahlvers, 2007). Recent work by Lakens, Semin, and Foroni (2012) supports and further specifies the significance of the metaphorical association between black and white and negativity and positivity, respectively. Across six experiments, the authors show that if white ideographs are not presented in relation to black ones, then the anchoring of light and dark or white and black with good and bad, respectively, is not manifested. Thus, this association relies on the activation of the interdependence by means of the metaphorical relationship. However, when the metaphorical relationship is not activated, the association between valence and brightness is absent.

Meier, Hauser, Robinson, Friesen, and Schjeldahl (2007) have shown that divine figures (i.e., God and the Devil) are anchored on a vertical dimension. Thus, when words related to God (e.g., *the Almighty*) and words related to "up" (e.g., *ascendant*) were classified together, participants were significantly faster (the same for words related to the Devil when presented with down-related concepts) than when words related to God had to be classified together with concepts related to "down" (Experiment 1). Participants were also faster to categorize God-related words when presented at the top (vs. bottom) of the screen, whereas the reverse was observed for Devil-related words (Experiment 2). Participants' memory for the vertical location of God- and Devil-like images also showed a metaphor-consistent bias (up for God; down for Devil). The authors showed that this metaphorical relation also influenced memory and social judgments. Namely, participants remembered photographs related to God as appearing more on the top of the monitor (vs. Devil-related photographs as appearing more on the bottom) when compared to neutral words (Experiment 3). Finally, participants rated strangers as more likely to believe in God when their images appeared in a high versus low vertical position.

Interpersonal Relationships and Ambient Temperature

Recent research has also documented the way affect is grounded by *physical features of the environment,* such as temperature, interpersonal distance, or scents in social judgment domains. The first empirical demonstration of such effects was provided by Williams and Bargh (2008a), who asked participants to hold a warm or a cold cup of coffee before receiving information about a hypothetical person described as *intelligent, skillful, industrious, determined, practical,* and *cautious.* When subsequently asked to provide their personality impression of this hypothetical person on several bipolar traits, participants who had held a warm cup of coffee rated the target as warmer than did participants who had held a cold cup of coffee. IJzerman and Semin (2009) have reported similar effects. Participants in a warmer room (relative to a colder room) reported higher social proximity to a target person.

Metaphors such as "icy stare" and "cold reception" as indicators of social exclusion have also been investigated (Zhong & Leonardelli, 2008). In two experiments, the authors observed that recalling a social exclusion experience led participants to estimate room temperature as lower than did recalling an inclusion experience. Furthermore, the induction of social exclusion through an online virtual interaction led participants to report greater desirability for warm foods and drinks. The finding that the recollection of social exclusion induces perceptions of lower temperature seems to question the unidirectionality from source (temperature) to target (sociability) postulated by the CMT (Lakoff & Johnson, 1999).

Williams and Bargh (2008b) showed that participants primed with spatially proximal coordinates reported stronger bonds to their family members and their hometown than those primed with distant coordinates. More recently, IJzerman and Semin (2010) have shown that inducing experiences of physical and verbal proximity gives rise to perceptions of higher temperature. Note that these results provide support for Zhong and Leonardelli's (2008) finding that feelings of social distance induce feelings of coldness and extend their research by finding that social proximity leads to perceptions of warmth.

Environmental odors also affect cognition and behavior across a variety of contexts. Scents were shown not only to enhance the mental accessibility of the behavioral concepts, such as cleaning, but also to influence affective judgments and morality related cognition and behavior, based on metaphorical associations. For instance, Holland, Hendriks, and Aarts (2005) demonstrated that participants in a cleaning scent condition were faster in identifying cleaning-related words, listed more cleaning activities, and kept their working table cleaner than did participants in the control condition without any scent. Other research has shown that human odors affect social interaction, including helping behavior (e.g., Baron, 1997) and attraction to others (cf. Demattè, Osterbauer, & Spence, 2007; Li, Moallem, Paller, & Gottfried, 2007). In a recent chapter, Semin and Garrido (2012) reported that environmental contexts characterized by warm temperature, close distance, and pleasant smells promote generalized positive sociability evaluations. In the presence of these environmental conditions, not only a social target but also uninvolved others, such as the experimenter, were rated as warmer, closer, and more friendly, in contrast to the ratings observed in the cold, distant, and unpleasant smell conditions.

Smelly Studies on Morality, Suspicion, and Cleansing Immorality

When we are suspicious, then, we often use the expression "Something smells fishy." Lee and Schwarz (2012) examined this metaphor and observed that the incidental exposure to fishy smells induced suspicion and undermined cooperation in a trust (Experiment 1) and a public goods game (Experiment 2). Socially induced suspicion enhanced the correct labeling of fishy smells but not other smells (Experiments 3a–3c), and heightened the sensitivity to detect even very low concentrations of fishy smells (Experiment 7).

Expressions such as a "clean conscience" or a "disgusting act" suggest a metaphorical association between *morality* and activities related to physical cleanliness (Lee & Schwarz, 2011). The first empirical evidence supporting this metaphorical association was provided by Zhong and Liljenquist (2006). Participants who recalled unethical (vs. ethical) behaviors from the past were more likely to generate more cleansing-related words, such as soap or shower, than participants who recalled ethical behaviors. Furthermore, participants who copied an unethical story rated the cleansing products more highly as compared to those who copied the ethical story. A final experiment showed that this linguistic association has behavioral consequences. Namely, after recalling an unethical behavior, 67% of the participants preferred receiving an antiseptic wipe rather than a pencil as a free gift.

The relationship between morality and physical cleanliness was further demonstrated by Lee and Schwarz (2010), who showed that people are more likely to purify specific body parts that are involved in the production of the moral transgression. Participants induced to perform an immoral action (lying) using their hands (by using e-mail) preferred a hand-washing product, whereas those lying via voice mail preferred a mouthwash.

Schnall, Benton, and Harvey (2008) found that activating the cognitive concept of cleanliness (e.g., *pure, washed, clean, immaculate*) influenced moral judgments, such that they became less severe, showing the bidirectional nature of the metaphor that links cleanliness and morality. Furthermore, after experiencing a disgusting film clip, participants who engaged in cleaning behavior (e.g., washing one's hands) made less severe judgments of moral dilemmas than those who did not wash their hands after the disgusting film clip.

Power

Metaphorical references to someone with *high* status or on *top* of the hierarchy associate power with space. As Schubert (2005) suggests, when we think about power differences, we think about differences on the vertical dimension. Schubert's results indicate that instances of powerful groups (e.g., master) are classified faster when they appear above the powerless groups (e.g., servant) on a monitor. The reverse is reported for powerless groups, who were judged more quickly when they were presented below powerful groups. Additionally, participants were faster and more accurate when identifying powerful and powerless groups while making judgments using an upward or a downward movement, respectively. Moreover, Schubert verified that these effects were independent of the valence of powerful and powerless groups. Physical size was investigated as another dimension underlying the metaphorical representation of power. Schubert, Walduzs, and Giessner (2009) observed that it took less time to judge a powerful group as powerful when it was written in a larger font (vs. smaller font). The reverse was true for judgments of powerless groups.

Research by Lakens, Semin, and Foroni (2011), however, suggests that power is not simply structured in space in absolute terms, but that *relational differences* in power moderate the vertical representation of the powerful *above* the powerless. In a set of experiments the authors used either both powerful and powerless stimuli in the experimental task (i.e., manipulating power *within* participants), or only powerful or only powerless stimuli (i.e., manipulating power *between* participants). While in the former case the relative differences in power were salient and strengthened the vertical spatial structuring of power differences, in the latter, relative differences in power were absent, and the tendency to structure power differences in vertical space was no longer observed.

Weight and Importance

Another instance of metaphorical representation that has been investigated is *importance* as *weight*. Jostmann, Lakens, and Schubert (2009) have shown that holding a heavy versus a light clipboard increased judgments of the value of foreign currencies, as well as the perceived importance of fair decision-making procedures. Similar results were subsequently reported by Ackerman, Nocera, and Bargh (2010), who observed that participants provided with a job application on a heavy clipboard rated the job candidate as better and as displaying a more serious interest in the position than those holding a lighter clipboard. Furthermore, participants using the heavy clipboard rated their own accuracy on the task as more important than did participants using the light clipboard. Male participants holding a heavy clipboard also allocated more money to social issues.

Time

The metaphorical representation of time is one of the better-studied research domains, showing the intimate connection of the cognitive representation of time with the representation of space (e.g., a *short* break, a *long* vacation). Our culture is abundant with spatial representations of time, as in the case of clocks, sundials, and hourglasses, just to name a few. Our language is also full of examples that depict time, its order, and duration with spatial references (Clark, 1973; Lakoff & Johnson, 1980). Based on expressions such as "the past is behind" and "the future is ahead," Boroditsky (2000) explored whether spatial priming consistent with either an ego-moving (the agent is moving in time), or a time-moving schema would affect how people interpret ambiguous temporal statements. For example, in English the statement *The meeting that was scheduled for next Wednesday was moved forward 2 days* can be disambiguated differently if we take the perspective of the agent moving in time (space) or if we assume time itself as moving. Over 70% of the participants in the study responded in a prime-consistent manner.

Interestingly, spatial metaphors of time are culturally determined. In Western cultures, people think of the past as being to the left, and the future as being to the right. Indeed, when talking about time, we make spatial gestures to the left in the case of references to the past and to the right when referring to the future (e.g., Casasanto & Lozano, 2006; Núñez & Sweetser, 2006). Recently, Blom and Semin (2013) showed that hand–arm movements (HAMs) in relation to the architecture of the body (left or right axis) influence temporal judgments. Left HAMs to the left of the body led participants to perceive an event retrieved memory as more distant, and right HAMs to the right of the body led them to perceive the event as closer in time.

Other studies have shown that when participants are asked to push a key on one side or the other in response to time-related stimuli (e.g., past, future), they are faster when past-related stimuli appear on the left and future-related stimuli appear on the right (e.g., Ishihara, Keller, Rossetti, & Prinz, 2008; Vallesi, McIntosh, & Stuss, 2011; Wegner & Pratt, 2008). These compatibility effects between time-related stimuli and the spatial position (left or right) of response keys are also shown when participants categorize the temporal meaning of past and future words upon auditory presentation to the left or right ear (Ouellet, Santiago, Funes, & Lupiáñez, 2010; Ouellet, Santiago, Israeli, & Gabay, 2010; Santiago, Lupiáñez, Pérez, & Funes, 2007). Recently, Lakens, Semin, and Garrido (2011) demonstrated the visuospatial anchoring of time, showing that words related to the past (e.g., yesterday) were placed significantly to the left of midpoint and words related to the future (e.g., tomorrow) to the right of midpoint on a horizontal line. Furthermore, when past and future referent words were presented with equal loudness to both ears, participants disambiguated future words to the right ear and the past words to the left ear (see Farias, Garrido, & Semin, 2013, for a similar demonstration of the relation between political concepts and the horizontal space).

The left–past and the right–future spatial pattern, however, is not a universal one; rather, it is culture-specific, and in all likelihood shaped by writing direction (e.g., Nachshon, 1985). Research to date has shown time to be represented also front to back or back to front, right to left (e.g., Boroditsky, 2000). For example, Fuhrman and Boroditsky (2010) found that whereas English speakers tend to arrange temporal sequences from left to right, the opposite is true for Hebrew speakers. Boroditsky and Gaby (2010) also report that people of Pormpuraaw (an Australian Aboriginal community) arranged time according to *cardinal directions*. This and other research showing the cultural variations in the spatial anchoring of time reveals both the generality and relativity of how the abstract concept of time is understood. While the spatial anchoring of time seems to be a general phenomenon, the spatial referents that ground time vary considerably across cultures.

Concluding Notes to Abstract Concepts and the Evidence

The questions we posed earlier with respect to the grounding of concrete concepts reemerge even more strongly in the case of abstract concepts. Do these studies and their theoretical basis provide any evidence for abstract concepts being grounded in the sensorimotor system? Does the CMT-based research on which we have reported here constitute a theory that clearly identifies a sensorimotor basis for abstract concepts such as love, affect, trust?

CMT has inspired a substantial amount of psychological research, particularly in cognitive and social psychology. Yet one of the main criticisms leveled at CMT is that it lacks, as Murphy (1996, 1997) pointed out, a process model of how representations would be used in understanding and thought. Indeed, it is possible to marshal the same concern about most of the research we reviewed earlier. That is, the research is predominantly about representation with no process assumptions. Elucidating the processes involved in how metaphors shape inferences and judgment presents an important challenge. Moreover, metaphorical expressions for diverse domains arise from the similarities between "preexisting conceptual structures"; thus, there is a structural similarity between the concept of "journey" and the concept of "love," and the respective components of each concept can be projected in a systematic manner. This means, according to Murphy, that metaphorical expression about certain domains does not necessarily reflect the influence of the metaphor on the representation. The argument here is that the metaphor does not establish the relationship between source and target but that all concepts (source and target) are directly represented to start off with. A key issue is whether these metaphors simply reflect linguistic convention or they actually represent how people think (e.g., Murphy, 1997).

However, an alternative view to be found in a classical representational perspective (e.g., Landauer & Dumais, 1997) suggests that the meanings of new words are anchored in the meanings of other words, associated with the new words, or that co-occur with the new words. Accordingly, meaning is the result of associations between linguistic units that can be revealed by statistical computations of large bodies of text. These computational models of word co-occurrences have been successful in predicting human performance (Burgess

& Lund, 2000). Indeed, these models and the computational data they have advanced can be taken as evidence for a purely symbolic, system-based representation of meaning (cf. Louwerse & Jeuniaux, 2008). Similar objects occupy similar contexts. For instance, knives, forks, and cutlery are generally to be found together in the kitchen, as are pans and pots. The co-occurrence of these words in their context will be a possible way to map their meanings in context. Indeed, Louwerse and Zwaan (2009) showed that the spatial distance between pairs of U.S. cities can be derived from their distributions across texts.

This computational approach could also be adopted to examine the degree to which results from research that has examined different metaphors about space, size, or brightness, and both the classification and judgment of, for example, valence- and power-related stimuli are linguistically reproducible. Thus, the metaphorical association between a concrete and an abstract domain may reflect a naturally occurring correlation between a concrete and a more abstract characteristic. This could likely be the case for size and power (Schubert et al., 2009). Size is a cue to power in the animal world, and to physical power in humans. The same rationale may apply to upper vertical positions, as height is correlated with size and lying down is an act of submission in many animal species. These co-occurrences are likely to be reflected in language, but are they in any way grounded in sensory systems or have the regularities been abstractions from our linguistic ecology?

The recurrent question of whether abstract concepts are grounded in the sensorimotor system or are represented in amodal symbolic system remains open, and the evidence is still ambiguous. Thus, our field is in need of a general theory for the processes that ground abstract *and* concrete concepts.

CONCLUDING COMMENTS

It is undoubtedly the case that symbolic representation distances itself from sensorimotor experience. This is highlighted in a classic study by Boysen, Berntson, Hannan, and Cacioppo (1996), who conducted a reverse contingency study with five chimpanzees that had training in counting and numerical skills. The chimpanzees were presented with two arrays of different amounts of candy or two Arabic numerals. One array always contained more than the other. The chimpanzees always selected the array with the higher number of candies. The critical condition in this experiment was the application of a reversed reinforcement contingency. In this condition, the selected array of candy was removed and the subject received the nonselected candies (or the number of candies represented by the nonselected Arabic numeral). The chimpanzees were unable to maximize their reward by selecting the smaller array when candies were used as array elements. They simply could not learn the reverse contingency rule. However, when Arabic numerals were substituted for the candy arrays, all animals showed an immediate shift to a more optimal response strategy. They selected the lower Arabic numeral and received the larger reward. Once symbols (Arabic numerals) were substituted for the appetitive stimulus, the chimpanzees were able to learn an "abstract" rule.

> The ability of symbols to encompass selective features or attributes of their real-world referents may constitute an important advantage of symbolic representations. Symbols may permit an organism to efficiently process selected information and adaptively respond on the basis of that knowledge structure while minimizing potential interference from lower level evaluative mechanisms. (Boysen et al., 1996, p. 85)

This is indeed one of the main functions of representing a sensorimotor experience symbolically: distancing oneself from the immediacy of the experience. Language endows us with ability to travel in time, to construct alternative realities, to represent a multitude of possible and impossible states, but these creative "experiments" are only possible to the extent that we can distance ourselves from the immediacy of our here and now. However, these apparent "flights of fantasy" have at least two experiential or sensorimotor anchors. The first—as in the case of the chimpanzees noted earlier—is that the abstract symbol does not detract from the appetitive referent that motivates the continuation of making choices again and again over hundreds of trials (cf. Boysen et al., 1996). The second is that the symbolically driven actions are sensorimotor executions that yield candies, with larger amounts obtained and consumed!

The current controversy, often cast in terms of concrete versus abstract concepts and their grounding, is about the relative operation of two interlocking processes as far as concepts and cognitive processes are concerned. Concepts, namely, linguistic expressions, are undoubtedly symbolic, but they maintain different degrees of proximity to sensorimotor processes. In other words, they are both modal and amodal. The important question is whether to develop and advance a model that highlights the relative role played by modal and amodal processes in different situated performances. In essence, the resolution of the embodiment dilemma is not a competition between modal and amodal models, but in advancing an explication of when and how much each process is operative in human cognitive processes.

REFERENCES

Ackerman, J. M., Nocera, C. C., & Bargh, J. A. (2010). Incidental haptic sensations influence social judgments and decisions. *Science, 328*, 1712–1715.

Aziz-Zadeh, L., Wilson, S., Rizzolatti, G., & Iacoboni, M. (2006). A comparison of premotor areas activated by action observation and action phrases. *Current Biology, 16*, 1818–1823.

Baron, R. A. (1997). The sweet smell of helping: Effects of pleasant ambient fragrance on prosocial behavior in shopping malls. *Journal of Personality and Social Psychology*, *23*, 498–503.

Barsalou, L. W. (1999a). Perceptual symbol systems. *Behavioral and Brain Sciences, 22*, 577–660.

Barsalou, L. W. (1999b). Language comprehension: Archival memory or preparation for situated action? *Discourse Processes, 28*, 61–80.

Barsalou, L. W. (2008). Grounded cognition. *Annual Review of Psychology*, *59*, 617–645.

Barsalou, L. W., Santos, A., Simmons, W. K., & Wilson, C. D. (2008). Language and simulation in conceptual processing. In M. de Vega, A. M. Glenberg, & A. C. Graesser (Eds.), *Symbols, embodiment, and meaning* (pp. 245–283). Oxford, UK: Oxford University Press.

Blom, S., & Semin, G. R. (2013). Moving events in time: Time referent hand–arm movements influence perceived temporal distance to past events. *Journal of Experimental Psychology: General, 142*(2), 319–322.

Borghi, A. M. (2005). Object concepts and action. In D. Pecher & R. A. Zwaan (Eds.), *Grounding cognition: The role of perception and action in memory, language, and thinking* (pp. 8–34). Cambridge, UK: Cambridge University Press.

Borghi, A. M., Glenberg, A. M., & Kaschak, M. P. (2004). Putting words in perspective. *Memory and Cognition*, *32*, 863–873.

Boroditsky, L. (2000). Metaphoric structuring: Understanding time through spatial metaphors. *Cognition*, *75*, 1–18.

Boroditsky, L., & Gaby, A. (2010). Remembrances of times East: Absolute spatial representations of time in an Australian Aboriginal community. *Psychological Science, 21*, 1635–1639.

Boulenger, V., Roy, A. C., Paulignan, Y., Deprez, V., Jeannerod, M., & Nazir, T. A. (2006). Cross-talk between language processes and overt motor behavior in the first 200 ms of processing. *Journal of Cognitive Neuroscience, 18*, 1607–1615.

Boysen, S. T., Berntson, G. G., Hannan, M. B., & Cacioppo, J. T. (1996). Quantity-based interference and symbolic representations in chimpanzees (*Pan troglodytes*). *Journal of Experimental Psychology: Animal Behavior Processes*, *22*, 76–86.

Bub, D. N., & Masson, M. E. J. (2010). On the nature of hand–action representations evoked during written sentence comprehension. *Cognition, 116*, 394–408.

Buccino, G., Riggio, L., Melli, G., Binkofski, F., Gallese, V., & Rizzolatti, G. (2005). Listening to actionrelated sentences modulates the activity of the motor system: A combined TMS and behavioral study. *Brain Research: Cognitive Brain Research*, *24*, 355–363.

Burgess, C., & Lund, K. (2000). The dynamics of meaning in memory. In E. Dietrich & A. B. Markman (Eds.), *Cognitive dynamics: Conceptual and representational change in humans and machines* (pp. 117–156). Mahwah, NJ: Erlbaum.

Casasanto, D., & Dijkstra, K. (2010). Motor action and emotional memory. *Cognition*, *115*, 179–185.

Casasanto, D., & Lozano, S. (2006). Metaphor in the mind and hands. In *Proceedings of the 28th Annual Meeting of the Cognitive Science Society* (pp. 142–147). Vancouver: Cognitive Science Society.

Chomsky, N. (1957). *Syntactic structures.* Paris: Mouton.

Clark, A. (1999). An embodied cognitive science? *Trends in Cognitive Sciences, 3,* 345–351.

Clark, H. H. (1973). Space, time, semantics, and the child. In T. E. Moore (Ed.), *Cognitive development and the acquisition of language* (pp. 28–64). New York: Academic Press.

Collins, J., Pecher, D., Zeelenberg, R., & Coulson, S. (2011). Modality switching in a property verification task: An ERP study of what happens when candles flicker after high heels click. *Frontiers in Psychology, 2,* 10.

Connell, L. (2007) Representing object colour in language comprehension. *Cognition, 102,* 476–485.

Crawford, L. E. (2009). Conceptual metaphors of affect. *Emotion Review, 1,* 129–139.

Crawford, L. E., Margolies, S. M., Drake, J. T., & Murphy, M. E. (2006). Affect biases memory of location: Evidence for the spatial representation of affect. *Cognition and Emotion, 20,* 1153–1169.

Damasio, A. (1989). The brain binds entities and events by multiregional activation from convergence zones. *Neural Computation, 1,* 123–132.

Damasio, A. (2010). *The self comes to mind: Constructing the conscious brain.* New York: Random House/Pantheon.

Decety, J., & Grèzes, J. (2006). The power of simulation: Imagining ones own and others behaviour [Special issue]. *Brain Research, 1079,* 4–14.

Demattè, M. L., Osterbauer, R., & Spence, C. (2007). Olfactory cues modulate facial attractiveness. *Chemical Senses, 32,* 603–610.

Dennett, D. (1969). *Content and consciousness.* London, UK: Routledge.

Dove, G. (2009). *Beyond perceptual symbols: A call for representational pluralism. Cognition, 110,* 412–431.

Dove, G. (2011). On the need for embodied and dis-embodied cognition. *Frontiers in Psychology, 1*(242), 1–13.

Farias, A. R., Garrido, M. V., & Semin, G. R. (2013). Converging modalities ground abstract categories: The case of politics. *PLoS ONE, 8*(4), e6097.

Fodor, J. (1975). *The language of thought.* New York: Crowell.

Fuhrman, O., & Boroditsky, L. (2010). Cross-cultural differences in mental representations of time: Evidence from an implicit non-linguistic task. *Cognitive Science, 34,* 1430–1451.

Gibbs, R. W. (1994). *The poetics of mind: Figurative thought, language, and understanding.* New York: Cambridge University Press.

Girardi, G., Lindemann, O., & Bekkering, H. (2010). Context effects on the processing of action-relevant object features. *Journal of Experimental Psychology: Human Perception and Performance, 36,* 330–340.

Glenberg, A. M. (1997). What memory is for. *Behavioral and Brain Sciences, 20,* 1–55.

Glenberg, A. M. (2008). Toward the integration of bodily states, language, and action. In G. R. Semin & E. R. Smith (Eds.), *Embodied grounding: Social, cognitive, affective, and neuroscientific approaches* (pp. 43–70). New York: Cambridge University Press.

Glenberg, A. M., & Kaschak, M. P. (2002). Grounding language in action. *Psychonomic Bulletin and Review, 9,* 558–565.

Glenberg, A. M., Sato, M., Cattaneo, L., Riggio, L., Palumbo, D., & Buccino, G. (2008). Processing abstract language modulates motor system activity. *Quarterly Journal of Experimental Psychology, 61,* 905–919.

Goldberg, R. F., Perfetti, C. A., & Schneider, W. (2006). Perceptual knowledge retrieval activates sensory brain regions. *Journal of Neuroscience, 26,* 4917–4921.

Goldman, A. I. (2006). *Simulating minds: The philosophy, psychology and neuroscience of mind reading.* New York: Oxford University Press.

Harnad, S. (1990). The symbol grounding problem. *Physica D: Nonlinear Phenomena, 42,* 335–346.

Hauk, O., Johnsrude, I., & Pulvermüller, F. (2004). Somatotopic representation of action words in human motor and premotor cortex. *Neuron, 41,* 301–307.

Hauk, O., & Pulvermüller, F. (2004). Neurophysiological distinction of action words in the fronto-central cortex. *Human Brain Mapping, 21,* 191–201.

Hauk, O., Shtyrov, Y., & Pulvermüller, F. (2006). The sound of actions as reflected by mismatch negativity: Rapid activation of cortical sensory–motor networks by sounds associated with finger and tongue movements. *European Journal of Neuroscience, 23,* 811–821.

Holland, R. W., Hendriks, M., & Aarts, H.

(2005). Smells like clean spirit: Nonconscious effects of scent on cognition and behavior. *Psychological Science, 16*, 689–693.

IJzerman, H., & Semin, G. R. (2009). The thermometer of social relations: Mapping social proximity on temperature. *Psychological Science, 10*, 1214–1220.

IJzerman, H., & Semin, G. R. (2010). Temperature perceptions as a ground for social proximity. *Journal of Experimental Social Psychology, 46*, 867–873.

Ishihara, M., Keller, P. E., Rossetti, Y., & Prinz, W. (2008). Horizontal spatial representations of time: Evidence for the STEARC effect. *Cortex, 44*, 454–461.

James, W. (1950). *The principles of psychology*. New York: Dover. (Original work published 1890)

Jostmann, N. B., Lakens, D., & Schubert, T. W. (2009). Weight as an embodiment of importance. *Psychological Science, 20*, 1169–1174.

Kan, I. P., Barsalou, L. W., Solomon, K. O., Minor, J. K., & Thompson-Schill, S. L. (2003). Role of mental imagery in a property verification task: fMRI evidence for perceptual representations of conceptual knowledge. *Cognitive Neuropsychology, 20*, 525–540.

Kaschak, M. P., & Glenberg, A. M. (2004). This construction needs learned. *Journal of Experimental Psychology: General, 133*, 450–467.

Klatzky, R. L., Pellegrino, J. W., McCloskey, B. P., & Doherty, S. (1989). Can you squeeze a tomato?: The role of motor representations in semantic sensibility judgments. *Journal of Memory and Language, 28*, 56–77.

Lakens, D., Semin, G. R., & Foroni, F. (2011). Why your highness needs the people: Comparing the absolute and relative representation of power in vertical space. *Social Psychology, 43*, 205–215.

Lakens, L., Semin, G. R., & Foroni, F. (2012). But for the bad, there would not be good. Conceptual opposition vs. mere association: Metaphoric grounding of valence. *Journal of Experimental Psychology: General, 141*(3), 584–594.

Lakens, L., Semin, G. R., & Garrido, M. V. (2011). The sound of time: Cross-modal convergence in the spatial structuring of time. *Consciousness and Cognition, 20*, 437–443.

Lakoff, G., & Johnson, M. (1980). *Metaphors we live by*. Chicago: University of Chicago Press.

Lakoff, G., & Johnson, M. (1999). *Philosophy in the flesh*. New York: Basic Books.

Landau, M. J., Meier, B. P., & Keefer, L. (2010). A metaphor-enriched social cognition. *Psychological Bulletin, 136*, 1045–1067.

Landauer, T. K., & Dumais, S. T. (1997). A solution to Plato's problem: The latent semantic analysis theory of acquisition, induction, and representation of knowledge. *Psychological Review, 104*, 211–240.

Lee, S. W. S., & Schwarz, N. (2010). Dirty hands and dirty mouths: Embodiment of the moral-purity metaphor is specific to the motor modality involved in moral transgression. *Psychological Science, 21*, 1423–1425.

Lee, S. W. S., & Schwarz, N. (2011). Wiping the slate clean: Psychological consequences of physical cleansing. *Current Directions in Psychological Science, 20*, 307–311.

Lee, S. W. S., & Schwarz, N. (2012). Bidirectionality, mediation, and moderation of metaphorical effects: The embodiment of social suspicion and fishy smells. *Journal of Personality and Social Psychology, 103*, 737–749.

Li, W., Moallem, I., Paller, K. A., & Gottfried, J. A. (2007). Subliminal smells can guide social preferences. *Psychological Science, 18*, 1044–1049.

Louwerse, M. M., & Jeuniaux, P. (2008). Language comprehension is both embodied and symbolic. In M. De Vega, A. M. Glenberg, & A. C. Graesser (Eds.), *Embodiment and meaning: A debate* (pp. 309–326). Oxford, UK: Oxford University Press.

Louwerse, M. M., & Zwaan, R. A. (2009). Language encodes geographical information. *Cognitive Science, 33*, 51–73.

Machery, E. (2007). Concept empiricism: a meth odological critique. *Cognition, 104*, 19–46.

Machery, E. (2010). Précis of d*oing without concepts*. *Mind and Language, 25*, 602–611.

Mahon, B. Z., & Caramazza, A. (2008). A critical look at the embodied cognition hypothesis and a new proposal for groundal conceptual content. *Journal of Physiology, 102*, 59–70.

Marques, J. F. (2006). Specialization and semantic organization: Evidence for multiple semantics linked to sensory modalities. *Memory and Cognition, 34*, 60–67.

Martin, A. (2007). The representation of object concepts in the brain. *Annual Review of Psychology, 58*, 25–45.

Masson, M. E. J., Bub, D. N., & Warren, C. M. (2008). Kicking calculators: Contribution of embodied representations to sentence comprehension. *Journal of Memory and Language, 59*, 256–265.

Meier, B. P., Hauser, D. J., Robinson, M. D., Friesen, C. K., & Schjeldahl, K. (2007). What's "up" with God? Vertical space as a representation of the divine. *Journal of Personality and Social Psychology, 93*, 699–710.

Meier, B. P., & Robinson, M. D. (2004). Why the sunny side is up: Associations between affect and vertical position. *Psychological Science, 15*, 243–247.

Meier, B. P., & Robinson, M. D. (2006). Does "feeling down" mean seeing down?: Depressive symptoms and vertical selective attention. *Journal of Research in Personality, 40*, 451–461.

Meier, B. P., Robinson, M. D., & Caven, A. J. (2008). Why a Big Mac is a good mac: Associations between affect and size. *Basic and Applied Social Psychology, 30*, 46–55.

Meier, B. P., Robinson, M. D., & Clore, G. L. (2004). Why good guys wear white: Automatic inferences about stimulus valence based on color. *Psychological Science, 15*, 82–87.

Meier, B. P., Robinson, M. D., Crawford, L. E., & Ahlvers, W. J. (2007). When "light" and "dark" thoughts become light and dark responses: Affect biased brightness judgments. *Emotion, 7*, 366–376.

Murphy, G. L. (1996). On metaphoric representation. *Cognition, 60*, 173–204.

Murphy, G. L. (1997). Reasons to doubt the present evidence for metaphoric representation. *Cognition, 62*, 99–108.

Nachshon, I. (1985). Directional preferences in perception of visual stimuli. *International Journal of Neuroscience, 25*, 161–174.

Núñez, R. E., & Sweetser, E. (2006). With the future behind them: Convergent evidence from Aymara language and gesture in the crosslinguistic comparison of spatial construals of time. *Cognitive Science, 30*, 401–450.

Ouellet, M., Santiago, J., Funes, M. J., & Lupiáñez, J. (2010). Thinking about the future moves attention to the right. *Journal of Experimental Psychology: Human Perception and Performance, 36*, 17–24.

Ouellet, M., Santiago, J., Israeli, Z., & Gabay, S. (2010). Is the future the right time? *Experimental Psychology, 57*, 308–314.

Palma, T. A., Garrido, M. V., & Semin, G. R. (2011). Grounding person memory in space: Does spatial anchoring of behaviors improve recall? *European Journal of Social Psychology, 41*, 275–280.

Pecher, D., Van Dantzig, S., Zwaan, R. A., & Zeelenberg, R. (2009). Language comprehenders retain implied shape and orientation of objects. *Quarterly Journal of Experimental Psychology, 62*, 1108–1114.

Pecher, D., Zeelenberg, R., & Barsalou, L. W. (2003). Verifying different-modality properties for concepts produces switching costs. *Psychological Science, 14*, 119–124.

Pezzulo, G., Barca, L., Bocconi, A. L., & Borghi, A. M. (2010). When affordances climb into your mind: Advantages of motor simulation in a memory task performed by novice and expert rock climbers. *Brain and Cognition, 73*, 68–73.

Pulvermüller, F. (1999). Words in the brain's language. *Behavioral and Brain Sciences, 22*, 253–279.

Pulvermüller, F., Härle, M., & Hummel, F. (2000). Neurophysiological distinction of semantic verb categories. *NeuroReport, 11*, 2789–2793.

Pulvermüller, F., Shtyrov, Y., & Ilmoniemi, R. J. (2005). Brain signatures of meaning access in action word recognition. *Journal of Cognitive Neuroscience, 17*, 884–892.

Santiago, J., Lupiáñez, J., Pérez, E., & Funes, M. J. (2007). Time (also) flies from left to right. *Psychonomic Bulletin and Review, 14*, 512–516.

Schnall, S., Benton, J., & Harvey, S. (2008). With a clean conscience: Cleanliness reduces the severity of moral judgments. *Psychological Science, 19*, 1219–1222.

Schubert, T. W. (2005). Your highness: Vertical positions as perceptual symbols of power. *Journal of Personality and Social Psychology, 89*, 1–21.

Schubert, T. W., Waldzus, S., & Giessner, S. R. (2009). Control over the association of power and size. *Social Cognition, 27*, 1–19.

Searle, J. R. (1980). Minds, brains, and programs. *Behavioral and Brain Sciences, 3*, 417–457.

Semin, G. R., & Garrido, M. V. (2012). A systemic approach to impression formation: From verbal to multimodal processes. In J. Forgas, K. Fiedler, & C. Sedikides (Eds.), *Social thinking and interpersonal behavior* (pp. 81–100). New York: Psychology Press.

Semin, G. R., Garrido, M. V., & Palma, T. A. (2012). Socially situated cognition: Recasting social cognition as an emergent phenomenon. In S. Fiske & N. Macrae (Eds.), *Sage handbook of social cognition* (pp. 135–165). London: Sage.

Semin, G. R., Garrido, M. V., & Palma, T. A.

(2013). Interfacing body, mind, the physical, and social world: Socially situated cognition. In D. E. Carlston (Ed.), *The Oxford handbook of social cognition*. New York: Oxford University Press.

Semin, G. R., & Smith, E. (2013). Socially situated cognition in perspective. *Social Cognition, 31,* 125–146.

Shtyrov, Y., Hauk, O. & Pulvermüller, F. (2004). Distributed neuronal networks for encoding category-specific semantic information: the mismatch negativity to action words. *European Journal of Neuroscience, 19,* 1083–1092.

Simmons, W. K., Hamann, S. B., Harenski, C. N., Hu, X. P., & Barsalou, L. W. (2008). fMRI evidence for word association and situated simulation in conceptual processing. *Journal of Physiology, 102,* 106–119.

Smith, E. R., & Semin, G. R. (2004). Socially situated cognition: Cognition in its social context. *Advances in Experimental Social Psychology, 36,* 53–117.

Solomon, K. O., & Barsalou, L. W. (2004). Perceptual simulation in property verification. *Memory & Cognition, 32,* 244–259.

Stanfield, R. A., & Zwaan, R. A. (2001). The effect of implied orientation derived from verbal context on picture recognition. *Psychological Science, 12,* 153–156.

Taylor, L. J., & Zwaan, R. A. (2008). Motor resonance and linguistic focus. *Quarterly Journal of Experimental Psychology, 61,* 896–904.

Tettamanti, M., Alkadhi, H., Moro, A., Perani, D., Kollias, S., & Weniger, D. (2002). Neural correlates for the acquisition of natural language syntax. *NeuroImage, 17,* 700–709.

Tettamanti, M., Buccino, G., Saccuman, M. C., Gallese, V., Danna, M., Scifo, P., et al. (2005). Listening to action-related sentences activates fronto-parietal motor circuits. *Journal of Cognitive Neuroscience, 17*(2), 273–281.

Tversky, B., Morrison, J. B., Franklin, N., & Bryant, D. (1999). Three spaces of spatial cognition. *The Professional Geographer, 51,* 516–524.

Vallesi, A., McIntosh, A. R., & Stuss, D. T. (2011). Over-recruitment in the aging brain as a function of task demands: Evidence for a compensatory view. *Journal of Cognitive Neuroscience, 23,* 801–815.

Van Dantzig, S., Pecher, D., Zeelenberg, R., & Barsalou, L. W. (2008). Perceptual processing affects conceptual processing. *Cognitive Science, 32,* 579–590.

Vermeulen, N., Niedenthal, P. M., & Luminet, O. (2007). Switching between sensory and affective systems incurs processing costs. *Cognitive Science, 31,* 183–192.

Weger, U. W., & Pratt, J. (2008). Time flies like an arrow: Space–time compatibility effects suggest the use of a mental timeline. *Psychonomic Bulletin and Review, 15,* 426–430.

Williams, L. E., & Bargh, J. A. (2008a). Experiencing physical warmth promotes interpersonal warmth. *Science, 322,* 606–607.

Williams, L. E., & Bargh, J. A. (2008b). Keeping one's distance: The influence of spatial distance cues on affect and evaluation. *Psychological Science, 19,* 302–308.

Wilson, M. (2002). Six views of embodied cognition. *Psychonomic Bulletin and Review, 9,* 625–636.

Wu, L. L., & Barsalou, L. W. (2009). Perceptual simulation in conceptual combination: Evidence from property generation. *Acta Psychologica, 132,* 173–189.

Zhong, C. B., & Leonardelli, G. J. (2008). Cold and lonely: Does social exclusion literally feel cold? *Psychological Science, 19,* 838–842.

Zhong, C. B., & Liljenquist, K. (2006). Washing away your sins: Threatened morality and physical cleansing. *Science, 313,* 1451–1452.

Zwaan, R. A., Radvansky, G. A. (1998). Situation models in language and memory. *Psychological Bulletin, 123,* 162–185.

Zwaan, R. A., Stanfield, R. A., & Yaxley, R. H. (2002). Language comprehenders mentally represent the shapes of objects. *Psychological Science, 13,* 168–171.

Zwaan, R. A., & Taylor, L. J. (2006). Seeing, acting, understanding: Motor resonance in language comprehension. *Journal of Experimental Psychology: General, 135,* 1–11.

CHAPTER 37

Dual Experiences, Multiple Processes

Looking Beyond Dualities for Mechanisms of the Mind

David M. Amodio

When considering the vast array of psychological experiences and behaviors, William James noted that "their variety and complexity is such as to leave a chaotic impression on the observer" (1890, p. 1). Indeed. The human mind is so complex that, ironically, it eludes comprehension by our own human minds; to gain insight into the psyche, simplification is needed. It is interesting, then, that psychologists' attempts to explain the human mind and behavior are dominated by theories invoking only two processes. From Descartes' duality of the mind and body and Freud's id and superego (the duality behind the ego) to modern dual-process models of implicit versus explicit processes and automaticity versus control, dualities abound in psychological theory. Why is there such a strong tendency to explain the complexity of the mind in terms of dualities? And, to the extent that dual-process accounts are limited, are there alternative theoretical approaches that provide better explanations of social cognitive phenomena? The first question—on why psychologists are drawn to dualities—is a fundamental philosophical question of the mind, with an answer that is sure to be abstruse and elusive (Dennett, 1991; Levine, 1983). In this chapter, I address the second question of whether there are better alternatives.

At the outset of this chapter, it is useful to distinguish between two general types of dual-process models. One type tends to pertain to a specific question about psychological function; these are typically narrowly focused, well-specified, and, as such, not intended to explain other psychological functions. For example, consider dual-process theories of attribution, which explain the way we form trait inferences about a person from his or her behavior. Several influential theories were developed to distinguish between two components of attribution, such as internal versus external causes (Heider, 1958) or the dual stages of identifying a behavior and then interpreting its meaning (Trope, 1986). Hence, these are described as "dual-process" theories. To the extent that a psychological question pertains to two specific processes, then a dual-process model is entirely appropriate. Indeed, by the same token, several other theories of attribution have specified three processes (e.g., Gilbert, Pelham, & Krull, 1988; Kelley, 1967; Quattrone, 1982; Weiner, 1986) or more (Jones & Davis, 1965), as defined by the theorist's question. The components of these models typically refer to psychological operations—computations of the mind that contribute to the response of interest. Among these highly-specified models, the fact that many include two components does not seem to reflect a special emergent feature of mental structure, but rather the particular way in which a theoretical question is framed.

A second type of dual-process model is more general in its applicability, proposed to encompass a broader set of psychological functions. These include, for example, dual-process models of automaticity versus control (Shiffrin & Schneider, 1977), implicit versus explicit processing (Greenwald & Banaji, 1995), similarity-based versus rule-based processing (Sloman, 1996), System 1 versus System 2 (Kahneman & Frederick, 2002; Stanovich, 1999), and to lesser extents, models of systematic versus heuristic processing (Chaiken, 1980) and central versus peripheral processing (Petty & Cacioppo, 1986). Unlike the highly-specified models I described earlier, this type of dual-process model includes approaches that may be applied to many different psychological phenomena. However—and critically—whereas the more specific dual-process models describe the *operations* of each process, these broader dual-process models often describe *attributes* of a psychological process, such as whether it occurs quickly or is subject to awareness. It is this type of dual-process theory that represents the general theme of dualities in theories of the mind—the same that inspired Descartes and Freud—and is the subject of this chapter.

In this chapter, I discuss two examples of broad, dual-process frameworks that have been influential in the field of social psychology: the implicit–explicit and automatic–controlled dichotomies. After discussing some key limitations of these approaches to understanding social cognition and self-regulation, respectively, I describe alternative, multiprocess theoretical models that provide more precise, more functional, and more generative explanations of social cognition and behavior. My overarching position is that while these broad dual-process frameworks have been successful in providing intuitive descriptions of psychological phenomena and framing broad theoretical questions, a focus on such dualities can obscure the underlying psychological mechanisms we seek to elucidate.

MECHANISMS OF IMPLICIT SOCIAL COGNITION

In recent years, dual-process theories concerning implicit and explicit processes have become prominent and have been applied to a wide range of social cognitive phenomena (Greenwald & Banaji, 1995). The terms *implicit* and *explicit* refer to conscious and nonconscious forms of processing, following research in the memory literature (e.g., Jacoby & Witherspoon, 1982; Schacter, 1987). *Explicit* refers to having awareness of a particular process or response, such as when forming an impression, coming to a decision, or performing an action. *Implicit* simply refers to a lack of awareness regarding a response or its underlying cause. Importantly, the implicit–explicit distinction describes a property of a process but not its operation. Amodio and Ratner (2011a) described implicit processes as "the 'dark matter' of the mind—the mental processes that operate in the absence of conscious awareness." Like the dark matter in outer space, implicit processes are believed to exist only because the causes of so many behaviors are not available to our conscious awareness. In this sense, *implicit* refers to the negative space between explainable behaviors. It is the modern black box that cognitive psychologists have, for decades, sought to illuminate. Thus, to say a process is implicit does not explain its operation or function. Indeed, because the terms *implicit* and *explicit* merely describe a property of a psychological response, and not the process itself, one could argue that the implicit–explicit dichotomy does not necessarily imply a meaningful dual-process framework.

How does one begin to explore a psychological process that operates implicitly? Although the process may unfold without awareness, it is reasonable to assume that an implicit response reflects a form of cognition that is rooted in existing associations in memory (Greenwald & Banaji, 1995). Indeed, most psychological theories assume that implicit effects reflect associative processes in memory, usually as part of a dual-process model that distinguishes forms of implicit and explicit processes (Smith & DeCoster, 2000; Sloman, 1996). These models propose that implicit processes reflect a single system of symbolic or connectionist representations of information in memory, whereas explicit processes reflect a different system of propositional knowledge (e.g., beliefs) that is consciously accessible (e.g., Gawronski & Bodenhausen, 2006). In these models, information may be stored in a complex network of concepts with associative links varying in strength, along which activity spreads from one concept to others. These models were designed, in part, to explain semantic priming effects in social cognition, such as when a "primed" trait concept influences subsequent impressions of a person without the perceiver's awareness (Higgins, Rholes, & Jones, 1977). Such single-system models of implicit processes have been invoked to account for a wide range of social cognitive effects involving attitudes, semantic concepts (e.g., traits or stereotypes), and affective responses.

Dual-process models of implicit–explicit social cognition have been very influential, generating novel and sophisticated theories of mental processes while providing an intuitive metaphor of the mind. But, the benefits of these dual-process accounts are balanced by some critical limitations. For example, associative models have difficulty explaining noncognitive phenomena, such as emotion and motivation, and few, if any, of the models developed in the field of social cognition correspond with emerging multisystem models of neural function related to implicit learning and memory (Poldrack & Foerde, 2007). Most importantly, because associative models represent a metaphor of information processing that is conceptually disembodied from physiological processes of the brain and behavior, it is difficult for them to address the mechanisms through which mental processes interface with behavior (Barsalou, 2008; Smith & Semin, 2004). A common criticism of the connectionist approach, by comparison, is that connectionist models can explain anything in an infinite regress of processing units, but without necessarily corresponding to how the human mind and brain actually work. For these reasons, current dual-process models of implicit social cognition may be limited in their ability to explain an adequate range of implicitly operating mechanisms and their influences on behavior.

Beyond Dual Processes: The Memory Systems Model of Implicit Social Cognition

An alternative to dual-process models of implicit social cognition is suggested by recent developments in the cognitive neuroscience literature on learning and memory. Early research on the neural basis of learning and memory began with a dual-process, implicit–explicit analysis, most famously with the case of the patient known by the initials "HM." HM suffered an extreme form of epilepsy, and as a last-resort treatment, doctors surgically removed significant portions of the bilateral temporal lobes of his brain, including the hippocampus, amygdala, and parahippocampal gyrus. HM recovered, but with a striking impairment: He could no longer form long-term episodic memories, and he showed severe impairment in recollection of explicit memories from before his surgery (Scoville & Milner, 1957). Nevertheless, he retained intact capacities for several other forms of learning and memory, such as motor skills and habits, as well as some aspects of semantic associations (e.g., factual knowledge). Thus, he lost his explicit memory while retaining many implicit processes. One outcome of HM's case is that researchers paid more attention to the different types of capacities that were spared and that appeared to operate implicitly.

In the wake of cases like HM's, a large body of human and animal research began to identify several different forms of implicit learning and memory associated with distinct neural substrates (Figure 37.1; Squire & Zola, 1996). It is now known that implicit learning and memory processes encompass a wide range of capacities, such as semantic priming, perceptual priming, fear conditioning, instrumental and reward conditioning, and the learning of skills and habits. The dissociations between these processes have been illuminated through studies of neurological patients, selective animal lesions, and careful behavioral experimentation. That is, in most cases, a lesion of a brain region linked to one form of memory causes the specific impairment of that form of memory without affecting other capacities. Not surprisingly, this approach was heavily influenced

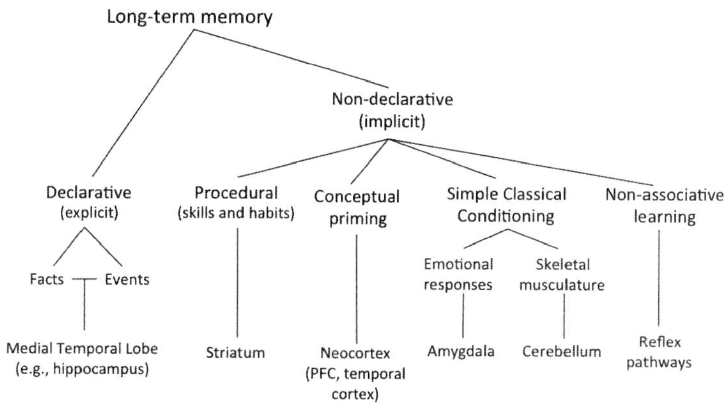

FIGURE 37.1. A memory systems model of distinctive functions and their putative neural substrates. Adapted from Squire and Knowlton (1994). Copyright by The MIT Press. Adapted by permission.

by research on nonhuman animals—a subject model that does not permit inferences about awareness and therefore does not lend itself to consciousness-based explanations. It is for this reason, perhaps, that animal researchers have focused more directly on functional mechanisms than on whether a process is subject to awareness.

Critically, for the purpose of this chapter, this body of work illustrates that "implicit" is not one thing. This idea stands in contrast to the tendency of many dual-process models in social cognition to assume that *implicit* refers to a single, associative form of cognitive processing. More importantly, this body of work has shifted the focus from characterizing mental processes as implicit or explicit to understanding the different functional characteristics of these implicit systems. It is notable that although this memory systems perspective is prominent in cognition and cognitive neuroscience, it has not yet been widely incorporated into theories of social cognition (cf. Amodio, 2008; Amodio & Devine, 2006; Amodio & Ratner, 2011a; also see Carlston, 1994, for a related approach). Nevertheless, this perspective may provide an important theoretical advance beyond current dual-process conceptualizations of implicit processes. In what follows, I highlight three distinct memory systems that all operate implicitly yet support very different functions in cognition and behavior.

Semantic Associative Memory

As I noted earlier, most contemporary models of implicit social cognition are based on theories of associative learning and memory (McClelland & Rumelhart, 1985). These associations refer to semantic information that is organized in networks linking cognitive concepts. According to these models, implicit associations are learned slowly over the course of repeated stimulus pairings (Sloman, 1996) and may be extinguished after repeated exposure to a concept in the absence of its prior associate (Smith & DeCoster, 2000). This general form of learning underlies the associative networks that form the basis of most contemporary models of implicit social cognition.

In the brain, implicit semantic processes have been associated with activity in the left prefrontal cortex (PFC) and temporal lobe, in conjunction with broader neocortical networks (Martin, 2007). Complex semantic networks guide actions, such as movement and speech, through a representational hierarchy that connects high-level representations of goals and response contingencies to lower-level motor plans, along a rostral-to-caudal axis of connectivity within the PFC (Badre & D'Esposito, 2009; Fuster, 2004). In social cognition research, semantic memory systems are thought to govern high-level social cognitive processes such as trait impressions and stereotype formation (Smith & DeCoster, 2000), which are often expressed in verbal behavior (Amodio & Devine, 2006). Although the expression of semantic associations may become explicit, the mechanisms producing these responses operate implicitly.

Fear Conditioning

Classical fear conditioning is a widely studied mechanism for learning threat-related associations and affective responses, and it functions very differently than the type of associative learning and memory implicated in most dual-process models of social cognition. *Classical conditioning* refers to the process of learning to associate a neutral conditioned stimulus (CS) with an aversive or rewarding unconditioned stimulus (US). Fear conditioning may be described as a reactive form of aversive conditioning, in the sense that it concerns a learned association between a neutral stimulus and an affectively charged outcome (e.g., as opposed to semantic associative learning, which concerns the association between two concepts). Although this process is often described as a form of association, it is more accurately described as a process of learning an adaptive whole-body response to a potentially threatening outcome. In this way, the fear conditioning process is different than the evaluative conditioning process often examined in social cognition studies of humans.

Fear conditioning is subserved by the amygdala and associated subcortical structures. The amygdala receives sensory input very early in the processing stream and can promote a wide range of responses, including those relevant to fear as well as reward. Fear-conditioned associations, specifically, are processed by the amygdala's central nucleus, and expressed primarily in the form of autonomic arousal, attentional vigilance, and the inhibition of action (e.g., freezing; LeDoux, 2000). In human social interactions, such responses may be manifested in anxious feelings, and in awkward and inhibited behaviors such as averted gaze, disfluent speech, closed body posture, and interpersonal distance (Amodio & Devine, 2006; Dovidio, Kawakami, & Gaertner, 2002; McConnell & Leibold, 2001).

Importantly, key characteristics of classical fear conditioning distinguish it from the learning of semantic associations in social cognition models. For example, unlike slowly learned implicit semantic associations, fear-conditioned associations are acquired rapidly, often after a single CS–US pairing (LeDoux, 2000) and may be expressed independently of explicit awareness or semantic associations (Bechara et al., 1995). Furthermore, the extinction of fear-conditioned associations (i.e., to CS-alone presentations) occurs very slowly with new learning, yet traces of the conditioned association can result in rapid reconditioning (Bouton, 1994; but see Schiller et al., 2010). These properties are very different from those typically ascribed to the learning and unlearning of implicit conceptual associations in traditional sociocognitive models. Furthermore, the fear conditioning literature offers well-delineated pathways for behavioral expression, whereas traditional implicit social cognition models do not typically address the mechanistic link from cognition to behavior.

Instrumental Learning and Memory

Instrumental learning and memory systems concern associations between an action and an outcome; thus, these systems are often linked to theories of motivation and reward processes. Instrumental associations are learned following repeated reinforced stimulus–action pairings, independently of explicit awareness of such pairings. Instrumental responses may reflect goals or habits. Whereas goal-directed (reward) responses are acquired and modified rapidly following changes in feedback contingencies, habit-like responses develop incrementally and may be extinguished very slowly after feedback is decoupled from a particular response (Yin & Knowlton, 2006).

The instrumental memory system has been associated with the striatum and related basal ganglia structures, which have strong recursive connections with the PFC (via the caudate nucleus) and with motor areas (via the putamen) that coordinate goal-directed and habit-based responses (Alexander, DeLong, & Strick, 1986). Hence, as with fear conditioning, the pathways for behavioral expression of instrumental associations are well delineated. Furthermore, the characteristics of instrumental learning and memory differ from those of other learning and memory systems in critical ways.

Interactions among Memory Systems

So far, I have highlighted distinctions between different forms of implicit memory that underlie social cognition. However, research is beginning to shed light on how these memory systems interact with each other, working in competition or in concert to produce complex behaviors (Foerde, Knowlton, & Poldrack, 2006; Foerde & Shohamy, 2011). Indeed, behavioral tasks used to assess implicit associations likely engage a blend of these systems. For example, implicit attitudes assessed by sequential priming tasks may reflect a combination of semantic associations (e.g., with good vs. bad concepts), threat- or reward-related associations, and instrumental associations (e.g., reinforced and habitual actions). Implicit learning and memory processes also interact with explicit processes. For example, explicit episodic and semantic memory systems play important roles in the formation and representation of complex goals and in the contextual effects that modulate implicit processes (Poldrack & Packard, 2003). Clearly, much of our behavior is guided by explicit goals and information that is communicated explicitly between individuals. But although these goals may be explicit, the mechanisms that guide goal pursuit usually operate implicitly. In this way, most of our behaviors involve the coordination of multiple implicit and explicit processes. A consideration of these processes and their interplay will help to clarify the nature of implicit social cognition and its effect on behavior. By contrast, an emphasis on dual-process frameworks could obscure these efforts.

Role of Memory Systems in Social Cognition

In the previous section, I described some of the chief characteristic functions of different implicit memory systems. But how do these relate to social cognitive phenomena addressed by popular dual-process theories? Although theories of implicit social cognition have historically focused on a single mode of implicit processing, hints of multiple modes of implicit processing have been prevalent in the literature (e.g., Carlston, 1994; Lieberman, 2000; Wood & Neal, 2007). Conceptual distinctions among cognition, affect, and behavior, which roughly correspond to the three implicit memory systems described in the previous section, have guided research on attitudes and social processes for nearly a century. These distinctions are especially pronounced in the intergroup bias literature, in which researchers often use sequential priming tasks to examine associations between social group targets and semantic concepts (i.e., stereotypes), evaluations, affect, and approach/avoidance responses (Amodio & Mendoza, 2010). Although these responses likely reflect different underlying processes, they have traditionally been interpreted as reflecting a single underlying system that corresponds closely with a semantic memory system. For example, implicit evaluation—a complex construct that combines cognitive, affective, and behavioral processes—is often assumed to reflect a single underlying system of semantic association, yet it most likely reflects a combination of the memory system functions described here.

Dissociable Mechanisms Underlying Implicit Social Cognition

The memory systems model posits that implicit social cognitive responses reflect different underlying memory systems, and although these systems typically work in concert and appear blended in overt responses, they should be theoretically dissociable. In an early test of this idea, my colleagues and I proposed that long-held distinctions between implicit attitudes and stereotypes might, in part, reflect different underlying memory systems for affective versus semantic (i.e., cognitive) associations (Amodio, Harmon-Jones, & Devine, 2003). This research was motivated, in part, by findings that claimed to show evidence of "affective priming" using only reaction time tasks that assess the strength of word associations. Although it was clear that such tasks assess semantic associations, including those representing evaluations (e.g., semantic associations between an object and the concept of "good" or "bad"), it was unclear that such tasks could provide evidence for an affective association. Given the long history of considering affective forms of prejudice in the intergroup literature, it was important for us to know whether implicit forms of bias revealed by priming tasks might also have an affective component.

When considering potential affective substrates for implicit racial bias, the fear conditioning system mechanism appeared to be an excellent candidate, as it could respond rapidly to stimuli and did not require conscious awareness. Indeed, soon after we began this line of research, two functional magnetic resonance imaging (fMRI) papers were published that suggested an association between amygdala activity and implicit racial bias (Hart et al., 2000; Phelps et al., 2000). In Amodio et al. (2003), we used the startle-eyeblink method to index the rapid activation of the amygdala's central nucleus—the part of the amygdala that is specifically involved in fear conditioning—and observed larger startle-eyeblink responses among White participants in response to Black than White faces. We argued that this pattern reflected a uniquely affective form of implicit racial attitudes, driven by a fear conditioning mechanism that could not be explained by semantic systems. Subsequent fMRI studies have replicated this pattern of amygdala response and related it to behavioral measures of implicit prejudice (Cunningham et al., 2004).

As a more direct test of the memory systems hypothesis that implicit stereotype and affective responses to race are dissociable, Amodio and Devine (2006) used separate behavioral tasks to assess subjects' implicit stereotyping and evaluative associations with white versus black Americans. The stereotyping measure was designed to assess semantic associations that were equated on valence, whereas the evaluative bias measure was designed to pick up on general affective and evaluative associations that were unrelated to stereotypes. That is, the stereotyping measure was intended to pick up on a semantic memory system but not affective systems (i.e., fear conditioning or instrumental learning systems). By contrast, the evaluative measure was intended to pick up primarily on an affective memory system rooted in fear conditioning (although, given the task structure, it could also pick up on aspects of instrumental learning or semantic associations with valence categories; Gilbert, Swencionis, & Amodio, 2012). Across three studies, these measures of implicit stereotyping and evaluation were not significantly correlated, yet they predicted different types of intergroup behavior (as described in the following section), suggesting independent underlying processes.

In a more recent test of the memory systems model (Amodio & Hamilton, 2012), we hypothesized that intergroup anxiety—a response associated with activity in the amygdala and related neural circuits—would selectively increase the activation of some forms of implicit bias but not others. Because implicit affective forms of racial bias have been linked to the amygdala, a substrate of fear conditioning, we predicted that anxiety associated with an interracial interaction would increase white participants' degree of evaluative racial bias. By contrast, the neural systems involved in anxiety are not directly connected to regions linked to associative semantic memory, so we did not expect intergroup anxiety to modulate activity of stereotype-based semantic racial associations.

Indeed, this pattern emerged in our experiment: White participants who thought they were going to interact with a black experimenter reported greater anxiety than those anticipating an interaction with a white experimenter. Importantly, those in the black interaction condition exhibited stronger racial bias on a measure of implicit evaluation than those in the white interaction condition, but scores on an implicit stereotyping measure, which held valence constant, did not differ by condition. Furthermore, self-reported anxiety was associated with implicit evaluation but not implicit stereotyping among participants in the interracial interaction condition. Together, these findings provide additional support for a memory systems model of implicit social cognition, and in doing so, present a novel theoretical analysis of how intergroup social anxiety affects the activation of implicit racial associations. It is notable that, to my knowledge, no existing dual-process model would have predicted this particular pattern.

Predicting Behavior

A limitation of existing dual-process accounts of implicit social cognition is that they do not explain the path from implicit processes to behavior. The memory systems model provides an important advance in this regard by offering specific predictions, based on neural structure and function, for how different types of implicit associations may be expressed in different ways through different channels of behavior (Amodio, 2008; Amodio & Ratner, 2011a). For example, fear-conditioned associations are expressed primarily as increased autonomic arousal, freezing, and passive avoidance. Thus, implicit affective associations linked to threat in a human social interaction should produce similar behaviors, characterized by anxiety-related nonverbals and interpersonal distance. By contrast, semantic effects are typically expressed in higher-level representations of impressions and social goals, and should be expressed in verbal responses and overt judgments, and in more instrumental behaviors. Indeed, this pattern was observed by Amodio and Devine (2006) in a set of double-dissociation studies conducted in the context of interracial interactions. For example, subjects' implicit attitudes toward blacks predicted how far they sat from the belongings of their African American study partner in a row of chairs (significantly above any effect of implicit stereotyping), whereas implicit stereotyping predicted their expectations for their partners' performance on a series of exams (significantly above any effect of implicit attitudes). Interestingly, past findings of implicit effects on behavior generally corroborate the memory systems model's predictions, such that greater implicit evaluative bias predicted more uncomfortable and/or less friendly social behavior (e.g., Dovidio et al., 2002), whereas implicit stereotype associations predicted stereotype-relevant judgments (Devine, 1989). The memory systems approach provides a multiprocess theoretical framework to account for these patterns, whereas existing dual-process models do not.

Changing Implicit Associations

Producing change in implicit associations has been the most challenging goal of implicit social cognition research. A consideration of the distinct learning characteristics among memory systems promises to clarify models of implicit change, and the memory systems model suggests that interventions can be tailored to the specific characteristics of the underlying memory systems. Although such interventions have not yet been tested directly, existing research suggests that repeated exposure to countervailing semantic concepts may be effective in weakening stereotype associations (e.g., Kawakami, Dovidio, Moll, Hermsen, & Russin, 2000), but such associations are more difficult to alter when they involve affect (Rydell & McConnell, 2006). Other research has shown that extensive training of approach behaviors toward outgroup faces, which likely involves instrumental learning, can lessen negative behavioral responses to outgroups (Kawakami, Phills, Steele, & Dovidio, 2007). Furthermore, changes in one system of memory can influence another and, in some cases, compete for expression in behavior (Poldrack & Packard, 2003). These observations are not easily accommodated by existing dual-process models that assume a single system of implicit associations.

Summary

Many dual-process models are, at their cores, theories about implicit versus explicit forms of processing, with awareness being the defining feature of the process. However, awareness refers only to a descriptive attribute of the process; it does not describe a mechanism or function. As such, the implicit–explicit distinction does not truly constitute a dual-process model. My goal in this section has been to present the memory systems model as an example of a theoretical approach that moves beyond a focus on properties of awareness and addresses specific psychological mechanisms and functions. Research on memory systems also illustrates the multiprocess nature of the mind. Although a researcher may choose to focus on a subset of processes to address a particular question, it may be useful to acknowledge the roles of the broader set of processes in the context of a larger integrated model of psychological function.

MULTIPROCESS APPROACHES TO CONTROL

Unlike the concepts of "implicit" and "explicit," which are defined as the property of conscious accessibility (Cohen &

Squire, 1980; Schacter, 1987; Squire, 1992), the concepts of automaticity and control in social cognition refer primarily to intentionality; that is, to the mechanisms that guide intentional and unintentional responses (Bargh, 1994); however, some usages refer to specific operations that occur automatically or with control (Shiffrin & Schneider, 1977). Automatic responses are triggered externally, such as through a subliminal priming procedure, much like the "ideomotor" response described by James and developed most notably by Bargh (1982, 1989). Controlled responses, by comparison, are triggered internally, driven by one's goals and intentions (Wegner & Bargh, 1998).

Despite these conceptual distinctions, the constructs of implicit–explicit and automaticity–control are often used interchangeably. This is likely because the features of these two constructs correspond in some salient ways. For example, automatic responses are often triggered without one's conscious awareness, and, as a consequence, "automatic" is often equated with "implicit." However, an automatic response need not be nonconscious; a person may be aware of what triggered his or her unintentional response (Amodio & Mendoza, 2010; Bargh, 1994; Hall & Payne, 2010). Similarly, control is often described as requiring conscious deliberation; therefore, it is often equated with awareness. This, too, is an inaccurate description, as some forms of controlled processing are known to occur without conscious deliberation (e.g., Amodio, 2010; Amodio et al., 2004; Mendoza, Gollwitzer, & Amodio, 2010; Schmidt, Crump, Cheesman, & Besner, 2007; Shiffrin & Schneider, 1977). For example, using event-related potentials (ERPs) to measure rapid neural responses, Amodio et al. (2004) demonstrated that the initiation of controlled processing occurs rapidly following a cue for control. This activation occurred too quickly to reflect conscious deliberation, and prior research has shown that this neural process operates independently of conscious awareness (Berns, Cohen, & Mintun, 1997; Niewenhuis, Ridderinkhof, Blom, Band, & Kok, 2001). Thus, it is useful to distinguish automaticity and control from issues of awareness when considering their utility as an organizing framework of dual processes.

Automaticity and Control Each Represent Multiple Processes

Automatic and controlled processes are often conceptualized as two components of a dual process. But unlike the implicit–explicit distinction, which refers descriptively to the property of awareness, automaticity and control refer to two sets of complex mechanisms that operate at multiple levels of cognition and are expressed through multiple channels of response. The tendency to view automaticity and control as two sides of a dual process can mask the important mechanisms that underlie their complex functions.

In the previous section, I outlined different types of implicit processes, which are also relevant to different mechanisms through which an automatic response may be triggered and enacted. In this section, I focus on the different mechanisms that contribute to control. The idea that control involves multiple components is not new in social psychology (Wilson & Brekke, 1994; Wegener & Petty, 1997), though it may still be underappreciated. Similarly, research on motivation has long distinguished between stages of goal pursuit that are relevant to the process of action control, ranging from goal formation, commitment, and planning, to effort mobilization and implementation (e.g., Heckhausen & Gollwitzer, 1987; Gollwitzer, 2012).

Models such as these illustrate that control involves multiple components with different functions, and that an understanding of these components provides a clearer account of behavior and the specific ways in which control may succeed or fail. More recently, researchers have begun to investigate more specific cognitive and neural mechanisms involved in the process of control. Here, I briefly describe some of the key components of control that have been examined in this line of research.

Conflict Monitoring

How is control initiated in the first place? This is a long-standing question in social psychology, about which dual-process theories are generally silent (but see Monteith, 1993; Wegner, 1994). I became interested in this question because it promised to elucidate a puzzle in the intergroup bias literature: In prior work, my colleagues and I observed two general patterns of behavior among low-prejudice individuals, which related to their internal and external motivations to respond without prejudice (Amodio et al., 2003; Devine, Plant, Amodio, Harmon-Jones, & Vance, 2002). Although these two groups of egalitarians—one dubbed "good regulators," the other dubbed "poor regulators" by Amodio, Devine, and Harmon-Jones (2008)—held similarly positive attitudes toward black Americans and showed genuine internal motivation to respond without prejudice (Plant & Devine, 1998), they differed in their ability to regulate their implicit behavioral and physiological responses to black outgroup members. This pattern was not easily explained by existing dual-process models and, as such, we could not begin to develop intervention strategies to enhance control among those who were less effective.

At the time I was thinking about these issues, new theories were emerging in the cognitive neuroscience literature that directly addressed the question of how control is initiated. These theories noted that corrective control is needed when behavior begins to deviate from one's intentions. Such cases reflect a conflict between one's intended response and some alternative tendency or bias. In order for corrective control to be engaged, this conflict must be detected as the response unfolds. Cognitive neuroscience research on response conflict tasks, such as the color-naming Stroop (1935) task, had observed characteristic patterns of brain activity during high-conflict trials, such as when the meaning of a word (e.g., *red*) conflicts with one's goal to name the ink color in which the word appears (e.g., the color blue), in comparison to low-conflict trials (*red* appearing in the color red; Carter et al., 1998; MacDonald, Cohen, Stenger, & Carter, 2000). These studies revealed that activity in the anterior cingulate cortex (ACC) was particularly strong during response conflict trials. In light of these findings, Botvinick, Braver, Barch, Carter, and Cohen (2001) proposed that the ACC supports a *conflict monitoring* function, such that it is involved in detecting conflict between alternative motor impulses. Furthermore, when conflict arises, the ACC signals structures in a different region of the brain, the PFC, which is involved in implementing one's intended response over other competing tendencies (Kerns et al., 2004). Thus, these researchers posited a distinction between neural processes involved in detecting the need for control (vis-à-vis response conflict) and the implementation of control—two distinct components of controlled processing.

This model of conflict monitoring was adapted by Amodio et al. (2004) to address the question of why egalitarians vary in their control of intergroup responses. Measures of brain activity (electroencephalography [EEG]), collected while participants completed a stereotype priming task, revealed that ACC activity was stronger on task trials that required greater control than on trials that did not require control (Amodio et al., 2004). Furthermore, these results dissociated the neural detection of conflict from the process of implementing control in behavior. That is, we observed significant activation of the ACC, indicating the detection of conflict, independent of whether subsequent response control was successful or unsuccessful (i.e., on both the N2 and error-related negative ERP components, respectively). This suggested that the process of detecting the need for control was independent of the implementation of control.

In subsequent work, we addressed our original question about why the two types of egalitarians—good regulators and poor regulators—differed in their ability to control their expressions of intergroup bias. Examining ACC activity as an indicator of conflict monitoring, we found that the "poor regulators" often failed to control because they had trouble detecting the need for control, and not because they had trouble implementing control (Amodio et al., 2008; see also Study 2 in Amodio et al., 2003). This finding suggested that interventions designed to enhance control among these individuals should focus on strategies for detecting the need for control rather than on strategies for selecting or implementing an intended response. In a separate line of research, we examined responses that are made in response to social pressure, in which external social cues moderate the regulation of bias. We found that detecting the need for control on the basis of an external social cue requires additional neurocognitive processes, linked to the medial frontal cortex and its role in mentalizing (Amodio & Frith, 2006), in addition to the ACC-based mechanism for detecting conflict based on internal cues (Amodio, Kubota, Harmon-Jones, & Devine, 2006). This finding helped to explain why externally motivated behaviors can be especially difficult to regulate.

Implementation of Control

Once conflict is detected, controlled processes must be implemented. Cognitive neuroscience research suggests that when conflict is detected, the ACC signals regions of the PFC involved in response control (Miller & Cohen, 2001). These PFC regions primarily target motor responses—indeed, the PFC is thought to be an extension of motor cortex that evolved to support higher-level cognitive representations (e.g., of complex goals), and PFC subregions are connected in a hierarchical fashion that feed back to motor structures (Badre & D'Esposito, 2009). Although the PFC is interconnected with regions throughout the brain, the predominance of its connections with motor regions comports with research showing that people are often most effective in controlling their behavioral responses, yet often ineffective at directly regulating their emotions and thoughts (e.g., Gross & Levenson, 1993; Wegner, Schneider, Carter, & White, 1987; see Amodio & Ratner, 2011b, for a review of this topic). Thus, a consideration of PFC function and connectivity can shed light on the specific mechanisms of control.

Cognitive neuroscience research on PFC function suggests at least three forms of motor control linked to separate underlying neural mechanisms. One form of control concerns the implementation of goal-directed actions—motor responses that reflect an intended action. The implementation of goal-directed behaviors involves bidirectional connections between the PFC and the striatum (i.e., the frontostriatal loop), which operate in concert with thalamic and midbrain processes (Middleton & Strick, 2000; Yin & Knowlton, 2006). This type of goal-directed action control tends to involve left-lateralized PFC activity, at least among right-handed research subjects. Left PFC activity has also been associated with action control in contexts such as regulating intergroup behaviors (Amodio, 2010; Amodio, Devine, & Harmon-Jones, 2007), obtaining rewards (Pizzagalli, Sherwood, Henriques, & Davidson, 2005), and instrumental aggression (Harmon-Jones & Sigelman, 2001).

A second form of motor control is active inhibition—the intentional stopping of a response. Active inhibition has been linked to right PFC activity, particularly in the right inferior frontal cortex (Aron, Robbins, & Poldrack, 2004). Much of the research on this form of control has examined responses on the stop-signal or go/no-go tasks (for a review, see Aron, 2011). Tasks such as these include simple cues for action and stopping, and they are designed to probe basic domain-general mechanisms of inhibitory control. However, response-stopping tasks have also been used to probe responses to social stimuli. For example, the Go/No-Go Association Task of the Implicit Association Test (IAT) has been used to assess implicit social attitudes, and behavior on this task likely relies on inhibitory control processes. Furthermore, in fMRI studies of social perception, greater activity in the right inferior PFC is sometimes observed (e.g., when responding to an outgroup member, in comparison with responding to an ingroup member); thus, one can speculate that responses to outgroup faces, as compared with ingroup faces, in these studies might reflect participants' attempts to withhold a potentially race-biased response (Lieberman, Hariri, Jarcho, Eisenberger, & Bookheimer, 2005; Mitchell, Ames, Jenkins, & Banaji, 2009). It is notable that inhibitory control may be involved in what I described earlier as "implemental control" (i.e., goal-directed action), in the sense that a prepotent response may be inhibited while the intended response is implemented (as in "override" models of control). However, in "race" models of control (Logan, Cowan, & Davis, 1984), in which two response tendencies compete for expression in behavior, inhibitory control is not necessary for the successful implementation of a controlled response. Thus, it is useful to distinguish between these two forms of control.

A third form of motor control pertains to eye movements, although it is rarely discussed in the social cognition literature. Oculomotor networks constitute an important interface between perception and action in the context of control, and the control of eye movements is associated with activity in dorsal regions of the PFC (Brodmann's Area 8) that are referred to as the "frontal eye-fields." Given the field's renewed interest in the role of attention and perception in mechanisms of control (e.g., Amodio, 2010; Ofan, Rubin, & Amodio, 2011), I expect that this form of control will receive greater attention from social cognitive theorists in the near future. Importantly, these three forms of motor control usually operate in concert, as suggested by their integrated neural connections and complementary functions.

It is notable that other recent theories of control have implicated multiple processes. In particular, the quadruple-process (quad) model of automaticity and control distinguishes between two components of controlled processing (Conrey, Sherman, Gawronski, Hugenberg, & Groom, 2005; Sherman et al., 2008). According to this model, one component is *discriminability* (D), which refers to the ability to determine a correct (i.e., intentional) response. A second component is *overcoming bias* (OB), which refers to success at overcoming a countervailing automatic tendency. Some efforts have been made to relate the quad model to underlying neural processes (e.g., Beer et al., 2008; Gonsalkorale, Sherman, Allen, Klauer, & Amodio, 2011), but more research is needed to determine the relation between parameters of the quad model and specific neural systems governing automaticity and control.

Models of PFC anatomy and function also highlight the effects of control on sensory and perceptual processes—aspects of control that have only recently begun to receive attention in social psychology (e.g., Amodio, 2010; Ratner & Amodio, 2013; Ofan et al., 2011, 2013). Through dense connections to the thalamus and other sensory structures (Barbas & Zikopoulos, 2007), the PFC is believed to play a role in selecting motivationally relevant sensory signals while suppressing irrelevant information, in the service of task goals. The PFC continues to modulate the perception of sensory inputs through connections to visual and auditory association cortices (Medalla, Lera, Feinberg, & Barbas, 2007). For example, in an fMRI study of visual processing, efforts to ignore a visual stimulus were associated with reduced activity in the visual association regions, and this effect was driven by activity in the left PFC (Gazzaley et al., 2007). Additionally, studies of pain regulation revealed that PFC activity is associated with changes in the perception of pain (Salomons, Johnstone, Backonja, Shackman, & Davidson, 2007; Wager et al., 2004). These findings suggest that control regions of the PFC function to regulate sensory and perceptual processes, presumably in the service of facilitating goal-driven responses. These aspects of control represent promising directions for future social cognition research on control.

In summary, findings from the cognitive neuroscience literature have helped to expand and refine social cognitive models of control, already far beyond the single-system view of control assumed in many dual-process approaches. This expanded view of control has begun to shift the field's attention away from phenomenological properties of automaticity and control, such as their degree of implicitness or intentionality, toward functional accounts of these processes that are more useful for understanding social cognitive mechanisms and behavior (Amodio & Ratner, 2011b; Henke, 2010).

CONCLUSIONS

Classic dualisms in psychology, such as those proposed by Descartes and Freud, have been largely discarded by contemporary psychologists, yet dualistic thinking is alive and well in the form of many modern dual-process theories. It is true that dual-process theories have been enormously successful in framing general patterns of psychological responses and in generating much research. Dual-process models that describe the operations of specific processes, selected from a broader set of processes, have been particularly useful in comparison with general dual-process frameworks that refer only to a characteristic property of a process. However, nearly all dual-process models are limited in a critical regard: The mind is not composed of dual processes. Indeed, the brain comprises several different interacting systems with uniquely different functions, and the range of human behaviors cannot be explained by a simple dual-process account.

A focus on dualities places an unnecessary constraint on how we think about the mind and behavior. Given the emerging knowledge on multiple systems in the mind and brain, general dual-process theories may be limited because they are misspecified—that is, they do not correspond well with known behavioral patterns or neurocognitive systems—or because they are too highly specified, concerned with a particular process in a circumscribed context. In order to advance our understanding of the mechanisms that drive human behavior, theorists will likely need to move beyond dualistic frameworks to consider the multisystem models that more closely comport with neural structure, psychological function, and behavior.

One nevertheless continues to wonder: Why is there a preponderance of dual-process theories in the psychological literature? Why have ancient philosophers and contemporary psychologists alike viewed the mind as operating in terms of dualities? These are interesting questions, regardless of whether they can be answered. At the outset of this chapter, I noted that the dualism of consciousness dominates the human experience. Just as it dominates our experience, it likely dominates our attempt at understanding the inner workings of our minds and the causes of our behaviors. Rather ironically, psychologists themselves are subject to the limitations of the very thing they hope to elucidate. Given the eminence of consciousness in human experience, it is not surprising that psychological theories are also dominated by the divide between what we can observe and what we cannot (i.e., *the explanatory gap*; Levine, 1983). Indeed, in a recent *word cloud* analysis of the most common phrases used in social and personality psychology, the term *implicit* was among the most prominent, following only *behavior* and *perception* (Hirsch, 2010). The irresistible tendency to see the world in terms of awareness may indeed explain the continued popularity of dual-process models in psychology. However, if neurocognitive function is not organized in terms of dualities, then dualistic constructs, such as those built on the conscious–nonconscious dichotomy, may prove to be red herrings—diversions away from the true mechanisms of the mind we hope to discover.

While the limitations of the dual-process approach are increasingly recognized, they are being addressed by emerging multiprocess models of the mind and brain. In this chapter, I have described two major research areas—implicit social cognition and self-regulation—in which multiprocess models offer more refined explanations than prior dual-process explanations. As our understanding of psychological function advances, and as findings from social psychology are increasingly integrated with those in neuroscience and other related fields, multiprocess models may begin to replace the dual-process approaches that are still prominent today. Dual-process views are unlikely to disappear completely, though—after all, psychologists are still humans, and the conscious–unconscious duality will continue to loom large in our theories of the mind, just as it does in our everyday experiences. Although the tendency to see dualities will likely persist as long as humans are still doing psychology, the emergence of brain-based multiprocess theories of social cognition are enabling psychologists to look beyond dualities to understand mechanisms of the mind.

REFERENCES

Alexander, G. E., DeLong, M. R., & Strick, P. L. (1986). Parallel organization of functionally segregated circuits linking basal ganglia and cortex. *Annual Review of Neuroscience*, 9, 357–381.

Amodio, D. M. (2008). The social neuroscience of intergroup relations. *European Review of Social Psychology, 19,* 1–54.

Amodio, D. M. (2010). Coordinated roles of motivation and perception in the regulation of intergroup responses: Frontal cortical asymmetry effects on the P2 event-related potential and behavior. *Journal of Cognitive Neuroscience, 22,* 2609–2617.

Amodio, D. M. & Devine, P. G. (2006). Stereotyping and evaluation in implicit race bias: Evidence for independent constructs and unique effects on behavior. *Journal of Personality and Social Psychology*, 91, 652–661.

Amodio, D. M., Devine, P. G., & Harmon-Jones, E. (2007). A dynamic model of guilt: Implications for motivation and self-regulation in the context of prejudice. *Psychological Science, 18*, 524–530.

Amodio, D. M., Devine, P. G., & Harmon-Jones, E. (2008). Individual differences in the regulation of intergroup bias: The role of conflict monitoring and neural signals for control. *Journal of Personality and Social Psychology, 94*, 60–74.

Amodio, D. M., & Frith, C. D. (2006). Meeting of minds: The medial frontal cortex and social cognition. *Nature Reviews Neuroscience, 7*, 268–277.

Amodio, D. M., & Hamilton, H. K. (2012). Intergroup anxiety effects on implicit racial evaluation and stereotyping. *Emotion, 12*, 1273–1280.

Amodio, D. M., Harmon-Jones, E., & Devine, P. G. (2003). Individual differences in the activation and control of affective race bias as assessed by startle eyeblink responses and self-report. *Journal of Personality and Social Psychology, 84*, 738–753.

Amodio, D. M., Harmon-Jones, E., Devine, P. G., Curtin, J. J., Hartley, S. L., & Covert, A. E. (2004). Neural signals for the detection of unintentional race bias. *Psychological Science, 15*, 88–93.

Amodio, D. M., Kubota, J. T., Harmon-Jones, E., & Devine, P. G. (2006). Alternative mechanisms for regulating racial responses according to internal vs. external cues. *Social Cognitive and Affective Neuroscience, 1*, 26–36.

Amodio, D. M., & Mendoza, S. A. (2010). Implicit intergroup bias: Cognitive, affective, and motivational underpinnings. In B. Gawronski & B. K. Payne (Eds.), *Handbook of implicit social cognition* (pp. 353–374). New York: Guilford Press.

Amodio, D. M., & Ratner, K. G. (2011a). A memory systems model of implicit social cognition. *Current Directions in Psychological Science, 20*, 143–148.

Amodio, D. M., & Ratner, K. (2011b). Mechanisms for the regulation of intergroup responses: A social neuroscience analysis. In J. Decety & J. T. Cacioppo (Eds.), *Handbook of social neuroscience* (pp. 729–741). New York: Oxford University Press.

Aron, A. R. (2011). From proactive to reactive and selective control: Developing a richer model for stopping inappropriate responses. *Biological Psychiatry, 69*, 55–68.

Aron, A. R., Robbins, T. W., & Poldrack, R. A. (2004). Inhibition and the right inferior frontal cortex. *Trends in Cognitive Sciences, 8*, 170–177.

Badre, D., & D'Esposito, M. (2009). Is the rostro-caudal axis of the frontal lobe hierarchical? *Nature Reviews Neuroscience, 10*, 659–669.

Barbas, H. & Zikopoulos, B. (2007). The prefrontal cortex and flexible behavior. *The Neuroscientist, 13*, 532–545.

Bargh, J. A. (1982). Attention and automaticity in the processing of self-relevant information. *Journal of Personality and Social Psychology, 49*, 1040–1053.

Bargh, J. A. (1989). Conditional automaticity: Varieties of automatic influence in social perception and cognition. In J. S. Uleman & J. A. Bargh (Eds.), *Unintended thought* (pp. 3–51). New York: Guilford Press.

Bargh, J. A. (1994). The four horsemen of automaticity: Awareness, intention, efficiency, and control in social cognition. In R. S. Wyer, Jr., & T. K. Srull (Eds.), *Handbook of social cognition* (2nd ed., pp. 1–40). Hillsdale, NJ: Erlbaum.

Barsalou, L. W. (2008). Grounded cognition. *Annual Review of Psychology, 59*, 617–645.

Bechara, A., Tranel, D., Damasio, H., Adolphs, R., Rockland, C., & Damasio, A. R. (1995). Double dissociation of conditioning and declarative knowledge relative to the amygdala and hippocampus in humans. *Science, 269*, 1115–1118.

Beer, J. S., Stallen, M., Lombardo, M. V., Gonsalkorale, K., Cunningham, W. A., & Sherman, J. W. (2008). The Quadruple Process model approach to examining the neural underpinnings of prejudice. *NeuroImage, 43*, 775–783.

Berns, G. S., Cohen, J. D., & Mintun, M. A. (1997). Brain regions responsive to novelty in the absence of awareness. *Science, 276*, 1272–1275.

Botvinick, M. M., Braver, T. S., Barch, D. M., Carter, C. S., & Cohen, J. D. (2001). Conflict monitoring and cognitive control. *Psychological Review, 108*, 624–652.

Bouton, M. E. (1994). Conditioning, remembering, and forgetting. *Journal of Experimental Psychology: Animal Behavior Processes, 20*, 219–231.

Carlston, D. E. (1994). Associated Systems Theory: A systematic approach to the cognitive representation of persons and events. In R. S. Wyer (Ed.), *Advances in Social Cognition:*

Vol. 7. Associated systems theory (pp. 1–78). Hillsdale, NJ: Erlbaum.

Carter, C. S., Braver, T. S., Barch, D. M., Botvinick, M. M., Noll, D. C., & Cohen, J. D. (1998). Anterior cingulate cortex, error detection, and the online monitoring of performance. *Science, 280*, 747–749.

Chaiken, S. (1980). Heuristic versus systematic information processing and the use of source versus message cues in persuasion. *Journal of Personality and Social Psychology, 39*(5), 752–766.

Cohen, N. J., & Squire, L. R. (1980). Preserved learning and retention of pattern analyzing skill in amnesia: Dissociation of knowing how and knowing that. *Science, 210*, 207–210.

Conrey, F. R., Sherman, J. W., Gawronski, B., Hugenberg, K., & Groom, C. (2005). Separating multiple processes in implicit social cognition: The quad model of implicit task performance. *Journal of Personality and Social Psychology, 89*, 469–487.

Cunningham, W. A., Johnson, M. K., Raye, C. L., Gatenby, J. C., Gore, J. C., & Banaji, M. R. (2004). Separable neural components in the processing of Black and White faces. *Psychological Science, 15*, 806–813.

Dennett, D. C. (1991). *Consciousness explained.* Boston: Little, Brown.

Devine, P. G. (1989). Prejudice and stereotypes: Their automatic and controlled components. *Journal of Personality and Social Psychology, 56*, 5–18.

Devine, P. G., Plant, E. A., Amodio, D. M., Harmon-Jones, E., & Vance, S. L. (2002). The regulation of explicit and implicit racial bias: The role of motivations to respond without prejudice. *Journal of Personality and Social Psychology, 82*, 835–848.

Dovidio, J. F., Kawakami, K., & Gaertner, S. L. (2002). Implicit and explicit prejudice and interracial interaction. *Journal of Personality and Social Psychology, 82*, 62–68.

Foerde, K., & Shohamy, D. (2011). Feedback timing modulates brain systems for learning in humans. *Journal of Neuroscience, 31*, 13157–13167.

Foerde, K., Knowlton, B. J., & Poldrack, R. A. (2006). Modulation of competing memory systems by distraction. *Proceedings of the National Academy of Science, 103*, 11778–11783.

Fuster, J. M. (2004). Upper processing stages of the perception–action cycle. *Trends in Cognitive Sciences, 8*, 143–145.

Gawronski, B., & Bodenhausen, G. V. (2006). Associative and propositional processes in evaluation: An integrative review of implicit and explicit attitude change. *Psychological Bulletin, 132*, 692–731.

Gazzaley, A., Rissman, J., Cooney, J. W., Rutman, A., Seibert, T., Clapp, W., et al. (2007). Functional interactions between prefrontal and visual association cortex contribute to top-down modulation of visual processing. *Cerebral Cortex, 17*, 125–135.

Gilbert, D. T., Pelham, B. W., & Krull, D. S. (1988). On cognitive busyness: When person perceivers meet persons perceived. *Journal of Personality and Social Psychology, 54*, 733–740.

Gilbert, S. J., Swencionis, J. K., & Amodio, D. M. (2012). Evaluative vs. trait representation in intergroup social judgments: Distinct roles of anterior temporal lobe and prefrontal cortex. *Neuropsychologia, 50*(14), 3600–3611.

Gollwitzer, P. M. (2012). Mindset theory of action phases. In P. Van Lange, A. W. Kruglanski, & E. T. Higgins (Eds.), *Handbook of theories of social psychology* (pp. 526–545). London: Sage.

Gonsalkorale, K., Sherman, J. W., Allen, T. J., Klauer, K. C., & Amodio, D. M. (2011). Accounting for successful control of implicit racial bias: The roles of association activation, response monitoring, and overcoming bias. *Personality and Social Psychology Bulletin, 37*, 1534–1545.

Greenwald, A. G., & Banaji, M. R. (1995). Implicit social cognition: Attitudes, self-esteem and stereotypes. *Psychological Review, 102*, 4–27.

Gross, J. J., & Levenson, R. W. (1993). Emotional suppression: Physiology, self-report, and expressive behavior. *Journal of Personality and Social Psychology, 64*, 970–986.

Hall, D., & Payne, B. K. (2010). Unconscious attitudes, unconscious influence, and challenges to self-control. In Y. Trope, K. Ochsner, & R. Hassin (Eds.), *Self-control in society, mind, and brain* (pp. 221–242). New York: Oxford University Press.

Harmon-Jones, E., & Sigelman, J. (2001). State anger and prefrontal brain activity: Evidence that insult-related relative left prefrontal activation is associated with experienced anger and aggression. *Journal of Personality and Social Psychology, 80*, 797–803.

Hart, A. J., Whalen, P. J., Shin, L. M., McInerney, S. C., Fischer, H., & Rauch, S. L. (2000).

Differential response in the human amygdala to racial outgroup versus ingroup face stimuli. *NeuroReport, 11*, 2351–2355.

Heckhausen, H., & Gollwitzer, P. M. (1987). Thought contents and cognitive functioning in motivational vs. volitional states of mind. *Motivation and Emotion, 11*, 101–120.

Heider, F. (1958). *The psychology of interpersonal relations*. New York: Wiley.

Henke, K. (2010). A model for memory systems based on processing modes rather than consciousness. *Nature Reviews Neuroscience, 11*, 523–532.

Higgins, E. T., Rholes, W. S., & Jones, C. R. (1977). Category accessibility and impression formation. *Journal of Experimental Social Psycholgoy, 13*, 141–154.

Hirsch, J. B. (2010). 2009 in review: A year in social/personality psychology [blog post]. Retrieved from *www.psychologytoday.com/blog/mind-matter-meaning/201001/2009-in-review-year-in-socialpersonality-psychology*.

Jacoby, L. L., & Witherspoon, D. (1982). Remembering without awareness. *Canadian Journal of Psychology, 36*, 300–324.

James, W. (1890). *The principles of psychology*. New York: Holt.

Jones, E. E., & Davis, K. E. (1965). From acts to dispositions: the attribution process in social psychology. In L. Berkowitz (Ed.), *Advances in experimental social psychology* (Vol. 2, pp. 219–266), New York: Academic Press.

Kahneman, D., & Frederick, S. (2002). Representativeness revisited: Attribute substitution in intuitive judgement. In T. Gilovich, D. Griffin, & D. Kahneman (Eds.), *Heuristics and biases: The psychology of intuitive judgment* (pp. 49–81). Cambridge, UK: Cambridge University Press.

Kawakami, K., Dovidio, J. F., Moll, J., Hermsen, S., & Russin, A. (2000). Just say no (to stereotyping): Effects of training on the negation of stereotypic associations on stereotype activation. *Journal of Personality and Social Psychology, 78*, 871–888.

Kawakami, K., Phills, C. E., Steele, J. R., & Dovidio, J. F. (2007). (Close) distance makes the heart grow fonder: Improving implicit racial attitudes and interracial interactions through approach behaviors. *Journal of Personality and Social Psychology, 92*, 957–971.

Kelley, H. H. (1967). Attribution theory in social psychology. In D. Levine (Ed.), *Nebraska Symposium on Motivation* (Vol. 15, pp. 192–238). Lincoln: University of Nebraska Press.

Kerns, J. G., Cohen, J. D., MacDonald, A. W., Cho, R. Y., Stenger, V. A., & Carter, C. S. (2004). Anterior cingulate conflict monitoring and adjustments in control. *Science, 303*, 1023–1026.

LeDoux, J. E. (2000). Emotion circuits in the brain. *Annual Review of Neuroscience, 23*, 155–184.

Levine, J. (1983). Materialism and qualia: The explanatory gap. *Pacific Philosophical Quarterly, 64*, 354–361.

Lieberman, M. D. (2000). Intuition: A social cognitive neuroscience approach. *Psychological Bulletin, 126*, 109–137.

Lieberman, M. D., Hariri, A., Jarcho, J. M., Eisenberger, N. I., & Bookheimer, S. Y. (2005). An fMRI investigation of race-related amygdala activity in African-American and Caucasian-American individuals. *Nature Neuroscience, 8*, 720–722.

Logan, G. D., Cowan, W. B., & Davis, K. A. (1984). On the ability to inhibit responses in simple and choice reaction time tasks: A model and a method. *Journal of Experimental Psychology: Human Perception and Performance, 10*, 276–291.

MacDonald, A. W., Cohen, J. D., Stenger, V. A., & Carter, C. S. (2000). Dissociating the role of dorsolateral prefrontal cortex and anterior cingulate cortex in cognitive control. *Science, 288*, 1835–1837.

Martin, A. (2007). The representation of object concepts in the brain. *Annual Review of Psychology, 58*, 25–45.

McClelland, J. L., & Rumelhart, D. E. (1985). Distributed memory and the representation of general and specific information. *Journal of Experimental Psychology: General, 114*, 159–188.

McConnell, A. R., & Leibold, J. M. (2001). Relations among the Implicit Association Test, discriminatory behavior, and explicit measures of racial attitudes. *Journal of Experimental Social Psychology, 37*, 435–442.

Medalla, M., Lera, P., Feinberg, M., & Barbas, H. (2007). Specificity in inhibitory systems associated with prefrontal pathways to temporal cortex in primates. *Cerebral Cortex, 17*, 136–150.

Mendoza , S. A., Gollwitzer, P. M., & Amodio, D. M. (2010). Reducing the expression of implicit stereotypes: Reflexive control through implementation intentions. *Personality and Social Psychology Bulletin, 36*, 512–523.

Middleton, F. A., & Strick, P. L. (2000). Basal

ganglia and cerebellar loops: Motor and cognitive circuits. *Brain Research Reviews, 31*, 236–250.

Miller, E. K., & Cohen, J. D. (2001). An integrative theory of prefrontal cortex function. *Annual Review of Neuroscience, 24*, 167–202.

Mitchell, J. P., Ames, D. L., Jenkins, A. C., & Banaji, M. R. (2009). Neural correlates of stereotype application. *Journal of Cognitive Neuroscience, 21*, 594–604.

Monteith, M. J. (1993). Self-regulation of prejudiced responses: Implications for progress in prejudice reduction efforts. *Journal of Personality and Social Psychology, 65*, 469–485.

Nieuwenhuis, S., Ridderinkhof, K. R., Blom, J., Band, G. P. H., & Kok, A. (2001). Error-related brain potentials are differently related to awareness of response errors: Evidence from an antisaccade task. *Psychophysiology, 38*, 752–760.

Ofan, R. H., Rubin, N., &Amodio, D. M. (2011). Seeing race: N170 responses to race and their relation to automatic racial attitudes and controlled processing. *Journal of Cognitive Neuroscience, 23*, 3152–3161.

Ofan, R. H., Rubin, N., Amodio, D. M. (2013). Situation-based social anxiety enhances the neural processing of faces: Evidence from an intergroup context. *Social Cognitive and Affective Neuroscience*. [Epub ahead of print]

Payne, B. K. (2012). Control, awareness, and other things we might learn to live without. In S. T. Fiske & C. N. Macrae (Eds.), *Sage handbook of social cognition* (pp. 12–31). London: Sage.

Petty, R. E., & Cacioppo, J. T. (1986). The elaboration likelihood model of persuasion. In L. Berkowitz (Ed.), *Advances in experimental social psychology* (Vol 19, pp. 1123–1205). New York: Academic Press.

Phelps, E. A., O'Connor, K. J., Cunningham, W. A., Funayama, E. S., Gatenby, J. C., Gore, J. C., et al. (2000). Performance on indirect measures of race evaluation predicts amygdala activation. *Journal of Cognitive Neuroscience, 12*, 720–738.

Pizzagalli, D. A., Sherwood, R. J., Henriques, J. B., & Davidson, R. J. (2005). Frontal brain asymmetry and reward responsiveness: A source-localization study. *Psychological Science, 16*, 805–813.

Plant, E. A., & Devine, P. G. (1998). Internal and external motivation to respond without prejudice. *Journal of Personality and Social Psychology, 75*, 811–832.

Poldrack, R. A., & Foerde, K. (2007). Category learning and the memory systems debate. *Neuroscience and Biobehavioral Reviews, 32*, 197–205.

Poldrack, R. A., & Packard, M. G. (2003). Competition between memory systems: Converging evidence from animal and human studies. *Neuropsychologia, 41*, 245–251.

Quattrone, G. A. (1982). Overattribution and unit formation: When behavior engulfs the person. *Journal of Personality and Social Psychology, 42*, 593–607.

Ratner, K. G., & Amodio, D. M. (2013). Seeing "us vs. them": Minimal group effects on the neural encoding of faces. *Journal of Experimental Social Psychology, 49*, 298–301.

Rydell, R. J., & McConnell, A. R. (2006). Understanding implicit and explicit attitude change: A systems of reasoning analysis. *Journal of Personality and Social Psychology, 91*, 995–1008.

Salomons, T. V., Johnstone, T., Backonja, M. M., Shackman, A. J., & Davidson, R. J. (2007). Individual differences in the effects of perceived controllability on pain perception: Critical role of the prefrontal cortex. *Journal of Cognitive Neuroscience, 19*, 993–1003.

Schacter, D. L. (1987). Implicit memory: History and current status. *Journal of Experimental Psychology: Learning, Memory, and Cognition, 13*, 501–518.

Schiller, D., Monfils, M., Raio, C. M., Johnson, D., LeDoux, J. E., & Phelps, E. A. (2010). Blocking the return of fear in humans using reconsolidation update mechanisms. *Nature, 463*, 49–53.

Schmidt, J. R., Crump, M. J., Cheesman, J., & Besner, D. (2007). Contingency learning without awareness: Evidence for implicit control. *Consciousness and Cognition, 16*, 421–435.

Scoville, W. B., & Milner, B. (1957). Loss of recent memory after bilateral hippocampal lesions. *Journal of Neurology, Neurosurgery, and Psychiatry, 20*, 11–21.

Sherman, J. W., Gawronski, B., Gonsalkorale, K., Hugenberg, K., Allen, T. J., & Groom, C. J. (2008). The self-regulation of automatic associations and behavioral impulses. *Psychological Review, 115*, 314–335.

Shiffrin, R., & Schneider, W. (1977). Controlled and automatic human information processing: II. Perceptual learning, automatic attending, and a general theory. *Psychological Review, 84,* 127–190.

Sloman, S. A. (1996). The empirical case for two systems of reasoning. *Psychological Bulletin, 119,* 3–22.

Smith, E. R., & DeCoster, J. (2000). Dual process models in social and cognitive psychology: Conceptual integration and links to underlying memory systems. *Personality and Social Psychology Review, 4,* 108–131.

Smith, E. R., & Semin, G. R. (2004). Socially situated cognition: Cognition in its social context. *Advances in Experimental Social Psychology, 36,* 53–117.

Squire, L. R. (1992). Memory and the hippocampus: A synthesis from findings with rats, monkeys, and humans. *Psychological Review, 99,* 195–231.

Squire, L. R., & Knowlton, B. J. (1994). Structure and function of declarative and nondeclarative memory systems. In M. S. Gazzaniga (Ed.), *The cognitive neurosciences.* Cambridge, MA: MIT Press.

Stanovich, K. E. (1999). *Who is rational?: Studies of individual differences in reasoning.* Mahwah, NJ: Erlbaum.

Stroop, J. R. (1935). Studies of interference in serial verbal reactions. *Journal of Experimental Psychology, 18,* 643–662.

Trope, Y. (1986). Identification and inferential processes in dispositional attribution. *Psychological Review, 93,* 239–257.

Uleman, J. S. (2005). Introduction: Becoming aware of the new unconscious. In R. R. Hassin, J. S. Uleman, & J. A. Bargh (Eds.), *The new unconscious* (pp. 3–15). New York: Oxford University Press.

Wager, T. D., Rilling, J. K., Smith, E. E., Sokolik, A., Casey, K. L., Davidson, R. J., et al. (2004). Placebo-induced changes in fMRI in the anticipation and experience of pain. *Science, 303,* 1162–1167.

Wegener, D. T., & Petty, R. E. (1997). The flexible correction model: The role of naive theories of bias in bias correction. In M. P. Zanna (Ed.), *Advances in experimental social psychology* (Vol. 29, pp. 141–208). Mahwah, NJ: Erlbaum.

Wegner, D. M. (1994). Ironic processes of mental control. *Psychological Review, 101,* 34–52.

Wegner, D. M., & Bargh, J. A. (1998). Control and automaticity in social life. In D. T. Gilbert, S. T. Fiske., & G. Lindzey (Eds.), *The handbook of social psychology, Vols. 1 and 2* (4th ed., pp. 446–496). New York: McGraw-Hill.

Wegner, D. M., Schneider, D. J., Carter, S., & White, T. (1987). Paradoxical effects of thought suppression. *Journal of Personality and Social Psychology, 53,* 5–13.

Weiner, B. (1986). *An attributional theory of motivation and emotion.* New York: Springer-Verlag.

Wilson, T. D., & Brekke, N. (1994). Mental contamination and mental correction: Unwanted influences on judgments and evaluations. *Psychological Bulletin, 116,* 117–142.

Wood, W., & Neal, D. T. (2007). A new look at habits and the interface between habits and goals. *Psychological Review, 114,* 843–863.

Yin, H. H., & Knowlton, B. J. (2006). The role of the basal ganglia in habit formation. *Nature Reviews Neuroscience, 7,* 464–476.

CHAPTER 38

Rethinking Duality
Criticisms and Ways Forward

Melissa J. Ferguson, Thomas C. Mann, and Michael T. Wojnowicz

The chapters in this volume are undoubtedly replete with examples of philosophers' and social scientists' historical recognition of the dual nature of human thought. Writers from the classical era through modern times have noted many times over that human behavior seems to emerge from dueling forces in the psyche (Newell, 1973), and contemporary social and cognitive psychologists have conceptualized these two forces as mental systems that can be studied empirically. In this chapter, we raise conceptual and methodological concerns about dual-mode models in the social cognitive psychological literature. In our view, the problems that fall out of a dual-mode approach to social cognitive research may outweigh its advantages.

Going beyond these concerns, we suggest new ways forward, including a reconsideration of how to think of dissociations between outcomes, and ways to understand the involvement of motivation and control in human thought. We also consider ways to test models of process and advocate for a greater emphasis on testing the independent role of the operating conditions in which a phenomenon emerges.

CRITICISMS OF DUALITY

Nomenclature

Before addressing the evidence for dual-mode models, we first note that much of the social cognitive literature could be clarified with greater precision of terminology, particularly regarding the terms *system*, *process*, and *representation* (e.g., for more discussion, see Evans, 2008; Ferguson & Fukukura, 2012; Gigerenzer & Regier, 1996; Keren & Schul, 2009; Moors & De Houwer, 2006; Newstead, 2000). One of the biggest sources of confusion, it seems to us, is the widely variable application of the term *system* and its tendency to be interchanged with *process*. This leads to confusion within and outside the field, as scholars working in areas such as cognition, neuroscience, and perception attempt to map their conception of *system* onto ours (and cannot).

Additionally, the terms *process* and *representation* are defined in typical ways that do not capture their complexity in the cognitive sciences literature. Whereas the use of *process* in the social psychological literature usually refers to associative versus rule-based operations (e.g., for definitions of these terms, see Chomsky, 1980, 1986; Hahn & Chater, 1998; Pylyshyn, 1980; Searle, 1980; Sloman, 1996; Smith, Langston, & Nisbett, 1992), the concept of representation usually refers to distributed versus symbolic (i.e., for definitions see e.g., Barsalou, 2008; Hahn & Chater, 1998; Sloman, 1996).And, these types of representation are often confounded with these types of process, in that it is assumed that rule-based processing depends solely (e.g., Sloman, 1996; but see discussion in Hahn & Chater, 1998) or partially (Smith & DeCoster, 2000) on symbolic representations, while associative processing (based on similarity or contiguity) is assumed exclusively to involve distributed representations (e.g., Bassili & Brown; Smith & DeCoster, 2000; cf. Hahn & Chater, 1998; Mitchell, Ames, Jenkins, & Banaji, 2009). In the cognitive sciences literature, however, some have argued that associative versus rule-based processing is not inherently wedded to one type of representation, and intense debate on the capacities and plausibility of each type of representation continues (e.g., Barsalou, 1999, 2008; Dietrich & Markman, 2003; Fodor, 1981; Rumelhart, 1989; Van Gelder, 1990). There is also a widespread tendency to confound what a process *does* (e.g., associative versus rule-based operations) with characteristics of its operation (e.g., awareness, intention, speed, control; Gawronski & Bodenhausen, 2009; Lieberman, 2003; Moors & De Houwer, 2006; Sherman, 2006a; Sherman et al., 2008). These continuous operating characteristics cannot be combined to form discrete (dual) processes or systems (see Keren & Schul, 2009, Logan, 1985; Moors & De Houwer, 2006) and also do not reliably or strongly correlate with process or with each other (see Bargh, 1994). For example, although it is widely assumed that associative processing occurs without awareness or control, there is in fact surprisingly little evidence for this (e.g., Berry, Shanks, Li, Rains, & Henson, 2010; Berry, Shanks, Speekenbrink, & Henson, 2012; Gawronski, Bodenhausen, & Becker, 2007; Mitchell et al., 2009).

How Convincing Are the Dissociation Data Suggesting Dual-Mode Models?

The evidence on which many dual-mode models rely consists of dissociations in which one manipulation impacts a first outcome but not a second, and a different manipulation impacts the second outcome but not the first (e.g., Gawronski & Bodenhausen, 2006; Rydell & McConnell, 2006; Rydell, McConnell, Mackie, & Strain, 2006; Wilson, Lindsey, & Schooler, 2000; for a review, see Chaiken & Trope, 1999). Such dissociation evidence is widely used at both the cognitive and the brain level to argue for separable functional processes (Dunn & Kirsner, 2003). Dissociations are consistent with two different underlying processes, but the problem is that they are also consistent with, and cannot dismiss, a single underlying process or system (Bedford, 2003; Chater, 2003; Dunn & Kirsner, 2003; Kinder & Shanks, 2001; Plaut, 1995). Such dissociations conclusively show only that some potentially small processing component is differentially sensitive to one manipulation but not another. For instance, take Chater's (2003) example of peanut allergy versus prawn allergy (two natural "manipulations"): In the first case, consumption of peanuts produces a systemic reaction but consumption of prawns does not, and in the second case, the reverse pattern emerges. Yet this dissociation proves nothing about dual digestive or immune systems. We know instead that this dissociation is produced by differential sensitivity of a single immune system to different foods (Keren & Schul, 2009; see also the not-the-liver fallacy; Bedford, 2003).

It is also the case that any dissociation data that emerge from the use of two different measures (e.g., implicit attitude measure vs. a Likert scale) are inherently inconclusive with regard to the involvement of two different processes (or systems) given that the (likely many) differences between any two measures can be orthogonal to process (Cunningham & Zelazo, 2007; Payne, 2005; Payne, Burkley, & Stokes, 2008; Sloman, 1996), and given recent evidence demonstrating that any measure likely captures multiple types of processes (e.g., Bishara & Payne, 2009; Conrey, Sherman, Gawronski, Hugenberg, & Groom, 2005; Sherman, 2006b). It is also important to note that even if different measures enable outcomes that seem more compatible with rule-based versus associative processes (e.g., truth testing), such evidence is equally inconclusive. As even Sloman (1996) argued, in general, it is impossible to rely on responses that manifest "associative" or "rule-like" qualities to argue for underlying process. The robustness of rules allows for any "associative" response to be modeled in terms of rules (also see Kruglanski & Dechesne, 2006; Kruglanski, Erb, Pierro, Mannetti, & Chun, 2006). Similarly, recent work with connectionist systems, which have been held up as the hardware implementing associative processing (e.g., Sloman, 1996; Smith & DeCoster, 2000), have proven capable of modeling deductive syllogisms (Rogers & McClelland, 2004), causal reasoning (Read & Montoya, 1999), executive control (Rougier, Noelle, Braver, Cohen, & O'Reilly, 2005) and serial-like processing (Spivey, 2007) all of which are usually held to characterize the rule-based system. In other words, outcomes that seem based in similarity or contiguity can still be modeled with rules, and outcomes that seem based in rule-based classification independent of similarity/contiguity can also be modeled in an associative-like structure. Outcomes might vary in different instances not because of fundamentally distinct systems or processes, but because of different parameter values within a single process (e.g., Shanks & Berry, 2012; Kruglanski et al., 2006).

Sloman (1996) argues that the best evidence that can be marshaled in support of dual-systems theories comes in the form of simultaneous contradictory belief ("Criterion S"). This refers to a conscious sense that two conflicting responses are both appropriate, *at the same moment in time*. Despite its logic, Criterion S presents a number of problems. The criterion is an inference about process drawn from introspection, which has well-documented limitations (Nisbett & Wilson, 1977). Any number of systems or processes might interact in complex ways in producing a conscious experience, which introspection likely can only imperfectly tap. It is also possible that even if beliefs are simultaneous, they may be produced by the same system. For example, it may be the case that "simultaneous contradictory beliefs" never actually occur per se; rather, people alternate quickly between different reasoning outcomes and merely report these as simultaneous (Osman, 2004). Or, a conflict could emerge from two contradictory rule-like beliefs (e.g., Chater, 2009). Or instances of manifest conflicting beliefs might truly reflect ambiguity about the application of particular rules (Betsch & Fiedler, 1999; Gigerenzer & Regier, 1996) and by some accounts should be present in any complex system that has many rules from which to select in any instance (Kelso & Engstrøm, 2006). Finally, even if one wishes to maintain that a given system must have a single output for any input, it is not clear why this output could not consist of a conscious state of ambivalence.

Finally, theorists sometimes use dissociation of brain activation to make the case for dual systems (e.g., Cushman, Young, & Greene, 2010; Lieberman, Gaunt, Gilbert, & Trope, 2002; Satpute & Lieberman, 2006; Smith & DeCoster, 2000; Spunt & Lieberman, 2013). For example, in their generalized dual-systems model, Smith and DeCoster (2000) cite the role of the hippocampus in implementing a fast-learning, effortful, symbolic processing system, and draw on lesion research to demonstrate the independence of this system from a slower, effortless one localized elsewhere. Such evidence suffers from the same issues cited earlier, such as the inability of dissociation evidence to establish two independent systems (e.g., Dunn & Kirsner, 2003). In fact, dissociations are possible in the case of lesions within nonmodular systems (Plaut, 1995).

Other evidence that is problematic for notions of independent systems at the level of neural hardware comes from what Anderson (2010) terms *neural reuse*. Under Anderson's (2007a, 2007b, 2010) conception, new functions are implemented in the brain by drawing on dispersed areas of cortex that previously participated in other functioning, such that localized brain regions come to participate in a variety of functions. In other words, a particular function (e.g., syllogistic reasoning) would be implemented not by a *dedicated* section or circuit of cortex, but by a pattern of activity among cortical elements that each participate in other functions when active in other combinations. These findings make it difficult to substantiate evidence that particular brain areas are the exclusive domain of any one particular type of processing, and they cast further doubt on the idea that even apparent cortical dissociations support dual-systems claims.

WAYS FORWARD

We believe the dual-mode approach has gotten entrenched, and its tentative status due to controversial data and theory is thus often obscured. For example, some of the key assumptions on which many social cognitive dual-mode theories are based are undermined by empirical findings and conceptual argument. These examples also stand as critiques of dual-mode theory, but they additionally point to new ways to conceptualize some general issues in the literature. We consider below two examples of such assumptions, then consider alternative ways to explain dissociated outcomes and the role of motivation.

Rethinking Learning

One of the most widely agreed upon differences between associative and rule-based processing, or between "System 1" and "System 2," is the rate or ease of learning. System 1 (or, associative processing) and System 2 (or, rule-based processing) are commonly referred to as the "slow" versus "fast" learning systems, respectively (for a review, see Conrey & Smith, 2007; cf. Gawronski & Bodenhausen, 2006, 2011; Gawronski & Bodenhausen, 2006, 2007, 2011). Many dual-mode theories assume that associative processes are slow learning because they consist of processes in the implicit memory system, and the implicit memory system has been historically characterized as slow learning. Rule-based processing, on the other hand, is thought to be fast learning, because it is enabled by the explicit memory system, which in turn is thought to be fast learning. In the social psychological literature, associative (or implicit) processing is therefore assumed to enable learning about a new event or pairing only after a long time, and after a large amount of experience. Rule-based, or symbolic or explicit processes, on the other hand, are assumed to enable learning after a single trial.

It is important to note that this assumption of learning is one of the most central criteria of most dual-mode models. This is because much of the argument for the necessity (functionality) of two independent systems consists of human and nonhuman animals' purported needs for both fast and slow learning (see Sherry & Schacter, 1987, for a discussion of the imperative for independent fast and slow learning systems in humans and other species). Thus, the evolutionary or functional explanation for two separate systems is based directly on (incompatible) learning needs.

Despite the centrality of the assumption of differential learning rates in many dual-mode models, much work calls this assumption into question in ways that highlight both the need to move beyond such conceptions and, importantly, strategies for doing so. First, contrary to widespread assumptions in the social cognitive literature, many scholars argue that implicit memory is actually composed of various kinds of processes that have fundamentally different characteristics, including learning rate (see Amodio & Ratner, 2011; Poldrack & Foerde, 2007; Squire & Kandel, 1999). For example, whereas semantic memory is often characterized as slow to develop (McClelland, McNaughton, & O'Reilly, 1995), aversive as well as appetitive conditioning can be acquired across animal models and in humans very rapidly, sometimes in a single trial (e.g., Cahill & McGaugh, 1990; Fanselow, 1990; Garcia, Kimeldorf, & Koelling, 1955; Hermer-Vazquez et al., 2005; LeDoux, 2000; Lossner & Rose, 1983; Rutishauser, Mamelak, & Schuman, 2006; Yin & Knowlton, 2006). Amodio and Ratner (2011) argue that it is misleading to assume that implicit (associative, "System 1") processes in social psychological phenomena rely on a single system that is characterized by one kind of learning. This conception (existing largely outside of social psychological literature) of memory and learning then directly challenges one of the most commonly accepted assumptions of almost all dual-mode models (for an exception, see Gawronski & Bodenhausen, 2006, 2011).

In addition to the data showing that appetitive and aversive conditioning (i.e., often assumed to be based on associative processing) can happen rapidly, there also exists another type of evidence of fast learning. Studies from the social cognitive attitudes literature show that participants can develop implicit (or System 1, associative-based) attitudes toward objects on the basis of new verbal (propositionally based) information learned only minutes earlier (Ashburn-

Nardo, Voils, & Monteith, 2001; Castelli, Zogmaister, Smith, & Arcuri, 2004; Gawronski et al., 2007; Gawronski & LeBel, 2008; Gregg, Seibt, & Banaji, 2006). This is especially interesting given that such verbal instructions are often presumed to depend on System 2 processing (Epstein, 1994; Rydell & McConnell, 2006). Gregg and colleagues (2006), for instance, asked participants to suppose that two novel groups, the Niffites and the Luppites, comprised good versus evil people. In an Implicit Association Test (IAT; Greenwald, McGhee, & Schwartz, 1998) administered 1 or 2 minutes later, they showed greater implicit preference for whichever group was described as good.

Even more recent work shows that people can even rapidly *revise* newly formed implicit attitudes based on very little propositional information. Cone and Ferguson (2012) predicted that people should show revision in their newly formed implicit attitudes for minimally self-relevant novel objects. When participants were assigned to groups based on (a bogus) personality test, they showed an implicit preference toward their ingroup only minutes later, providing further evidence that implicit attitudes can form extremely rapidly. However, the authors then told some of them that there was a mistake in their ingroup assignment and they actually belonged to the *other* group. Their implicit attitudes nevertheless then immediately showed a significant shift toward the other group, showing fast revision. Whereas previous work had found no evidence of fast revision of attitudes toward fictional groups that had no relevance to participants, this recent work shows that such revision commonly occurs when the novel attitude objects have some minimal relevance, such as one's ingroup. We also demonstrated that *revised* implicit attitudes toward a novel object were just as strong as their newly formed attitudes had been, suggesting that the evidence for fast revision was not implicit ambivalence (Petty, Tormala, Briñol, & Jarvis, 2006).

In summary, evidence from two different literatures (conditioning in animals and humans; social cognitive attitudes in humans) points strongly against the slow learning claims for System 1 types of processes, at least in the realm of attitudes. This kind of evidence may be interpreted in various ways: It can be seen as casting doubt on the learning rates typically linked with the two different modes, casting doubt on the assumption that there are only two modes, or challenging the need for separate systems or processes altogether. Relative to the last possibility, although the evidence for two (relatively independent) memory systems has been seen as strong, there are tenable challenges. Not only is there a fair amount of criticism of the evidence for two memory systems (e.g., Hintzman, 1990; Howe, Rabinowitz, & Grant, 1993; Ostergaard, 1992; see Poldrack, 1996, for a review), but also researchers have started to examine computational models to test the claims of a single versus multiple systems. Shanks and Berry and their colleagues (Berry, Shanks, & Henson, 2008a, 2008b; Berry et al., 2012; Shanks & Berry, 2012; Shanks & Perruchet, 2002) have developed mathematical models of single memory systems based on signal detection theory (SDT), and have found strong support for a single- versus dual-memory system (see also Craik, 1983; Kolers & Roediger, 1984). This work (see Shanks & Berry, 2012) assumes that the dissociation data (from priming vs. recognition tasks) interpreted as support for separate implicit and explicit memory systems can be modeled using a simple SDT model that assumes a single process. One of the key ideas here is that in both priming (i.e., implicit) and recognition (i.e., explicit) tasks, there is the *same* underlying source of memory trace (one process), but the tasks differ in the type and amount of nonmemorial noise. They argue that dissociations between these types of tasks in fact emerge from these different types of noise that obscure to varying degrees the same underlying signal of the memory trace. The progression and implications of this work are obviously highly relevant for social cognitive theorizing.

In summary, we have outlined some evidence and theory that challenge one of the major foundations upon which most of the dual-mode theory is built, the existence of two memory systems and the different learning rate between them. What remains is a comprehensive examination of the conditions under which implicit attitudes and processes more generally show fast versus slow change (see Ferguson & Fukukura, 2012). For example, there are obviously differences in the types of manipulations that produce change on implicit versus explicit measures (e.g., see Gawronski & Bodenhausen, 2006), and the reasons for such dissociations remain unclear. Our point here is that we may not necessarily have to go to a dual-mode model in order to explain such differences. We have outlined the various nonprocess reasons that could potentially explain such dissociation data, and the burden is now on theorists to generate single-system alternatives to the current crop of dual-mode explanations.

Rethinking "Symbolic" Thought in "System 1"

Perhaps one of the strongest arguments for "System 2" processes and representations is that some kinds of cognition seem to require symbolic, syntactically structured thought, such as language, probability, logic, and math (Dietrich & Markman, 2003; Fodor & Pylyshyn, 1988). This debate has often centered on the requirements of language and its observed productivity, systematicity, and compositionality. In terms of productivity, whereas associative thought is assumed by many to be merely reproductive, in that it is limited to whatever we have experienced in the past, we must also have some form of thinking that is productive so as to be able to deal with totally novel situations. For instance, as Chomsky (1968) speculated, we can generate an infinite number of propositions (claims), and this unboundedness could not come from associative thought. *Systematicity* refers to the fact that our ability to understand that "Mary loves John" implies our ability to understand that "John loves Mary." And *compositionality* refers to the fact that our ability to understand that "Mary loves John" is a function of our understanding of its constituent parts, "Mary," "loves," and "John."

However, the claims that these characteristics can only be generated by rule-based thinking have been refuted in a number of ways, through either argument (Chalmers, 1990, 1993; Smolensky, 1988; Van Gelder, 1990) or examples of connectionist models that show these characteristics (Chalmers, 1990; Elman, 1990; Pollack, 1990; Smolensky, 1990). (Note that even Sloman, 1996, did not agree with the claim that associative processing is merely reproductive.) There is now an impressive body of evidence demonstrating, for example, that various characteristics of language can be modeled successfully with connectionist networks (e.g., Christiansen & Chater, 2001, 2009; McClelland, Plaut, Gotts, & Maia, 2003). Thus, the common claims that System 2 is more "verbal" or language-based seem unwarranted.

There are related and frequently asserted claims that only (conscious) rule-based processing could enable the reading of multiword phrases and abstract mathematics (e.g., Deutsch, Gawronski, & Strack, 2006; Greenwald & Liu, 1985, 1992; Baumeister & Masicampo, 2010; Morewedge & Kahneman, 2010; Winkielman, 2008; but see, e.g., Anderson, Spoehr, & Bennett, 1994). However, recent work challenges this assumption by showing that people can solve math problems and read multiword phrases nonconsciously (Sklar, Levy, Goldstein, Mandel, Maril, & Hassin, 2012). Sklar and colleagues used a recently developed method called continuous flash suppression (Tsuchiya & Koch, 2005), which consists of presentation of material (e.g., an equation) to one eye with a simultaneous presentation of rapidly changing masks (noise) to the other eye. The continuous flashes of noise to the one eye keep the static information to the other eye below conscious awareness, for up to 2 seconds. For nonconscious reading, Sklar and colleagues (2012) showed that participants were able to nonconsciously process whether the meaning of three-word sentences constituted a semantic violation (e.g., "I ironed coffee") or not ("I ironed clothes"). As for evidence of nonconscious arithmetic, when presented with equations (e.g., 2 + 3 + 5 = . . .), participants responded significantly faster to solutions of those equations (e.g., 10) than to nonsolutions (e.g., 11). The findings show that cognitive operations that classically are assumed to be uniquely enabled by rule-based thinking can occur nonconsciously.

These findings are a perfect example of how the notion of process (in this case, rule-based vs. associative) could potentially be confounded with a characteristic of the operation of the process (consciousness). To the extent that one believes that rule-based processing has to be conscious (confounding the two), these findings would indicate that the process at play here cannot be rule-based (and could, instead, be associative). However, if one believes, as we do, that the operating characteristics of a process are orthogonal to what it is the process is doing (following rules vs. operating by similarity and contiguity), then one would not necessarily believe that rule-based processing has to be accompanied by consciousness (e.g., Sloman, 1996). So, therefore, these data are agnostic about what the process is, and instead tell us simply that these outcomes that have been historically branded as consciousness-dependent (reading, doing math), however they are enabled or solved, can in fact operate without consciousness.

Rethinking Dissociated Outcomes

We noted earlier that many scholars interpret empirical dissociations across (implicit vs. explicit) behavioral measures as evidence for two different systems, or processes. We also noted that a dual-mode model is certainly consistent with such dissociation. But such evidence could also be consistent with a single-system/process model. What type of single-system model might explain such dissociations? Let's consider a prototypical case of dissociation in social psychology: the difference in attitudes toward racial/ethnic groups as a function of whether an implicit versus explicit measure is used. For example, when racial outgroup attitudes are measured after relatively short cognitive processing durations (e.g., on the IAT), they often appear negative, whereas when the same attitudes are measured after relatively long processing durations (e.g., through self-report), they often appear more positive, or egalitarian (e.g., Dovidio, Kawakami, & Gaertner, 2002).

The dual-mode interpretation of these data is that whereas the "fast" attitudes are explained by System 1, the endorsed responses are often explained by System 2 (or a combination of System 1 and System 2; see Gawronski & Bodenhausen, 2006; Strack & Deutsch, 2004). A single-system interpretation, on the other hand, comes from the mathematical modeling of dynamical systems (Hirsch & Smale, 1974). *Dynamical systems models* (technically, coupled differential equations) describe the dynamics of a group of multiple interacting components. Dynamical systems frequently exhibit a property of *self-organization* (e.g., Kelso 1995); that is, the system's components gradually assemble themselves from a disordered state into an ordered state, and they do so without a central executive directing those changes. The key idea here rests on the mathematical concept of an "attractor." To put the key concepts together, the dynamical system comprises multiple components that interact.The *state* of the system is a pattern of numbers that describe each component's value at some particular time. After the system has been externally perturbed, for example, by a stimulus, (this is called an *initial condition*), the "dynamics" describe how the system moves itself, toward particular states (called the *stable states* or "attractors" of the system).

In cognitive science, the brain has been considered a dynamical *system* by many theorists (e.g., Beer, 1995; Kelso, 1995; Spivey, 2007). The brain comprises multiple interacting components (brain regions, or neurons), and it is continuously perturbed by external forces (stimulation from sensory receptors), but it responds to these perturbations according to its own internal principles for componentwise interactions (the brain regions or neurons interact due to patterns of synaptic connectivity between spiking neurons; see, e.g., Hopfield, 1984; Izhikevich, 2007). Now what might an attractor be in the brain? Let's first illustrate the concept of an attractor in a simple one-dimensional system. Consider a "system" that is simply the height of a tennis ball above the ground. Imagine that someone drops a tennis ball from the Space Needle (650 ft. above the ground) with zero velocity. That state (of being 650 ft. above the ground) is highly unstable, and the ball is pushed to the ground (by the force of gravity). Thus, the "attractor" in that simple system is the ground (more specifically, the height of 0 ft.). Dynamical systems approaches to neural cognition extend this concept to the brain by considering it as a high-dimensional system whose components are neurons and whose state is, for example, the current firing rate of each neuron. The dynamical systems perspective observes that certain firing configurations could be highly unstable, because of the network effect of communication between neurons: Learned patterns of synaptic connectivity cause one neuron's firing to influence, whether directly or indirectly, the firing of other neurons in the network. Recurrent connectivity between neuronal regions, and or lateral inhibition, can cause the neural firing patterns eventually to "settle" or converge into certain predetermined, interpretable neural patterns (e.g., Wang, 2001). Thus, the brain is pushed into relatively stable firing patterns, representing relatively coherent, interpretable representations (e.g., "I see Professor Spivey," rather than "I see a person 40% likely to be Professor Spivey, 35% likely to be my brother-in-law, and so forth"; see Spivey, 2007). Indeed, there is evidence for the existence of attractors in many neural systems (e.g., the olfactory system: Mazor & Laurent, 2005; the hippocampus: Wills, Lever, Cacucci, Burgess, & O'Keefe, 2005; the prefrontal cortex: Durstewitz, Kelc, & Gunturkun, 1999; the lateral intraparietal (LIP) area: Ganguli et al., 2008).

What are the implications for attitudes toward groups of people? Dynamical systems can explain some basic dissociation phenomena (e.g., how early negative biases morph into personally endorsed positive decisions), without stipulating two deciders. Early biases may be exhibited as a single mental system transitions through multiple intermediate decision states en route to its finalized decision. This notion of intermediate tentative decision states is common in the mathematical modeling of neural decisions (see Bogacz, Brown, Moehlis, Holmes, & Cohen, 2006), even in the simple drift-diffusion models that accumulate sensory evidence over time. But the more neurobiologically detailed decision-making models are often endowed with recurrent feedback and/or lateral inhibition, two fundamental features of neurobiological processing (O'Reilly, 1998). These decision-making models are no longer just accumulators of evidence; they are now dynamical systems harboring attractors. That is, these dynamical systems do not stop processing when the incoming evidence is shut off; they gravitate automatically from certain regions of space (the "unstable" regions of space, usually representing blends of multiple decisions or interpretations) into other regions of space (the "stable" regions of space, usually representing coherent singular interpretations or decisions). Many detailed models of neural decision making incorporate these features: for example, the competing accumulator model (Usher & McClelland, 2001), the normalized recurrence model (Spivey, 2007), the recurrent neural circuit model (e.g., Wong & Wang, 2006), and the dynamical field theory model (Erlhagen & Schöner, 2002).

The important observation is that just as a bird can fly toward its nest through multiple pathways, a dynamical neural system can transition into its eventual decision (stable firing pattern) according to potentially very many different trajectories (its continuously evolving firing patterns over the preceding temporal period). Let us imagine from a macro-scale (as does normalized recurrence; Spivey, 2007) that the typical brain comprises a number of informational sources (personal memories, semantic information, emotional associations, future goals, etc.), each of which provides partial probabilistic support for a certain evaluative decision (e.g., liking vs. disliking white or black Americans). From a dynamical systems perspective, the decision is made when the conflict distributed across the cacophonous system is resolved into a single harmonious decision. A dynamical systems model (e.g., any of the ones listed earlier) describes the dynamics of this decision process; in particular, it describes how a certain initial set of conflicts across informational sources dynamically resolves into a decision. Let us first assume that, as self-reports suggest, white people in general possess greater overall informational support for "liking" rather "disliking" both black people and white people. However, let us further assume that, as IAT findings suggest, white people nevertheless harbor greater conflict among their information sources when they have to decide whether they like black people then when they do the same about white people. Then a stochastic dynamical systems model makes very particular predictions about the dynamics of the decision—qualitative predictions that can be "read off" the equations of the previous models (see, e.g., the introduction to Wojnowicz, Ferguson, Dale, & Spivey, 2009). In particular, such models predict that the decision would exhibit *deviation* (a general trend of moving through regions of decision space with greater input of dislike in the transitional moments of mental processing), *disorder* (brief excursions toward a dislike interpretation rather than a like interpretation), and *acceleration* (i.e., processing of the decision would accelerate over time; the simultaneous activation of multiple alternative decisions causes excess activation in the neural system, thus artificially slowing processing due to lateral inhibition).

The dynamical perspective on explicit attitude formation was supported by recent research analyzing hand movement trajectories taken by participants during their like versus dislike evaluations of racial groups (Wojnowicz et al., 2009). Participants were asked to click on "LIKE" or "DISLIKE" response boxes (in the upper corners of the computer screen) to report their evaluations of a series of stimuli. The key stimuli, "black people" and "white people" were embedded within a large set of distractor stimuli, such as "ice cream" and "Hitler." The results were that participants tended to select "LIKE" for both white people and black people. However, while participants were selecting "LIKE" for black people, their hands exhibited significant greater curvature toward the "DISLIKE" response box. Moreover, their hand movement patterns exhibited greater disorder and greater acceleration.

These results suggest that the dissociated measurements of racial evaluations (more specifically, the fact that among white participants a "black people" stimulus yields negative evaluations on IAT measures and positive evaluations on self-reports, whereas a "white people" stimulus yields positive evaluations on both) may be explained, at least in part, by the way in which a dynamical cognitive system processes high levels of conflict. According to dynamical systems theory, when a person must choose between two possible options, and when there is relatively high conflict distributed across multiple sources of informational support (memories of personal experiences, emotional associations, semantic knowledge, etc.), then the system will deliver relatively strong support for the nonendorsed option during early moments of mental processing. This is precisely what is observed in implicit measures of racial evaluation. Critically, this perspective can be interpreted as a single system or process. In particular, from the dynamical systems perspective, mental processing is described according to a single set of neurobiologically plausible principles that are common to many brain regions (O'Reilly, 1998), so there is no "ontological gulf" between two incommensurate systems (i.e., System 1 and System 2). That is, both the early implicit biases and the later endorsed decision are part and parcel of a single process—the dynamic evolution of a distributed parallel mental representation.

There is increasing research in social psychology that shows how a dynamical systems perspective can be applied to classical social psychological questions (for reviews, see Freeman & Ambady, 2010; Freeman, Dale, & Farmer, 2011). One important contribution is that this work allows an examination of real-time processing by using the motor movements of a hand, for example, as a proxy for ongoing cognition. This provides an incredibly fine-grained temporal profile of how decisions unfold in real time, and can reveal outcomes that differ from the typical implicit measures of response times (e.g., Song & Nakayama, 2006, 2008; Wojnowicz et al., 2009). However, another contribution is that this work can address the single- versus multiple-mode question. Whenever there are claims about how one system or process transitions to another (in a discrete or continuous fashion), the dynamical systems perspective and its associated methodological tools (mouse tracking, eye tracking) can directly test those claims. We view this as an exciting new direction in social cognition work, particularly given its applicability to theory about (the number of) systems and processes.

Rethinking Goals and Control

The dynamical systems perspective is also currently being used to help explain goal pursuit and executive control while invoking brain systems as interacting parallel distributed processing networks, although this work is more recent. Modeling the functionalities of goal pursuit and executive control generally require multiple brain systems (the prefrontal cortex, basal ganglia, posterior cortex, etc., are regions that have functionally meaningful specializations in terms of neuromodulation, connectivity patterns, firing rate stability, etc.), but at the same time, these multiple brain systems are well defined as parallel distributed processing networks, whose cognitive processing is characterized by interaction both inside and between brain regions, and conform to a single set of shared processing principles, such as distributed processing, lateral inhibition, and recurrent feedback (O'Reilly, 1998).

One major question is how people pursue distant goals through a parallel distributed processing network—an approach differing from that of some of the dual-mode theories that see the pursuit of distant goals as requiring inherently discrete logical rules in a serial processing system (e.g., Strack & Deutsch, 2004). As a solution to this problem, recent work in computational neuroscience has investigated how the basal ganglia serve as an "adaptive critic" of the rest of the brain, instantiating a type of learning known as reinforcement learning (e.g., Montague, Dayan & Sejnowski, 1996). The term *reinforcement learning,* unfortunately, sounds antiquated, conjuring up Skinner's no longer influential notion that higher-order cognition can be explained by very simple procedures for learning knee-jerk reactions to the environment. However, the label is misleading. Contemporary reinforcement learning approaches are relatively quite sophisticated (see Fukukura, Helzer, & Ferguson, 2013), and they demonstrate how "merely associative" stimulus–response mechanisms could subserve the complex, strategic pursuit of distant goals. According to this literature, brains contain an internal critic that tracks the "value" of transitions between various environmental states (or their cortical representations; see Montague et al., 1996). Whenever the person reaches a more highly valued state than expected, the critic sends out an internally manufactured dopaminergic reward signal. Using these dopaminergic reward signals, the "adaptive critic" (located in the basal ganglia) determines the value of being in a particular state. Using these value assessments, the adaptive critic trains the rest of the brain to choose behaviors that subserve a person's strategic goals, even when pursuing the goal will require repeated deliberation at multiple junctures deep into the future. What these findings mean, in effect, is that the frequently derided notion of stimulus–response associations can be actually quite intelligent. These associations are far more sophisticated than brutish knee-jerk reactions to immediate pleasure and pain; instead, the strength of these associations can capture, in a single quantity, complex information about how to maximize the expected value of an arbitrarily distant future. In fact, when stimulus–response associations are sculpted by an internal critic, they can guide an agent to successful performance even in penultimate logical, rule-based tasks, such as backgammon or chess games (see Sutton & Barto, 1998). Although assessing the value of an action in the face of such dynamic iterative stochastic loops is complicated, recent work in reinforcement learning has determined that it is possibly in theory (e.g., Houk, Adams, & Barto, 1995), and that the brain seems to be making such computations (e.g., Dayan & Daw, 2008).

Similar work has extended these findings to explain how the prefrontal cortex can subserve executive control functionalities, without depending upon explicit logical rules (Rougier et al., 2005) or employing a distinct form of computation (e.g., discrete logical symbolic thought). Aligning one's behavior with respect to transient goals is part of what is meant by psychological control —in particular by the capacity of "flexible top-down processing." O'Reilly and Frank (2006) argue that flexible top-down processing is subserved by the prefrontal cortex due to that region's distinct neurocomputational features. In particular, prefrontal cortical neurons are characterized (compared to, say, posterior cortical neurons) by their abilities (1) to actively maintain goal-related information, (2) to flexibly update representations in response to dopaminergic signals (of value), and (3) to send widespread feedback to the rest of the brain. In this way, the prefrontal cortex can strategically bias lower-level sensory representations or attentional resources in a way that subserves goal-related needs (e.g., Miller & Cohen, 2001). The way that this "flexible top-down processing" region can interactively influence the brain is described in O'Reilly and Frank's (2006) dynamic gating model of prefrontal control. Importantly, this model implements motivated control through multiple interacting parallel-processing brain regions, fundamentally characterized by interaction both inside and between brain regions. What justifies the use of the term *multiple* systems or brain regions is not distinct computational formats (i.e., symbolic vs. distributed representations) or a wall of separation between the systems (whereby communication is unclear), but rather the fact that the nature of the parallel distributed processing inside has important fundamental differences (neuromodulators, network centrality, etc.). Recent theoretical work on multiple interacting systems (Ferguson & Wojnowicz, 2011) has examined how this "multiple interacting systems" model of executive control could explain the social psychological phenomenon of evaluative readiness (Ferguson, 2008). The primary idea is that the prefrontal cortex serves to dynamically project the high-dimensional dynamics of the posterior cortical system in such a way that it best subserves motivational needs (see Ferguson & Wojnowicz, 2011).

CONCLUSION

We have outlined some criticisms of dual-mode theory, as well as ways to move beyond the criticisms. We now conclude by making two suggestions. The first is that, in our view, the question of rule-based versus associative processing can only be convincingly tested using computational model testing. Computational models consist of assigning computational programs that specify algorithms (e.g., rule-following) for cognitive functions. Critically, these computational programs are then runnable and can be tested for how they fit behavioral data. We view computational models as the most informative type of model testing (e.g., Hintzman, 1990; Newell, 1990; Sun, 2008), because they provide highly specified (both procedurally and conceptually) predictions that can be formally tested and compared with human (or animal) data. Most of the computational work in social psychology over the last few decades has consisted of connectionist models (Read & Monroe, 2008). There is almost no application of symbolic models such as Adaptive Character of Thought–Rational (ACT-R; Anderson, 1993; Anderson & Lebiere, 1998) or CLARION (Sun, Slusarz, & Terry, 2005), or hybrid models (e.g., Smolensky, 1988) to social psychological phenomena. This is possibly a missed opportunity given that social cognitive dual-process models strongly postulate rule-based processing (and/or symbolic representations).

Our second suggestion is to advocate for greater testing of the operating characteristics of a process—in other words, the dimensions such as awareness, resources, control, speed, and intention, according to which phenomena emerge (e.g., see Moors & De Houwer, 2006). In our view, such information is valuable, necessary, and informative, and might even be of greater interest to our field than the identification of rule-based versus associative processing. In fact, the operating characteristics that are studied most often in the context of dual-mode theories include awareness, intention, control, and effort. The common currency of subjective experience among these characteristics most often studied by social psychologists is undoubtedly no accident, and knowledge about the extent and nature of phenomena that can emerge outside of, or only with, our subjective consent or awareness will probably continue to be of interest to our field, and to those outside of it (e.g., Ross, Lepper, & Ward, 2010).

REFERENCES

Amodio, D. M., & Ratner, K. (2011). A memory systems model of implicit social cognition. *Current Directions in Psychologica Science, 20,* 143–148.

Anderson, J. R. (1993). *Rules of the mind.* Hillsdale, NJ: Erlbaum.

Anderson, J. R., Lebiere, C. (1998). *The atomic components of thought.* Mahwah, NJ: Erlbaum.

Anderson, M. L. (2007a). Evolution of cognitive function via redeployment of brain areas. *The Neuroscientist, 13,* 13–21.

Anderson, M. L. (2007b). The massive redeployment hypothesis and the functional topography of the brain. *Philosophical Psychology, 21,* 143–174.

Anderson, M. L. (2010). Neural reuse: A fundamental organizational principle of the brain. *Behavioral and Brain Sciences, 33,* 245–266.

Anderson, J. A., Spoehr, K. T., & Bennett, D. J. (1994). A study in numerical perversity: Teaching arithmetic to a neural network. In

D. S. Levine & M. Aparicio, IV (Eds.), *Neural networks for knowledge representation and inference* (pp. 311–335). Hillsdale, NJ: Erlbaum.

Ashburn-Nardo, L., Voils, C., & Monteith, M. (2001). Implicit associations as the seeds of intergroup bias: How easily do they take root? *Journal of Personality and Social Psychology, 81*, 789–799.

Bargh, J. A. (1994). The four horsemen of automaticity: Awareness, intention, efficiency, and control in social cognition. In R. S. Wyer, Jr., & T. K. Srull (Eds.), *Handbook of social cognition* (Vol. 2, pp. 1–40). Hillsdale, NJ: Erlbaum.

Barsalou, L. W. (1999). Perceptual symbol systems. *Behavioral and Brain Sciences, 22*, 577–660.

Barsalou, L. W. (2008). Grounded cognition. *Annual Review of Psychology, 59*, 617–645.

Bassili, J. N., & Brown, R. (2005). Implicit and explicit attitudes: Research, challenges and theory. In D. Albarracín, B. T. Johnson, & M. P. Zanna (Eds.), *Handbook of attitudes and attitude change* (pp. 543–574). Mahwah, NJ: Erlbaum.

Baumeister, R. F., & Masicampo, E. J. (2010). Conscious thought is for facilitating social and cultural interactions: How mental simulations serve the animal–culture interface. *Psychological Review, 117*, 945– 971.

Bedford, F. L. (2003). More on the not-the-liver fallacy: Medical, neuropsychological, and perceptual dissociations. *Cortex, 39*, 170–173.

Beer, R. D. (1995). A dynamical systems perspective on agent–environment interaction. *Artificial Intelligence, 72*(1–2), 173–215.

Berry, C. J., Shanks, D. R., & Henson, R. N. A. (2008a). A unitary signal-detection model of implicit and explicit memory. *Trends in Cognitive Sciences, 12*(10), 367–373.

Berry, C. J., Shanks, D. R., & Henson, R. N. A. (2008b). A single-system account of the relationship between priming, recognition, and fluency. *Journal of Experimental Psychology: Learning, Memory, and Cognition, 34*, 97–111.

Berry, C. J., Shanks, D. R., Li, S., Rains, L. S., & Henson, R. N. A. (2010). Can "pure" implicit memory be isolated?: A test of a single-system model of recognition and repetition priming. *Canadian Journal of Experimental Psychology, 64*, 241–255.

Berry, C. J., Shanks, D. R., Speekenbrink, M., & Henson, R. N. A. (2012). Models of recognition, repetition priming, and fluency: Exploring a new framework. *Psychological Review, 119*(1), 40–79.

Betsch, T., & Fiedler, K. (1999). Understanding conjunction effects: The role of implicit mental models. *European Journal of Social Psychology, 29*, 75–93.

Bishara, A. J., & Payne, B. (2009). Multinomial process tree models of control and automaticity in weapon misidentification. *Journal of Experimental Social Psychology, 45*(3), 524–534.

Bogacz, R., Brown, E., Moehlis, J., Holmes, P., & Cohen, J. D. (2006). The physics of optimal decision making: A formal analysis of models of performance in two-alternative forced-choice tasks. *Psychological Review, 113*(4), 700–765.

Cahill, L., & McGaugh, J. (1990). Amygdala complex lesions differentially affect retention of tasks using appetitive and aversive reinforcement. *Behavioral Neuroscience, 10*, 532–543.

Castelli, L., Zogmaister, C., Smith, E. R., & Arcuri, L. (2004). On the automatic evaluation of social exemplars. *Journal of Personality and Social Psychology, 86*, 373–387.

Chaiken, S., & Trope, Y. (Eds.). (1999). *Dual-process theories in social psychology.* New York: Guilford Press.

Chalmers, D. (1990). Why Fodor and Pylyshyn were wrong: The simplest refutation. In *Proceedings of the 12th Annual Conference of the Cognitive Science Society.* Hillsdale, NJ: Erlbaum.

Chalmers, D. (1993). *Connectionism and compositionality: Why Fodor and Pylyshyn were wrong. Philosophical Psychology*, 5–19.

Chater, N. (2003). How much can we learn from double dissociations. *Cortex, 39*, 167–169.

Chater, N. (2009). Rational and mechanistic perspectives on reinforcement learning. *Cognition, 113*, 350–364.

Chomsky, N. (1968). *Language and mind.* New York: Harcourt, Brace & World.

Chomsky, N. (1980). *Rules and representations.* New York: Columbia University Press.

Chomsky, N. (1986). *Knowledge of language: Its nature, origin, and use.* Westport, CT: Prager.

Christiansen, M. H., & Chater, N. (2001). Connectionist psycholinguistics: Capturing the empirical data. *Trends in Cognitive Sciences, 5*, 82–88.

Christiansen, M. H., & Chater, N. (2009). The myth of language universals and the myth of universal grammar. *Behavioral and Brain Sciences, 32,* 452–453.

Cone, J., & Ferguson, M. (2012). *Changing your implicit mind: On the rapid formation and revision of implicit attitudes.* Unpublished manuscript, Cornell University, Ithaca, NY.

Conrey, F. R., Sherman, J. W., Gawronski, B., Hugenberg, K., & Groom, C. (2005). Separating multiple processes in implicit social cognition: The quad model of implicit task performance. *Journal of Personality and Social Psychology, 89,* 469–487.

Conrey, F. R., & Smith, E. (2007). Attitude representation: Attitudes as patterns in a distributed, connectionist representational system. *Social Cognition, 25,* 718–735.

Craik, F. I. M. (1983). On the transfer of information from temporary to permanent memory. *Philosophical Transactions of the Royal Society of London Series B: Biological Sciences, 302* (1110), 341–359.

Cunningham, W. A., & Zelazo, P. D. (2007). Attitudes and evaluations: A social cognitive neuroscience perspective. *Trends in Cognitive Sciences, 11,* 97–104.

Cushman, F., Young, L., & Greene, J. D. (2010). Multi-system moral psychology. In J. Doris, G. Harman, S. Nichols, J. Prinz, W. Sinnott-Armstrong, & S. Stich (Eds.), *The Oxford handbook of moral psychology* (pp. 47–71). Oxford, UK: Oxford University Press.

Dayan, P., & Daw, N. D. (2008). Decision theory, reinforcement learning, and the brain. *Cognitive Affective and Behavioral Neuroscience, 8,* 429–453.

Deutsch, R., Gawronski, B., & Strack, F. (2006). At the boundaries of automaticity: Negation as reflective operation. *Journal of Personality and Social Psychology, 91*(3), 385–405.

Dietrich, E., & Markman, A. (2003). Discrete thoughts: Why cognition must use discrete representations. *Mind and Language, 18,* 95–119.

Dovidio, J. F., Kawakami, K., & Gaertner, S. L. (2002). Implicit and explicit prejudice and interracial interaction. *Journal of Personality and Social Psychology, 82*(1), 62–68.

Dunn, J. C., & Kirsner, K. (2003). What can we infer from double dissociations. *Cortex, 39,* 1–7.

Durstewitz, D., Kelc, M., & Gunturkun, O. (1999). A neurocomputational theory of the dopaminergic modulation of working memory functions. *Journal of Neuroscience, 19,* 2807–2822.

Elman, J. L. (1990). Representation and structure in connectionist models. In G. Altmann (Ed.), *Cognitive models of speech processing* (pp. 345–382). Cambridge, MA: MIT Press.

Epstein, S. (1994). Integration of the cognitive and psychodynamic unconscious. *American Psychologist, 49,* 709–724.

Erlhagen, W., & Schöner, G. (2002). Dynamic field theory of movement preparation. *Psychological Review, 109*(3), 545–572.

Evans, J. S. (2008). Dual-processing accounrs of reasonins, judgment, and social cognition, *Annual Review of Psychology, 59,* 255–278.

Evans, J. (2009). How many dual-process theories do we need?: One, two, or many? In J. Evans & K. Frankish (Eds.), *In two minds: Dual processes and beyond* (pp. 33–54). Oxford, UK: Oxford University Press.

Fanselow, M. S. (1990). Factors governing one trial contextual conditioning. *Animal Learning and Behavior, 18,* 264–270.

Ferguson, M. J. (2008). On becoming ready to pursue a goal you don't know you have: Effects of nonconscious goals on evaluative readiness. *Journal of Personality and Social Psychology, 95*(6), 1268–1294.

Ferguson, M. J., & Fukukura, J. (2012). Likes and dislikes: A social cognitive perspective. In S. Fiske & C. N. Macrae (Eds.), *Sage handbook of social cognition* (pp. 165–189). Los Angeles, CA: Sage.

Ferguson, M. J., & Wojnowicz, M. (2011). The when and how of evaluative readiness: A social cognitive neuroscience perspective. *Personality and Social Psychology Compass, 5,* 1018–1038.

Fodor, J. (1981). *RePresentations: Philosophical essays on the foundations of cognitive science.* Cambridge, MA: MIT Press.

Fodor, J. (1983). *Modularity of mind: An essay on faculty psychology.* Cambridge, MA: MIT Press.

Fodor, J., & Pylyshyn, Z. (1988). Connectionism and cognitive architecture: A critical analysis. In S. Pinker & J. Mehler (Eds.), *Connections and symbols* (pp. 3–71). Cambridge, MA: MIT Press.

Freeman, J. B., & Ambady, N. (2010). MouseTracker: Software for studying real-time mental processing using a computer mouse-tracking method. *Behavior Research Methods, 42,* 226–241.

Freeman, J. B., Dale, R., & Farmer, T. A. (2011).

Hand in motion reveals mind in motion. *Frontiers in Psychology, 2*, 59.

Fukukura, J., Helzer, E. G., & Ferguson, M. J. (2013). Prospection by any other name? A response to Seligman et al. *Perspectives on Psychological Science, 8*, 146–150.

Ganguli, S., Bisley, J. W., Roitman, J. D., Shadlen, M. N., Goldberg, M. E., & Miller, K. D. (2008). One-dimensional dynamics of attention and decision making in LIP. *Neuron, 58*(1), 15–25.

Garcia, J., Kimeldorf, D., & Koelling, R. (1955). Conditioned aversion to saccharin resulting from exposure to gamma radiation. *Science, 122*, 157–158.

Gawronski, B., & Bodenhausen, G. V. (2006). Associative and propositional processes in evaluation: An integrative review of implicit and explicit attitude change. *Psychological Bulletin, 132*, 692–731.

Gawronski, B., & Bodenhausen, G. V. (2007). Unraveling the processes underlying evaluation: Attitudes from the perspective of the APE Model. *Social Cognition, 25*, 687–717.

Gawronski, B., & Bodenhausen, G. V. (2009). Operating principles versus operating conditions in associative and propositional processes. *Behavioral and Brain Sciences, 32*, 207–208.

Gawronski, B., & Bodenhausen, G. V. (2011). The associative–propositional evaluation model: Theory, evidence, and open questions. *Advances in Experimental Social Psychology, 44*, 59–127.

Gawronski, B., Bodenhausen, G. V., & Becker, A. P. (2007). I like it, because I like myself: Associative self-anchoring and post-decisional change of implicit evaluations. *Journal of Experimental Social Psychology, 43*, 221–232.

Gawronski, B., & LeBel, E. P. (2008). Understanding patterns of attitude change: When implicit measures show change, but explicit measures do not. *Journal of Experimental Social Psychology, 44*, 1355–1361.

Gigerenzer, G., & Regier, T. (1996). How do we tell an association from a rule?: Comment on Sloman (1996). *Psychological Bulletin, 119*, 23–26.

Gregg, A., Seibt, B., & Banaji, M. (2006). Easier done than undone: Asymmetry in the malleability of implicit preferences. *Journal of Personality and Social Psychology, 90*, 1–20.

Greenwald, A. G. (1992). New Look 3: Reclaiming unconscious cognition. *American Psychologist, 47*, 766–779.

Greenwald, A. G., & Liu, T. J. (1985). Limited unconscious processing of meaning. *Bulletin of the Meetings of the Psychonomic Society, 23*, 292–313.

Greenwald, A. G., McGhee, D. E., & Schwartz, J. L. K. (1998). Measuring individual differences in implicit cognition: The Implicit Association Test. *Journal of Personality and Social Psychology, 74*, 1464–1480.

Hahn, U., & Chater, N. (1998). Similarity and rules: Distinct? Exhaustive? Empirically distinguishable? *Cognition, 65*, 197–230.

Hermer-Vazquez, L., Hermer-Vazquez, R., Rybinnik, I., Greebel, G., Keller, R., Xu, S., et al. (2005). Rapid learning and ?exible memory in "habit" tasks in rats trained with brain stimulation reward. *Physiology and Behavior, 84*, 753–759.

Hintzman, D. (1990). Human learning and memory: Connections and dissociations. *Annual Review of Psychology, 41*, 109–139.

Hirsch, M. W., & Smale, S. (1974). *Differential equations, dynamical systems, and linear algebra* (Vol. 3). New York: Academic Press.

Hopfield, J. J. (1984). Neurons with graded response have collective computational properties like those of two-state neurons. *Proceedings of the National Academy of Sciences, 81*(10), 3088–3092.

Houk, J. C., Adams, J. L., & Barto, A. G. (1995). A model of how the basal ganglia generate and use neural signals that predict reinforcement. In J. Houk, J. Davis., & D. Beiser (Eds.), *Models of information processing in the basal ganglia* (pp. 249–270). Cambridge, MA: MIT Press.

Howe, M., Rabinowitz, F., Grant, M. (1993). On measuring (in)dependence of cognitive processes. *Psychological Review, 100*, 737–747.

Izhikevich, E. M. (2007). *Dynamical systems in neuroscience: The geometry of excitability and bursting*. Cambridge, MA: MIT Press.

Kelso, J. A. S. (1995). *Dynamic patterns: The self-organization of brain and behavior*. Cambridge, MA: MIT Press.

Kelso, J. A. S., & Engstrøm, D. A. (2006). *The complementary nature*. Cambridge, MA: The MIT Press.

Keren, G., & Schul, Y. (2009). Two is not always better than one: A critical evaluation of two-system theories. *Perspectives on Psychological Science, 4*, 533–550.

Kinder, A., & Shanks, D. R. (2001). Amnesia and the declarative/nondeclarative distinction: A recurrent network model of classification, recognition, and repetition priming. *Journal of Cognitive Neuroscience, 13*, 648–669.

Kolers, P. A., & Roediger, H. L. (1984). Procedures of mind. *Journal of Verbal Learning and Verbal Behavior, 23*, 425–449.

Kruglanski, A. W., & Dechesne, M. (2006). Are associative and propositional processes qualitatively distinct?: A comment on Gawronski and Bodenhausen (2006). *Psychological Bulletin, 132*, 736–739.

Kruglanski, A. W., Erb, H.-P., Pierro, A., Mannetti, L., & Chun, W. Y. (2006). On parametric continuities in the world of binary either ors. *Psychological Inquiry, 17*, 153–165.

LeDoux, J. E. (2000). Emotion circuits in the brain. *Annual Review of Neuroscience, 23*, 155–184.

Lieberman, M. D. (2003). Reflective and reflexive judgment processes: A social cognitive neuroscience approach. In J. P. Forgas, K. R. Williams, & W. Von Hippel (Eds.), *Social judgments: Implicit and explicit processes* (pp. 44–67). New York: Cambridge University Press.

Lieberman, M. D., Gaunt, R., Gilbert, D. T., & Trope, Y. (2002). Reflection and reflexion: A social cognitive neuroscience approach to attributional inference. *Advances in Experimental Social Psychology, 34*, 199–249.

Logan, G. D. (1985). On the ability to inhibit simple thoughts and actions: II. Stop-signal studies of repetition priming. *Journal of Experimental Psychology: Learning, Memory and Cognition, 11*, 675–691.

Lössner, B., & Rose, S. P. (1983). Passive avoidance training increases fucokinase activity in right forebrain base of day-old chicks. *Journal of Neurochemistry, 41*(5), 1357–1363.

Mazor, O., & Laurent, G. (2005). Transient dynamics versus fixed points in odor representations by locust antennal lobe projection neurons. *Neuron, 48*(4), 661–673.

McClelland, J. L., McNaughton, B. L., & O'Reilly, R. C. (1995). Why there are complementary learning systems in the hippocampus and neocortex: Insights from the successes and failures of connectionist models of learning and memory. *Psychological Review, 102*, 419–457.

McClelland, J. L., Plaut, D. C., Gotts, S. J., & Maia, T. V. (2003). Developing a domain-general framework for cognition: What is the best approach? Commentary on a target article by Anderson and Lebiere. *Behavioral and Brain Sciences, 22*, 611–614.

Miller, E. K., & Cohen, J. D. (2001). An integrative theory of prefrontal cortex function. *Annual Review of Neurosciences, 24*, 167–202.

Mitchell, J. P., Ames, D. L., Jenkins, A. C., & Banaji, M. R. (2009). Neural correlates of stereotype application. *Journal of Cognitive Neuroscience, 21*, 594–604.

Montague, P. R., & Dayan, P., & Sejnowski, T. J. (1996). A framework for mesencephalic dopamine systems based on predictive hebbian learning. *Journal of Neuroscience, 16*(5), 1936–1947.

Moors, A., & De Houwer, J. (2006). Automaticity: A theoretical and conceptual analysis. *Psychological Bulletin, 132*, 297–326.

Morewedge, C. K., & Kahneman, D. (2010). Associative processes in intuitive judgment. *Trends in Cognitive Science, 14*(10), 435–440.

Newell, A. (1973). You can't play 20 questions with nature and win: Projective comments on the papers of this symposium. In W. G. Chase (Ed.), *Visual information processing* (pp. 283–308). New York: Academic Press.

Newell, A. (1990). *Unified theories of cognition.* Cambridge, MA: Harvard University Press.

Newstead, S. (2000). Are there two different types of thinking? *Behavioral and Brain Sciences, 23*, 690–691.

Nisbett, R. E., & Wilson, T. D. (1977). Telling more than we can know: Verbal reports on mental processes. *Psychological Review, 84*, 231–259.

O'Reilly, R. C. (1998). Six principles for biologically based computational models of cortical cognition. *Trends in Cognitive Sciences, 2*(11), 455–462.

O'Reilly, R. C., & Frank, M. J. (2006). Making working memory work: A computational model of learning in the prefrontal cortex and basal ganglia. *Neural Computation, 18*(2), 283–328.

Osman, M. (2004). An evaluation of dual-process theories of reasoning. *Psychonomic Bulletin and Review, 11*, 988–1010.

Ostergaard, A. L. (1992). A method for judging measures of stochastic dependence: Further comments on the current controversy. *Journal of Experimental Psychology: Learning, Memory, and Cognition, 18*, 413–420.

Payne, B. (2005). Conceptualizing control in social cognition: How executive functioning modulates the expression of automatic stereotyping. *Journal of Personality and Social Psychology, 89*(4), 488–503.

Payne, B., Burkley, M. A., & Stokes, M. B. (2008). Why do implicit and explicit attitude tests diverge? The role of structural fit. *Journal of Personality and Social Psychology, 94*(1), 16–31.

Petty, R. E., Tormala, Z. L., Briñol, P., & Jarvis, W. B. G. (2006). Implicit ambivalence from attitude change: An exploration of the PAST model. *Journal of Personality and Social Psychology, 90*, 21–41.

Plaut, D. C. (1995). Double dissociation without modularity: Evidence from connectionist neuropsychology. *Journal of Clinical and Experimental Neuropsychology, 17*, 291–321.

Poldrack, R. A. (1996). On testing for stochastic dissociations. *Psychonomic Bulletin and Review, 3*, 434–448.

Poldrack, R. A., & Foerde, K. (2007). Category learning and the memory systems debate. *Neuroscience and Biobehavioral Reviews, 32*, 197–205.

Pollack, J. B. (1990). Recursive Distributed Representations. *Artificial Intelligence* 46, 1, 77–105.

Pylyshyn, Z. (1980). Computation and cognition: Issues in the foundations of cognitive science. *Behavioral and Brain Sciences, 3*, 111–169.

Read, S. J., & Monroe, B. (2008). Computational models in personality and social psychology. *Handbook on computational cognitive modeling*. Cambridge University Press.

Read, S. J., & Montoya, J. A. (1999). An autoassociative model of causal learning and causal reasoning. *Journal of Personality and Social Psychology, 76*, 728–742.

Rogers, T. T., & McClelland, J. L. (2004). *Semantic cognition: A parallel distributed processing approach*. Cambridge, MA: MIT Press.

Ross, L., Lepper, M., & Ward, A. (2010). History of social psychology: Insights, challenges, and contributions to theory and application. In S. T. Fiske, D. T. Gilbert, & G. Lindzey (Eds.), *Handbook of social psychology* (Vol. 1, pp. 3–50). Hoboken, NJ: Wiley.

Rougier, N. P., Noelle, D. C., Braver, T. S., Cohen, J. D., & O'Reilly, R. C. (2005). Prefrontal cortex and flexible cognitive control: Rules without symbols. *Proceedings of the National Academy of Sciences USA, 102*(20), 7338–7343.

Rumelhart, D. E. (1989). Towards a microstructural account of human reasoning. In S. Vosniadou & A. Ortony (Eds.), *Similarity and analogical reasoning* (pp. 298–312). Cambridge, UK: Cambridge University Press.

Rutishauser, U., Mamelak, A. N., & Schuman, E. M. (2006). Single-trial learning of novel stimuli by individual neurons of the human hippocampus-amygdala complex. *Neuron, 49*, 805–813.

Rydell, R., & McConnell, A. R. (2006). Understanding implicit and explicit attitude change: A systems of reasoning analysis. *Journal of Personality and Social Psychology, 91*, 995–1008.

Rydell, R., McConnell, A. R., Mackie, D. M., & Strain, L. M. (2006). Of two minds: Forming and changing valence inconsistent implicit and explicit attitudes. *Psychological Science, 17*, 954–958.

Satpute, A. B., & Lieberman, M. D. (2006). Integrating automatic and controlled processing into neurocognitive models of social cognition. *Brain Research, 1079*, 86–97.

Searle, J. R. (1980). Minds, brains, and programs. *Behavioral and Brain Sciences, 3*(3), 417–457.

Shanks, D. R., & Berry, C. J. (2012). Are there multiple-memory systems?: Tests of models of implicit and explicit memory. *Quarterly Journal of Experimental Psychology, 65*, 1449–1474.

Shanks, D. R., & Perruchet, P. (2002). Dissociation between priming and recognition in the expression of sequential knowledge. *Psychonomic Bulletin and Review, 9*(2), 362–367.

Sherman, J. W. (2006a). Clearing up some misconceptions about the quad model. *Psychological Inquiry, 17*, 269–276.

Sherman, J. W. (2006b). On building a better process model: It's not only how many, but which ones and by which means. *Psychological Inquiry, 17*, 173–184.

Sherman, J., Gawronski, B., Gonsalkorale, K., Hugenberg, K., Allen, T., & Groom, C. (2008). The self-regulation of automatic associations and behavioral impulses. *Psychological Review, 115*, 314–335.

Sherry, D., & Schacter, D. (1987). The evolution of multiple memory systems. *Psychological Review, 94*, 439–454.

Sklar, A., Levy, N., Goldstein, A., Mandel, R., Maril, A., & Hassin, R. R. (2012). Uniquely human yet not conscious: Reading and doing arithmetic non-consciously. *Proceedings of the National Academy of Sciences USA, 109*(48), 19614–19619.

Sloman, S. (1996). The empirical case for two systems of reasoning. *Psychological Bulletin, 119*, 3–22.

Smith, E. E., Langston, C., & Nisbett, R. (1992). The case for rules in reasoning. *Cognitive Science, 16*, 1–40.

Smith, E. R., DeCoster, J. (2000). Dual-process models in social and cognitive psychology: Conceptual integration and links to underlying memory systems. *Personality and Social Psychology Review, 4*, 108–131.

Smolensky, P. (1988). On the proper treatment of connectionism. *Behavioral and Brain Sciences, 11*, 1–23.

Smolensky, P. (1990). In defense of PTC: Reply to continuing commentary. *The Behavioral and Brain Sciences. 13*, 407–411.

Song, J.-H., & Nakayama, K. (2006). Role of focal attention on latencies and trajectories of visually guided manual pointing. *Journal of Vision, 6*(9), 11.

Song, J.-H., & Nakayama, K. (2008). Target selection in visual search as revealed by movement trajectories. *Vision Research, 48*(7), 853–861.

Spivey, M. J. (2007). *The continuity of mind*. New York: Oxford University Press.

Squire, L. R., & Kandel, E. R. (1999). *Memory: From mind and molecules*. New York: Scientific American Library/Scientific American Books.

Spunt, R. P., & Lieberman, M. D. (2013). The busy social brain: Evidence for automaticity and control in the neural systems supporting social cognition and action understanding. *Psychological Science, 24*, 80–86.

Strack, F., & Deutsch, R. (2004). Reflective and impulsive determinants of social behavior. *Personality and Social Psychology Review, 8*, 220–247.

Sun, R. (Ed.). (2008). *The Cambridge handbook of computational psychology*. New York: Cambridge University Press.

Sun, R., Slusarz, P., & Terry, C. (2005). The interaction of the explicit and the implicit in skill learning: A dual-process approach. *Psychological Review, 112*, 159–192.

Sutton, R. S., & Barto, A. G. (1998). *Reinforcement learning: An introduction* (Vol. 1). Cambridge, UK: Cambridge University Press.

Tsuchiya, N., & Koch, C. (2005). Continuous flash suppression reduces negative afterimages. *Natural Neurosciences, 8*(8), 1096–1101.

Usher, M., McClelland, J. L. (2001). The time course of perceptual choice: The leaky, competing accumulator model. *Psychological Review, 108*(3), 550–592.

Van Gelder, T. (1990). Compositionality: A connectionist variation on a classical theme. *Cognitive Science, 14*, 355–384.

Van Gelder, T. (1995). What might cognition be, if not computation? *The Journal of Philosophy, 92*(7), 345–381.

Wang, X. J. (2001). Synaptic reverberation underlying mnemonic persistent activity. *Trends in Neurosciences, 24*(8), 455–463.

Wills, T. J., Lever, C., Cacucci, F., Burgess, N., & O'Keefe, J. (2005). Attractor dynamics in the hippocampal representation of the local environment. *Science, 308*(5723), 873–876.

Wilson, T., Lindsey, S., & Schooler, J. (2000). A model of dual attitudes. *Psychological Review, 107*, 101–126.

Winkielman, P. (2008). *Social cognition: The basis of human interaction*. New York: Psychology Press.

Wojnowicz, M., Ferguson, M. J., Dale, R., & Spivey, M. (2009). The self-organization of deliberate evaluations. *Psychological Science, 20*, 1428–1435.

Wong, K. F., & Wang, X. J. (2006). A recurrent network mechanism of time integration in perceptual decisions. *Journal of Neuroscience, 26*(4), 1314–1328.

Yin, H. H., & Knowlton, B. J. (2006). The role of the basal ganglia in habit formation. *Nature Reviews Neuroscience, 7*, 464–476.

Author Index

B

H

L

M

N

O

P

Q

R

S

T

U

V

W

Subject Index

D

E

F

G

Q

R

S